dentEssentials

High-Yield NBDE® Part I Review

FOURTH EDITION

KAPLAN MEDICAL

dentEssentials

High-Yield NBDE® Part I Review

FOURTH EDITION

Board Prep for First- and Second-Year Dental Students

Published by Kaplan Publishing, a division of Kaplan, Inc.
395 Hudson Street, 4th Floor
New York, NY 10014

Printed in the United States of America

10 9 8 7 6 5 4 3 2 1

ISBN-13: 978-1-60714-900-2

LEAD AUTHORS/EDITORS

Michael S. Manley, M.D.
Director, Basic Sciences and Step 1 Curriculum
Kaplan Medical

Leslie D. Manley, Ph.D.
Director, Basic Sciences and Step 1 Curriculum
Kaplan Medical

DENTAL ANATOMY EDITORS

Jeff Linfante, D.D.S.
Director of Dental Curriculum
Kaplan Medical

Ronald Salyk, D.D.S.
Morris Heights Health Center
Bronx, New York

CONTRIBUTORS

Thomas H. Adair, Ph.D.
Professor
Department of Physiology and Biophysics
University of Mississippi Medical Center

John Barone, M.D.
Anatomic and Clinical Pathologist

Stuart Bentley-Hibbert, M.D., Ph.D.
New York Presbyterian Hospital
Weill Cornell Medical Center

Steven R. Daugherty, Ph.D.
Director, Education and Testing
Kaplan Medical
and
Adjunct Professor
Rush Medical College

Douglas E. Fitzovich, Ph.D.
Professor of Physiology
DeBusk College of Osteopathic Medicine
Lincoln Memorial University

Beth Forshee, Ph.D.
Assistant Professor of Physiology
Lake Erie College of Osteopathic Medicine

Barbara Hansen, Ph.D.
Biochemistry Faculty
Kaplan Medical

Steven R. Harris, Ph.D
Associate Dean for Academic Affairs
Professor of Pharmacology
University of Pikeville
Kentucky College of Osteopathic Medicine

Robert F. Kissling III, M.D.

John A. Kriak, Pharm.D.
President/Chief Clinical Consultant, CAMMCO, LLC

Mary J. Ruebush, Ph.D.
Adjunct Professor of Medical Science, retired
Montana State University
Microbiology/Immunology Faculty, Kaplan Medical

Nancy Standler, M.D., Ph.D.
Department of Pathology
Valley View Medical Center
Intermountain Healthcare

Sam Turco, Ph.D.
Professor, Department of Biochemistry
University of Kentucky College of Medicine

James S. White, Ph.D.
Assistant Professor of Cell Biology
School of Osteopathic Medicine
University of Medicine and Dentistry of New Jersey
Adjunct Assistant Professor of Cell and Developmental Biology
University of Pennsylvania School of Medicine

Glenn C. Yiu M.D., Ph.D.
Clinical Fellow in Medicine
Harvard Medical School

Contents

(A more comprehensive list appears on the first page of each chapter.)

Introduction

The completion of the National Board Dental Examination Part I (NBDE Part I) is a milestone for dental students on their way to the practice of dentistry. The exam is one of several forms of evaluation used by the various licensing boards to assess the qualifications of an individual seeking the privilege to practice dentistry. NBDE Part I has been designed to test students' ability to understand both basic and dental science and to integrate this material into a problem-solving context.

The Examination

NBDE Part I is a comprehensive, computer-based exam that is administered in one day by Prometric, Inc. at Prometric Test Centers in the United States and Canada. It is comprised of 400 multiple-choice items, evenly distributed among the following disciplines:

- Anatomic Sciences
- Biochemistry/Physiology
- Microbiology/Pathology
- Dental Anatomy and Occlusion

Approximately 20% of the total number of questions are grouped into testlets. Testlets are presented in a case-based format, providing some background information on a patient within a given clinical scenario. The questions are developed around this information and have an interdisciplinary and clinical focus.

Candidates are given a total of 7 hours to complete the exam, divided into two sessions—morning and afternoon—with an optional lunch break in between.

NBDE I score results range from 49 to 99. The minimum passing score is 75. The two factors that affect a candidate's score are (1) the number of correct answers selected by the candidate, and (2) the score scale conversion for the exam.

Candidates who pass the exam will receive a **pass/fail** report. For remediation purposes, candidates who fail will receive a numerical score for each major discipline.

dentEssentials: Integrated Basic Science Review Book

The *dentEssentials* review book has been structured by organ system and is presented in a compact and concise manner. It focuses on the most relevant and important basic and dental science information in the form of reference charts and corresponding images. This design allows for a unique level of integration between the disciplines.

This book is divided into three sections.

- Section I presents the general principles of the basic science disciplines (biochemistry molecular biology, genetics, microbiology, immunology, embryology, and histology).
- Section II presents organ-specific information.
- Section III focuses on dental anatomy, occlusion, and histology.

Study Techniques

It is not recommended that you go back to your textbooks and begin the process of preparing for the NBDE by rereading them cover to cover and underlining every word on every page. This is not an efficient use of your time or an effective way to learn. Develop a plan and focus on the material most likely to be on the exam, narrowing down the amount of material you need to cover.

A good way to increase your retention and facilitate your recall of information is to be an active user of the material you are learning. Repetition makes memories. Each instance of recall produces a new memory trace, linking concepts and increasing the chance of recall of the information in the future. Recall actually changes the neuronal structures. To make information useful, it needs to be triangulated; it needs to be connected to other concepts and to experiences. It is important to remember that memorization should not be the primary goal during preparation; rather, you should develop the ability to process and apply the material in an integrated manner.

Begin the process of preparation by following the steps listed below:

- Assess your strengths and weaknesses, then rank the order of subjects from weak to strong.
- Start every study session with a list of specific goals.
- Personalize the review book. Use color highlighting, write margin notes, and summarize the topics you have learned.
- After reviewing the topics of the study session, imagine or actually try to teach the material and concepts to someone else.

As you get closer to the exam, read the *National Dental Board Examination Part I Guide*. This is provided by the ADA and is available online at **ada.org.**

On behalf of Kaplan Medical, we wish you the best of success in your studies and your dental career.

Section I

General Principles

Biochemistry

Chapter 1

Biochemistry

► Glycolysis

Glycolysis is a **cytoplasmic** pathway used by all cells to generate energy from glucose. **One** glucose molecule is converted into **2 pyruvate** molecules, generating a net of **2 ATPs** by substrate-level phosphorylation, and **2 NADHs**. When oxygen is present, NADH delivers electrons to the electron transport chain in mitochondria to generate ATP by oxidative phosphorylation. Under **anaerobic** conditions, lactate is generated and NADH is reoxidized to NAD^+.

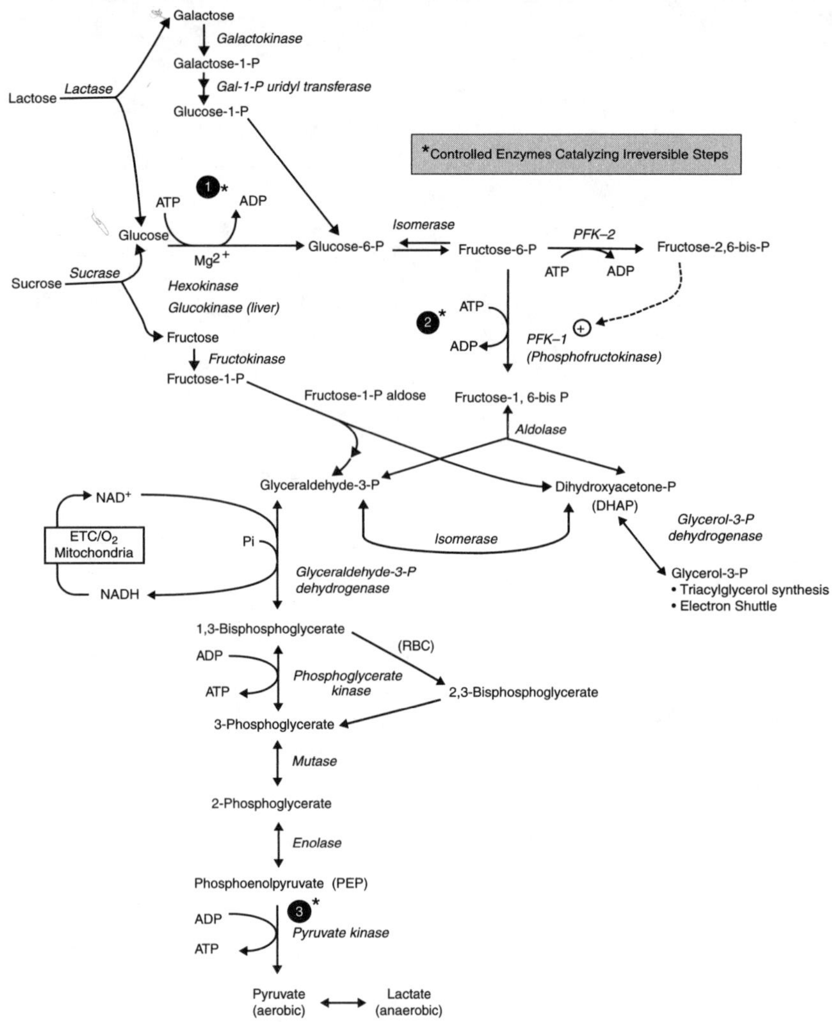

Regulation: Three irreversible steps

1

Hexokinase	Glucokinase*
Most tissues	Liver, β-islet cells
Low K_m	High K_m
⊖ G-6-P	Induced by insulin in liver

2

PFK-1	PFK-2
→ F-1,6-BP	→ F-2,6-BP
Rate-limiting step of glycolysis	Glycolysis regulator: ↑ glycolysis ↓ gluconeogenesis
⊕ AMP ⊕ F-2,6-BP† ⊖ ATP ⊖ Citrate	⊕ Insulin ⊖ Glucagon

3

Pyruvate kinase	
⊕ F-1,6-BP	⊖ ATP ⊖ Alanine†

*Glukokinase mutations may lead to a form of MODY.
†Liver specific

Glucose Transport

GLUT-1 and -3: basal uptake (most cells)

GLUT-2: storage (liver); glucose sensor (β-islet)

GLUT-4: ↑ by insulin (adipose, skeletal muscle); ↑ by exercise (skeletal muscle)

Disease Association	
Galactokinase deficiency	Galactosemia/galactosuria, cataracts in childhood (excess galactose is converted to galactitol via aldose reductase); Tx: no galactose in diet
Gal-1-P uridyl transferase deficiency	Same as above, but more severe with vomiting/diarrhea after milk ingestion, liver disease, lethargy, mental retardation; Tx: no galactose in diet
Fructokinase deficiency	Fructosuria; benign
Fructose-1-P aldolase B deficiency	Fructosuria, liver and proximal renal tubule disorder; Tx: no fructose in diet
Pyruvate kinase deficiency	Chronic hemolysis, ↑ 2,3-BPG and other glycolytic intermediates in the RBC, no Heinz bodies, autosomal recessive

Definition of abbreviations: MODY, mature-onset diabetes of the young; PFK, phosphofructokinase; RBC, red blood cell; Tx, treatment.

► The Citric Acid Cycle

The citric acid cycle **(tricarboxylic acid cycle)** is a **mitochondrial** pathway that occurs **only** under **aerobic conditions**. Each acetyl-CoA generated from pyruvate is used to produce **3 NADH**, **1 $FADH_2$**, and **1 GTP**. Both the NADH and $FADH_2$ deliver electrons to the electron transport chain (ETC) to generate ATP by oxidative phosphorylation.

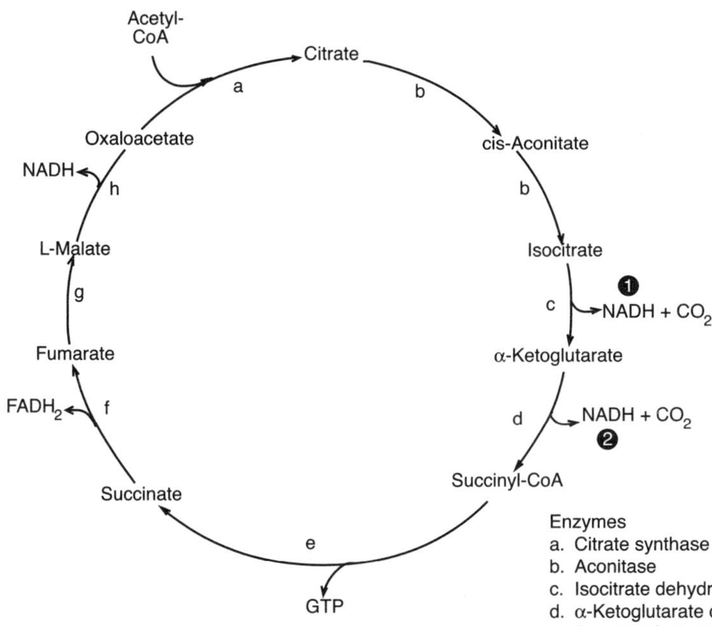

Enzymes
a. Citrate synthase
b. Aconitase
c. Isocitrate dehydrogenase
d. α-Ketoglutarate dehydrogenase
e. Succinyl-CoA thiokinase
f. Succinate dehydrogenase
g. Fumarase
h. Malate dehydrogenase

Regulation

❶ **Isocitrate dehydrogenase** (Rate-Limiting Step)	
⊕ ADP	⊖ ATP ⊖ NADH

❷ **α-Ketoglutarate dehydrogenase***	
	⊖ Succinyl CoA ⊖ ATP ⊖ NADH

*Similar to pyruvate dehydrogenase complex and uses the same cofactors

Links to Other Pathways

- **Gluconeogenesis** (malate shuttle)
- **Fatty acid synthesis** (citrate shuttle)
- **Amino acid synthesis** (oxaloacetate and α-ketoglutarate)
- **Heme synthesis** (succinyl CoA)

Stoichiometry of the Citric Acid Cycle

$$\text{Acetyl-CoA} + 3\ NAD^+ + FAD + GDP + P_i \rightarrow 2\ CO_2 + 3\ NADH + FADH_2 + GTP + CoA$$

The only net fate of acetyl-CoA as it proceeds through the citric acid cycle is conversion to CO_2. **The citric acid cycle is NOT a means to convert acetyl groups to glucose.** Humans lack the capacity to form glucose from acetyl-CoA.

► Oxidative Phosphorylation

Electron transport and the coupled synthesis of ATP are known as oxidative phosphorylation. The **electron transport chain (ETC)** is a series of carrier enzymes in the **inner mitochondrial membrane** that pass electrons, in a stepwise fashion, from NADH and $FADH_2$ to **oxygen**, the final electron acceptor. These carriers create a proton gradient across the inner membrane, which drives the F_0/F_1 ATP synthase, with a net production of **3 ATPs** per **NADH** and **2 ATPs** per **$FADH_2$**.

Electron Transport Chain

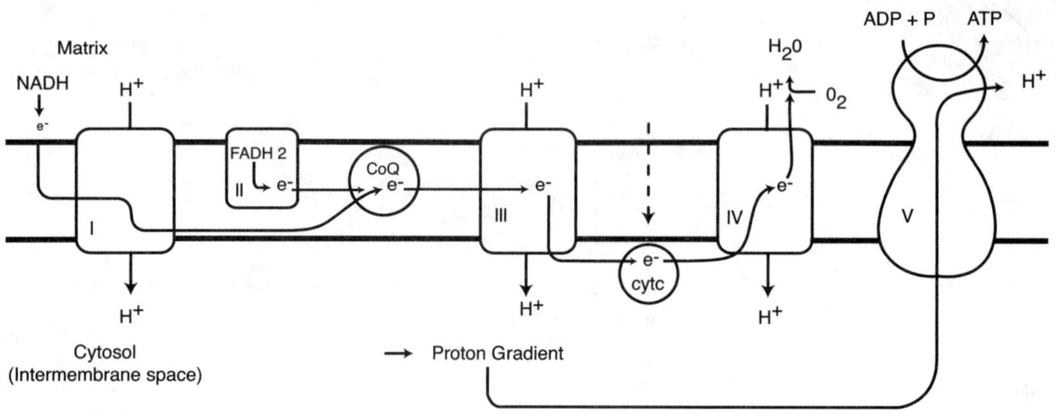

Complex I: NADH dehydrogenase Complex II: succinate dehydrogenase CoQ: coenzyme Q	Complex III: cytochrome b/c_1 Cyt C: cytochrome c Complex IV: cytochrome a/a_3 Complex V: F_oF_1ATP synthase

Clinical Correlation

Cyanide Poisoning

Blocks cytochrome a/a_3; cyanide from burning polyurethane (mattress/furniture stuffing); Tx: nitrites (creates methemoglobin, which binds cyanide)

Inhibitors

Inhibit ETC and O_2 consumption
Inhibit ATP synthesis

- Antimycin A, piscicide (Complex I)
- Cyanide (cyt oxidase)
- Rotenone, broad-spectrum insecticides, other pesticides (Complex 1)
- Oligomycin (F_o)

Uncouplers

Increase ETC and O_2 consumption
Decrease ATP synthesis
Produce heat

- 2,4-dinitrophenol (2,4-DNP)
- Salicylate (metabolite of aspirin)
- Uncoupling proteins (e.g., thermogenin)

▶ Pyruvate Metabolism

❶ **Lactate dehydrogenase:** *Anaerobic tissues:* converts pyruvate to lactate, reoxidizing cytoplasmic NADH to NAD^+.
Liver: converts lactate to pyruvate for gluconeogenesis or for metabolism to acetyl CoA

❷ **Pyruvate dehydrogenase:** generates acetyl-CoA for fatty acid synthesis and the citric acid cycle; complex of 3 enzymes

❸ **Pyruvate carboxylase:** produces oxaloacetate for gluconeogenesis and the citric acid cycle

❹ **Alanine aminotransferase (ALT, GPT):** *Muscle:* converts pyruvate to alanine to transport amino groups to the liver.
Liver: converts alanine to pyruvate for gluconeogenesis and delivers the amino group for urea synthesis

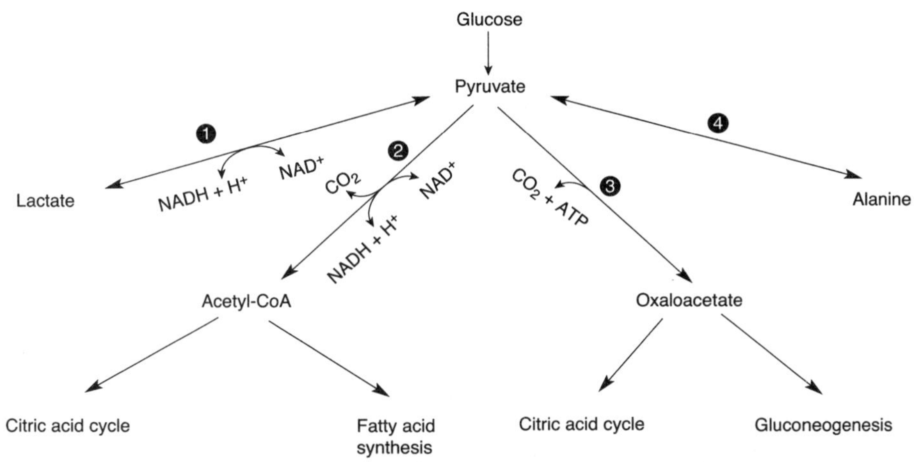

Regulation	
Pyruvate dehydrogenase (PDH)	
⊕ ADP	⊖ Acetyl-CoA
⊕ CoA	⊖ ATP
⊕ NAD^+	⊖ NADH
	⊖ glucagon

Cofactors: TPP (from thiamine), lipoic acid, CoA (from pantothenate), FAD (from riboflavin), NAD (from niacin)

Stoichiometry of Pyruvate Dehydrogenase

Pyruvate + NAD^+ + CoA → NADH + CO_2 + acetyl-CoA

Disease Association

Pyruvate Dehydrogenase Deficiency

Lactic acidosis, seizures, mental retardation, ataxia, spasticity

Cori Cycle

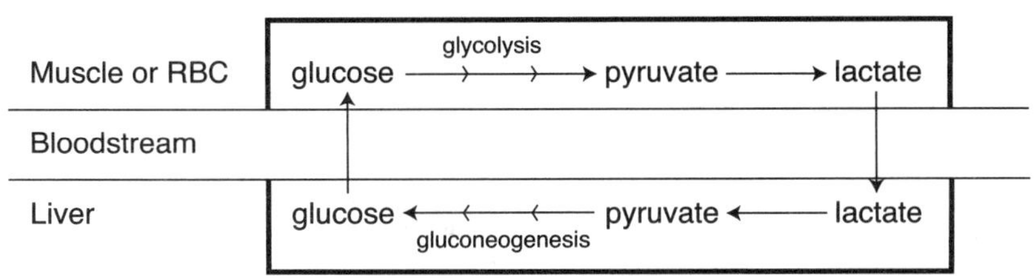

During fasting or exercise, lactate from RBCs or skeletal muscles is sent to the liver to make glucose that can be returned to the RBCs or muscle.

Definition of abbreviations: TCA, tricarboxylic acid; TPP, thiamine pyrophosphate.

► Hexose Monophosphate Shunt

The **hexose monophosphate (HMP) shunt** (pentose phosphate pathway) is a **cytosolic** pathway that uses **glucose-6-phosphate** to reduce NADP to NADPH, and synthesize **ribose-5-P**. NADPH is important for fatty acid and steroid biosynthesis, maintenance of reduced glutathione to protect against reactive oxygen species (ROS), and for bactericidal activity in polymorphonuclear leukocytes (PMNs). Ribose-5-P is required for nucleotide synthesis.

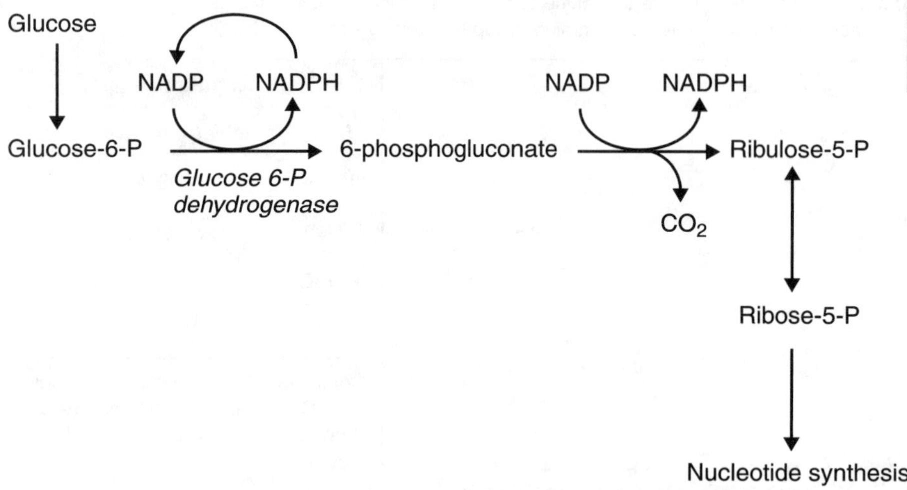

Regulation	
Glucose-6-P-dehydrogenase	
⊕ **$NADP^+$**	⊖ NADPH

Disease Association
Glucose-6-Phosphate Dehydrogenase Deficiency
Episodic self-limiting hemolytic anemia induced by infection and drugs (common) or chronic hemolysis (rare); X-linked recessive; female heterozygotes have ↑ resistance to malaria

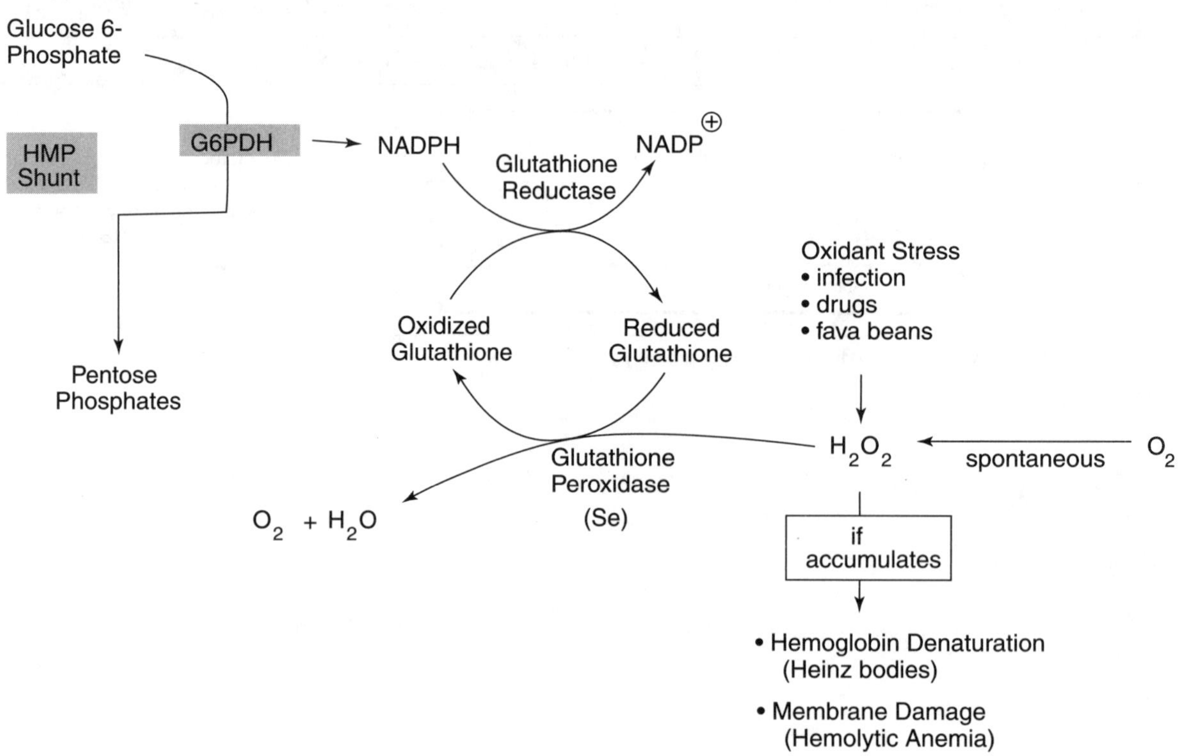

▶ Glycogenesis and Glycogenolysis

Glycogen is a branched polymer of glucose, stored primarily in liver and skeletal muscles, which can be mobilized during hypoglycemia (liver) or muscular contraction (muscles). Synthesis of glycogen (**glycogenesis**) is mediated by **glycogen synthase**, while its breakdown (**glycogenolysis**) is carried out by **glycogen phosphorylase**. Branching of the glycogen polymer occurs via a **branching enzyme**, which breaks an α-1,4-bond and transfers a block of glucosyl residues to create a new α-1,6-bond. This is reversed by a **debranching enzyme**.

Glycogen Metabolism

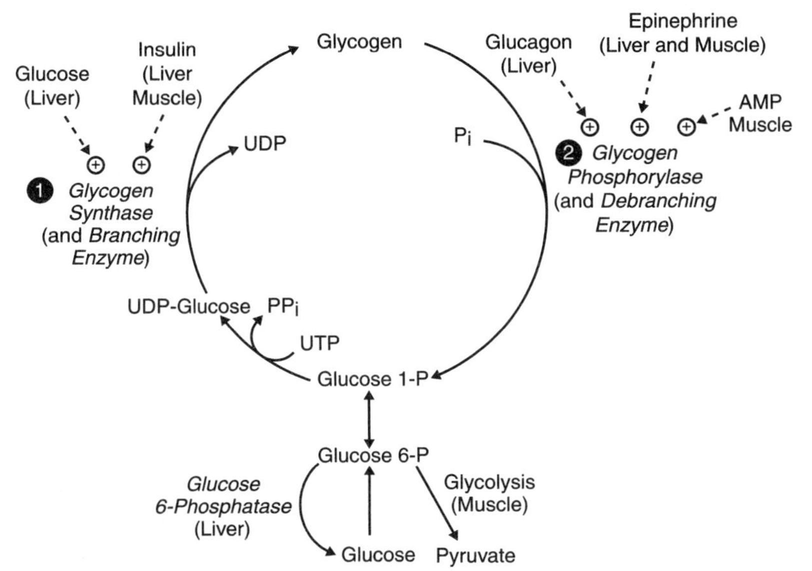

Regulation

❶ Glycogen synthase

Liver	Skeletal Muscle
⊕ Insulin	⊕ Insulin
⊕ Glucose	⊖ Epinephrine
⊖ Glucagon	
⊖ Epinephrine	

❷ Glycogen phosphorylase

Liver	Skeletal Muscle
⊕ glucagon	⊕ epinephrine
⊕ epinephrine	⊕ AMP
⊖ Insulin	⊕ Ca^{2+}
	⊖ ATP

Branching and Debranching Steps

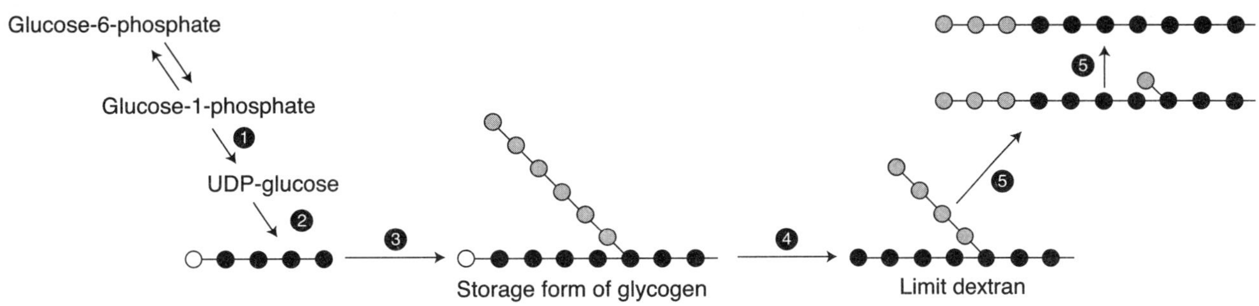

❶ UDP-glucose pyrophosphorylase

❷ Glycogen synthase

❸ Branching enzyme

❹ Glycogen phosphorylase

❺ Debranching enzyme

Glycogen Storage Diseases

Glycogen Storage Diseases	
Type I: von Gierke disease (↓ glucose-6-phosphatase)	Severe fasting hypoglycemia, lactic acidosis, hepatomegaly, hyperlipidemia, hyperuricemia, short stature
Type II: Pompe disease (↓ lysosomal-α-1,4-glucosidase)	Cardiomegaly, muscle weakness, death by 2 years
Type III: Cori disease (↓ glycogen debranching enzyme)	Mild hypoglycemia; liver enlargement
Type IV: Andersen disease (↓ branching enzyme)	Infantile hypotonia, cirrhosis, death by 2 years
Type V: McArdle disease (↓ muscle glycogen phosphorylase*)	Muscle cramps/weakness during initial phase of exercise, possible rhabdomyolysis and myoglobinuria
Type VI: Hers disease (↓ hepatic glycogen phosphorylase)	Mild fasting hypoglycemia, hepatomegaly, cirrhosis

*Also known as myophosphorylase

► Gluconeogenesis

Gluconeogenesis is a pathway for de novo synthesis of **glucose** from **C3 and C4 precursors** using both **mitochondrial** and **cytosolic** enzymes. Occurring only in liver, kidney, and intestinal epithelium, this pathway functions to provide glucose for the body, especially the brain and RBCs, which require glucose for energy (the brain can also use ketone bodies during fasting conditions). Gluconeogenesis occurs during fasting, as glycogen stores become depleted. Important substrates for gluconeogenesis are gluconeogenic **amino acids** (protein from muscle), **lactate** (from RBCs and muscle during anaerobic exercise), and **glycerol-3-P** (from triacylglycerol from adipose tissues).

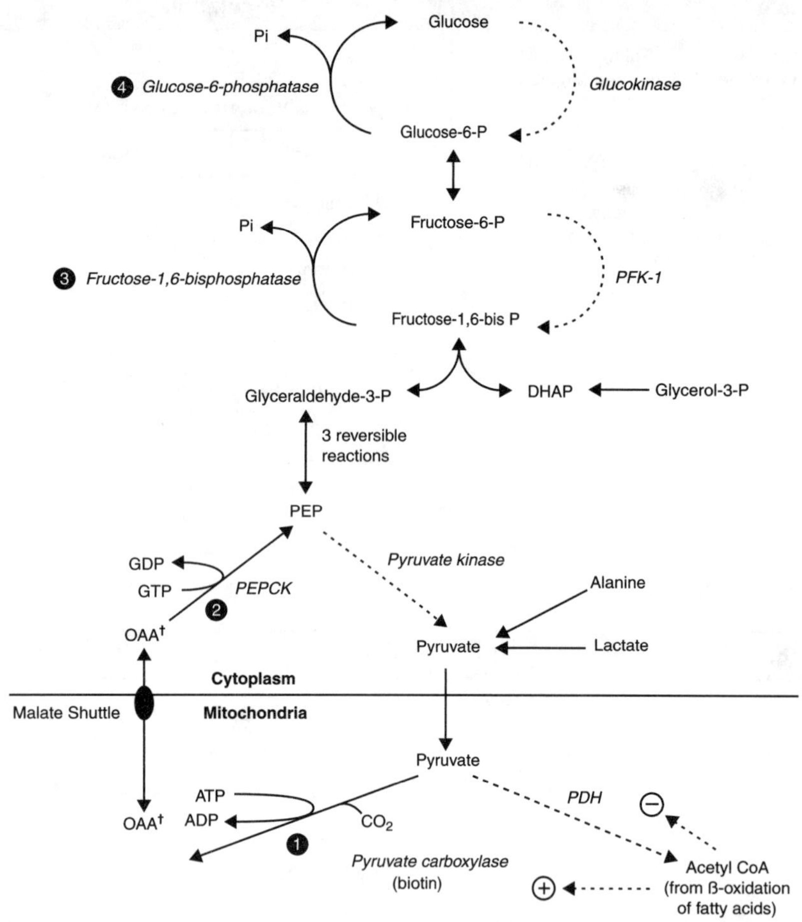

Regulation

Four **irreversible** steps:

❶ **Pyruvate carboxylase**	
Mitochondrial; requires biotin	
⊕ acetyl CoA	—

❷ **PEPCK**	
Cytosolic; requires GTP	
Induced by glucagon and cortisol	—

❸ **Fructose 1,6-bisphosphatase**	
Cytosolic	
⊕ ATP	⊖ AMP ⊖ F-2,6-BP‡ (from PFK2)

❹ **Glucose-6-phosphatase**
In endoplasmic reticulum; only in liver

‡Mediates insulin's inhibition and glucagon's stimulation of this enzyme

Disease Association

Glucose-6-Phosphatase Deficiency (von Gierke disease)

Severe hypoglycemia, lactic acidosis, hepatomegaly, hyperlipidemia, hyperuricemia, short stature

Alanine Cycle

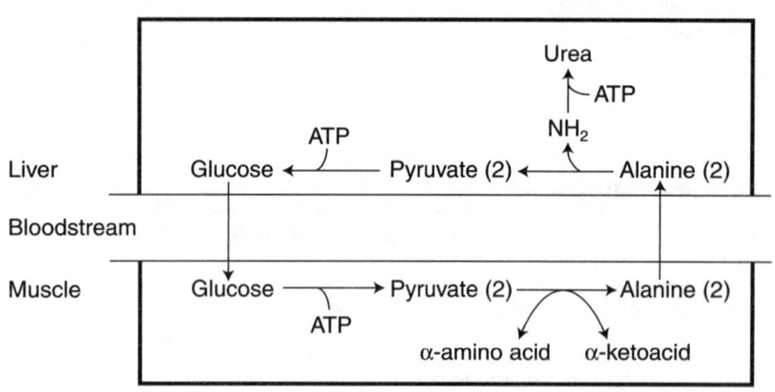

A pathway by which muscles release alanine to the liver, delivering both a gluconeogenic substrate (pyruvate) and an amino group for urea synthesis

Definition of abbreviations: PEPCK, phosphoenolpyruvate carboxykinase; PFK2, phosphofructokinase 2; RBC, red blood cell.

† OAA is not transported across the membrane directly. Instead, it is transported as malate in exchange for asparate via the malate shuttle.

► Amino Acid Structures

Hydrophobic Amino Acids

Nonpolar, Aliphatic Side Chains

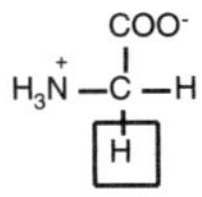

Glycine
Gly

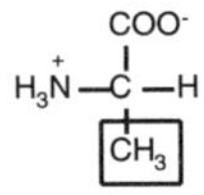

Alanine
Ala

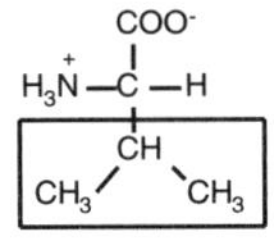

Valine
Val

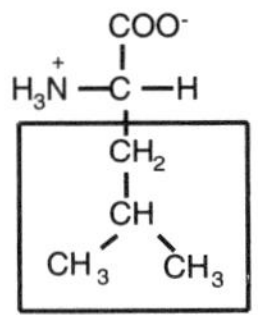

Leucine
Leu

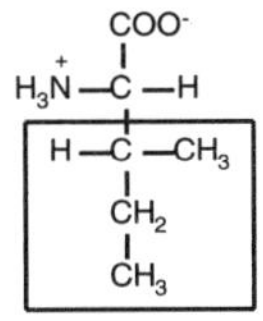

Isoleucine
Ile

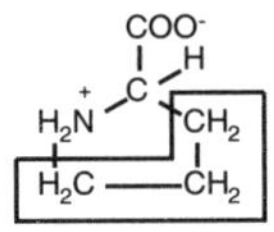

Proline
Pro

Aromatic Side Chains

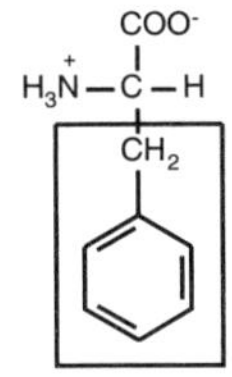

Phenylalanine
Phe

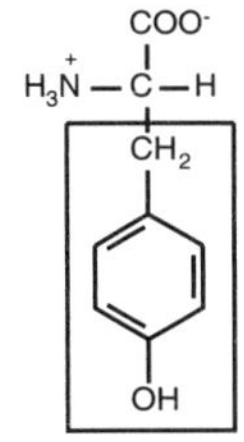

Tyrosine
Tyr

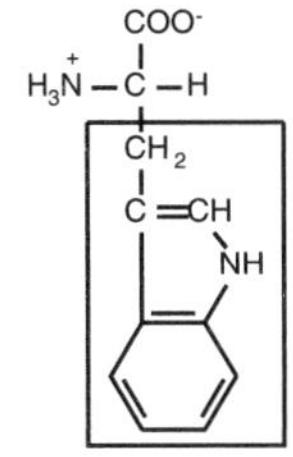

Tryptophan
Trp

Hydrophilic Amino Acids

Positively Charged R Groups

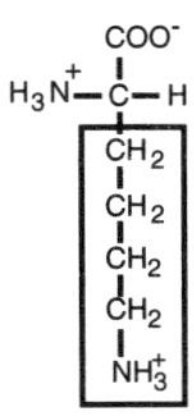

Lysine
Lys

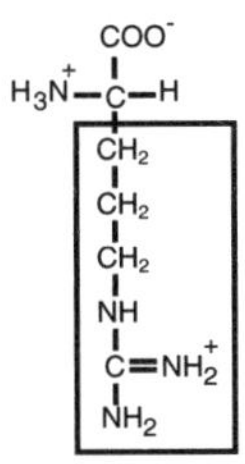

Arginine
Arg

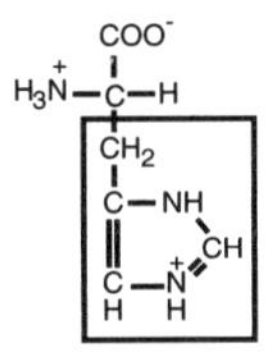

Histidine
His

Polar, Uncharged R Groups

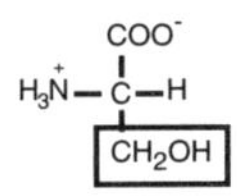

Serine
Ser

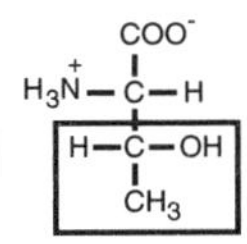

Threonine
Thr

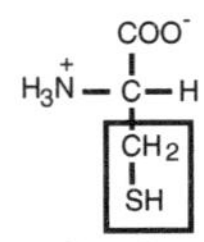

Cysteine
Cys

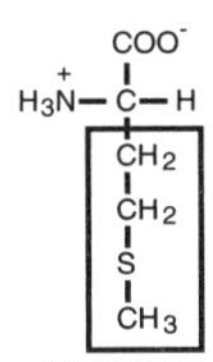

Methionine
Met

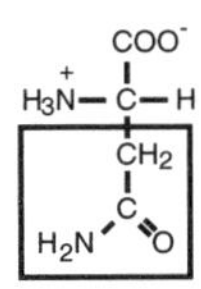

Asparagine
Asn

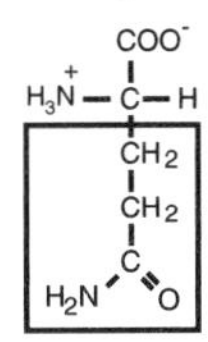

Glutamine
Gln

Negatively Charged R Groups

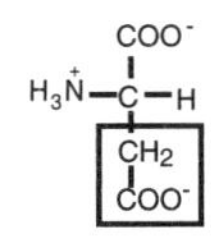

Aspartate
Asp

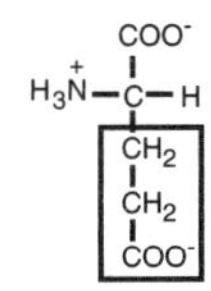

Glutamate
Glu

► Amino Acid Derivatives

Besides being the building blocks of proteins, amino acids are also precursors for various chemicals, such as **hormones**, **neurotransmitters**, and other small molecules.

Amino Acid	Product
Tyrosine	Thyroid hormones (T_3, T_4); melanin; catecholamines (dopamine, epinephrine)

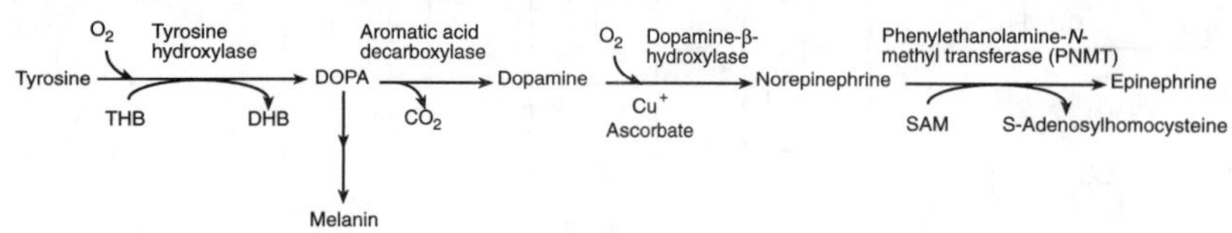

Tryptophan	Serotonin (5-HT); melatonin; NAD; NADP

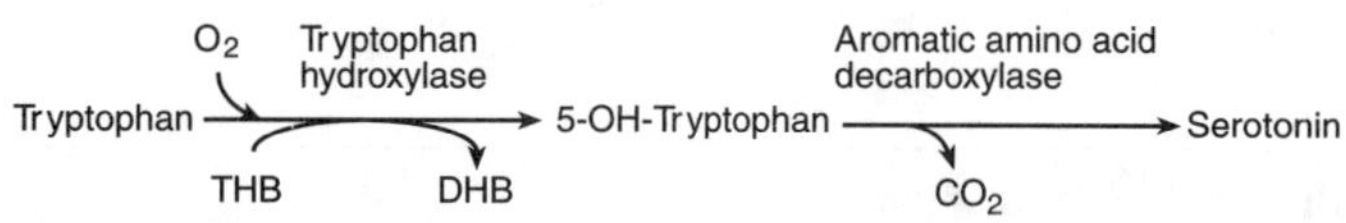

Glycine	Heme

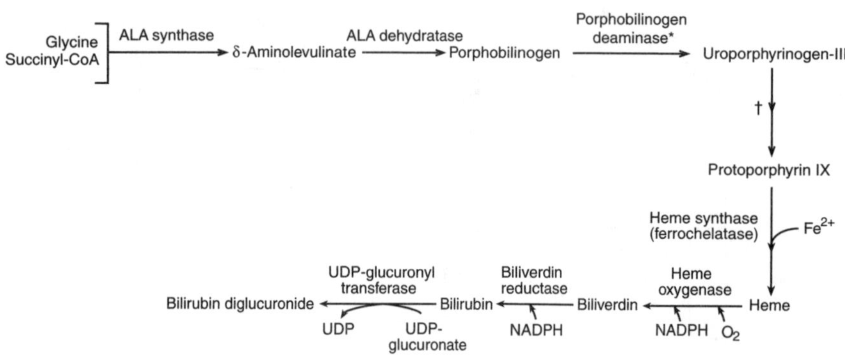

Glutamate	γ-aminobutyric acid (GABA)

Glutamate $\xrightarrow{\text{Glutamate decarboxylase}}$ γ-Aminobutyric acid (GABA)

Arginine	Nitric oxide (NO)

⊕ Ca^{2+}

Arginine + O_2 $\xrightarrow{\text{NO synthase}}$ Nitric oxide + citrulline (NADPH → $NADP^+$)

Histidine	Histamine

Histidine $\xrightarrow{\text{Histidine decarboxylase}}$ Histamine

Methionine	S-adenosylmethionine (SAM; methylating agent)
Arginine, glycine, SAM	Creatine

Disease Association

Albinism

Tyrosine hydroxylase (type I) or tyrosine transporter (type II) deficiency; ↓ pigmentation of skin, eyes, and hair, ↑ risk of skin cancer, visual defects

Carcinoid Syndrome

↑ **Serotonin** excretion from gastrointestinal neuroendocrine tumors (carcinoid tumors); cutaneous flushing, venous telangiectasia, diarrhea, bronchospasm, cardiac valvular lesions

Acute Intermittent Porphyria

Porphobilinogen deaminase* deficiency; episodic expression, acute abdominal pain, anxiety, confusion, paranoia, muscle weakness, no photosensitivity, port-wine urine in some patients, urine excretion of ALA and PBG; autosomal dominant; onset at puberty, 15% penetrance, variable expression; more common in women

Porphyria Cutanea Tarda

Uroporphyrinogen decarboxylase† deficiency; photosensitivity, skin inflammation, and blistering; cirrhosis often associated; autosomal dominant; late onset

Lead Poisoning

Inhibits **ALA dehydratase** and **ferrochelatase**; microcytic sideroblastic anemia; basophilic stippling of erythrocytes; headache, nausea, memory loss, abdominal pain, diarrhea (lead colic), lead lines in gums, neuropathy (claw hand, wrist-drop), ↑ urine excretion of ALA; Tx: dimercaprol and EDTA

Hemolytic Crisis

Jaundice due to ↑ bilirubin from severe hemolysis; ↓ hemoglobin; ↑ reticulocytes; may result from:
(1) G6PD deficiency hemolysis
(2) Sickle cell crisis
(3) Rh disease of newborn

UDP-Glucuronyl Transferase Deficiency

Jaundice due to low bilirubin conjugation; may result from:
(1) Crigler-Najjar syndromes
(2) Gilbert syndrome
(3) Physiologic jaundice of newborn, especially premature infants

* Also known as hydroxymethylbilane synthase; †an enzyme in the pathway between Uroporphyrinogen-III and Protoporphyrin IX.

► Amino Acid Synthesis and Metabolism

Amino acids are required for protein synthesis. Although some amino acids can be synthesized de novo (**nonessential**), others (**essential**) must be obtained from the digestion of dietary proteins. Nonessential amino acids are synthesized from intermediates of glycolysis and the citric acid cycle or from other amino acids. Degradation of amino acids occurs by transamination of the amino group to **glutamate**, while the remaining carbon skeletons of the amino acids may be oxidized to $CO_2 + H_2O$, or reverted to citric acid cycle intermediates for conversion to glucose (**glucogenic**) or ketones (**ketogenic**).

Genetic Deficiencies of Amino Acid Metabolism

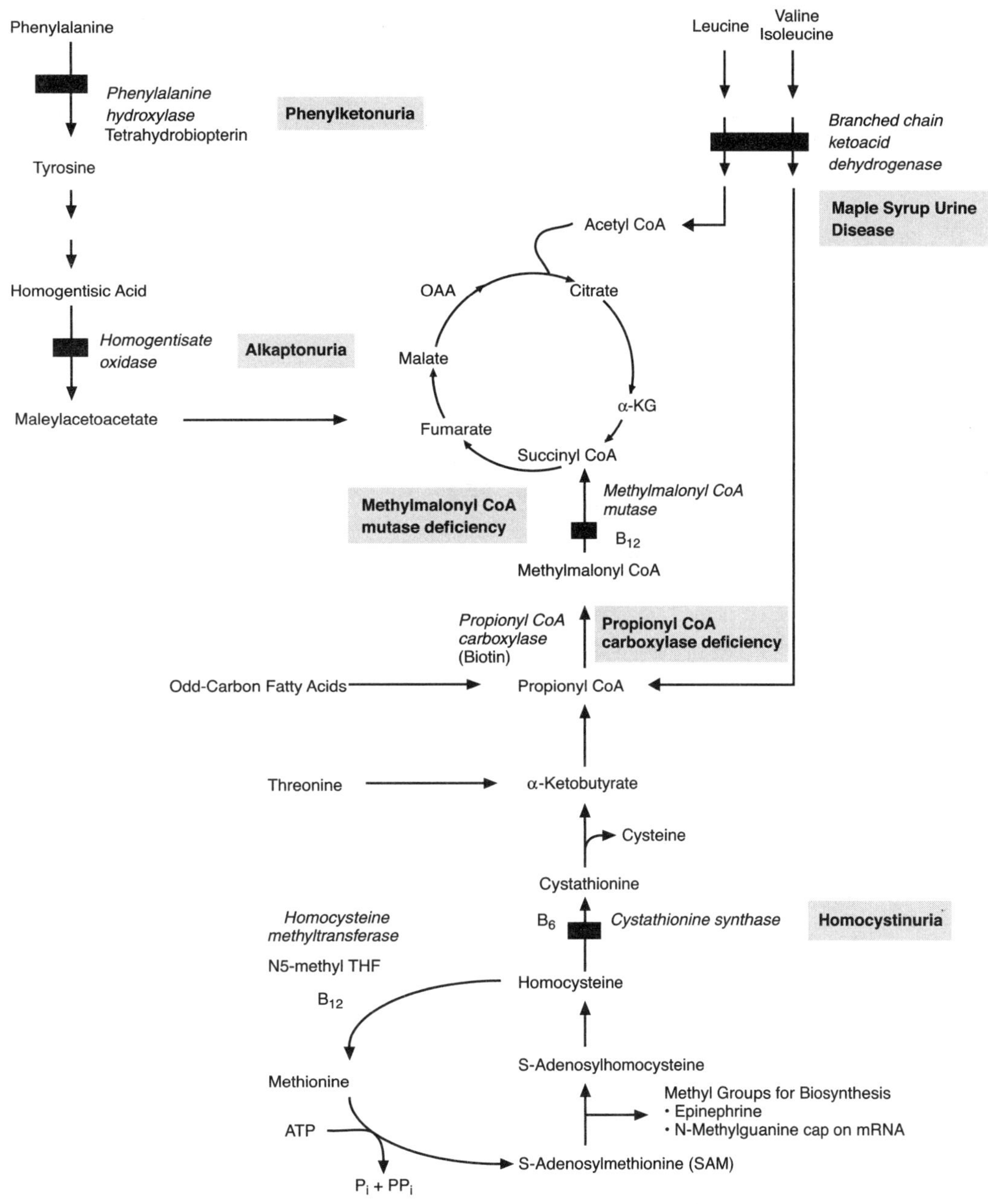

(Continued)

► Amino Acid Synthesis and Metabolism (*Cont'd.*)

Precursors for Nonessential Amino Acids

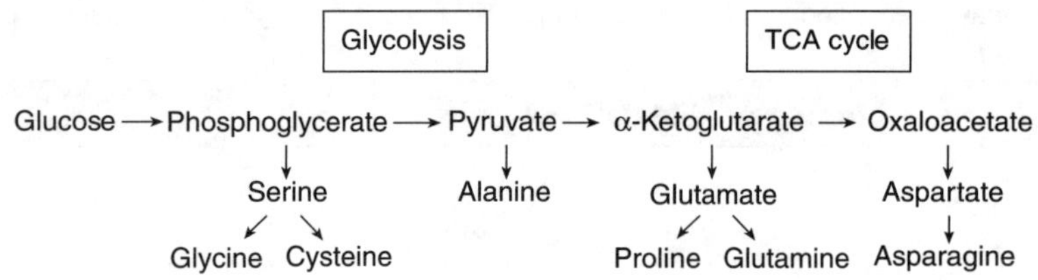

Essential Amino Acids*

Arginine†	Methionine
Histidine	Phenylalanine
Isoleucine	Threonine
Leucine	Tryptophan
Lysine	Valine

***Mnemonic:** PVT. TIM HALL; †essential during periods of growth and pregnancy

Transfer of α-Amino Groups to α-Ketoglutarate

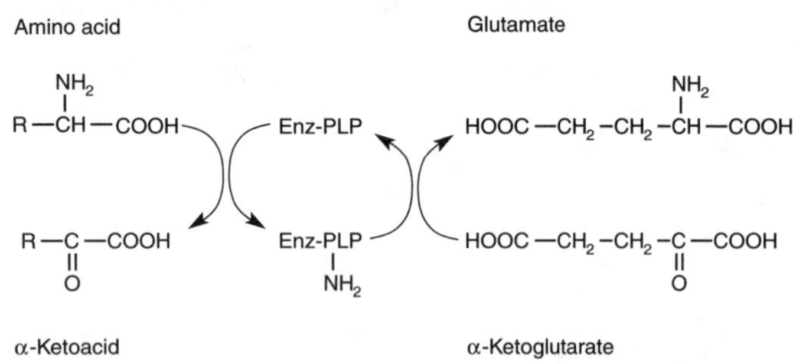

Glucogenic and Ketogenic Amino Acids

Ketogenic	Ketogenic and Glucogenic	Glucogenic
Leucine Lysine	Phenylalanine Tyrosine Tryptophan Isoleucine Threonine	All others

Disease Association

Hartnup disease	Transport protein defect with ↑ excretion of neutral amino acids; symptoms similar to pellagra; autosomal recessive
Phenylketonuria	Phenylalanine hydroxylase or dihydrobiopterin reductase deficiency → buildup of phenylalanine; tyrosine becomes essential; musty body odor, mental retardation, microcephaly, autosomal recessive; Tx: ↓ phenylalanine in diet; avoid aspartame (Nutrasweet®)
Alkaptonuria	Homogentisate oxidase deficiency (for tyrosine degradation); ↑ homogentisic acid in blood and urine (darkens when exposed to air), ochronosis (dark pigment in cartilage), arthritis in adulthood
Homocystinuria	↑ homocystine in urine. Classic homocystinuria, caused by a deficiency in cystathionine synthase, is associated with dislocated lens, deep venous thrombosis, stroke, atherosclerosis, mental retardation, and Marfan-like features. Deficiency of pyridoxine, folate, or vitamin B_{12} can produce a mild homocystinemia with elevated risk of atherosclerosis (previously listed symptoms absent). Methionine synthase (homocysteine methyltransferase) deficiency is extremely rare and is associated with megaloblastic anemia and mental retardation.
Cystinuria	Transport protein defect with ↑ excretion of lysine, arginine, cystine, and ornithine; excess cystine precipitates as kidney stones; Tx: acetazolamide
Maple syrup urine disease	Branched-chain ketoacid dehydrogenase deficiency; branched-chain ketoacidosis from infancy; weight loss, lethargy, alternating hypertonia/hypotonia, maple syrup odor of urine; ketosis/coma/death if untreated; Tx: ↓ valine, leucine, isoleucine in diet
Propionyl-CoA carboxylase deficiency **Methylmalonyl-CoA mutase deficiency**	Neonatal ketoacidosis from blocked degradation of valine, isoleucine, methionine, threonine, and odd-carbon fatty acids; Tx: ↓ these amino acids in diet *Propionyl-CoA carboxylase deficiency:* neonatal metabolic acidosis; hyperammonemia; elevated propionic acid, hydroxypropionic acid, and methylcitrate; poor feeding, vomiting, lethargy, coma *Methylmalonyl-CoA mutase deficiency:* symptoms similar to propionyl CoA carboxylase deficiency, but accumulating metabolites differ (↑ methylmalonic acid)

Definition of abbreviation: PLP, pyridoxal-phosphate, formed from vitamin B_6.

► Urea Cycle

Amino acids transported to the liver are transaminated to glutamate, which undergoes deamination to produce **NH_4^+** or transamination to make **aspartate**. Both of these are used for synthesis of urea in the liver for excretion via the **urea cycle**.

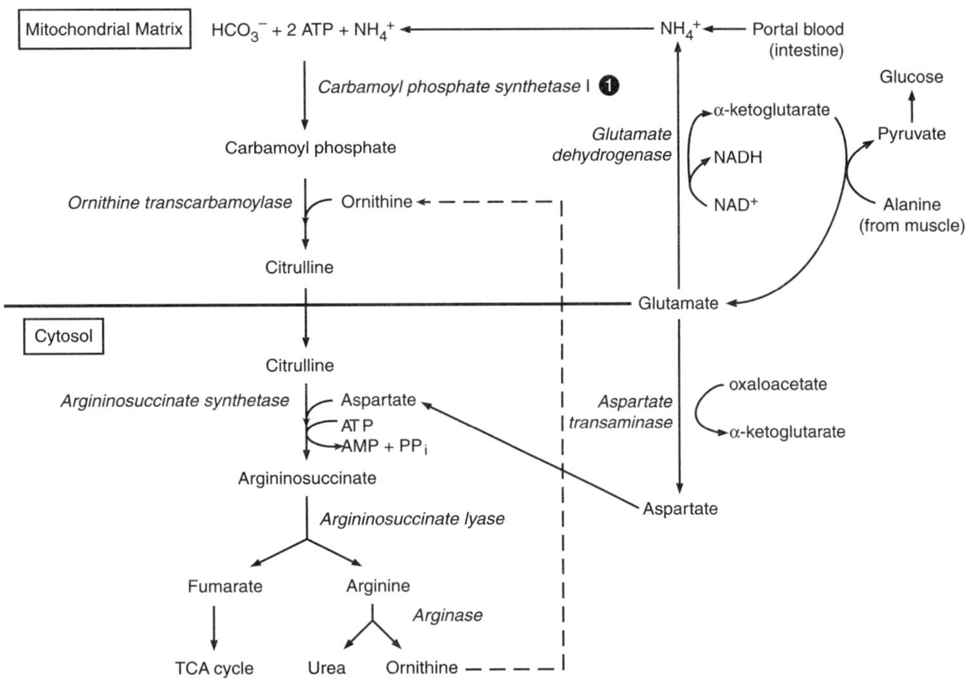

Regulation
❶ **Carbamoyl phosphate synthase I**

⊕ *N*-acetylglutamate*

*High protein diet → ↑ glutamate in mitochondria → ↑ *N*-acetylglutamate

Disease Association	
Carbamoyl Phosphate Synthetase Deficiency	**Ornithine Transcarbamoylase Deficiency**
↑ [NH_4^+]; hyperammonemia	↑ [NH_4^+]; hyperammonemia
↑ blood glutamine	↑ blood glutamine
↓ BUN	↓ BUN
No increase in uracil or orotic acid	Uracil and orotic acid ↑ in blood and urine*
Cerebral edema	Cerebral edema
Lethargy, convulsions, coma, death	Lethargy, convulsions, coma, death

*OTC deficiency: ↑ carbamoyl-P stimulates pyrimidine synthesis, causing ↑ orotic acid and uracil

► Lipid Synthesis and Metabolism

Fatty acids are synthesized from excess glucose in the liver and transported to adipose tissues for storage. Fatty acid **synthesis** occurs in the **cytosol** and involves the transport of **acetyl-CoA** from the mitochondria via the **citrate shuttle**, carboxylation to **malonyl CoA**, and linking together 2 carbons per cycle to form long fatty acid chains. Synthesis stops at **C_{16} palmitoyl-CoA**, requiring **7 ATP** and **14 NADPH**. Metabolism of fatty acids occurs by **β-oxidation**, which takes place in **mitochondria**, and involves transport of fatty acids from the cytosol via the **carnitine shuttle**, then oxidative removal of 2 carbons per cycle to yield **1 NADH**, **1 $FADH_2$**, and **1 acetyl-CoA**.

Fatty Acid Synthesis and Oxidation

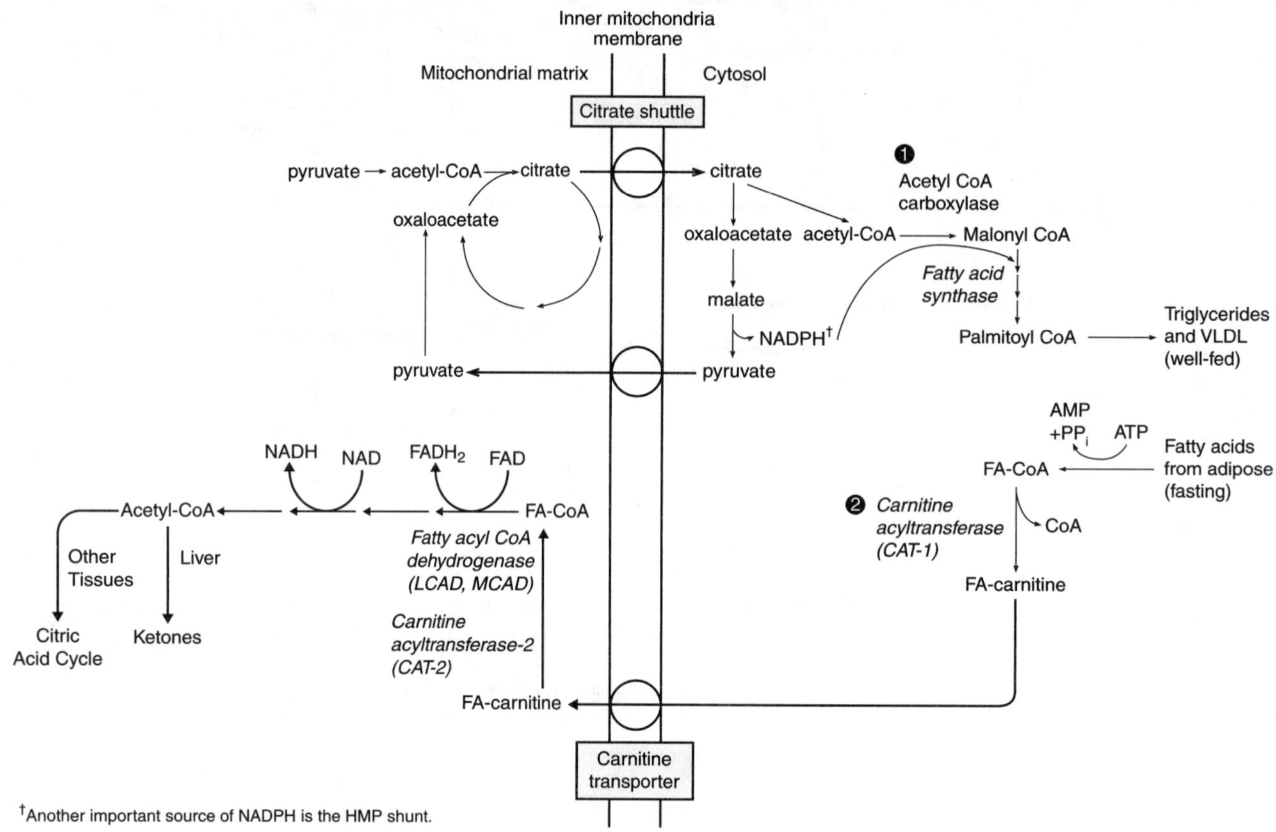

†Another important source of NADPH is the HMP shunt.

Triacylglycerols (triglycerides), the storage form of fatty acids, are formed primarily in the liver and adipose tissues by attaching **3 fatty acids** to a **glycerol-3-P**. Triacylglycerols are transported from liver to adipose as VLDL. Fatty acids from the diet are transported as chylomicrons. Both are digested by lipoprotein lipase (induced by insulin) in the capillaries of adipose and muscle. Fatty acids may be mobilized from triacylglycerols in adipose by hormone-sensitive lipase. Free fatty acids are delivered to tissues for beta oxidation.

Regulation		
❶ Acetyl-CoA carboxylase		**❷ Carnitine acyltransferase-1 (CAT-1)**
Rate-limiting for fatty acid synthesis; requires biotin		**Rate-limiting for fatty acid oxidation**
⊕ insulin ⊕ citrate	⊖ glucagon ⊖ palmitoyl-CoA	⊖ malonyl-CoA

Disease Association	
Myopathic CAT-2/CPT-2 Deficiency	**Medium Chain Acyl-Dehydrogenase (MCAD) Deficiency**
Muscle aches/weakness, myoglobulinuria provoked by prolonged exercise, ↑ muscle triacylglycerols	Fasting hypoglycemia, no ketone bodies, dicarboxylic acidemia, C8–C10 acyl carnitines in blood, vomiting, coma, death; Tx: give IV glucose, avoid fasting, maintain high carb/low fat diet, including short chain FAs, which can be metabolized

(Continued)

► Lipid Synthesis and Metabolism (*Cont'd.*)

Triacylglycerol (Triglyceride) Synthesis

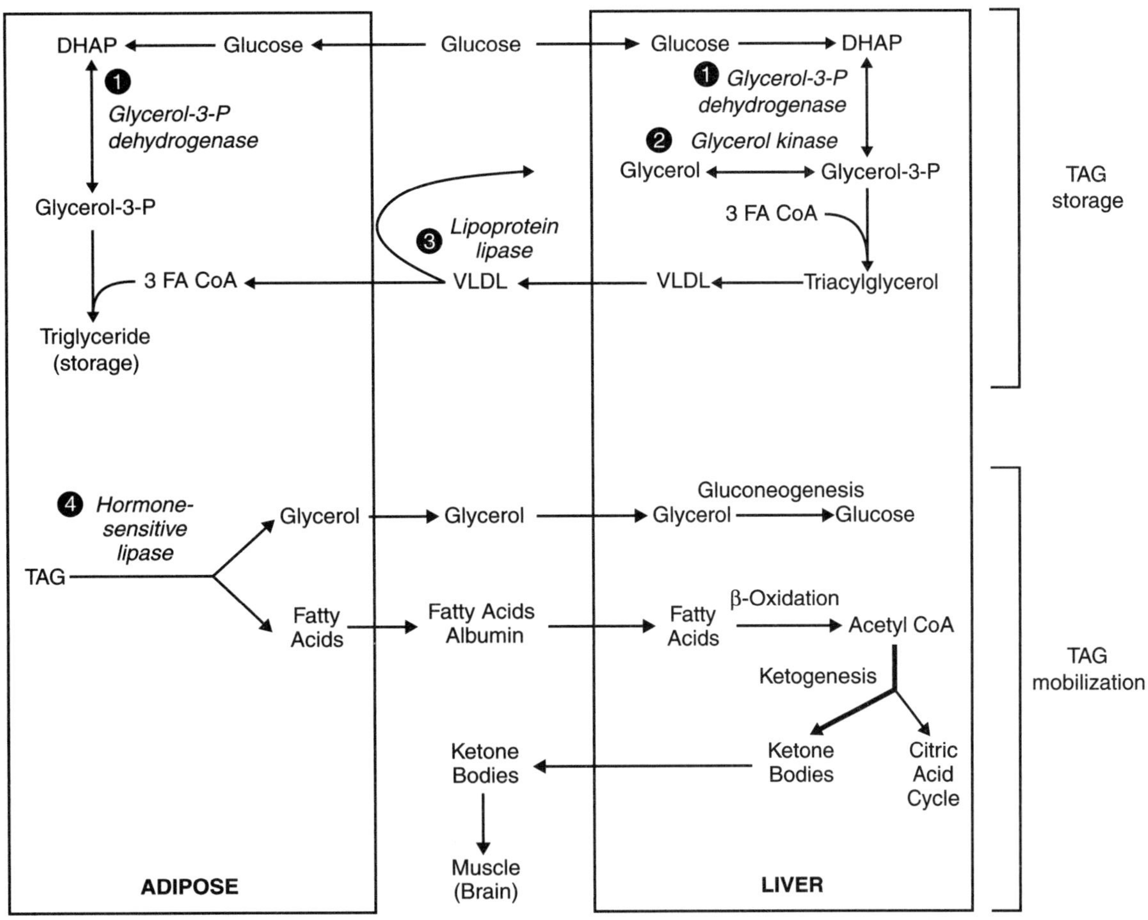

Notes	
❶ Glycerol-3P-dehydrogenase (adipose, liver) **❷ Glycerol kinase (liver only)**	Triacylglycerol synthesis from fatty acids
❸ Lipoprotein lipase	Located on luminal membrane of endothelial cells in adipose tissue

Regulation			
❸ Lipoprotein Lipase		**❹ Hormone sensitive lipase**	
Digests TGL in VLDL and chylomicrons. Fatty acids enter adipose		Mobilizes fatty acids from triacylglycerols	
Induced by insulin ⊕ ApoC-II	Repressed by ↓ insulin	⊕ Epinephrine Induced by cortisol	⊖ insulin

Definition of abbreviations: CAT, carnitine acyltransferase (a.k.a. CPT, carnitine palmitoyl transferase); L/MCAD, long/medium chain acyl-dehydrogenase; TAG, triacylglycerols.
Diabetic ketoacidosis results from overactive hormone-sensitive lipase often in the context of stress, trauma, or infection.

▶ Ketone Body Metabolism

During fasting, the liver converts excess acetyl-CoA from beta-oxidation of fatty acids into two ketone bodies, **acetoacetate** and **β-hydroxybutyrate**, which can be used by muscle and brain tissues. Ketosis represents a normal and advantageous response to fasting/starvation, whereas ketoacidosis is a pathologic condition associated with diabetes and other diseases.

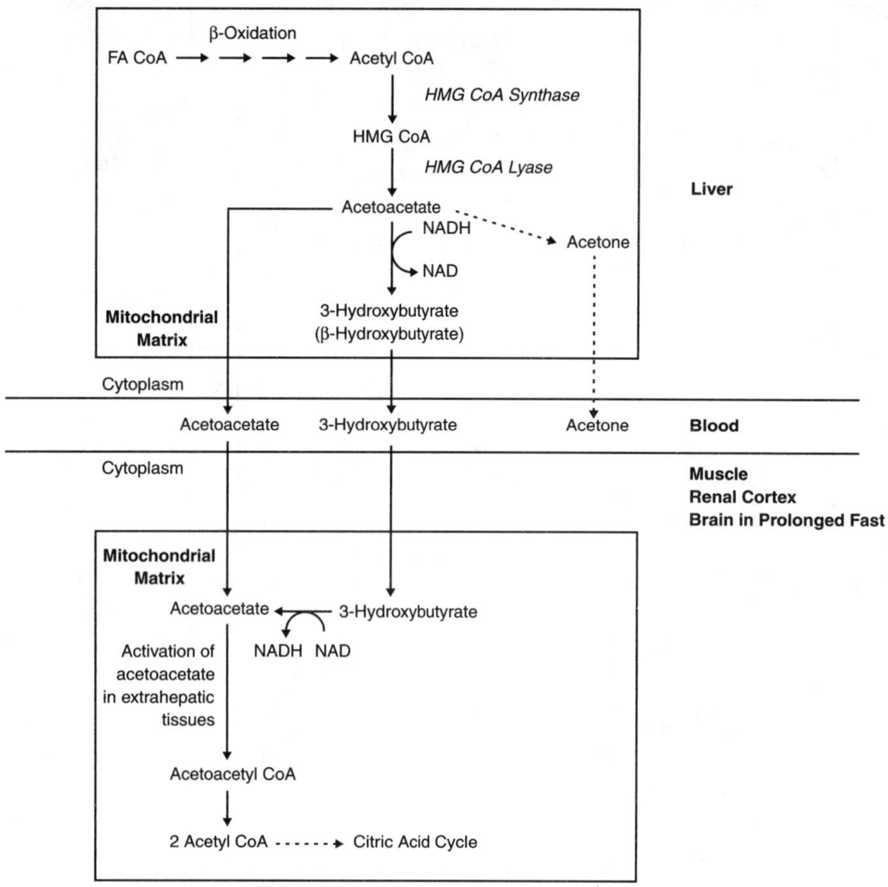

Disease Association
Diabetic Ketoacidosis
Excess ketone bodies in blood associated with type 1 diabetes mellitus not adequately managed with insulin, or precipitated by infection or trauma. Characterized by polyuria, dehydration, CNS depression and coma, sweet fruity breath (acetone). With the prevalence of obesity and stressful environments, ketoacidosis is now becoming more prevalent in type 2 diabetics, e.g., a diabetic in ketoacidosis cannot be assumed to be type 1.
Alcoholic Ketoacidosis
Excess ketone bodies due to high NADH/NAD ratio in liver; symptoms same as above *Note:* In either type of ketoacidosis, 3-hydroxybutyrate (β-hydroxybutyrate) is the predominant ketone body formed (not detected by the urine test). Measure 3-hydroxybutyrate to more accurately evaluate ketoacidosis.

▶ Cholesterol Synthesis

Cholesterol is obtained from diet (about 20%) or synthesized de novo (about 80%). Synthesis occurs primarily in the liver for storage and bile acid synthesis, but also in adrenal cortex, ovaries, and testes for steroid hormone synthesis. Cholesterol may also be esterified into **cholesterol esters** by acyl-cholesterol acyl-transferase (**ACAT**) in cells for storage.

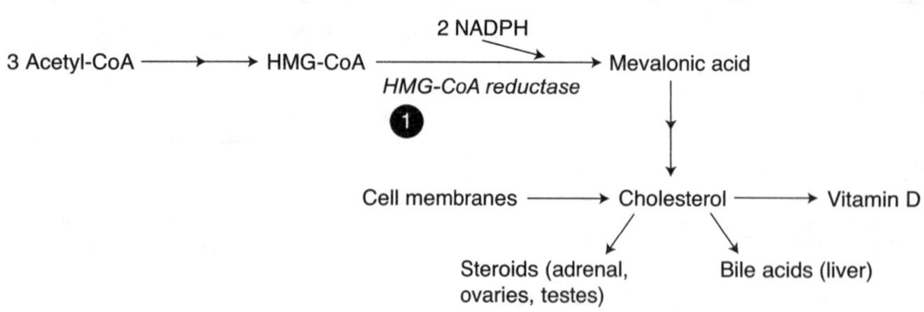

Regulation	
❶ HMG-CoA reductase	
Rate-limiting step	
⊕ insulin	⊖ glucagon
⊕ thyroxine	⊖ cholesterol

Pharmacology
HMG-CoA Inhibitors ("Statins"), e.g., lovastatin, pravastatin
↓ LDL; used for hypercholesterolemia; side effects: myopathy, liver dysfunction

▶ Lipoprotein Transport and Metabolism

Free fatty acids are transported by serum albumin, whereas neutral lipids (triacylglycerols and cholesterol esters) are transported by **lipoproteins**. Lipoproteins consist of a hydrophilic shell and a hydrophobic core and are classified by their density into **chylomicrons**, **VLDL**, **LDL**, and **HDL**.

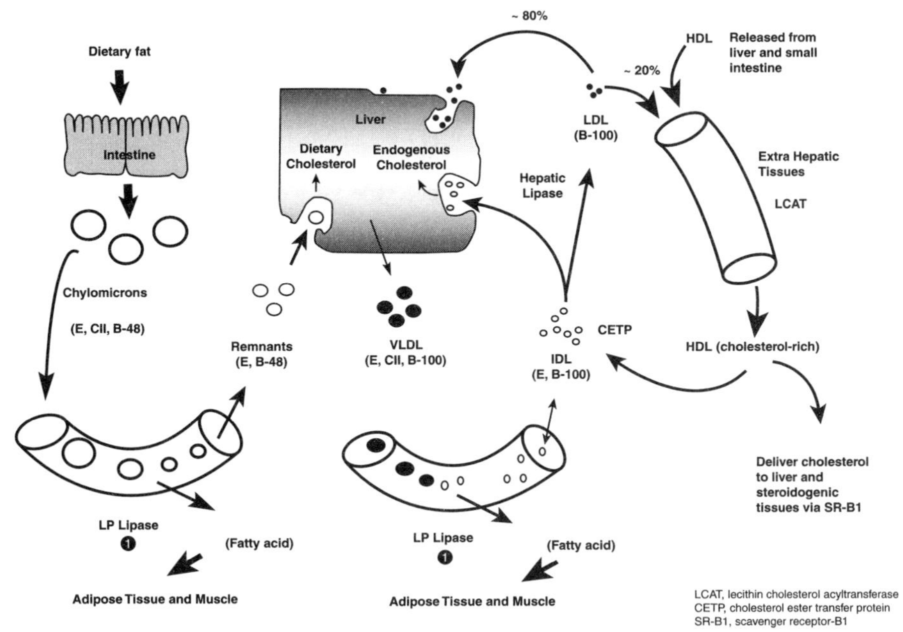

Classes of Lipoproteins and Important Apoproteins			
Lipoprotein	**Functions**	**Apoproteins**	**Functions**
Chylomicrons	Transport dietary triglyceride and cholesterol from intestine to tissues	apoB-48 apoC-II apoE	Secreted by epithelial cells Activates lipoprotein lipase Uptake by liver
VLDL	Transports triglyceride from liver to tissues	apoB-100 apoC-II apoE	Secreted by liver Activates lipoprotein lipase Uptake of remnants by liver
LDL	Delivers cholesterol into cells	apoB-100	Uptake by liver and other tissues via LDL receptor (apoB-100 receptor)
IDL (VLDL remnants)	Picks up cholesterol from HDL to become LDL Picked up by liver	apoE	Uptake by liver
HDL	Picks up cholesterol accumulating in blood vessels Delivers cholesterol to liver and steroidogenic tissues via scavenger receptor (SR-B1) Shuttles apoC-II and apoE in blood	apoA-1	Activates LCAT to produce cholesterol esters

Regulation

❶ Lipoprotein lipase

Hydrolyzes fatty acids from triacylglycerols from chylomicrons and VLDL

Induced by insulin
⊕ ApoC-II

Hyperlipidemias

Type I Hypertriglyceridemia

Lipoprotein lipase deficiency; ↑ triacylglycerols and chylomicrons; orange-red eruptive xanthomas, fatty liver, acute pancreatitis, abdominal pain after fatty meal; autosomal recessive

Type II Hypercholesterolemia

LDL receptor deficiency; ↑ risk of atherosclerosis and CAD, xanthomas of Achilles tendon, tuberous xanthomas on elbows, xanthelasma (lipid in eyelid), corneal arcus, homozygotes die <20 years; autosomal dominant

Pharmacology

Cholestyramine/Colestipol

↑ Elimination of bile salts leads to ↑ LDL receptor expression, leading to ↓ LDL; for hypercholesterolemia; side effect: GI discomfort

Gemfibrozil/Clofibrate ("Fibrates")

↑ elimination of VLDL leads to ↓ triacylglycerols and ↑ HDL; for hypertriglyceridemia; side effect: muscle toxicity ; acts via PPAR-α to induce LP lipase gene

Nicotinic Acid

↓ VLDL synthesis leads to ↓ LDL; for hypercholesterolemia and hypertriglyceridemia; side effects: GI irritation; hyperuricemia, hyperglycemia, flushing, pruritus

Definition of abbreviations: CAD, coronary artery disease; CETP, cholesterol ester transfer protein; HDL, high-density lipoprotein; LCAT, lecithin-cholesterol acyl transferase; LDL, low-density lipoprotein; PPAR, peroxisome proliferator-activated receptor; SR-B1, scavenger receptor B1; VLDL, very-low-density lipoprotein.

▶ Lysosomal Storage Diseases

Disease	Deficiency and Accumulated Substrate	Features	
Tay-Sachs disease	↓ Hexosaminidase A ↑ GM_2 ganglioside *(whorled membranes in lysosomes)*	• Psychomotor retardation • Cherry red spots in macula • Onset in 1st 6 mos.; death <2 years	AR*
Niemann-Pick disease	↓ Sphingomyelinase ↑ Sphingomyelin *(zebra bodies in lysosomes)*	• Hepatosplenomegaly • Microcephaly • Mental retardation • Foamy macrophages • Neonatal onset	AR
Gaucher disease	↓ β-glucocerebrosidase ↑ Glucocerebroside	• Three clinical subtypes; type 1 is most common • Hepatosplenomegaly • Bone involvement, including fractures and bone pain • Neurologic defects (rare, types 2 and 3) • Mental retardation • Gaucher cells (enlarged macrophages with fibrillary cytoplasm)	AR*
Fabry disease	↓ α-galactosidase A ↑ Ceramide trihexoside	• Renal failure • Telangiectasias • Angiokeratomas • Peripheral neuropathy with pain in extremities	XR
Metachromatic leukodystrophy	↓ arylsulfatase A ↑ sulfatide	• Ataxia • Dementia • Seizures	AR
Hurler syndrome (MPSI)	↓ α-L-iduronidase ↑ dermatan sulfate ↑ heparan sulfate	• Coarse facial features • Corneal clouding • Hepatosplenomegaly • Skeletal deformities • Upper airway obstruction • Recurrent ear infections • Hearing loss • Hydrocephalus • Mental retardation • Death <10 years	AR
Hunter syndrome (MPSII)	↓ L-iduronate-2-sulfatase ↓ dermatan sulfate ↑ heparan sulfate	• Both mild and severe forms • Severe similar to Hurler but retinal degeneration instead of corneal clouding, aggressive behavior, and death <15 years • Mild form compatible with long life	XR
Krabbe disease	↓ galactocerebrosidase ↑ galactocerebroside	• Defective myelin sheaths • Peripheral neuropathy • Severe seizures	AR

▶ Eicosanoid Metabolism

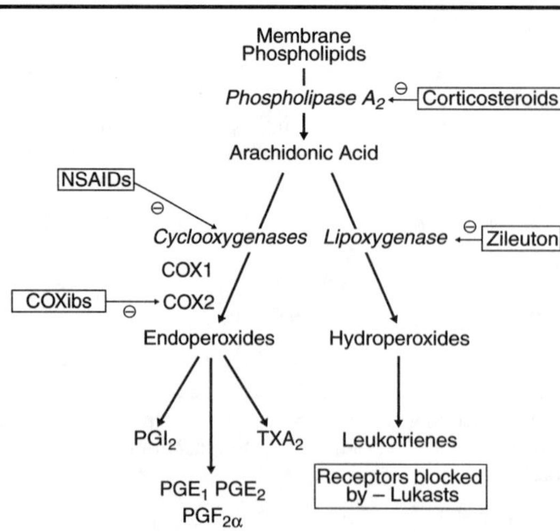

Definition of abbreviations: AR, autosomal recessive; COX, cyclooxygenase; NSAIDs, nonsteroidal anti-inflammatory drugs; XR, X-linked recessive.
*Common in Ashkenazi Jews

► Enzyme Kinetics

Whereas the thermodynamic equilibrium of a chemical reaction is determined by its **free energy** (ΔG), the rate at which the reaction reaches equilibrium is determined by its **activation energy** ($\Delta G^{\ddagger}$). Enzymes increase the rate of a reaction by reducing the energy of activation without affecting the equilibrium constant.

Michaelis-Menten Equation	Lineweaver-Burk Equation
$V = \frac{V_{max}\,[S]}{K_m + [S]}$ V = initial rate or velocity of reaction [S] = substrate concentration V_{max} = maximum rate of enzyme K_m = substrate concentration at $V_{max}/2$	$\frac{1}{V} = \frac{K_m}{V_{max}}\,\frac{1}{[S]} + \frac{1}{V_{max}}$ Reciprocal form of the Michaelis-Menten equation to achieve a straight line plot

In a typical enzyme-catalyzed reaction, the enzyme (E) is thought to bind reversibly to a substrate (S), forming a complex (ES), from which the product (P) dissociates as the reaction proceeds.

$$E + S \leftrightarrow E - S \rightarrow E + P,$$

where E is the enzyme, S is the substrate and P is the reaction product

The rate of a reaction as determined by both the concentration of enzyme (E) and substrate (S) is described by the **Michaelis-Menten equation**.

Michaelis-Menten Plot

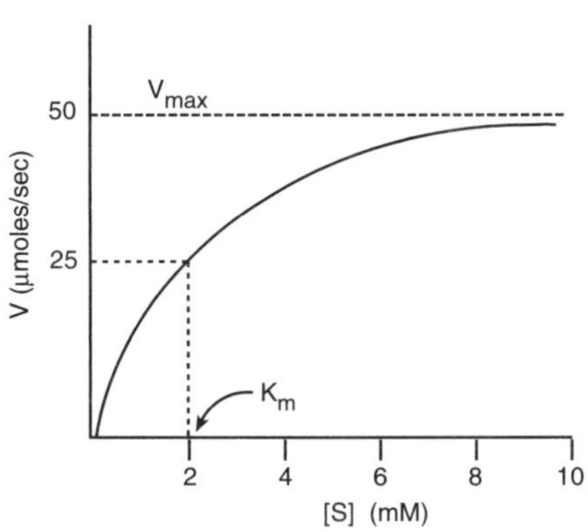

Lineweaver-Burk Plot

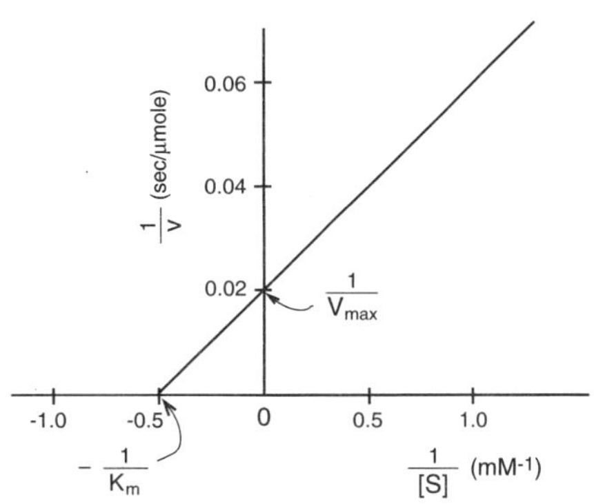

Classes of Inhibitors

Competitive, Reversible

(often substrate analogs that compete for the enzyme's binding site)

V_{max}: no effect
K_m: ↑

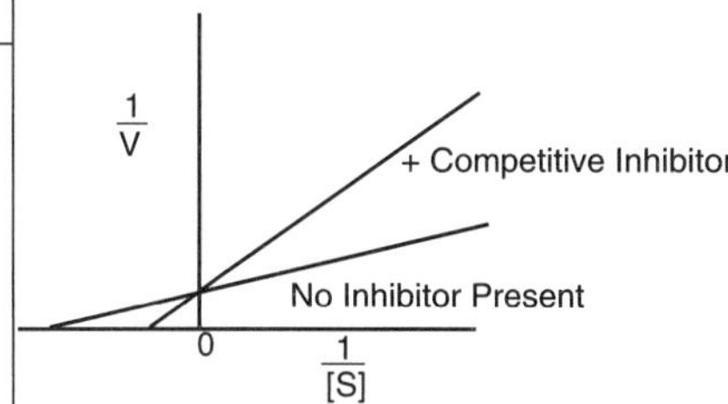

Noncompetitive, Reversible

(bind outside active site but affects enzyme activity, possibly allosterically)

V_{max}: ↓
K_m: no effect

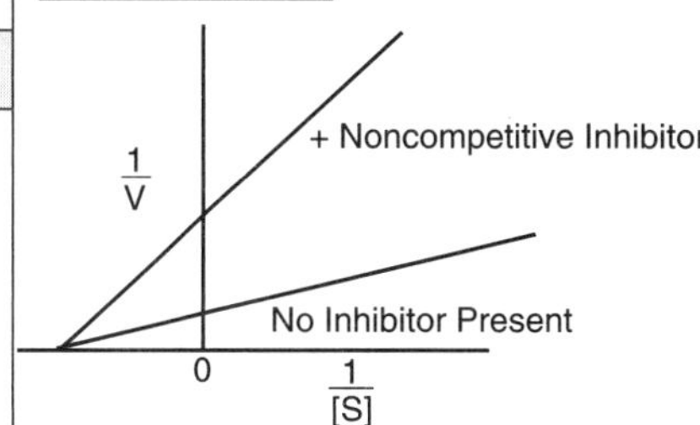

Irreversible (Inactivator)

(binds and inactivates enzyme permanently)

V_{max}: ↓
K_m: no effect

► Water-Soluble Vitamins

Vitamin or Coenzyme	Enzyme	Pathway	Deficiency
Biotin	Pyruvate carboxylase Acetyl-CoA carboxylase Propionyl-CoA carboxylase	Gluconeogenesis Fatty acid synthesis Odd-carbon fatty acids, Val, Met, Ile, Thr	Causes (rare): excessive consumption of raw eggs (contain avidin, a biotin-binding protein) Alopecia (hair loss), bowel inflammation, muscle pain
Thiamine (B_1)	Pyruvate dehydrogenase α-Ketoglutarate dehydrogenase Transketolase	PDH TCA cycle HMP shunt	Causes: alcoholism (alcohol interferes with absorption) Wernicke (ataxia, nystagmus, ophthalmoplegia) Korsakoff (confabulation, psychosis) High-output cardiac failure (wet beri-beri)
Niacin (B_3) NAD(H) NADP(H)	Dehydrogenases	Many	Pellagra may also be related to deficiency of tryptophan (corn major dietary staple), which supplies a portion of the niacin requirement Pellagra: diarrhea, dementia, dermatitis, and, if not treated, death
Folic acid THF	Thymidylate synthase Purine synthesis enzymes	Thymidine (pyrimidine) synthesis Purine synthesis	Causes: alcoholics and pregnancy (body stores depleted in 3 months) Homocystinemia with risk of deep vein thrombosis and atherosclerosis Megaloblastic (macrocytic) anemia Deficiency in early pregnancy causes neural tube defects in fetus
Cyanocobalamin (B_{12})	Homocysteine methyltransferase Methylmalonyl-CoA mutase	Methionine, SAM Odd-carbon fatty acids, Val, Met, Ile, Thr	Causes: pernicious anemia. Also in aging, especially with poor nutrition, bacterial overgrowth of terminal ileum, resection of the terminal ileum secondary to Crohn disease, chronic pancreatitis, and, rarely, vegans, or infection with *Diphyllobothrium latum* Megaloblastic (macrocytic) anemia Progressive peripheral neuropathy
Pyridoxine (B_6) PLP	Aminotransferases (transaminase): AST (SGOT), ALT (SGPT) δ-Aminolevulinate synthase	Protein catabolism Heme synthesis	Causes: isoniazid therapy Sideroblastic anemia Cheilosis or stomatitis (cracking or scaling of lip borders and corners of the mouth) Convulsions
Riboflavin (B_2) FAD(H_2)	Dehydrogenases	Many	Corneal neovascularization Cheilosis or stomatitis (cracking or scaling of lip borders and corners of the mouth) Magenta-colored tongue
Ascorbate (C)	Prolyl and lysyl hydroxylases Dopamine β-hydroxylase	Collagen synthesis Catecholamine synthesis Absorption of iron in GI tract	Causes: diet deficient in citrus fruits and green vegetables Scurvy: poor wound healing, easy bruising (perifollicular hemorrhage), bleeding gums, increased bleeding time, painful glossitis, anemia
Pantothenic acid CoA	Fatty acid synthase Fatty acyl CoA synthetase Pyruvate dehydrogenase α-Ketoglutarate dehydrogenase	Fatty acid metabolism PDH TCA cycle	Rare

Definition of abbreviations: ALT, alanine aminotransferase; AST, aspartate aminotransferase; CoA, coenzyme A; FAD(H_2), flavin adenine dinucleotide; HMP, hexose monophosphate shunt; NAD(H); nicotinamide adenine dinucleotide; NADP(H), nicotinamide adenine dinucleotide phosphate; PDH, pyruvate dehydrogenase; PLP, pyridoxal phosphate, SAM, S-adenosylmethionine; TCA, tricarboxylic acid cycle; THF, tetrahydrofolate.

► Lipid-Soluble Vitamins

Vitamin	Important Functions	Deficiency
D (cholecalciferol)	In response to hypocalcemia, helps normalize serum calcium levels	Rickets (in childhood): skeletal abnormalities (especially legs), muscle weakness After epiphysial fusion: osteomalacia
A (carotene)	Retinoic acid and retinol act as growth regulators, especially in epithelium Retinal is important in rod and cone cells for vision	Night blindness, metaplasia of corneal epithelium, dry eyes, bronchitis, pneumonia, follicular hyperkeratosis
K	Carboxylation of glutamic acid residues in many Ca^{2+}-binding proteins, importantly coagulation factors II, VII, IX, and X, as well as proteins C and S	Easy bruising, bleeding Increased prothrombin time, increased INR Associated with fat malabsorption, long-term antibiotic therapy, breast-fed newborns, infants of mothers who took anticonvulsants during pregnancy
E (α-tocopherol)	Antioxidant in the lipid phase; protects membrane lipids from peroxidation and helps prevent oxidation of LDL particles thought to be involved in atherosclerotic plaque formation	Hemolysis, neurologic problems, retinitis pigmentosa

Molecular Biology, Genetics, and Cell Biology

Chapter 2

► Nucleic Acid Structure

Nucleic acids, including **DNA** and **RNA**, are assembled from **nucleotides**, which contain a five-carbon sugar, a nitrogenous base, and phosphate. The sugar may be **ribose** (RNA) or **deoxyribose** (DNA). The base can be a **purine** (adenine or guanine) or **pyrimidine** (cytosine, uracil, thymidine). Phosphate groups link the 3′ carbon of one sugar to the 5′ carbon of the next, forming phosphodiester bonds. Base sequences are conventionally written in a **5′ → 3′** direction. Nucleotides lacking phosphate groups are called **nucleosides**. In prokaryotes and eukaryotes, RNA is generally single-stranded, while DNA is generally double-stranded in an **antiparallel** orientation, with two hydrogen bonds between base pairs **A and T** and three between **G and C**. Nuclear DNA forms a **double-helix**, which undergoes **supercoiling** via **topoisomerase** activity, and is generally associated with **histones** and other proteins to form **nucleosomes**, the basic packaging unit of **chromatin**.

Hydrogen Bonding in DNA

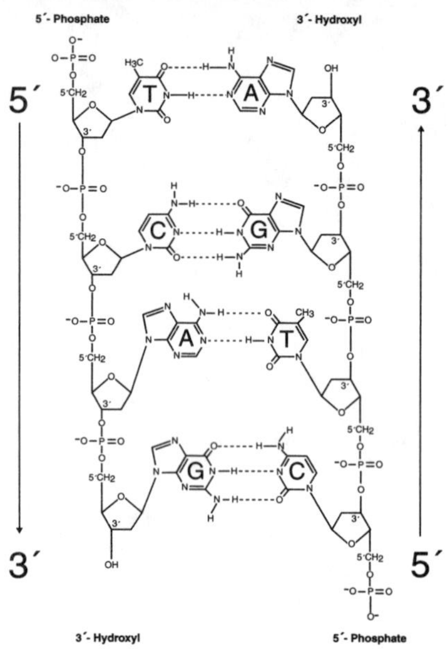

The B-DNA Double Helix

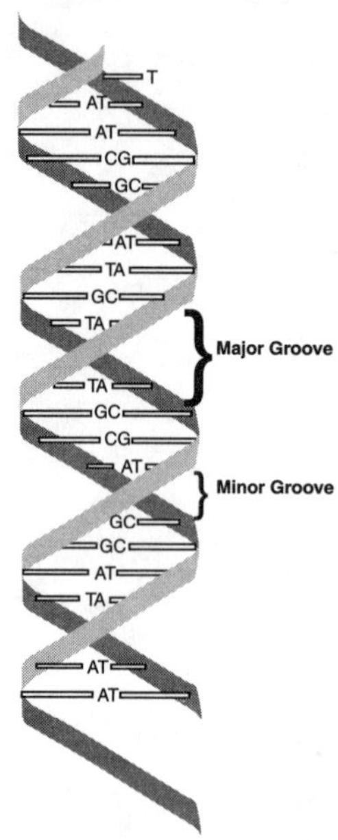

Nomenclature

Base	Nucleoside	Nucleotide
Adenine	Adenosine	Adenylate Adenosine monophosphate (AMP)
Guanine	Guanosine	Guanylate Guanosine monophosphate (GMP)
Cytosine	Cytidine	Cytidylate Cytidine monophosphate (CMP)
Thymine	Thymidine	Thymidylate Thymidine monophosphate (TMP)
Uracil	Uridine	Uridylate Uridine monophosphate (UMP)

Eukaryotic Chromatin Structure

Disease Association

Antihistone antibodies are characteristic of drug-induced SLE. Drugs include **hydralazine** and **procainamide**.

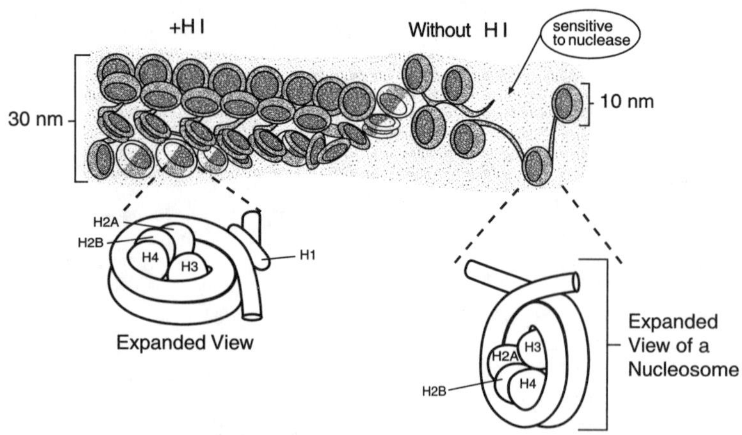

5-Carbon Sugar

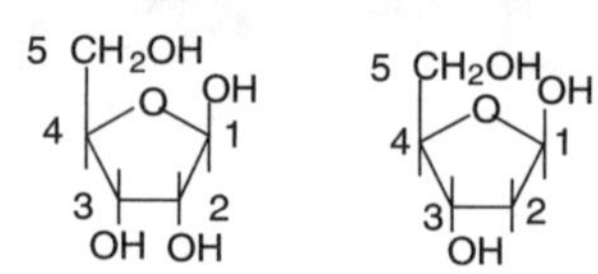

Ribose **2-Deoxyribose**

Nitrogenous Bases

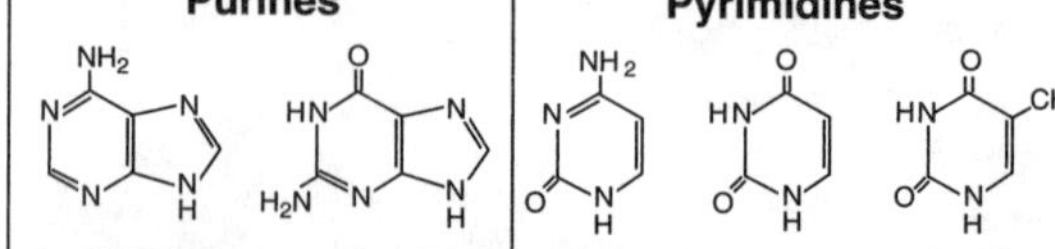

Chromatin

Euchromatin	Heterochromatin
Loosely packed	Tightly packed
Transcriptionally active	Transcriptionally inactive

▶ Nucleotide Synthesis and Salvage

Nucleotides for DNA and RNA synthesis can be generated by de novo synthesis or salvage pathways, both of which require **PRPP** generated from ribose-5-phosphate derived from the HMP shunt. **De novo synthesis** occurs mainly in the liver and generates new purine and pyrimidine bases from precursors. In contrast, **salvage pathways** reuse preformed bases derived from nucleotides during normal RNA turnover or released from dying cells or transported from the liver. Ribonucleotides are converted to deoxyribonucleotides for DNA synthesis by **ribonucleotide reductase**. Antineoplastic drugs that target ribonucleotide reductase (hydroxyurea), or an enzyme in the dTMP branch of pyrimidine synthesis (5-FU), or reduction of folate (methotrexate) preferentially inhibit DNA synthesis without compromising RNA synthesis and gene expression. Excretion of purine bases occurs in the form of **uric acid** from the kidneys.

De Novo Purine Synthesis

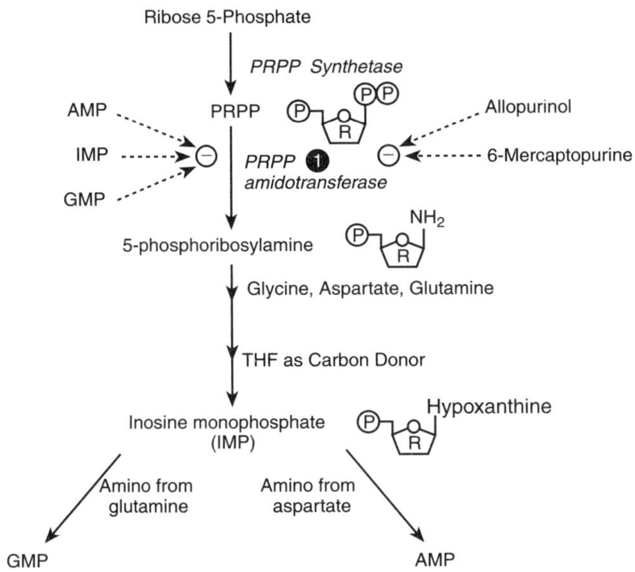

Regulation

❶ PRPP amidotransferase

⊖ AMP, IMP, GMP

De Novo Pyrimidine Synthesis

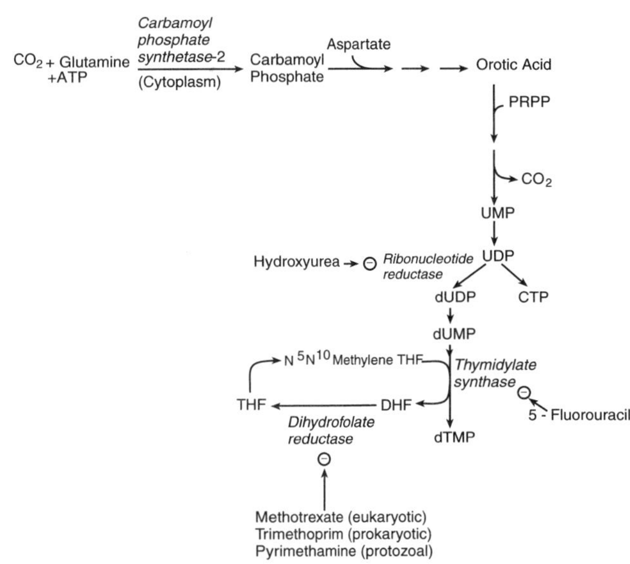

Purine Analogs

Allopurinol
- Inhibits PRPP amidotransferase
- Treatment of gout
- Inhibits xanthine oxidase

6-mercaptopurine; 6-thioguanine
- Inhibits PRPP amidino-transferase
- Antineoplastic

Pyrimidine Analogs

5-fluorodeoxyuridine;
5-bromodeoxyuridine
- Inhibit thymidylate synthase
- Antineoplastic

Folic Acid Analogs

Methotrexate; aminopterin
- Inhibit eukaryotic DHFR
- Antineoplastic

Trimethoprim
- Inhibits bacterial DHFR
- Antibacterial

Pyrimethamine
- Inhibits protozoal DHFR
- Antiprotozoal

Hydroxyurea

- Inhibits ribonucleotide reductase
- Antineoplastic

Definition of abbreviations: AMP, adenosine monophosphate; dTMP, deoxythymidine monophosphate; 5-FU, 5-flurouracil; IMP, inosine monophosphate; dUDP, deoxyuridine diphosphate; CTP, cytosine triphosphate; THF, tetrahydrofolate.

(*Continued*)

► Nucleotide Synthesis and Salvage (*Cont'd.*)

Purine Salvage Pathway and Excretion

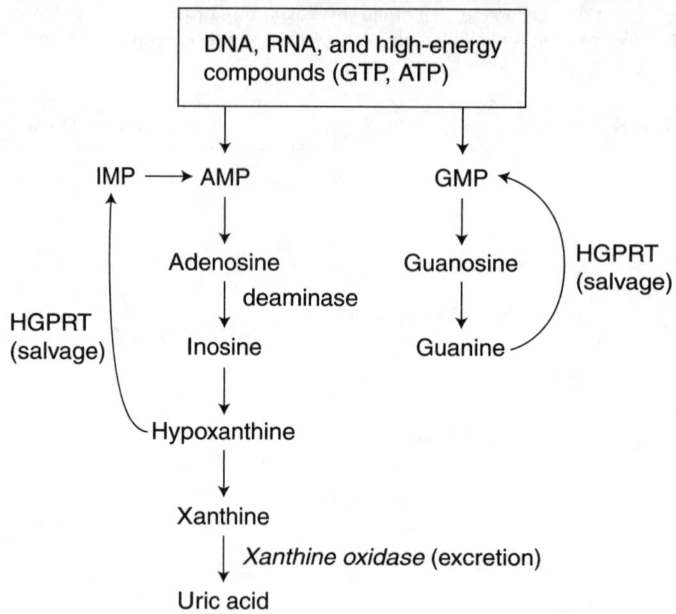

Definition of abbreviations: DHFR, dihydrofolate reductase; HGPRT, hypoxanthine-guanine phosphoribosyl pyrophosphate transferase; NSAID, nonsteroidal anti-inflammatory drug; PRPP, phosphoribosylpyrophosphate; THF, tetrahydrofolate; SCID, severe combined immunodeficiency disorder.

Disease Association
Adenosine Deaminase Deficiency
• SCID (no B- or T-cell function) • Multiple infections in children • Autosomal recessive • Tx: enzyme replacement, bone marrow transplant
Gout
↑ production or ↓ excretion of uric acid by kidneys
Lesch-Nyhan Syndrome
• HGPRT deficiency • Mental retardation (mild) • Spastic cerebral palsy • Self-mutilation • Hyperuricemia • X-linked recessive

► DNA Replication

DNA replication involves the synthesis of new DNA molecules in a 5′ → 3′ direction by **DNA polymerase** using the double-stranded DNA template. One strand (**leading strand**) is made continuously, while the other (**lagging strand**) is synthesized in segments. **Prokaryotic** chromosomes are closed, double-stranded circular DNA molecules with a single origin of replication that separates into two replication forks moving away in opposite directions. **Eukaryotic** chromosomes are double-stranded and linear with multiple origins of replication.

DNA Replication by a Semiconservative, Bidirectional Mechanism

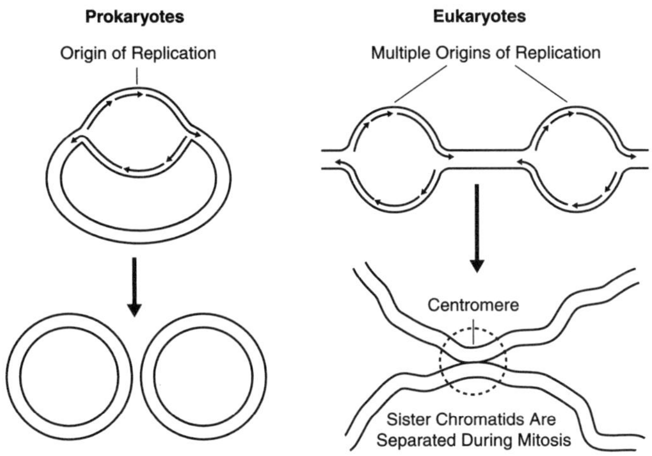

Events at the Replication Fork

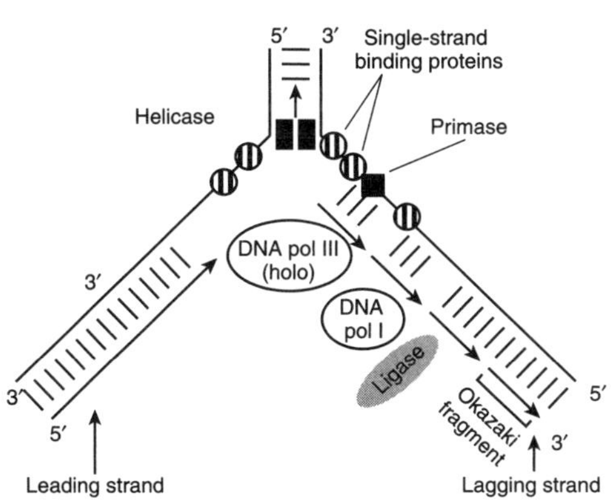

Regulation

	Prokaryote	Eukaryote
Recognizing replication origin	dna A	Unknown
Unwinding double helix	Helicase	Helicase
Strand stabilization	SSB	SSB
RNA primer synthesis	Primase	Primase
Leading strand synthesis	DNA pol III	DNA pol α and δ
Lagging strand synthesis	DNA pol III	DNA pol α
RNA primer removal	DNA pol I (5′→ 3′ exonuclease)	RNase H
Replacing RNA with DNA	DNA pol I	Unknown
Joining of Okazaki fragments	DNA ligase	DNA ligase
Removing positive supercoils ahead of replication fork	DNA topo II (DNA gyrase)	DNA topo II
Telomere synthesis	Not required	Telomerase

Pharmacology

Pyrimidine Analogs

Cytosine arabinoside
- Incorporation stops chain elongation
- Antineoplastic

Definition of abbreviations: DNA, deoxyribonucleic acid; DNA pol, DNA polymerase; DNA topo, DNA topoisomerase; RNA, ribonucleic acid; SSB, single-stranded DNA-binding protein.

► DNA Repair

DNA sequence and structure may be altered either during replication or by exposure to chemicals or radiation. Mutations include point mutations such as the **substitution** of one base with another. Substitution mutations in the third position of a codon **(wobble position)** are usually benign because several codons code for the same amino acid. Other types of mutations include (1) deletion or addition of one or two nucleotides (frameshift mutations), (2) large segment deletions (e.g., unequal crossover during meiosis), (3) mutations of 5′ or 3′ splice sites, or (4) triplet repeat expansion, which can lead to a longer, more unstable protein product (e.g., Huntington disease).

Damage	Cause	Recognition/ Excision Enzyme	Repair Enzymes
Thymine dimers (G_1)	UV radiation	Excision endonuclease (deficient in xeroderma pigmentosum)	DNA polymerase DNA ligase
Cytosine deamination (G_1)	Spontaneous/ chemicals	Uracil glycosylase AP endonuclease	DNA polymerase DNA ligase
Apurination or apyrimidination (G_1)	Spontaneous/ heat	AP endonuclease	DNA polymerase DNA ligase
Mismatched base (G_2)	DNA replication errors	A mutation on one of two genes, *hMSH2* or *hMLH1*, initiates defective repair of DNA mismatches, resulting in a condition known as hereditary nonpolyposis colorectal cancer—HNPCC.	DNA polymerase DNA ligase

Types of Mutations

Transition: A:T → G:C or G:C → A:T
Transversion: A:T → T:A or G:C → C:G

Silent	No change in AA	Sub
Missense	Change AA to another	Sub
Nonsense	Early stop codon	Sub or Ins/Del
Frameshift	Misreading of all codons downstream	Ins/Del

DNA Repair Defects

Xeroderma Pigmentosum

(defect in nucleotide excision-repair)

- Extreme UV sensitivity
- Excessive freckling
- Multiple skin cancers
- Corneal ulcerations
- Autosomal recessive

Ataxia Telangiectasia

(defect in ATM gene product, a member of PI-3 kinase family involved in mitogenic signal transduction, detection of DNA damage, and cell cycle control)

- Sensitivity to ionizing radiation
- Degenerative ataxia
- Dilated blood vessels
- Chromosomal aberrations
- Lymphomas
- Autosomal recessive

HNPCC

(defect in mismatch repair; usually hMSH2 or hMLH1 gene)

- Colorectal cancer
- ⅔ occur in right colon
- Autosomal dominant
- Part of Lynch syndrome (a multi-cancer syndrome)

Definition of abbreviations: AA, amino acid; HNPCC, hereditary nonpolyposis colorectal cancer; Ins/Del, insert or deletion; Sub, substitution.

► Transcription and RNA Processing

Transcription involves the synthesis of an RNA in a 5′ → 3′ direction by an RNA polymerase using DNA as a template. An important class of RNA is messenger RNA (mRNA). Initiation of transcription occurs from a promoter region, which is the binding site of RNA polymerase, and stops at a termination signal. In **prokaryotes**, a single mRNA transcript can encode several genes **(polycistronic)**, and no RNA processing is required, allowing transcription and translation to proceed simultaneously. In **eukaryotes**, all mRNAs are **monocistronic**, but often include coding segments **(exons)** interrupted by noncoding regions **(introns)**. Eukaryotic mRNAs must therefore undergo extensive processing, including a 5′ cap, a 3′ tail, and removal of introns followed by exon splicing. Ribosomal RNA (rRNA) and transfer RNA (tRNA) are also produced by transcription.

Prokaryotic Transcription

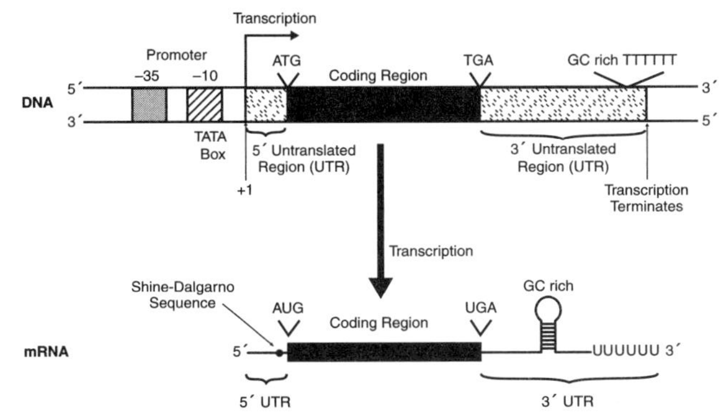

Eukaryotic Transcription and Processing

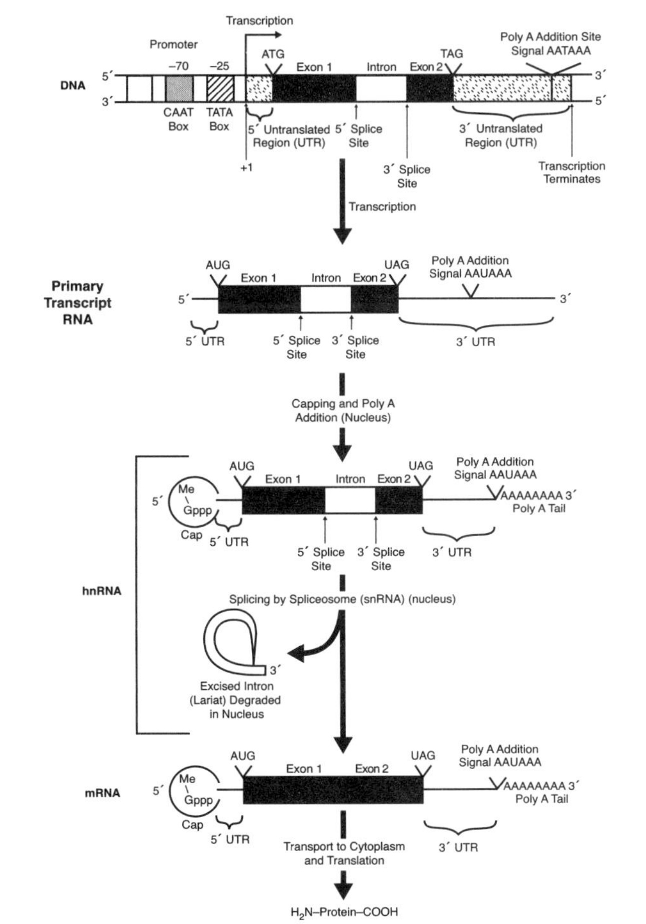

Properties

	Prokaryote	Eukaryote
Gene regions	May be polycistronic Continuous coding	Always monocistronic Exons and introns
RNA polymerase	Core enzyme: $\alpha 2\beta\beta'$	RNA pol I: rRNA RNA pol II: mRNA, snRNA RNA pol III: tRNA, 5S rRNA
Initiation	Promoter (–10) TATAAT and (–35) sequence; sigma initiation subunit	Promoter (–25) TATA and (–70) CAAT; transcription factors (TFIID) bind promoter
Termination	Stem loop and UUUU or stem loop and rho factor	Not well characterized
Postprocessing	None	5′ cap (7-MeG) 3′ tail (poly-A) Intron removal and exon splicing in pre-mRNA

Types of RNA

mRNA	Messenger RNA carries sequence info from DNA to ribosomes to be translated
rRNA	Ribosomal RNA is a component of ribosomes
tRNA	Transfer RNA carries amino acids to ribosomes for protein synthesis
snRNA	Small nuclear RNA plays role in RNA processing

Regulation of Gene Expression

Transcription initiation	Transcription factors bound to enhancer or silencer DNA regions affect transcription
Splicing	Alternative splicing of primary transcript yields variants of protein products
mRNA degradation	Various RNA-binding proteins determine stability of mRNA

Definition of abbreviations: hnRNA, heterogeneous nuclear RNA; 7-MeG, 7-methylguanosine; RNA pol, RNA polymerase; UTR, untranslated region.

► Protein Translation

Translation involves the synthesis of protein from mRNA templates in **ribosomes** (complexes of proteins and ribosomal RNAs [**rRNA**]). Protein synthesis begins from an initiation codon (**AUG** = methionine) and ends at a stop codon (**UAA**, **UGA**, or **UAG**). Elongation involves transfer RNAs (**tRNA**), which have an anticodon region at one end to recognize the codon on the mRNA and an amino acid attached at the other end for covalent linkage to the growing polypeptide chain. Several ribosomes can simultaneously transcribe an mRNA, forming a polyribosome, or **polysome**.

tRNA

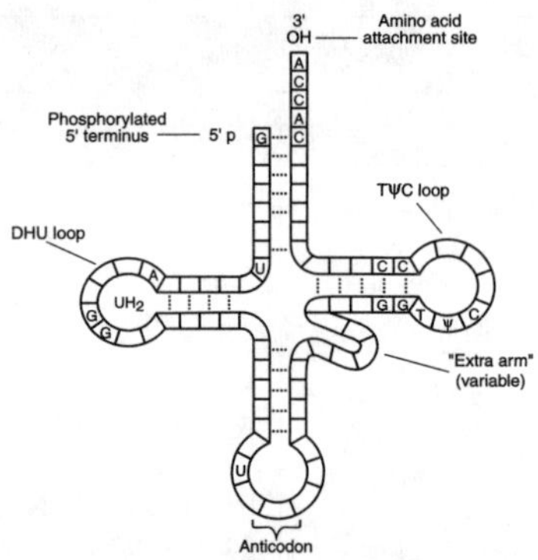

Genetic Code

Second base

First base	U	C	A	G	Third base
U	UUU, UUC: Phe UUA, UUG: Leu	UCU, UCC, UCA, UCG: Ser	UAU, UAC: Tyr UAA: Stop UAG: Stop	UGU, UGC: Cys UGA: Stop UGG: Trp	U C A G
C	CUU, CUC, CUA, CUG: Leu	CCU, CCC, CCA, CCG: Pro	CAU, CAC: His CAA, CAG: Gln	CGU, CGC, CGA, CGG: Arg	U C A G
A	AUU, AUC, AUA: Ile AUG: Start/fMet	ACU, ACC, ACA, ACG: Thr	AAU, AAC: Asn AAA, AAG: Lys	AGU, AGC: Ser AGA, AGG: Arg	U C A G
G	GUU, GUC, GUA, GUG: Val	GCU, GCC, GCA, GCG: Ala	GAU, GAC: Asp GAA, GAG: Glu	GGU, GGC, GGA, GGG: Gly	U C A G

Properties

	Prokaryote	Eukaryote
Ribosomes	30S + 50S = 70S	40S + 60S = 80S
Initiation	30S binds to Shine-Dalgarno sequence; fMet	40S associates with 5′ cap on mRNA; Met
Termination	Protein released at stop codon	

Formation of Aminoacyl-tRNA

Step I $ATP + NH_2{-}CH(R){-}COOH \longrightarrow NH_2{-}CH(R){-}C(=O){\sim}AMP + PP_i$

Step 2 $NH_2{-}CH(R){-}C(=O){-}AMP + tRNA \longrightarrow NH_2{-}CH(R){-}C(=O){-}tRNA + AMP$

Sum $NH_2{-}CH(R){-}COOH + ATP + tRNA \longrightarrow NH_2{-}CH(R){-}C(=O){-}tRNA + AMP + PP_i$

Polyribosome

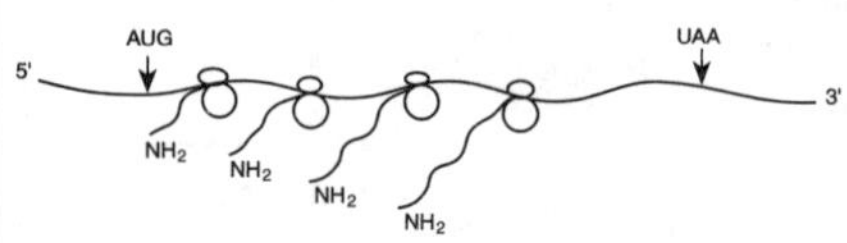

Steps In Translation

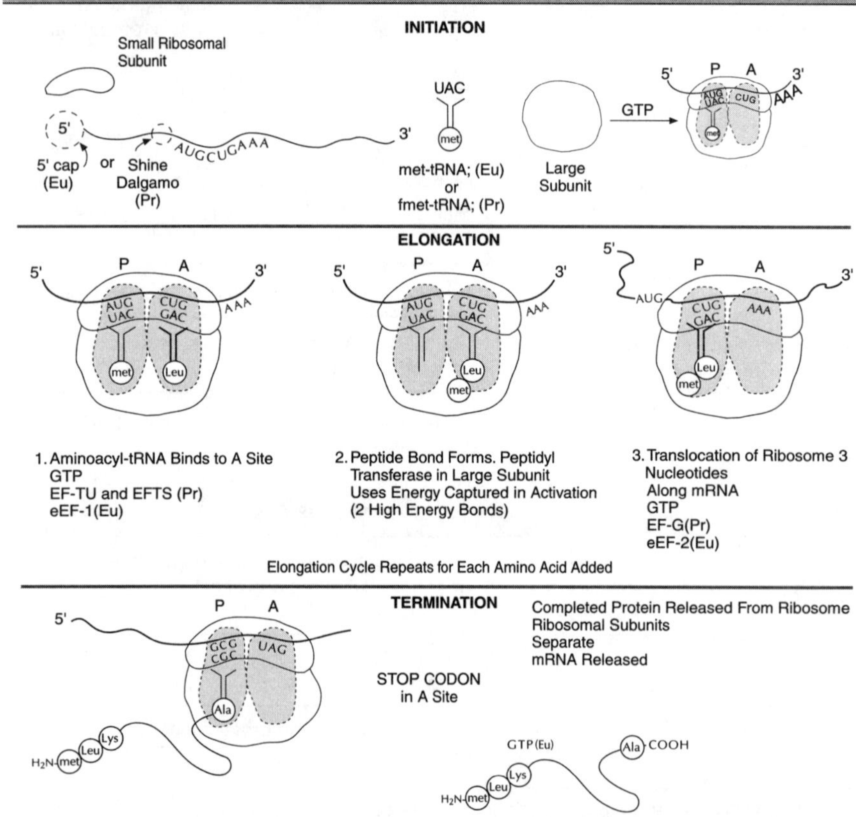

Pharmacology

Tetracyclines

(tetracycline, doxycycline, minocycline)

- Prevent binding of aminoacyl-tRNA to ribosome
- For *Chlamydia*, *Mycoplasma*, *H. pylori*, *Rickettsia*, *Brucella*, *Vibrio*, and acne
- Prophylaxis in chronic bronchitis
- Bacteriostatic
- Phototoxicity, GI distress, tooth discoloration, ↓ bone growth in children

Linezolid

- Blocks initiation complex formation
- For VRSA, VRE, drug-resistant pneumococci
- Headache, GI distress

Aminoglycosides

(streptomycin, gentamicin, neomycin)

- Cause misreading at initiation
- Accumulates intracellular via O_2-dependent uptake; anaerobes are resistant
- For gram ⊖ rods, enterococci
- Bactericidal
- Nephrotoxicity, ototoxicity

Macrolides

(erythromycin, clarithromycin, azithromycin)

- Interfere with translocation
- For gram ⊕ cocci, *Chlamydia*, *Mycoplasma*, *Ureaplasma*, *Legionella*, *Campylobacter*
- Bacteriostatic
- GI distress, inhibits P450, auditory dysfunction at high doses

Clindamycin

- Interferes with translocation
- For gram ⊕ cocci, *B. fragilis*
- Pseudomembranous colitis

Chloramphenicol

- Inhibits ribosomal peptidyl transferase
- For *Salmonella*, *B. fragilis*, *Rickettsia*, and bacterial meningitis (used as backup)
- Bacteriostatic
- Bone marrow suppression; aplastic anemia, "gray baby" syndrome (neonates), optic neuritis (children)

Definition of abbreviations: AA, amino acid; EF-2, elongation factor 2; fMet, formylmethionine; Met, methionine; VRE, vancomycin-resistant enterococci; VRSA, vancomycin-resistant *Staphylococcus aureus*.

▶ Post-Translational Modifications

Whereas cytoplasmic proteins are translated on free cytoplasmic ribosomes, secreted proteins, membrane proteins, and lysosomal enzymes have an ***N*-terminal hydrophobic signal sequence** and are translated on ribosomes associated with the rough endoplasmic reticulum (RER). After translation, proteins acquire more complex structures by being folded with the help of molecular **chaperones**. Misfolded proteins are targeted for destruction by **ubiquitin** and digested in cytoplasmic protein-digesting complexes called **proteasomes**.

Co- and Postranslational Covalent Modifications	
Glycosylation	Addition of oligosaccharides
Phosphorylation	Addition of phosphate groups by protein kinases
γ-carboxylation (vitamin K dependent)	Creation of Ca^{2+} binding sites
Prenylation	Addition of farnesyl/geranyl lipid groups to peripheral membrane proteins
Mannose phosphorylation	Addition of phosphates onto mannose residues to target protein to lysosomes

Protein Structure	
Primary	Amino acid sequence
Secondary	α-Helix or β-sheets
Tertiary	Higher order 3D structure
Quaternary	Multiple subunits

Synthesis of Secretory, Membrane, and Lysosomal Proteins

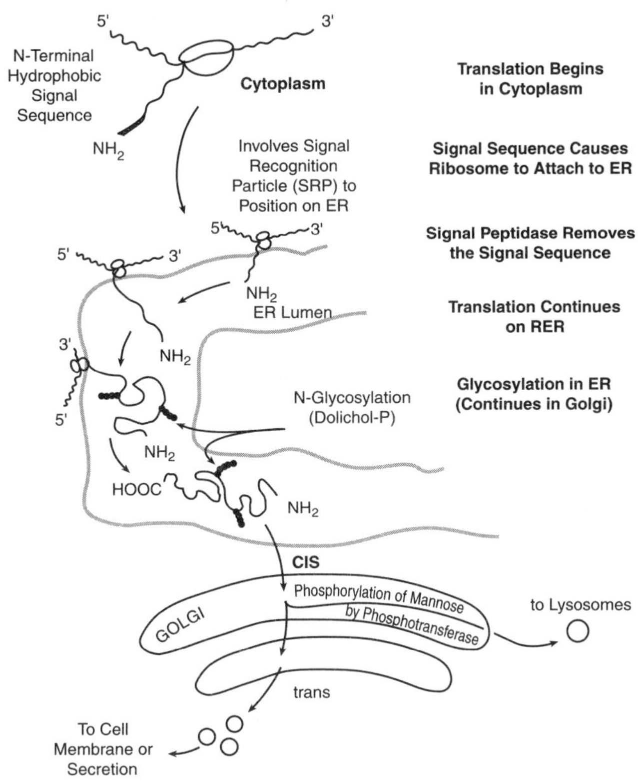

Disease Association

I-Cell Disease

(defect in mannose phosphorylation, causing lysosomal enzyme release into extracellular space and accumulation of undigested substrates in cell)

- Coarse facial features, gingival hyperplasia, macroglossia
- Craniofacial abnormalities, joint immobility, club-foot, claw-hand, scoliosis
- Psychomotor and growth retardation
- Cardiorespiratory failure
- Death in first decade
- 10–20-fold increase in lysosomal enzyme activity in serum

► Collagen Synthesis

Collagen is a structural protein composed of a triple helix of amino acid chains containing a repeating tripeptide Gly-X-Y-Gly-X-Y, where the unique amino acids **hydroxyproline** and **hydroxylysine** are frequently found in the X position. Hydroxylation of proline and lysine requires ascorbate (vitamin C), deficiency of which leads to scurvy.

Synthesis of Collagen

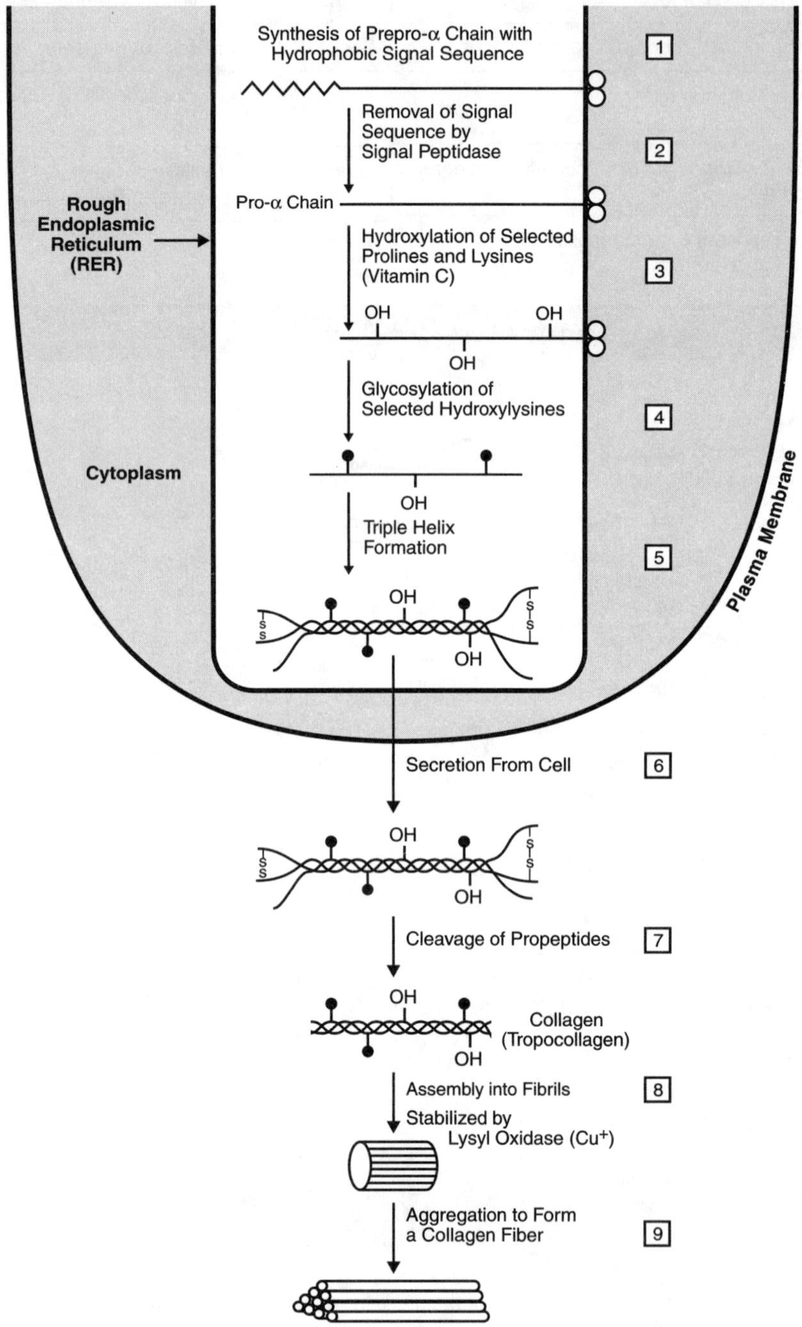

Disease Association

Scurvy

(reduced hydroxylation due to ascorbate/vitamin C deficiency)

- Petechiae, ecchymoses
- Loose teeth, bleeding gums
- Poor wound healing
- Poor bone development

Osteogenesis Imperfecta

(collagen gene mutations)

- Skeletal deformities
- Fractures
- Blue sclera

Ehlers-Danlos Syndrome

(collagen and lysine hydroxylase gene mutations)

- Hyperextensible, fragile skin
- Hypermobile joints, dislocations
- Varicose veins, ecchymoses

Menkes Disease

(deficient cross-linking secondary to copper deficiency)

- Depigmented (steely) hair
- Arterial tortuosity, rupture
- Cerebral degeneration
- Osteoporosis, anemia
- Mutation in gene for an ATP-dependent copper transport protein
- X-linked recessive

► Recombinant DNA

Recombinant DNA technology allows DNA fragments to be copied, manipulated, and analyzed in vitro. Eukaryotic DNA fragments may be **genomic DNA** containing both introns and exons, or **complementary DNA (cDNA)**, which is reverse-transcribed from mRNA and contains exons only. DNA fragments may be amplified by **polymerase chain reaction (PCR)**, cut with specific **restriction endonucleases**, and ligated into a **DNA vector**. These vectors can then be used for further manipulation or amplification of the DNA to produce genomic DNA or cDNA (expression) libraries, to generate recombinant proteins, or for incorporation into humans (**gene therapy**) or other animals (**transgenic animals**).

Formation of a Recombinant Plasmid

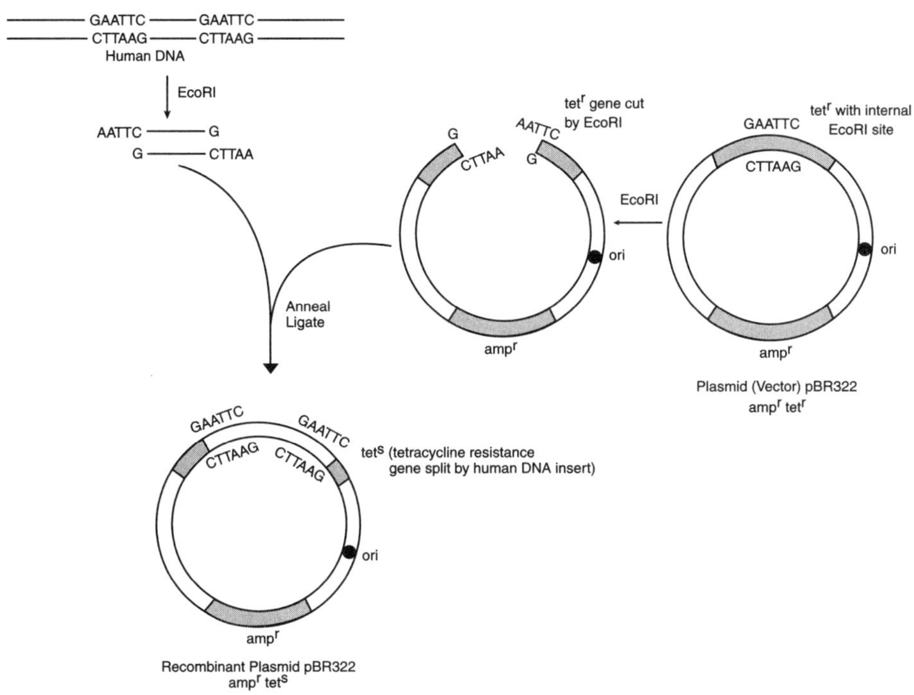

Polymerase Chain Reaction

- Amplifies large amounts of DNA from even just one DNA molecule
- Used for recombinant DNA manipulation, genetic testing, or disease screening
- Can be used to make cDNA from mRNA with reverse transcriptase (RT-PCR)

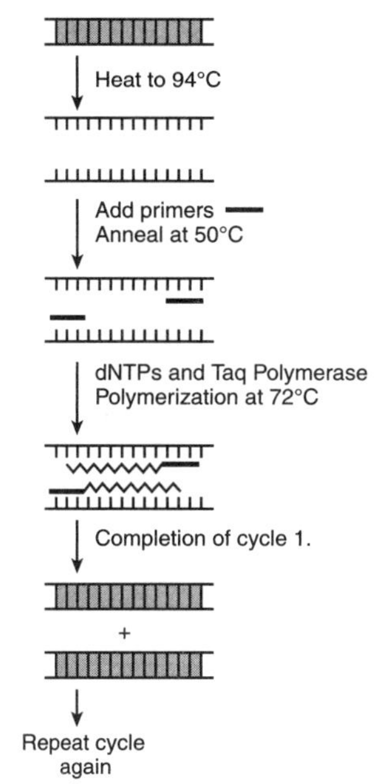

(Continued)

► Recombinant DNA (*Cont'd.*)

Screening a DNA Library

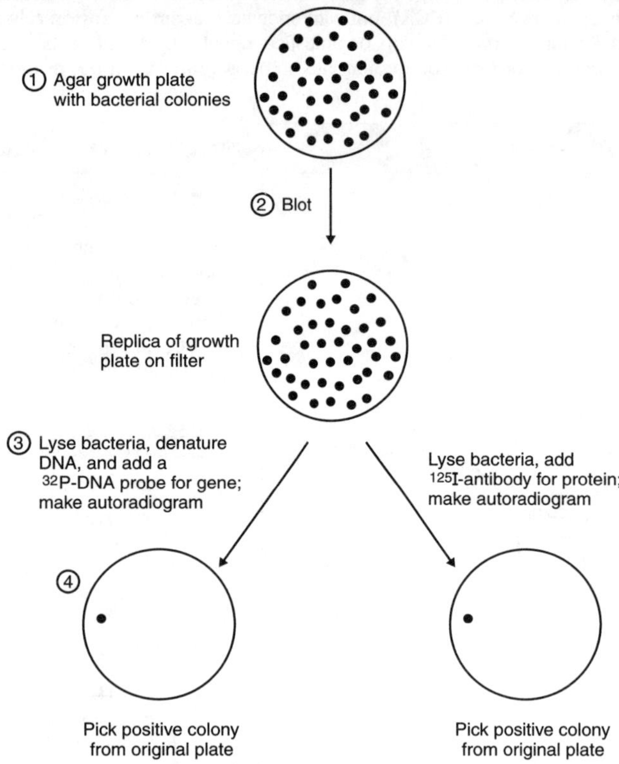

Restriction Endonucleases

- Recognizes palindromes in dsDNA and cuts, leaving sticky or blunt ends
- Used to make restriction maps of DNA or to produce fragments for manipulation

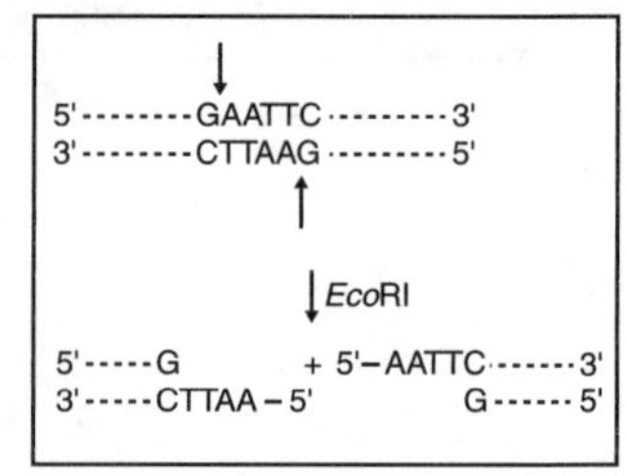

Sticky Ends

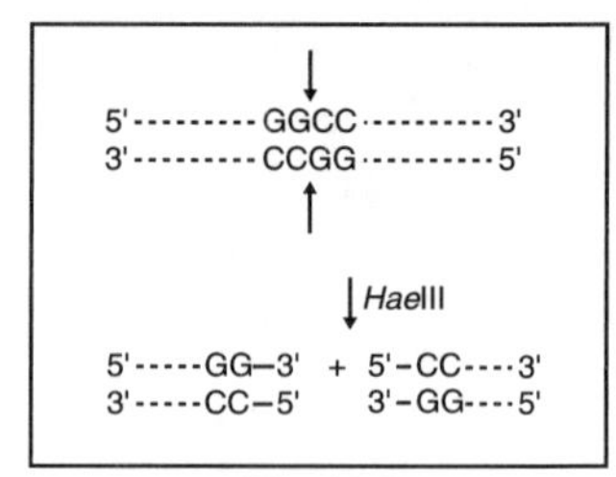

Blunt Ends

Incorporation of Cloned DNA

Cloned DNA Fragments

Gene Therapy (Somatic)

Cloned gene inserted into DNA of selected somatic cells

Gene not passed to offspring

Vector used to introduce cloned gene into host DNA/nuclei
- retrovirus
- adenovirus
- liposome

Examples
- SCID (severe combined immuno-deficiency); interleukin receptor gene
- Cystic fibrosis; CFTR gene

Transgenic Animals (Germ Line)

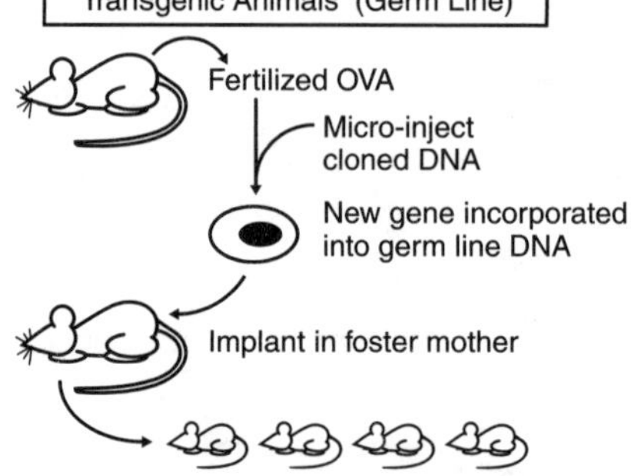

Offspring are transgenic
New gene inserted is a transgene
Design animal model for human disease this way

DNA Vectors

Circular, self-replicating DNA to carry and amplify DNA fragments in bacteria or yeast

Size	Vector
~100–12 kb	**Plasmid** Bacterial; restriction sites, replication origin, selection marker (e.g., antibiotic resistance)
~10–25 kb	**Phage** Packaging virus that infects bacteria; e.g., lambda (λ)
Up to 45 kb	**Cosmid** Plasmids with λ cloning sites
Up to 10 Mb	**BAC, YAC** Bacterial or yeast artificial chromosomes

Definition of abbreviation: dsDNA, double-stranded DNA.

► Genetic Testing

The presence of specific DNA, RNA, and proteins can be identified by first separating these molecules by **gel electrophoresis**, transferring to a membrane by **blotting**, and finally detecting with radioactive nucleic acid probes (for DNA and RNA) or antibodies (for proteins). Direct detection in cells or tissues can also be performed using similar tools to identify mRNA (**in situ hybridization**) or proteins (**immunostaining**). In vitro detection of proteins can also be achieved by enzyme-linked immunosorbent assay (**ELISA**). Using these methods of detection, diversity between individuals or genetic mutations manifested by different restriction endonuclease sites (restriction fragment length polymorphisms [**RFLP**]) or expansion of highly repetitive sequences (e.g., **satellites**, **minisatellites**, and **microsatellites**) may be employed for genetic testing.

	DNA	RNA	Protein
Separation	Gel electrophoresis		
Blotting (probe)	Southern (^{32}P-DNA)	Northern (^{32}P-DNA)	Western (^{125}I or antibody)
Other detection	—	In situ hybridization	Immunostaining or ELISA

	Repeated Unit	Length of Repeat
Satellites	20–175 bp	0.1–1 Mb
Minisatellites	20–70 bp	Up to 20 kb
Microsatellites	2–4 bp	<150 bp

Sickle Cell Disease (Southern Blot; RFLP)

*Mst*II restriction digest of patient sample, followed by Southern blotting using a probe against β-globin gene, allows identification of either the normal or sickle allele.

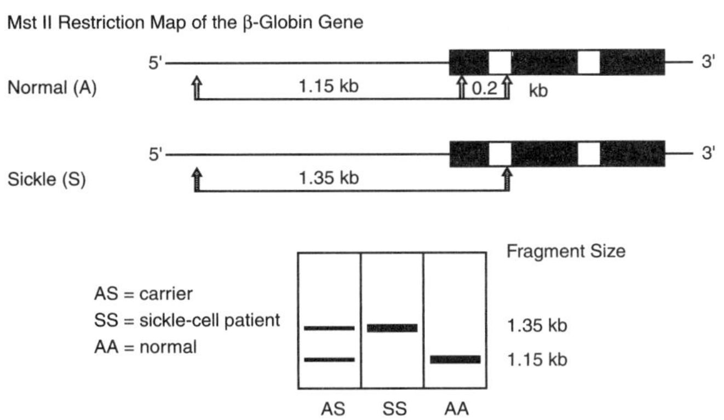

Paternity Testing (PCR; STRs or Microsatellites)

PCR amplification of STRs or microsatellite sequences can be used to match the banding pattern to each parent. The child should share one allele with each parent.

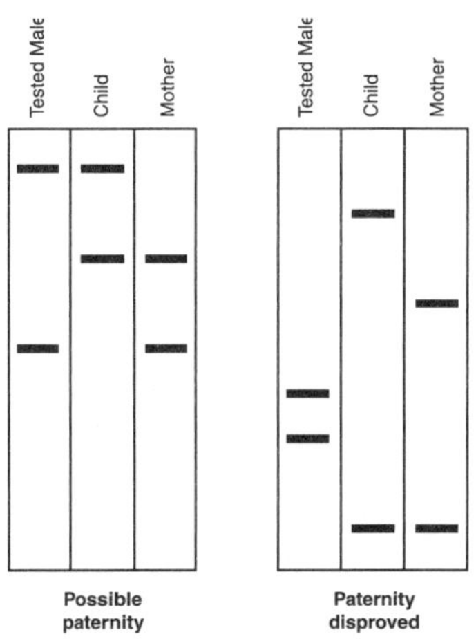

Cystic Fibrosis (PCR; ASO Dot Blot)

The most common CF mutation, ΔF508, can be detected by comparing PCR product sizes by gel electrophoresis or hybridization with allele-specific oligonucleotide (ASO) probes on a dot blot (a simplified form of Southern blot with no electrophoresis required).

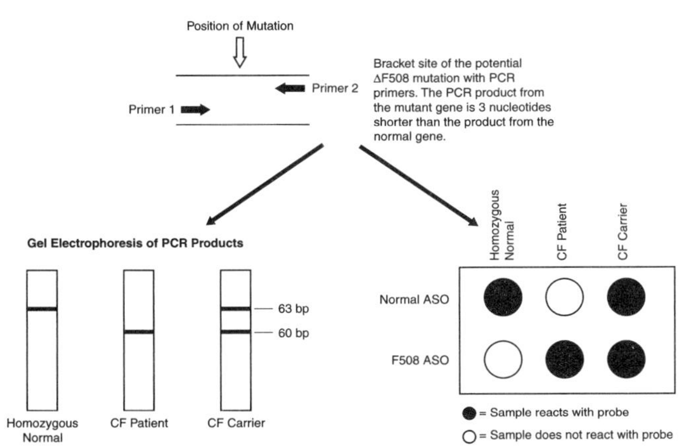

HIV Detection (ELISA and Western Blot)

Serum antibodies to HIV are first detected by ELISA and then confirmed by Western blot.

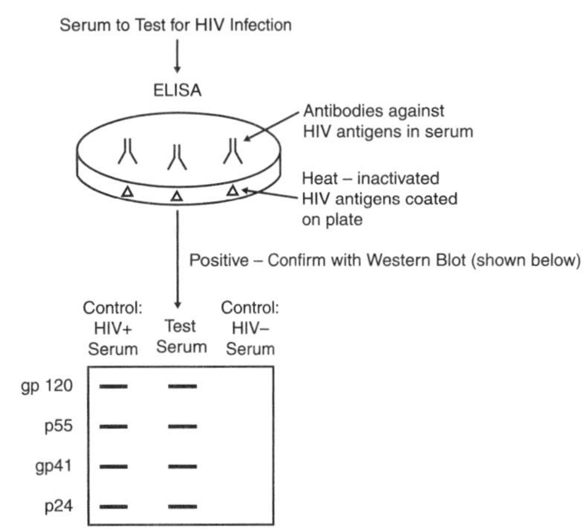

Definition of abbreviation: STR, short tandem repeats

► Patterns of Inheritance

Autosomal Dominant

- Affected individuals have an affected parent
- Either sex affected
- Variable to late onset (may be delayed to adulthood)
- Often encode structural proteins

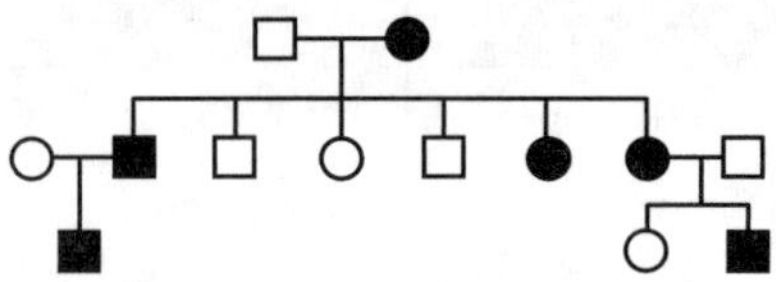

- **Familial hypercholesterolemia**
- **Huntington disease**
- **Neurofibromatosis**
- **Marfan syndrome**
- **von Hippel-Lindau disease**

Autosomal Recessive

- Affected individuals usually have unaffected (carrier) parents
- Either sex affected
- Early uniform onset (infancy/childhood)
- Often encode catalytic proteins

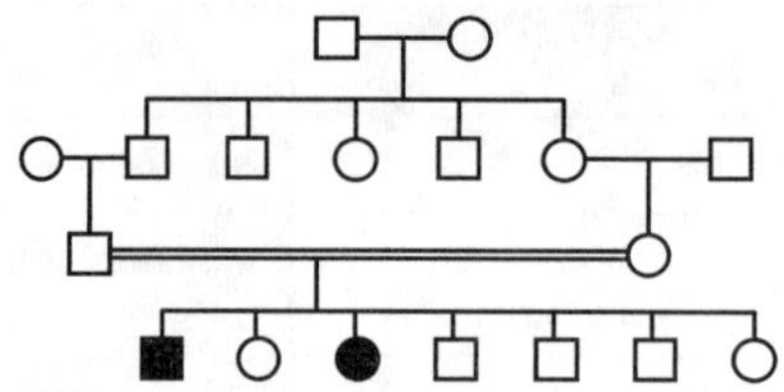

- **Sickle cell anemia**
- **Cystic fibrosis**
- **Phenylketonuria (PKU)**
- **Kartagener syndrome**

Pedigree Analysis

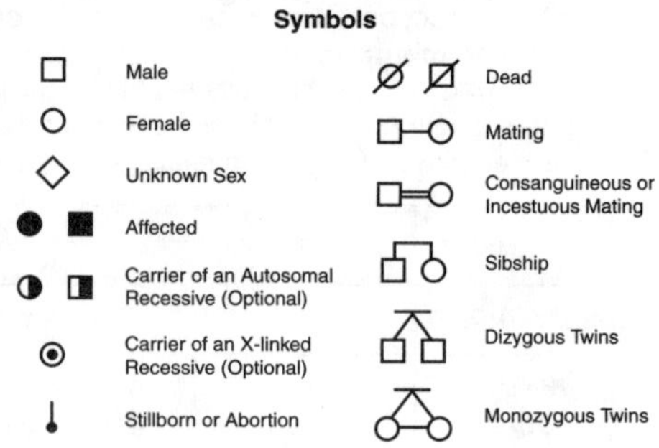

X-Linked Dominant

- Affected individuals have an affected parent
- Either sex affected
- No male-to-male transmission
- Females often have more mild and variable symptoms than males

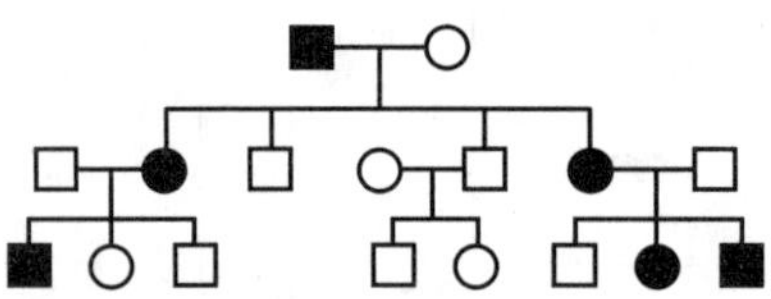

- **Fragile X syndrome**
- **Hypophosphatemic rickets**

X-Linked Recessive

- Affected individuals usually have unaffected (carrier) parents
- Usually affect males only
- No male-to-male transmission
- Female carriers sometimes show mild symptoms (manifesting heterozygote)

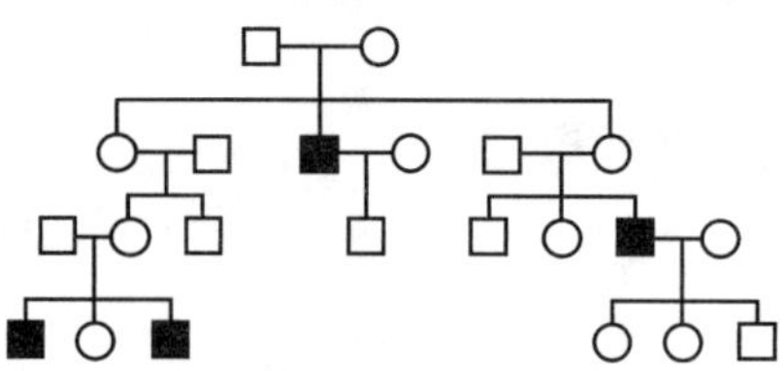

- **Duchenne muscular dystrophy**
- **Lesch-Nyhan syndrome**
- **G6PD deficiency**
- **Hemophilia A and B**

Mitochondrial Inheritance

- Inherited maternally because only mother contributes mitochondria during conception
- Either sex affected
- Usually neuropathies and myopathies because brain and muscle are highly dependent on oxidative phosphorylation

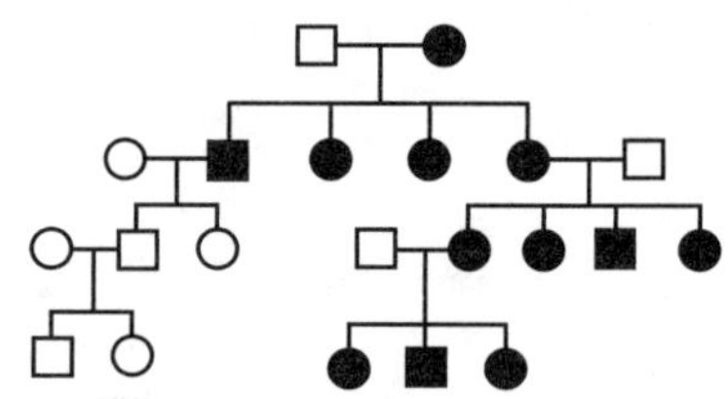

- **Leber hereditary optic neuropathy**
- **MELAS: m**itochondrial **e**ncephalomyopathy, **l**actic **a**cidosis, and **s**troke-like episodes
- **Myoclonic epilepsy** with ragged red muscle fiber

Decision Tree for Determining Mode of Inheritance*

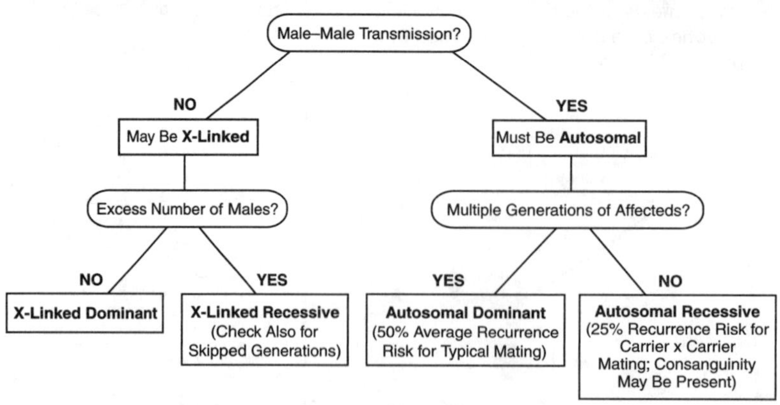

Definition of abbreviation: G6PD, glucose-6-phosphate dehydrogenase.

**Note:* If transmission occurs only through affected mothers and never through affected sons, the pedigree is likely to reflect mitochondrial inheritance.

▶ Single-Gene Disorders

Neurofibromatosis (NF) Type 1 (von Recklinghausen Disease)

(mutation in NF1 *tumor-suppressor gene on chromosome 17)*

- Multiple neurofibromas
- Café-au-lait spots (pigmented skin lesions)
- Lisch nodules (pigmented iris hamartomas)
- Increased risk of meningiomas and pheochromocytoma
- 90% of NF cases
- Autosomal dominant

Neurofibromatosis (NF) Type 2 (Bilateral Acoustic Neurofibromatosis)

(mutation in NF2 *tumor-suppressor gene on chromosome 22)*

- Bilateral acoustic neuromas
- Neurofibromas and café-au-lait spots
- Increased risk of meningiomas and pheochromocytoma
- 10% of NF cases
- Autosomal dominant

Marfan Syndrome

(mutation of fibrillin gene on chromosome 15)

- Skeletal abnormalities (tall build with hyperextensible joints)
- Subluxation of lens
- Cardiovascular defects (cystic medial necrosis, dissecting aortic aneurysm, valvular insufficiency)
- Autosomal dominant

von Hippel-Lindau Disease

(mutation in tumor-suppressor gene on chromosome 3)

- Hemangioblastomas in CNS and retina
- Renal cell carcinoma
- Cysts in internal organs
- Autosomal dominant

Cystic Fibrosis

(mutation in CFTR *chloride channel gene on chromosome 7q, leading to thick secretion of mucus plugs)*

- Recurrent pulmonary infections (*P. aeruginosa* and *S. aureus*)
- Pneumonia, bronchitis, bronchiectasis
- Pancreatic insufficiency; steatorrhea
- Fat-soluble vitamin deficiency
- Male infertility
- Biliary cirrhosis
- Meconium ileus
- Most common mutation: ΔF508
- Dx: ↑ NaCl in sweat; PCR and ASO probes
- Tx: *N*-acetylcysteine, respiratory therapy, enzyme replacement, vitamin supplement, inhaled bronchodilator, antibiotics
- Autosomal recessive

Features

Variable expression— differences in severity of symptoms for same genotype; allelic heterogeneity can contribute to variable expression

Incomplete penetrance— some individuals with disease genotype do not have disease phenotype

Delayed age of onset— individuals do not manifest phenotype until later in life

Pleiotropy— single disease mutation affects multiple organ systems

Locus heterogeneity— same disease phenotype from mutations in different loci

Anticipation— earlier age of onset and increased disease severity with each generation

Imprinting— symptoms depend on whether mutant gene was inherited from father or mother; due to different DNA methylation patterns of parents (e.g., Prader-Willi versus Angelman syndrome)

Definition of abbreviations: ASO, allele-specific oligonucleotides; CFTR, cystic fibrosis transmembrane conductance regulator; CNS, central nervous system; Dx, diagnosis; PCR, polymerase chain reaction; Tx, treatment.

► Chromosomal Abnormalities

Aneuploidy refers to having a chromosome number that is not a multiple of the haploid number. It is the most common type of chromosomal disorder, and its incidence is related to increasing maternal age. Most arise from a **nondisjunction** event, when chromosomes fail to segregate during cell division. Nondisjunction during either phase of meiosis usually leads to spontaneous abortion, but sometimes results in live birth, often with severe physical deformities and mental retardation. Trisomies are the most common genetic cause of pregnancy loss. Nondisjunction during mitosis in the developing embryo can lead to cells in a single individual carrying different karyotypes, a condition known as **mosaicism**. Based on the **Lyon hypothesis**, females are naturally mosaics for genes on the X chromosome because one X chromosome in every cell is randomly inactivated to form a **Barr body**. Fluorescence in situ hybridization (FISH) can detect DNA sequences to identify deletions, translocations, and aneuploidies.

Nondisjunction During Meiosis I

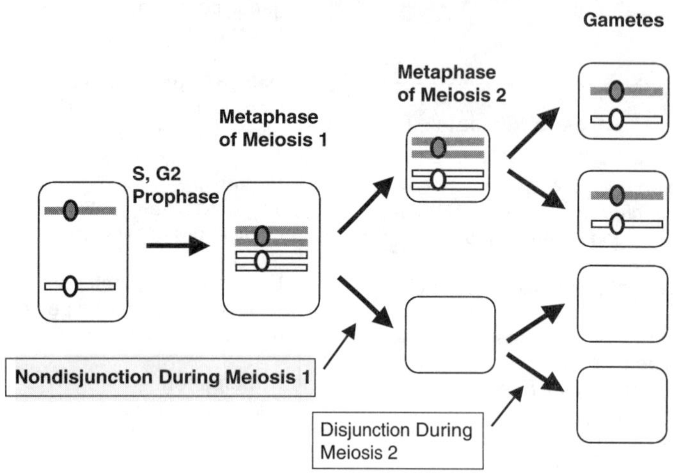

This figure shows the result of nondisjunction of one homologous pair (for example, chromosome 21) during meiosis 1. All other homologs segregate (disjoin) normally in the cell. Two of the gametes are diploid for chromosome 21. When fertilization occurs, the conception will be a trisomy 21 with Down syndrome. The other gametes with no copy of chromosome 21 will result in conceptions that are monosomy 21, a condition incompatible with a live birth.

Nondisjunction During Meiosis II

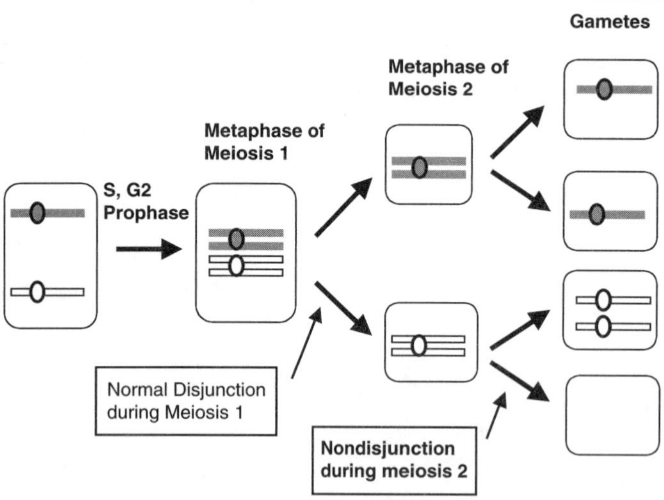

This figure shows the result of nondisjunction during meiosis 2. In this case, the sister chromatids of a chromosome (for example, chromosome 21) fail to segregate (disjoin). The sister chromatids of all other chromosomes segregate normally. One of the gametes is diploid for chromosome 21. When fertilization occurs, the conception will be a trisomy 21 with Down syndrome. One gamete has no copy of chromosome 21 and will result in a conception that is a monosomy 21. The remaining two gametes are normal haploid ones.

Autosomal Trisomies

Trisomy 21 (Down Syndrome)

- Most common chromosomal disorder
- Epicanthal folds, brachycephaly, flat nasal bridge, low-set ears, and short, broad hands with single transverse palmar crease
- Mental retardation
- Early-onset Alzheimer disease
- Congenital septal defects in heart
- ↑ risk of acute leukemia
- Incidence: 1/800 births (1/25 if age >45 years)
- 95% nondisjunction; 4% Robertsonian translocation

Trisomy 18 (Edwards Syndrome)

- Intrauterine growth retardation
- Mental retardation
- Failure to thrive
- Short sternum, small pelvis, rocker-bottom feet
- Cardiac, renal, and intestinal defects
- Usually death <1 year
- Incidence: 1/8,000 births

Trisomy 13 (Patau Syndrome)

- Microcephaly and abnormal brain development
- Cleft lip and palate, polydactyly
- Cardiac dextroposition and septal defects
- Incidence: 1/25,000 births

Sex Chromosome Aneuploidy

Turner Syndrome (45,XO)

- Short stature, webbed neck, shield chest
- Primary amenorrhea, infertility
- Coarctation of aorta
- Incidence: 1/6,000 female births

Klinefelter Syndrome (47,XXY)

- Eunuchoid body with lack of male secondary sex characteristics
- Hypogonadism, testicular atrophy
- Incidence: 1/2,000 male births

XYY Syndrome

- Excessively tall with severe acne
- ↑ risk of behavioral problems
- Incidence: 1/1,000 male births

► Other Chromosomal Abnormalities

In addition to aneuploidy, large segments of chromosomes may also undergo structural aberrations, including deletions, inversions, and translocations. **Deletions** occur when a chromosome loses a segment because of breakage. **Inversions** are rearrangements of the gene order within a single chromosome due to incorrect repair of two breaks. An inversion that includes a centromere is called a **pericentric** inversion, while one that does not involve the centromere is **paracentric**. Finally, **translocations** involve exchange of chromosomal material between nonhomologous chromosomes. **Reciprocal translocations** result when two nonhomologous chromosomes exchange pieces, while **Robertsonian translocations** involve any two acrocentric chromosomes that break near the centromeres and rejoin with a fusion of the q arms at the centromere and loss of the p arms.

Reciprocal Translocation

When one parent is a reciprocal translocation carrier:

- Adjacent segregation produces unbalanced genetic material and a likely loss of pregnancy
- Alternate segregation produces a normal haploid gamete (and diploid conception) or a liveborn who is a phenotypically normal translocation carrier

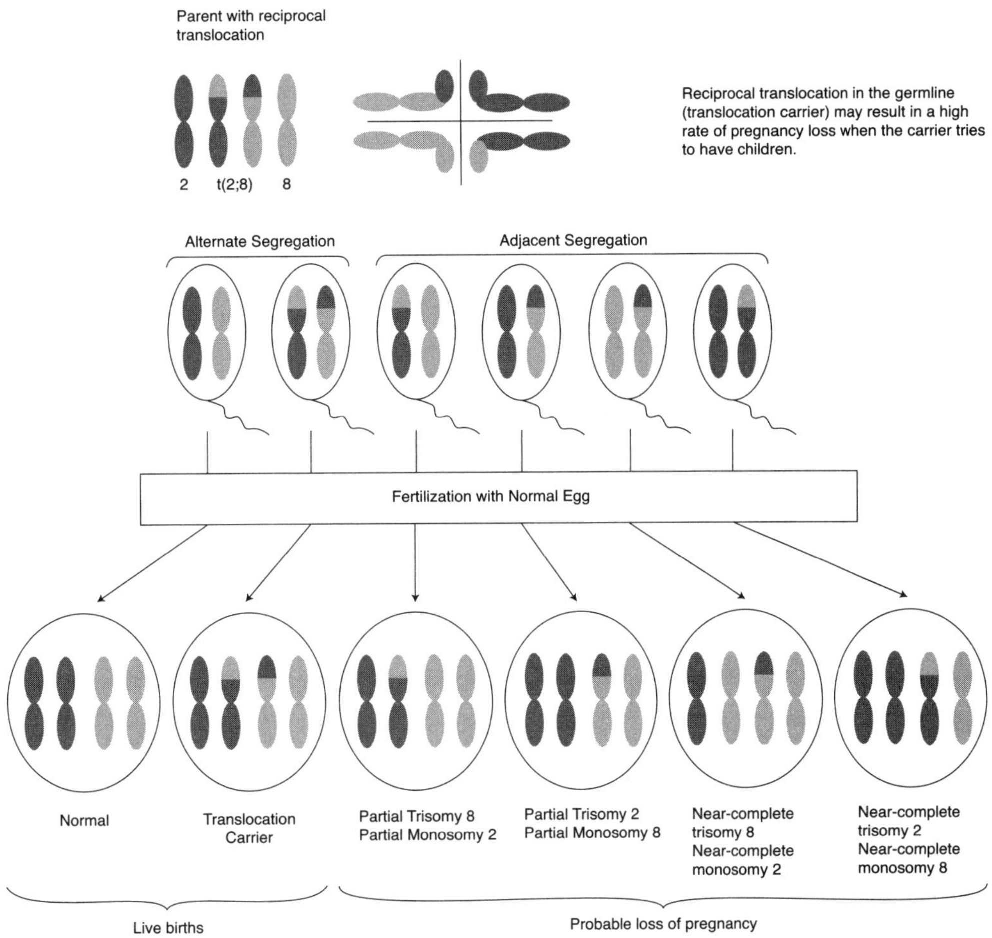

Reciprocal Translocations in Somatic Cells May Result in Cancer

t(9;22)	CML, ALL	*bcr-abl* fusion produces a fusion protein with tyrosine kinase activity.
t(8;14)	Burkitt lymphoma	*c-myc* oncogene (chromosome 8) placed near Ig heavy chain locus. Activating Ig heavy chain gene activates *c-myc.*
t(11;14)	Mantle cell lymphoma	*bcl-1* (chromosome 11) encodes cyclin D. Translocation places *bcl-1* near Ig heavy chain locus (chromosome 14).

Definition of abbreviations: ALL, acute lymphocytic leukemia; CML, chronic myelogenous leukemia.

(Continued)

► Other Chromosomal Abnormalities *(Cont'd.)*

Consequences of a Robertsonian Translocation in One Parent

Approximately 5% of Down syndrome cases result from a Robertsonian translocation affecting chromosomes 14 and 21. When a translocation carrier (in this case, a male) produces gametes, the translocation can segregate with the normal 14 or the normal 21. Although adjacent segregation usually results in pregnancy loss, it can result in a **trisomy 21**. Alternate segregation produces a normal haploid gamete (and diploid conception) or a liveborn who is a phenotypically normal translocation carrier.

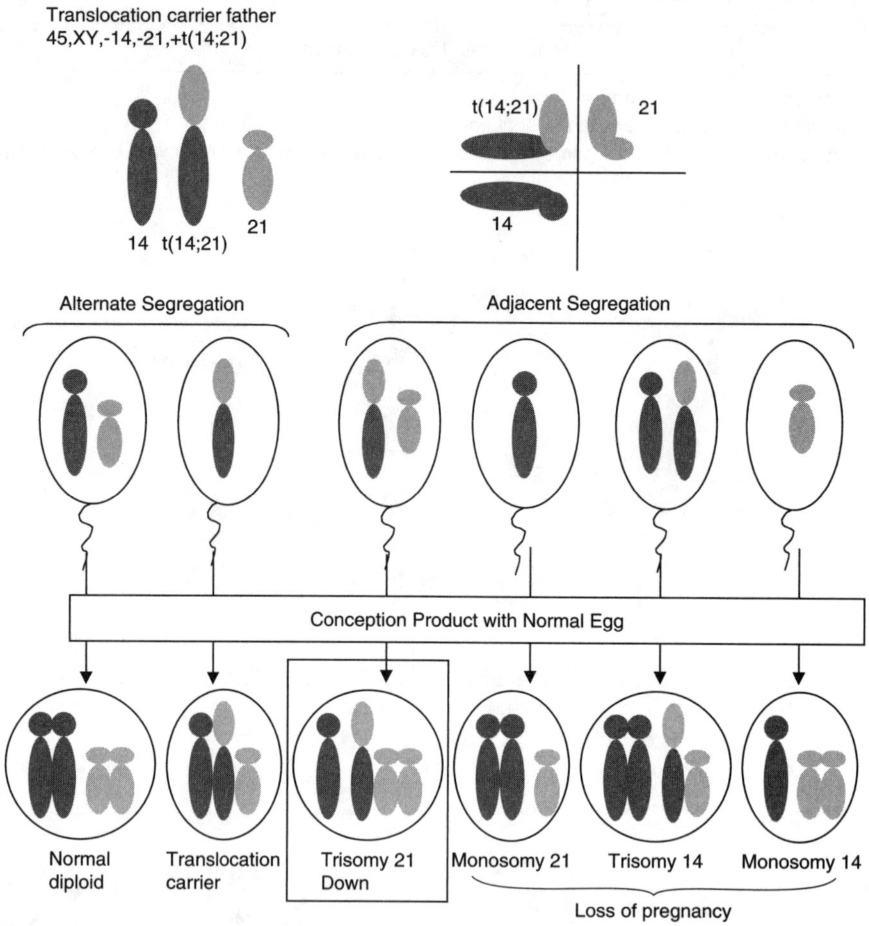

Down syndrome (nondisjunction during meiosis)	Down syndrome (parent carries a Robertsonian translocation)
• 47,XX,+21 or 47,XY,+21 • No association with prior pregnancy loss • Older mother • Very low recurrence rate	• 46,XX,-14,+t(14;21), or 46,XY,-14,+t(14;21) • *May* be associated with prior pregnancy losses • *May* be a young mother • Recurrence rate 10–15% if mom is translocation carrier; 1–2% if dad is translocation carrier

▶ Additional Diseases Resulting from Chromosomal Abnormalities

Disease	Abnormality	Characteristics
Cri-du-chat syndrome	Terminal or interstitial deletion of 5p	• Mental retardation • **Cat-like cry** • Microcephaly, low-set ears, micrognathia • Epicanthal folds
DiGeorge syndrome	Deletion of 22q11	• Hereditary absence of thymus and parathyroid glands due to **abnormal development of 3rd and 4th pharyngeal pouches** • T-cell deficiency • Cardiac outflow tract abnormalities • Abnormal facies • Hypoparathyroidism
Wilms tumor	Deletion of 11p13	• Malignant urinary tract tumors • □ diagnosed by age 4 • Tx: surgical removal
Angelman syndrome	Deletion of 15q11-q13 in **mother**	• **"Happy puppet" syndrome** • Always smiling but lacks speech • Hyperactive, hypotonic • Mental retardation, seizures • Dysmorphic facial features • Ataxic, puppet-like gait
Prader-Willi syndrome	Deletion of 15q11-q13 in **father**	• **Short stature** and **obese** with small hands and feet • **Hyperphagia** • Dysmorphic facial features • Mental retardation ***NOTE:*** **Angelman** and **Prader-Willi** are both examples of the effects of a deletion in an area affected by imprinting. A minority of cases are caused by uniparental disomy.

▶ Population Genetics

The **Hardy-Weinberg equilibrium** states that under certain conditions, if the population is large and randomly mating, the genotypic frequencies of the population will remain stable from generation to generation.

Hardy-Weinberg Conditions

1. No mutations
2. No selection against a genotype
3. No migration or immigration of the population
4. Random mating

If: frequency of A allele = p

frequency of a allele = q

Then: allele frequencies can be expressed as:

$$p + q = 1$$

genotypic frequencies at that locus can be expressed as:

$$p^2 + 2pq + q^2 = 1$$

where p^2 = frequency of genotype AA

$2pq$ = frequency of genotype Aa

q^2 = frequency of genotype aa

Factors Affecting Equilibrium

Natural Selection

Increases frequencies of genes that promote survival or fertility (e.g., malaria protection in sickle cell heterozygotes)

Genetic Drift

Gene frequency change due to finite population size

Gene Flow

Gene exchange between different populations

Linkage Disequilibrium

Preferential association of an allele at one locus with another allele at a nearby locus more frequently than by chance alone

► Subcellular Organelles

In contrast to simple prokaryotic cells that have a cell wall but no membrane-bound nucleus or organelles, eukaryotic cells are, in general, larger and lack a cell wall, but are composed of various subcellular membranous organelles with distinct functions.

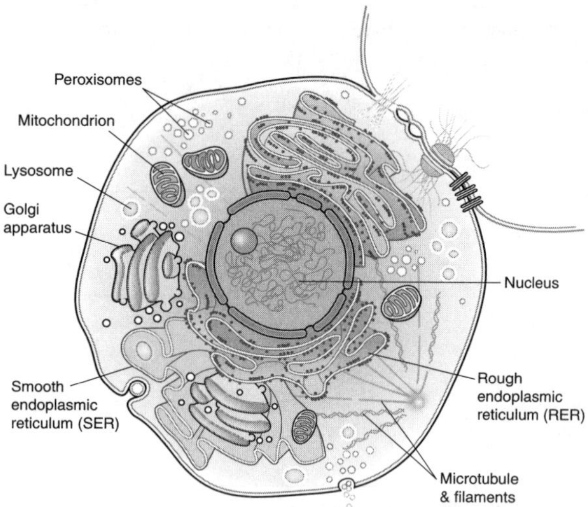

Prokaryotic	Eukaryotic
Small (1–10 μm)	Large (10–100 μm)
Thick, rigid cell wall	No cell wall
No membrane-bound organelles	Various subcellular membranous organelles
Non-membrane–bound nucleoid region	Nucleus with double-membrane envelope

Proteasome

- Small complexes of proteolytic enzymes in cytosol
- Digest (usually misfolded) proteins that are marked with ubiquitin
- Peptides produced are presented along with MHC I at the cell surface

Nucleus

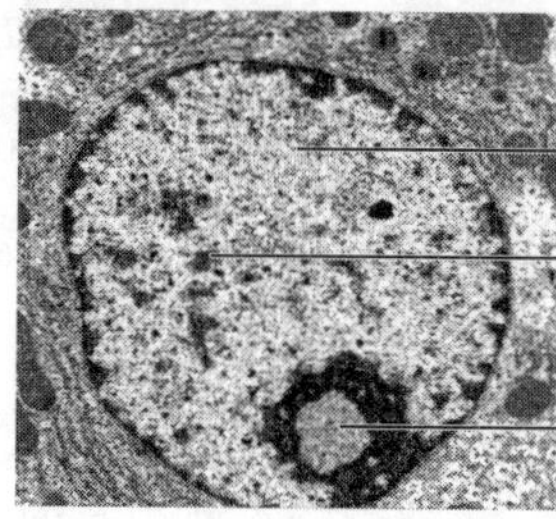

- Site of **DNA replication and transcription**
- Enclosed by nuclear envelope
- Contains **nucleolus** (site of ribosome synthesis); no membrane surrounds the nucleolus
- Contains DNA packaged with histones to form **chromatin**

Rough Endoplasmic Reticulum (RER)

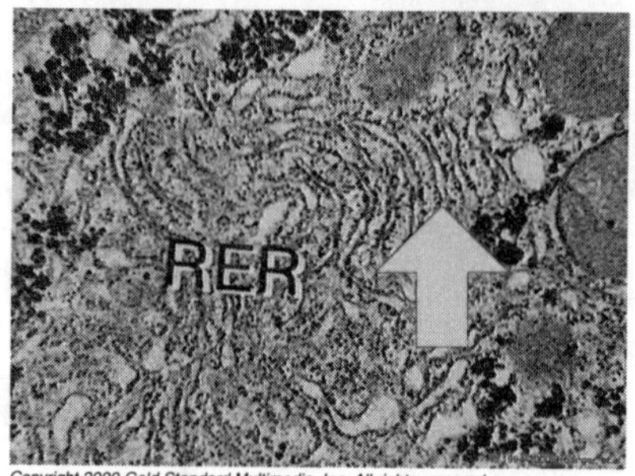

- Contains **ribosomes** for synthesizing proteins destined for RER, SER, Golgi, lysosomes, cell membrane, and secretion
- Cotranslational modifications, including ***N*-linked glycosylation** (proteins synthesized on free ribosomes are not usually glycosylated)

Ribosomes

- Site of **protein synthesis**
- Composed of ribosomal RNA (rRNA) and proteins forming large 60S + small 40S subunits
- Single mRNA simultaneously translated by several ribosomes is a **polysome**

Types of Ribosomes	
RER-Bound	**Free Cytosolic**
Proteins for RER, SER, Golgi apparatus, lysosomes, cell membrane, and secretion	Cytosolic, mitochondrial, nuclear, and peroxisomal proteins

(*Continued*)

► Subcellular Organelles (*Cont'd.*)

Golgi Apparatus

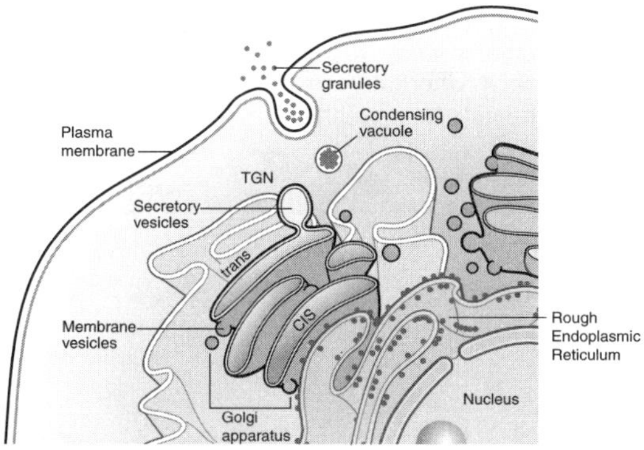

- Site of **post-translational modifications and protein sorting**
- Consists of disk-shaped cisternae in stacks
- ***Cis* (forming) face** associated with RER
- ***Trans* (maturing) face** oriented toward plasma membrane

Smooth Endoplasmic Reticulum (SER)

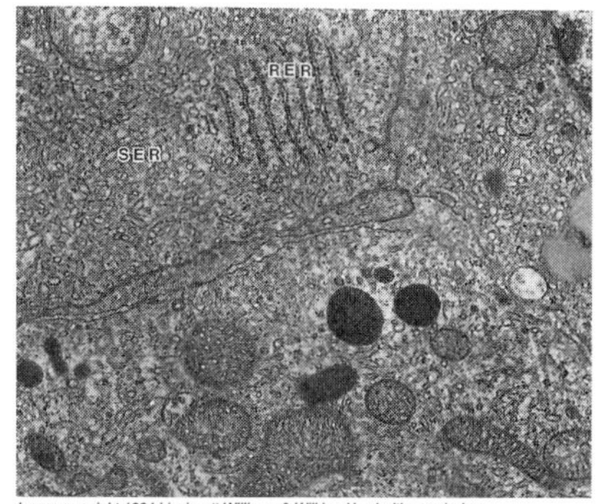

- Involved in detoxification reactions, including **phase I hydroxylation** (via cytochrome P450) and **phase II conjugation** (addition of polar groups)
- Synthesis of phospholipids, lipoproteins, and sterols
- Sequesters Ca^{2+}; known as **sarcoplasmic reticulum** in striated and smooth muscle cells

Mitochondria

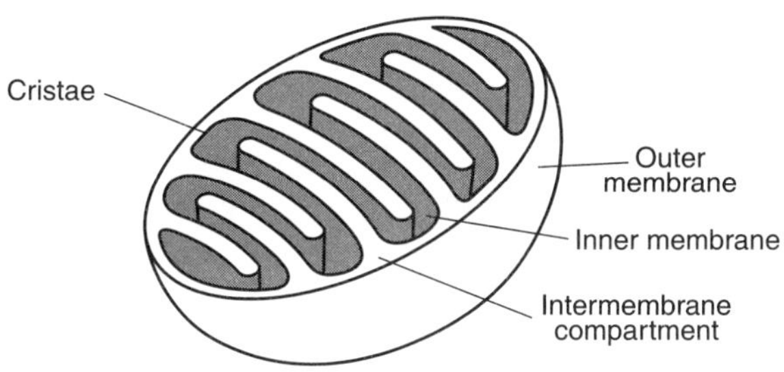

- Major function is ATP synthesis
- Similar to bacteria in size and shape; self-replicating
- Contain their own double-stranded circular DNA
- Smooth, permeable outer membrane; heavily infolded, impermeable inner membrane

Lysosomes

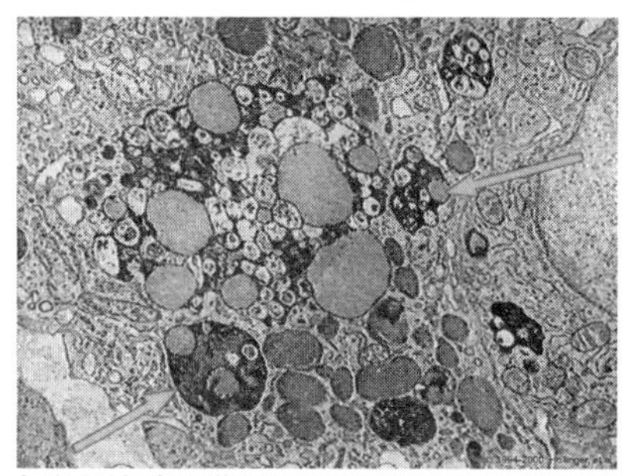

- Enzymatic degradation of extracellular or intracellular macromolecules
- Primary lysosome fuses with phagosomes or cellular organelles to form secondary lysosomes
- Acidic hydrolytic enzymes with optimal activity at pH 5
- Degradation of intracellular organelles known as **autophagy**

Endosomes

- Formed from endocytosed vesicles acquired by receptor-mediated endocytosis involving **clathrin-coated pits**
- Can fuse with primary lysosomes to form secondary lysosomes to degrade extracellular materials
- Exogenous peptides presented on membrane with MHC II on antigen presenting cells

Peroxisomes

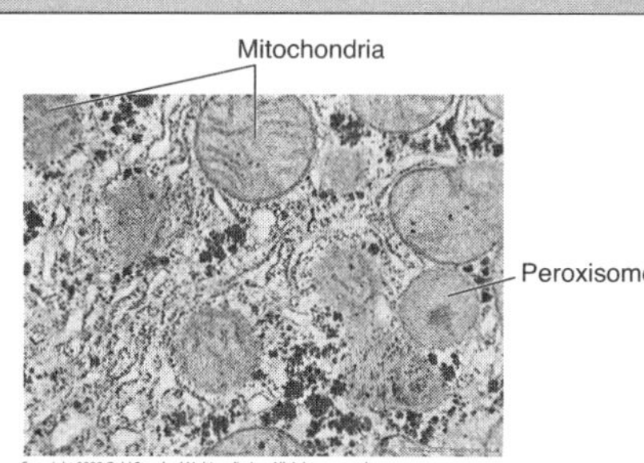

- Synthesis and degradation of hydrogen peroxide
- β-oxidation of very long chain fatty acids ($>C_{24}$)
- Phospholipid exchange reactions
- Bile acid synthesis

▶ Plasma Membrane

The **plasma membrane** of a cell is a bilayer of lipids and proteins. The lipids include phospholipids, unesterified cholesterol, and glycolipids and are **amphipathic** (polar head to interact with aqueous environment, and nonpolar tail to interact with the bilayer interior). Proteins may act as adhesion molecules, receptors, transporters, channels, or enzymes. Proteins embedded in the bilayer are **integral proteins**, whereas those loosely associated with the membrane are **peripheral proteins**. In general, ***N*-glycosylation** of proteins and lipids is associated with location on the external surface, whereas ***N*-myristoylation, prenylation**, and **palmitoylation** of proteins are associated with location on the cytoplasmic face of the plasma membrane.

Structure of Biologic Membranes

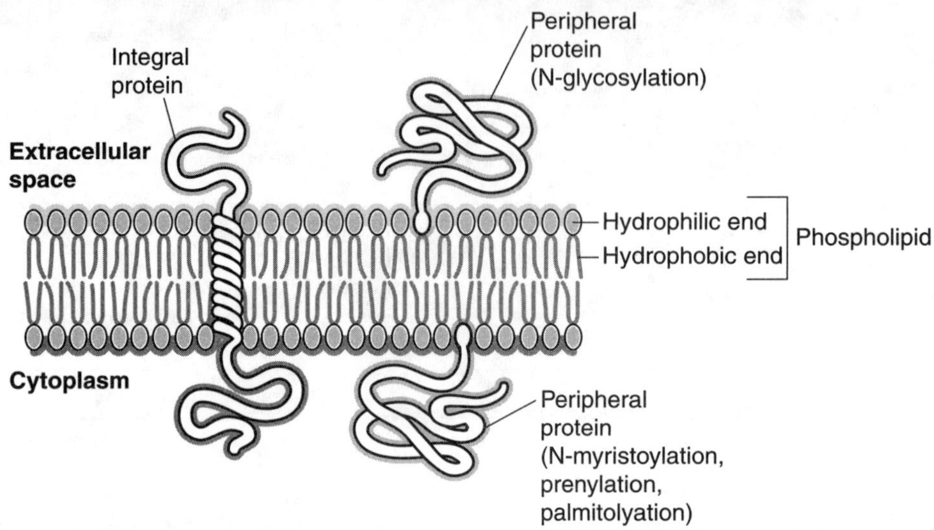

Types of Integral Membrane Proteins

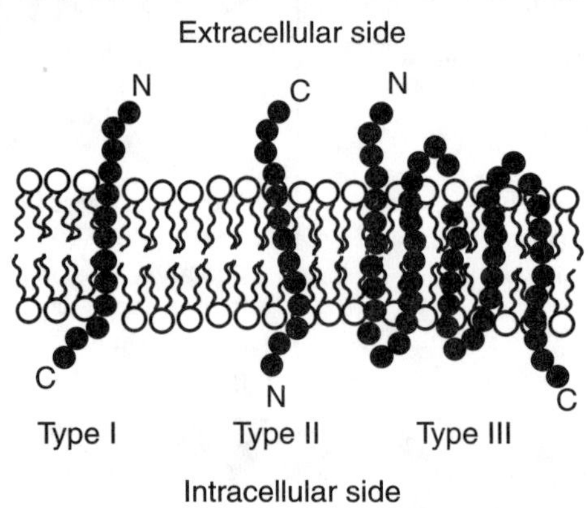

Types of Transport

Simple Diffusion	Facilitated Diffusion	Active Transport
• Movement of highly permeable molecules from a region of higher to lower concentration • e.g., O_2, CO_2, NO	• Passage of poorly permeable molecules from a region of higher to lower concentration via a carrier • e.g., glucose transporter	• Movement of molecules from a region of lower to higher concentration with *1)* energy expenditure via ATP hydrolysis, or *2)* cotransport using another molecule's chemical gradient • e.g., *1)* Na^+/K^+ pump, Ca^{2+}-ATPase • e.g., *2)* Na^+/glucose symporter

► Cytoskeleton

The cytoskeleton consists of a supportive network of tubules and filaments in the cytoplasm of eukaryotic cells. It is a dynamic structure responsible for cellular movement, changes in cell shape, and the contraction of muscle cells. It also provides the machinery for intracellular movement of organelles. The cytoskeleton is composed of three types of supportive structures: **microtubules*, intermediate filaments**, and **microfilaments**.

Microtubules*	Intermediate Filaments	Microfilaments
Tubulin (hollow cylindrical polymer of tubulin dimers)	• **Keratin** (epithelium) • **Vimentin** (nonepithelial) • **Neurofilament** (neurons)	**Actin** (double-stranded polymer twisted in helical pattern)
	Function	
• Movement of chromosomes in mitosis or meiosis • Intracellular transport via motor proteins • Ciliary and flagellar motility	Structural	• Structural • Muscle contraction via interaction with myosin

Axoneme Structure

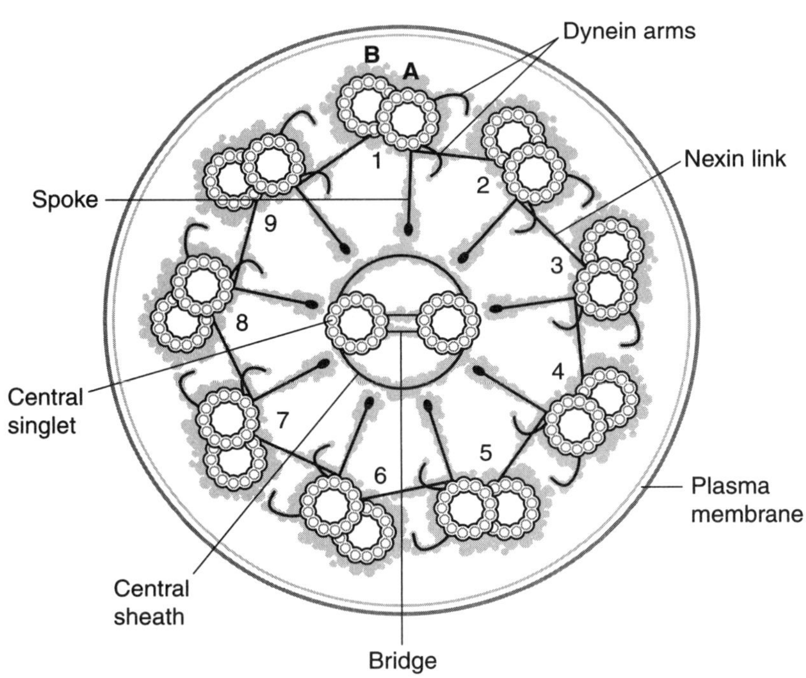

Motor Proteins

Kinesins for ⊖ → ⊕ anterograde direction

Dyneins for ⊕ → ⊖ retrograde direction

Disease Association

Chediak-Higashi Syndrome

(defect in microtubule polymerization in leukocytes)

- Recurrent pyogenic infections of respiratory tract and skin
- Partial albinism
- Photophobia, nystagmus, peripheral neuropathy, motor dysfunction, seizures
- Presents early in childhood

Kartagener Syndrome

(immotile cilia due to defect in axonemal proteins, such as dynein arms)

- Chronic cough, rhinitis, and sinusitis
- Situs inversus
- Fatigue and headaches
- Male infertility from immotile spermatozoa
- Autosomal recessive

Pharmacology

Colchicine

- Inhibits tubulin polymerization
- Used for gout

Vincristine/Vinblastine

- Inhibits tubulin polymerization
- Antineoplastic

Taxol

- Promotes tubulin polymerization
- Antineoplastic

*Microtubules are polarized structures with assembly/disassembly occurring at the ⊕ ends, which are oriented toward the cell's periphery.

► Cell Adhesion

A cell must physically interact via cell surface molecules with its external environment, whether it be the extracellular matrix or **basement membrane**. The basement membrane is a sheet-like structure underlying virtually all epithelia, which consists of **basal lamina** (made of type IV collagen, glycoproteins [e.g., laminin], and proteoglycans [e.g., heparin sulfate]), and **reticular lamina** (composed of reticular fibers). Cell junctions anchor cells to each other, seal boundaries between cells, and form channels for direct transport and communication between cells. The three types of junctional complexes include **anchoring, tight,** and **gap junctions**.

Cell Junctions

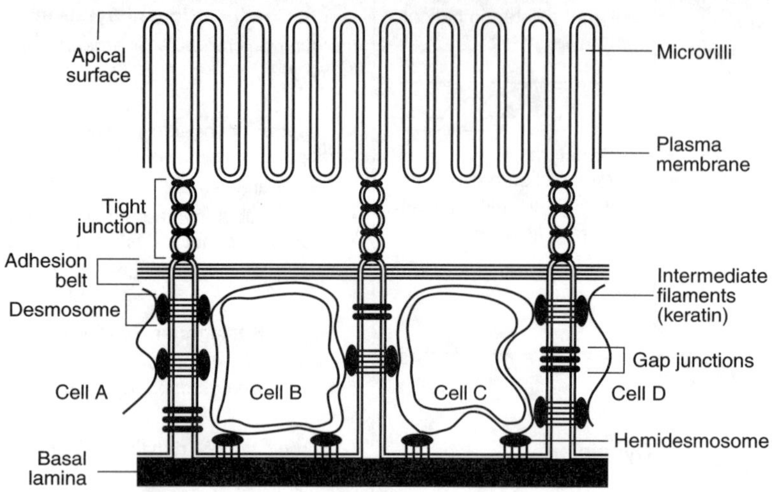

Anchoring Junctions	Tight Junctions	Gap Junctions
• **Adherens junction (zonula adherens)**—band-like junction near apical region for attachment to adjacent epithelial cells, forming an "adhesion belt" • **Desmosome (macula adherens)**—juxtaposition of two disk-shaped plaques from adjacent cells, with IFs radiating away from the plaques; **hemidesmosomes** anchor cells to the extracellular matrix	**Tight junction (zonula occludens)**—fusion of apposed cell membranes 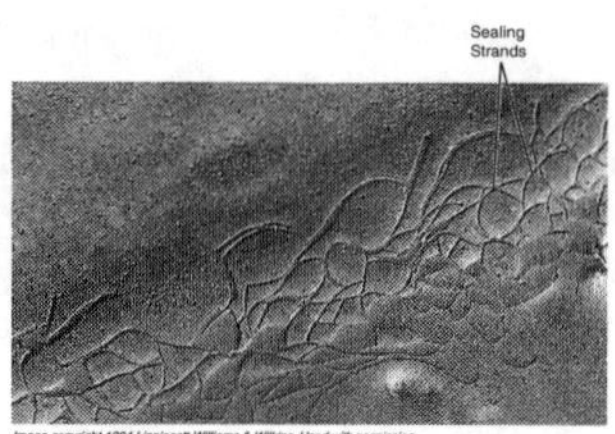	**Gap junctions**—direct passage for small particles and ions between cells via **connexon** channel proteins 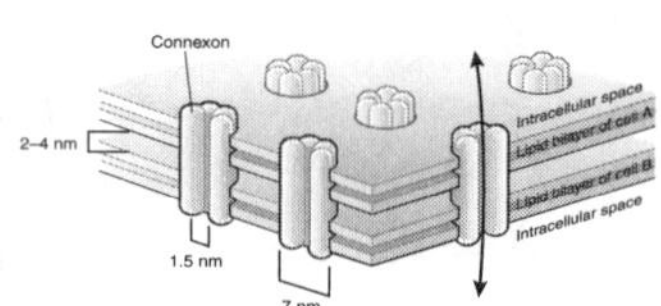
Function		
For structural integrity of large sheets of tissues (e.g., providing tensile strength of epithelial tissues); adhesion belt also allows epithelial tissue contractions	Provides a tight seal to prevent fluid leak between compartments (e.g., between intestinal lumen and intestinal villi)	Allows direct intercellular communications (e.g., allowing ions to pass for synchronous firing of cardiac pacemaker cells)

Extracellular Matrix

Proteoglycans
- 90–95% carbohydrate; 5–10% protein
- Forms hydrated gel for embedding fibrous proteins
- Provides shock absorption and lubrication

Collagen
- Triple helix of polypeptide chains rich in glycine and proline
- Collagens I–III: fibrous form for structure
- Collagen IV: sheet-like meshwork specific to basal lamina

Elastin
- Cross-linked fibers rich in glycine and proline
- Provides elasticity to tissues (e.g., lungs and large arteries)

Fibronectin
- Large, fibrous protein with disulfide crosslinks
- Provides adhesion between cells and extracellular matrix

Laminin
- Three polypeptide chains in shape of a cross and connected by disulfide bonds
- Major glycoprotein in basal lamina
- Provides adhesion between cells and extracellular matrix

Disease Association

Pemphigus Vulgaris
(autoantibodies against desmosomal proteins in skin cells)
- Painful flaccid bullae (blisters) in oropharynx and skin that rupture easily
- Postinflammatory hyperpigmentation
- Treatment: corticosteroids

Bullous Pemphigoid
(autoantibodies against basement-membrane hemidesmosomal proteins)
- Widespread blistering with pruritus
- Less severe than pemphigus vulgaris
- Rarely affects oral mucosa
- Can be drug induced (e.g., middle-aged or elderly patient on multiple medications)
- Treatment: corticosteroids

Definition of abbreviations: IF, intermediate filament.

▶ Cell Cycle

The cell cycle consists of the mitosis phase (M), the presynthetic gap (G_1), the DNA synthesis phase (S), and the postsynthetic gap (G_2). Mitosis is the shortest phase, consisting of **prophase, metaphase, anaphase**, and **telophase**. Both G_1 and G_2 phases are variable in duration, with most cells spending much of their time in a stable, nondividing G_0 phase. Cells in G_2 have twice the amount of DNA as those in G_1.

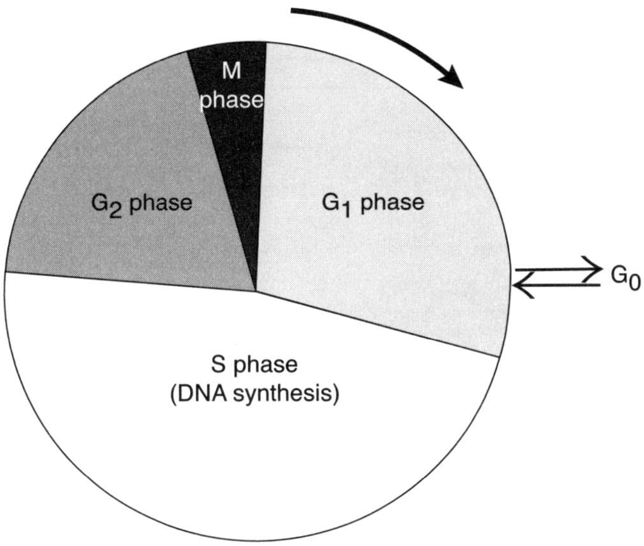

Phases of Mitosis	
Prophase 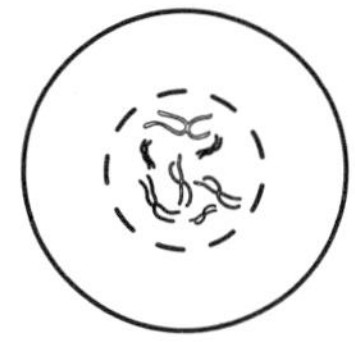	• Chromosomes coil • Nuclear envelope disappears • Spindle apparatus forms
Metaphase 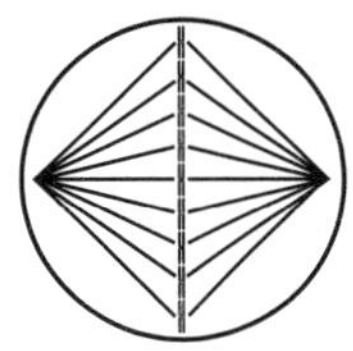	Chromosomes align
Anaphase 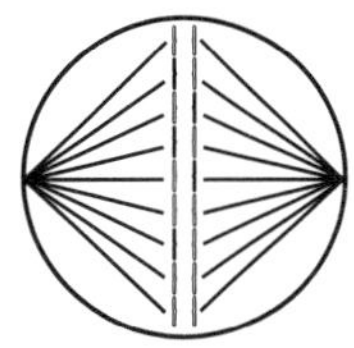	Chromatids separate
Telophase 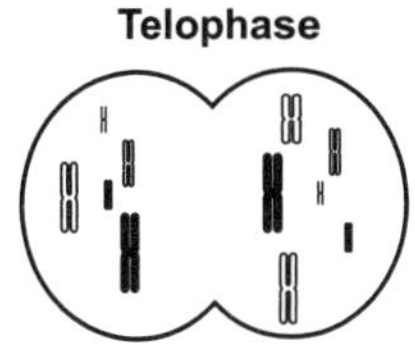	• Chromosomes uncoil • Nuclear envelope reappears • Spindle apparatus disassemble • Cell divides in two (cytokinesis)

Regulators of the Cell Cycle	
Cyclins	**Cyclin** levels rise and fall with stages of cell cycle.
CDKs	**Cyclin-dependent kinases** with various substrates promote cell-cycle progression.
APC	**Anaphase-promoting complex** triggers chromatid separation; degrades M-phase cyclins.
SPF	**S-phase promoting factor** includes CDKs and cyclins, which prepare cell for DNA replication.
MPF	**M-phase/maturation-promoting factor** includes CDKs and cyclins, which promote assembly of mitotic spindle and nuclear envelope breakdown.
p53	**p53** is a tumor suppressor that blocks cell cycle if DNA is damaged.
RB	**Retinoblastoma susceptibility protein** is a substrate of CDKs that promotes cell division.
p21	**p21** is a CDK inhibitor that also blocks cell-cycle progression.

Disease Association

Retinoblastoma

(mutation in the RB1 tumor-suppressor gene on chromosome 13)

- Most common childhood eye tumor
- Leukocoria (white reflex in pupil)
- Strabismus
- "Two-hit model" of carcinogenesis:
  1) inherited mutation of one allele
  2) somatic mutation of second allele

► Cell Signaling

In order to act on a cell, external molecules, such as hormones and neurotransmitters, must interact with a **receptor**. In general, small hydrophobic molecules (e.g., cortisol, sex hormones, thyroid hormone, and retinoids) can readily penetrate the plasma membrane to bind **intracellular receptors**, which often act as transcription factors to affect gene expression. Most other molecules bind to cell surface receptors, which include **ion-channel–linked receptors** (e.g., transmitter-gated channels), **G-protein–linked receptors** (the largest family), and **enzyme-linked receptors** (e.g., tyrosine kinase receptors). These cell surface receptors usually transmit their signal via a number of downstream **second messengers**, leading to a **signal transduction cascade**. One exception is the gaseous **nitric oxide** (NO), which readily diffuses across the plasma membrane to activate soluble **guanylate cyclase**, generate **cGMP**, and promote smooth muscle relaxation.

G-Protein–Coupled Receptor Systems

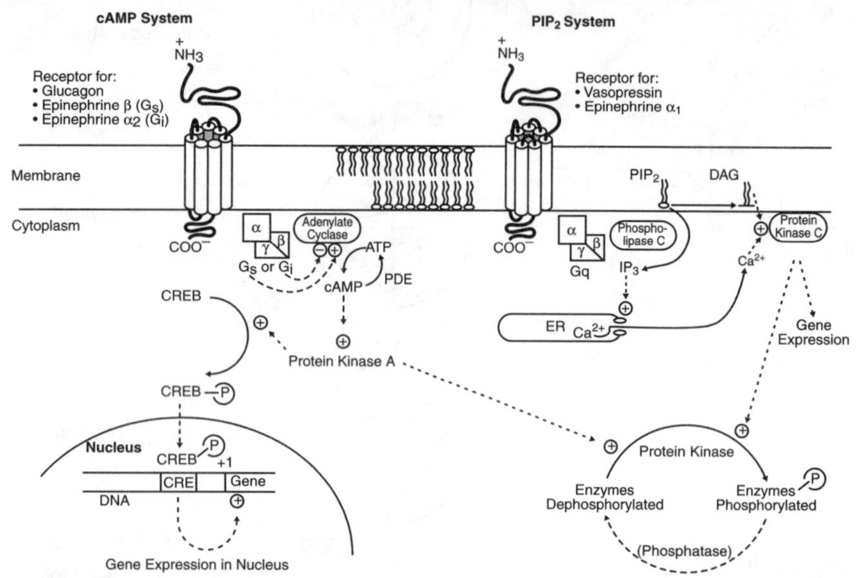

Trimeric G Protein Cycle

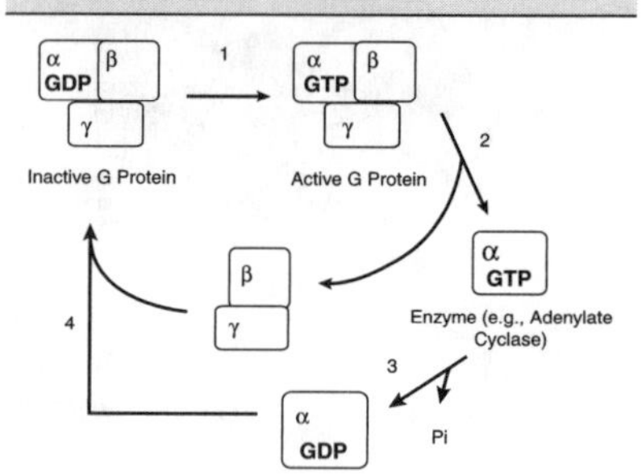

Tyrosine Kinase Receptor

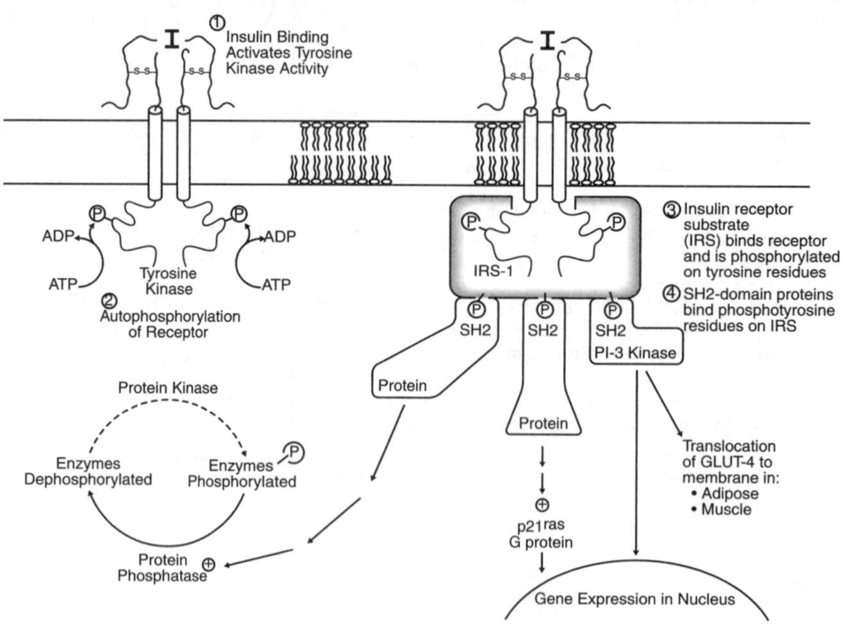

Definition of abbreviations: See next page.

(*Continued*)

▶ Cell Signaling *(Cont'd.)*

Guanylate Cyclase

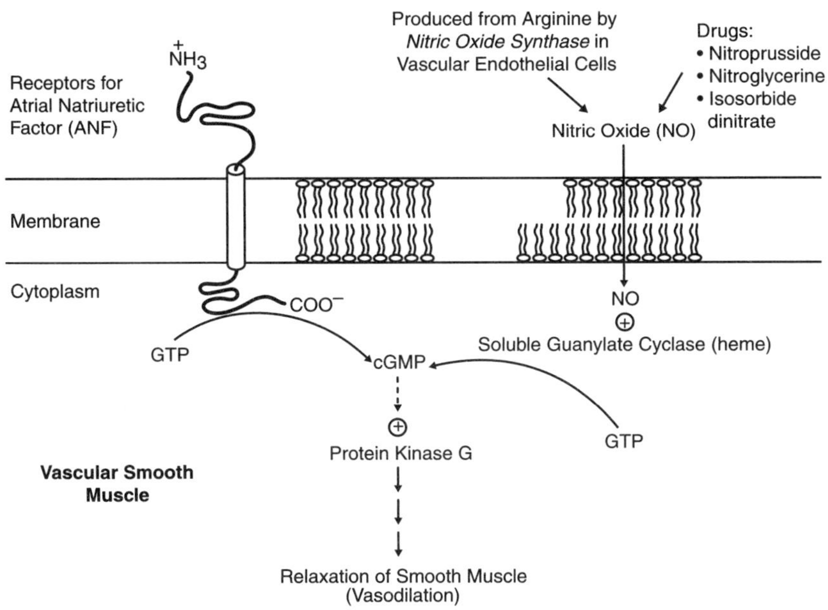

Pharmacology

Nitrates	Sildenafil
(nitroglycerin, nitroprusside, isosorbide dinitrate) • Converted to NO, which activates guanylate cyclase, leading to ↑ in cGMP. cGMP causes smooth muscle relaxation of blood vessels. • For angina and pulmonary edema • Adverse effects: headache, hypotension	• Inhibits cGMP-dependent phosphodiesterase (PDE5), leading to cGMP buildup, causing smooth muscle relaxation and dilation of blood vessels leading to the corpus cavernosum • For erectile dysfunction and Raynaud phenomenon • Adverse effects: headache, hypotension

Examples of Receptors

Adrenergic Receptors

- α_1 (G_q)—smooth muscle contraction
- α_2 ($G_{i/o}$)—inhibits NT release
- β_1 (G_s)—↑ heart rate and contractility
- β_2 (G_s)—smooth muscle relaxation

Muscarinic Acetylcholine Receptors

- M_1 (G_q)—affects CNS, PNS, gastric parietal cells
- M_2 ($G_{i/o}$)—↓ heart rate and contractility
- M_3 (G_q)—stimulates glandular secretions
- M_4 ($G_{i/o}$)—CNS only; role unclear
- M_5 (G_q)—role unclear

Dopamine Receptors

- D_1 (G_s)—smooth muscle relaxation; natriuresis; CNS effects
- D_2 ($G_{i/o}$)—inhibits sympathetic transmitter release; CNS effects
- D_3 ($G_{i/o}$)—similar to D_2
- D_4 ($G_{i/o}$)—similar to D_2
- D_5 (G_s)—similar to D_1

Vasopressin Receptors

- V_1 (G_q)—smooth muscle contraction
- V_2 (G_s)—↑ H_2O reabsorption in kidney

Other Receptors

- Insulin (TK)—↑ glycogen synthesis; ↓ glycogenolysis
- Glucagon (G_s)—↑ glycogenolysis; ↓ glycogen synthesis
- IGF (TK)—↑ proliferation of various cell types
- PDGF (TK)—↑ proliferation of connective tissue, glial, and smooth muscle cells
- EGF (TK)—↑ proliferation of mesenchymal, glial, and epithelial cells
- ANF (GC)—smooth muscle relaxation; ↑ Na^+ and H_2O excretion in kidney
- NO (GC)—smooth muscle relaxation

Definition of abbreviations: ANF, atrial natriuretic factor; ATP, adenosine triphosphate; cGMP, cyclic guanosine monophosphate; DAG, diacylglycerol; EGF, epidermal growth factor; ER, endoplasmic reticulum; GC, guanylate cyclase–coupled receptor; $G_{i/o}$, cAMP-inhibiting GPCR; G_q, PLC-activating GPCR; G_s, cAMP-activating GPCR; IGF, insulin-like growth factor; PDE, phosphodiesterase; PDGF, platelet-derived growth factor; PIP_2, phosphoinositol biphosphate; PLC, phospholipase C; NO, nitric oxide; TK, tyrosine kinase receptor.

Immunology

Chapter 3

Overview of the Immune System

► Characteristics of Innate versus Adaptive Immunity

The immune system can be divided into **two** complementary arms: the **innate** (native, natural) immune system and the **adaptive** (acquired, specific) immune system. These two arms work in concert with each other through soluble substances, such as antibodies, complement, and cytokines.

Characteristics	Innate	Adaptive
Specificity	For structures shared by groups of microbes	For specific antigens of microbial and nonmicrobial agents
Diversity	Limited	**High**
Memory	No	**Yes**
Self-reactivity	No	No
Components	**Innate**	**Adaptive**
Anatomic and chemical barriers	Skin, mucosa, chemicals (lysozyme, interferons α and β), temperature, pH	Lymph nodes, spleen, mucosal-associated lymphoid tissues
Blood proteins	**Complement**	**Antibodies**
Cells	**Phagocytes and NK cells**	**Lymphocytes** (other than NK cells)

► Overview of the Immune Response

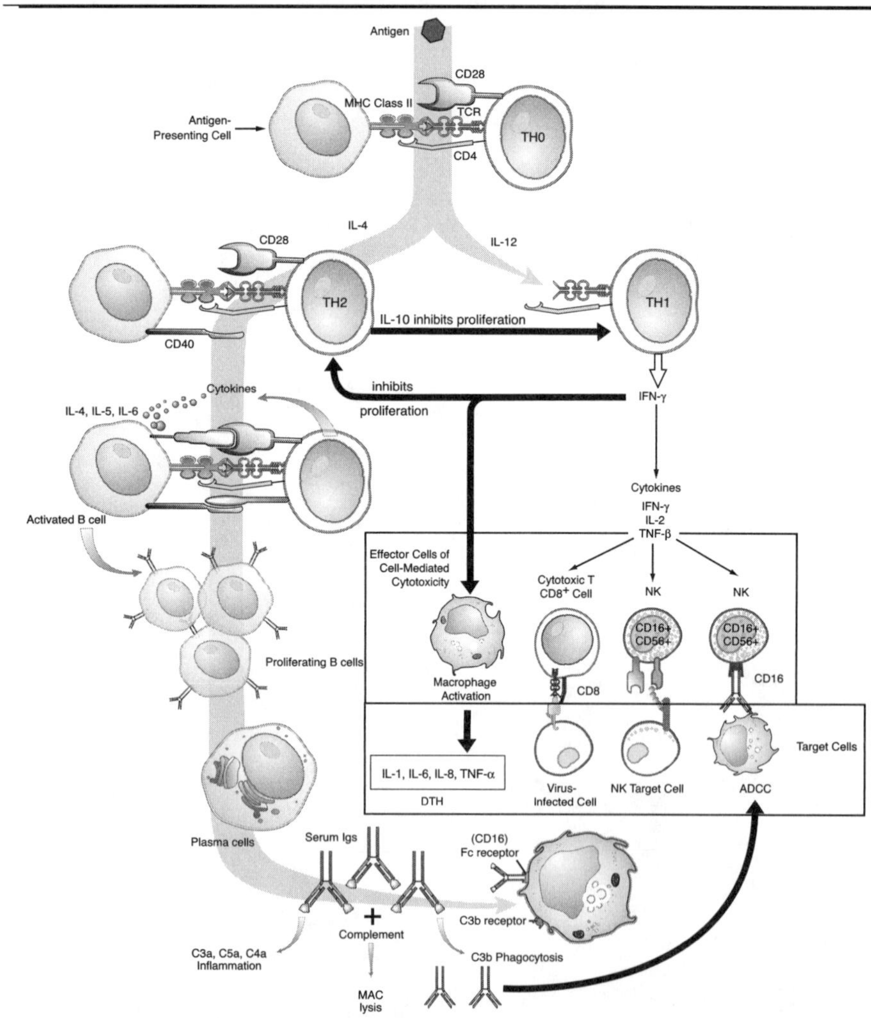

- Foreign materials are processed and presented to TH cells in the MHC class II groove.
- Extracellular pathogens stimulate production of TH2 cells, which provide the CD40L costimulatory signal and cytokines to induce B cells to differentiate into plasma cells, which produce antibody. Antibody may assist in phagocytosis (**opsonization**) or complement-mediated lysis.
- Intracellular pathogens stimulate production of TH1 cells, which stimulate the effector cells of cell-mediated immunity.
- Macrophages are induced to become more effective intracellular killers of the bacteria they ingest.
- Cytotoxic T cells kill virus-infected cells by recognition of peptides presented in the MHC class I molecule.
- Natural killer (NK) cells kill cells devoid of MHC class I that are infected with some viruses or have undergone malignant transformation.
- In antibody-dependent cell-mediated cytotoxicity (ADCC), abnormal surface molecules on infected or transformed cells are recognized by antibodies and targeted for extracellular lysis by NK cells, eosinophils, neutrophils, or macrophages.

Definition of abbreviations: MHC, major histocompatibility complex; TCR, T cell receptor; TH, T helper.

▶ Cells of the Immune System

Myeloid Cell	Location	Identifying Features	Function
Monocyte 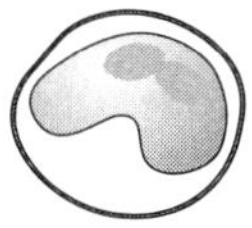	Bloodstream, 0–900/µL	**Kidney bean-shaped nucleus, CD 14 (endotoxin receptor) positive**	**Phagocytic**, differentiate into tissue macrophages
Macrophage 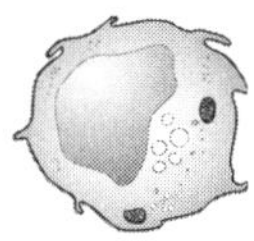	Tissues	Ruffled membrane, cytoplasm with vacuoles and vesicles (CD14+)	**Phagocytosis**, secretion of **cytokines**
Dendritic cell 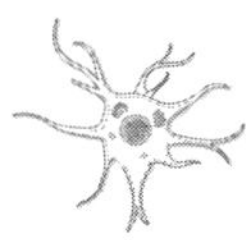	Epithelia, tissues	Long, cytoplasmic arms	**Antigen capture**, transport, and presentation (There are also plasmacytoid dendritic cells that look like plasma cells and produce interferon-α.)
Neutrophil 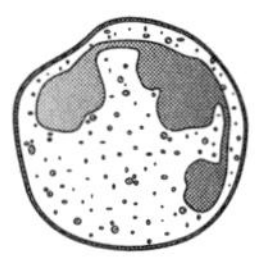	Bloodstream, 1,800–7,800/µL	**Multilobed** nucleus; **small pink** granules	**Phagocytosis** and activation of bactericidal mechanisms
Eosinophil 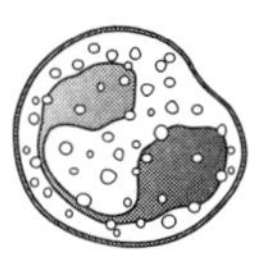	Bloodstream, 0–450/µL	**Bilobed** nucleus; **large pink** granules	**Killing of antibody-coated parasites**
Basophil 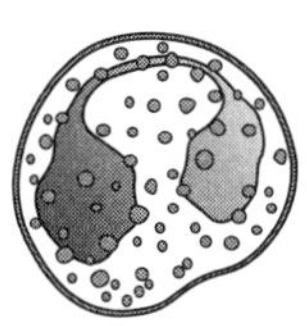	Bloodstream, 0–200/µL	**Bilobed** nucleus; **large blue** granules	**Nonphagocytic**, release pharmacologically active substances during **allergy**
Mast cell 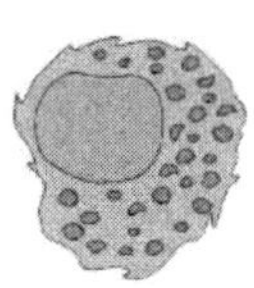	Tissues, mucosa, and epithelia	**Small** nucleus; **cytoplasm** packed with **large blue** granules	Release of granules containing histamine, etc., during **allergy**

(Continued)

► Cells of the Immune System *(Cont'd.)*

Lymphoid Cell	Location	Identifying Features	Function
Lymphocyte 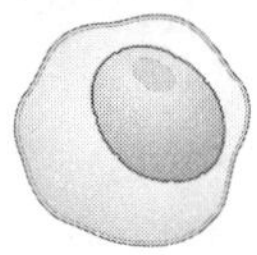	Bloodstream, 1,000–4,000/μL, lymph nodes, spleen, submucosa, and epithelia	**Large, dark** nucleus, small rim of cytoplasm	**B cells produce antibody** **TH (CD3+CD4+) cells regulate immune responses** **Cytotoxic T cells (CTLs: CD3+CD8+) kill altered or infected cells**
Natural killer (NK) lymphocyte 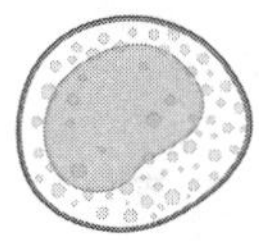	Bloodstream, ≤10% of lymphocytes	**Lymphocytes** with **large cytoplasmic** granules, **CD16+CD56+**	**Kill tumor/virus cell** targets or antibody-coated target cells
Plasma cell 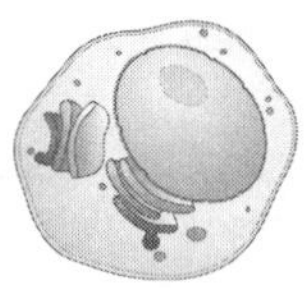	Lymph nodes, spleen, mucosal-associated lymphoid tissues, and bone marrow	**Small dark** nucleus, **intensely staining Golgi** apparatus	End cell of B-cell differentiation, **produce antibody**

► CHARACTERISTICS OF LYMPHOID CELLS
Comparison of B- and T-lymphocyte Antigen Receptors

Property	B-Cell Antigen Receptor	T-Cell Antigen Receptor
Idiotypes/lymphocyte	1	1
Isotypes/lymphocyte	2 (**IgM and IgD**)	1 (α/β)
Is secretion possible?	**Yes**	**No**
Number of combining sites/molecules	2	1
Mobility	**Flexible** (hinge region)	**Rigid**
Signal transduction molecules	Ig-α, Ig-β, **CD19, CD21**	**CD3**

► Generation of Receptor Diversity in B and T Lymphocytes

Mechanism	Cell in Which Expressed
Existence in genome of multiple V, D, J segments	B and T cells
VDJ recombination (gene segments are selected and recombined randomly to generate unique variable domains)	B and **T cells**
N-nucleotide addition (TdT adds nucleotides randomly where V, D, and J are joined)	**B cells (only heavy chain), T cells (both chains)**
Combinatorial association of heavy and light chains	B and T cells
Somatic hypermutation (mutations in variable domain coding occur during blastogenesis, and natural selection causes affinity maturation)	**B cells only,** after **Ag stimulation**

Definition of abbreviation: Tdt, terminal deoxyribonucleotidyl transferase.

► Human Major Histocompatibility Complex (MHC) Summary

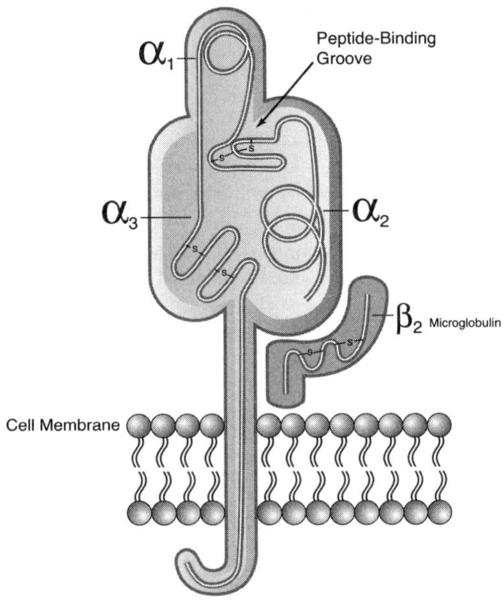

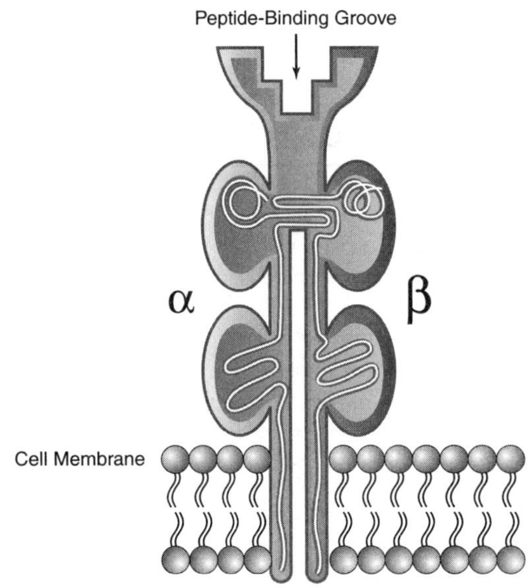

	MHC Class I	MHC Class II
Names	HLA-A, HLA-B, HLA-C	HLA-DP, HLA-DQ, HLA-DR
Tissue distribution	**All nucleated cells**, platelets	**B and T lymphocytes, antigen-presenting cells**
Recognized by	Cytotoxic T cells **(CD8+)**	Helper T cells **(CD4+)**
Peptides bound	Endogenously **synthesized**	Exogenously **processed**
Function	**Elimination of abnormal (infected) host cells** by cytotoxic T cells	**Presentation of foreign antigen** to helper T cells
Invariant chain	No	**Yes**
β_2-microglobulin	**Yes**	No

► Examples of HLA-Linked Immunologic Diseases

Disease	HLA Allele
Rheumatoid arthritis	DR4
Insulin-dependent diabetes mellitus	DR3/DR4
Multiple sclerosis, Goodpasture syndrome	DR2
Systemic lupus erythematosus	DR2/DR3
Ankylosing spondylitis, psoriasis, inflammatory bowel disease, Reiter syndrome	B27
Celiac disease	DQ2 or DQ8
Graves disease	B8

► Superantigens
(Staphylococcal Enterotoxins, Toxic-Shock Syndrome Toxin-1, and Streptococcal Pyrogenic Exotoxins)

- Superantigens cross-link the variable β domain of a T-cell receptor to an α chain of a class II MHC molecule.
- They cause life-threatening **overproduction of inflammatory cytokines (IL-1, IL-6, IFN-γ, and TNF-α)**.
- **Endotoxin** acts by direct stimulation of macrophages to produce IL-1, IL-6, and TNF-α in the absence of TH participation.

► T-Helper Cells

- Naive TH cells (THO) differentiate into TH1 cells when a strong initial innate immune response leads to production of IL-12 from macrophages or IFN-γ from NK cells.
- Differentiation of a THO cell into a TH2 cell occurs in the absence of an innate immune response. TH1 cells secrete cytokines that stimulate cell-mediated immunity (CMI). TH2 cells produce cytokines that stimulate humoral immunity (HMI). IFN-γ, produced by TH1, inhibits TH2. IL-4 and IL-10, produced by TH2, inhibit TH1.
- TH17 cells increase inflammation and produce IL-17.
- T_{reg} cells decrease inflammation and produce IL-10.
- T cells that are exposed to antigen presenting cells in the absence of costimulatory signals will become anergic.

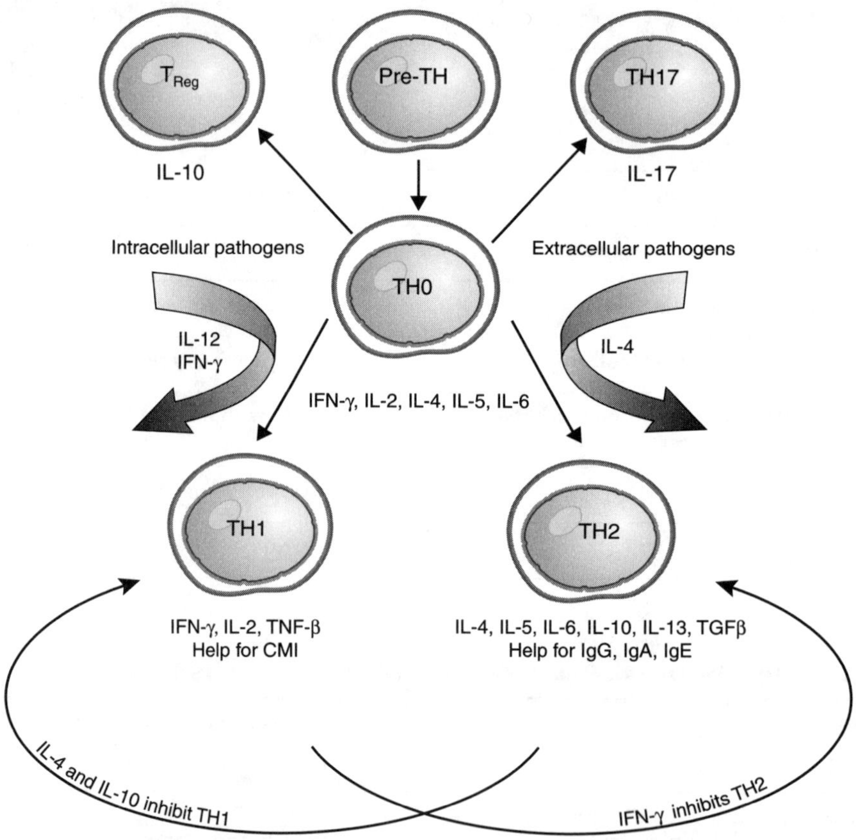

► Effector Cells in Cell-Mediated Immunity

Effector Cell	CD Markers	Antigen Recognition	MHC Recognition Required for Killing	Effector Molecules
CTL	TCR, CD3, **CD8**, CD2	**Specific**, TCR	Yes, **class I**	**Perforin, cytokines** (TNF-β, IFN-γ)
NK cell	**CD16, CD56,** CD2	ADCC: specific by IgG, otherwise recognizes lectins	No, **MHC I recognition inhibits**	**Perforin, cytokines** (TNF-β, IFN-γ)
Macrophage	**CD14**	**Nonspecific**	No	**Intracellular** mechanisms

► Key CD Markers

CD Designation	Cellular Expression	Known Functions
CD2 (LFA-2)	T cells, thymocytes, NK cells	Adhesion molecule
CD3	**T cells**, thymocytes	Signal transduction by the TCR
CD4	**TH cells**, thymocytes, monocytes, and macrophages	Coreceptor for **MHC class II** TH-cell activation, **receptor for HIV**
CD8	**CTLs**, some thymocytes	Coreceptor for **MHC class I**–restricted T cells
CD14 (LPS receptor)	Monocytes, macrophages, granulocytes	Binds LPS
CD16 (Fc receptor)	**NK cells**, macrophages, mast cells	Immune complex-induced cellular activation, ADCC
CD19 and 20	**B cells**	Coreceptor with CD21 for B-cell activation
CD21 (CR2, C3d receptor)	Mature B cells, follicular dendritic cells	Receptor for complement fragment C3d, forms coreceptor complex with CD19, **Epstein-Barr virus** receptor
CD25	Activated TH cells and T_{Reg}	Alpha chain of IL-2 receptor
CD28	T cells	T-cell receptor for costimulatory molecule B7
CD40	B cells, macrophages, dendritic cells, endothelial cells	Binds CD40L, **starts isotype switch**
CD56	**NK cells**	Not known

Definition of abbreviations: ADCC, antibody-dependent cell-mediated cytotoxicity; CTL, cytotoxic T lymphocytes; LPS, endotoxin (lipopolysaccharide); NK, natural killer; TCR, T-cell receptor.

► Cytokines

Cytokine	Source	Activity
Interleukin-1	Monocytes, macrophages	Stimulates cells, **endogenous pyrogen**
Interleukin-2	TH cells	**Induces proliferation**, enhances activity
Interleukin-3	TH cells, NK cells	Supports growth and differentiation of **myeloid cells**
Interleukin-4	TH2 cells	Stimulates activation, differentiation, class switch to IgG1 and **IgE**
Interleukin-5	TH2 cells	Stimulates proliferation and differentiation, class switch to **IgA**; in bone marrow, stimulates eosinophil production
Interleukin-6	Monocytes, macrophages, TH2 cells	Second endogenous pyrogen, promotes differentiation into plasma cells, **induces acute phase response**
Interleukin-7	Primary lymphoid organs	**Stimulates progenitor B- and T-cell production in bone marrow**
Interleukin-8	Macrophages, endothelial cells	**Chemokine** (chemotactic for neutrophils)
Interleukin-10	**TH2 cells**	Suppresses cytokine production of TH1 cells; diminishes inflammation
Interleukin-11	Bone marrow stroma	↑ platelet count
Interleukin-12	Macrophages	**Stimulates CMI**
Interleukin-17	TH17 cells	↑ inflammation and tissue damage associated with some autoimmune diseases
Interferon-α and -β	Leukocytes, fibroblasts	**Inhibits viral protein synthesis** by acting on uninfected cells
Interferon-γ	**TH1**, CTLs, NK cells	**Stimulates CMI, Inhibits TH2**, increases expression of class I and II MHC
Tumor necrosis factor-α and -β	CMI cells	Enhances CMI
Granulocyte and granulocyte-monocyte colony-stimulating factors (G-CSF and GM-CSF)	Macrophages and TH cells	Induce proliferation in bone marrow; counteract neutropenia following ablative chemotherapy

Definition of abbreviation: CMI, cell-mediated immunity.

► The Basic Structure of Immunoglobulin

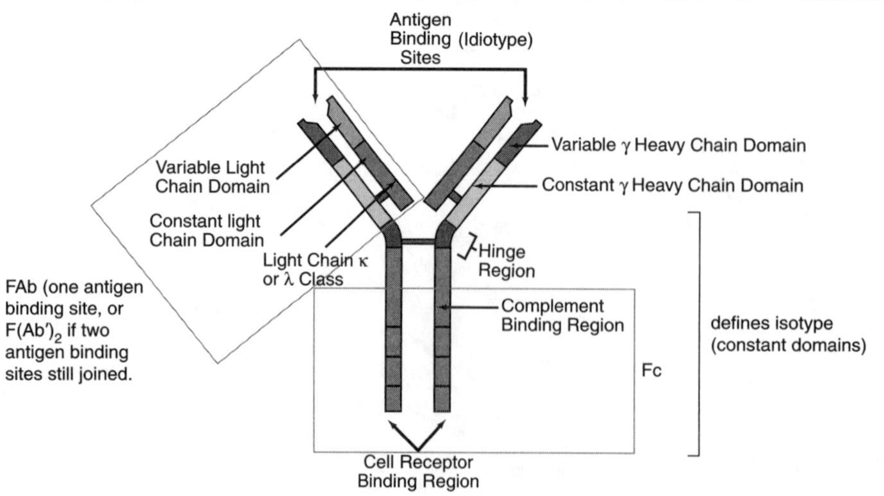

Immunoglobulin Epitopes

Allotype—polymorphic differences between members of species (see lines in Fc region)

Isotype—determinants common to constant domains of heavy and light chains

Idiotype—determinants unique to the antigen combining site

▶ Summary of the Biologic Functions of the Antibody Isotypes

	IgM	IgG	IgA	IgD	IgE
Heavy chain	μ	γ	α	δ	ε
Adult serum levels	40–345 mg/dL	650–1,500 mg/dL	75–390 mg/dL	Trace	Trace
Functions					
Complement activation, classic pathway	+	+	–	–	–
Opsonization	–	+	–	–	–
Antibody-dependent, cell-mediated cytotoxicity (ADCC)	–	+	–	–	–
Placental transport	–	+	–	–	–
Naive B-cell antigen receptor	+	–	–	+	–
Memory B-cell antigen receptor (one only)	–	+	+	–	+
Trigger mast cell granule release	–	–	–	–	+

▶ Precipitation of Ab-Ag Complexes

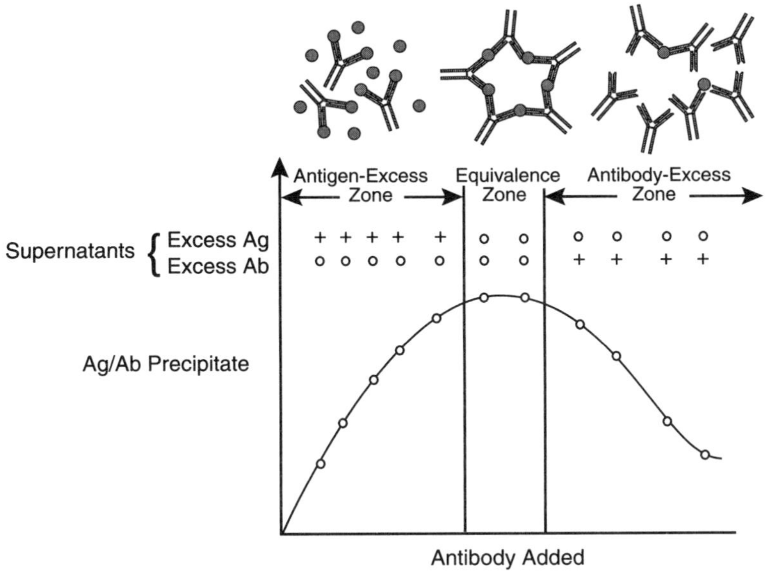

Prozone phenomenon—formation of suboptimal amount of precipitate in antibody excess (secondary syphilis)

Window period (hepatitis B)—the equivalence zone for HBsAg/HBsAb combination

Inflammation

► Acute Inflammation

Acute inflammation is an immediate response to injury, associated with redness, heat, swelling, pain, and loss of function. Understand the sequence of events of acute inflammation (extravasation, chemotaxis, phagocytosis, intracellular killing) and how these events set the stage for the subsequent adaptive immune response.

Hemodynamic changes	• Transient initial vasoconstriction, followed by massive dilation (mediated by histamine, bradykinin, and prostaglandins) • Increased vascular permeability (due to endothelial cell contraction and/or injury)—histamine, serotonin, bradykinin, leukotrienes (e.g., LTC_4, LTD_4, LTE_4) • Blood stasis due to increased viscosity allows neutrophils to marginate
Cellular response	• **Neutrophils:** (segmented) polymorphonuclear leukocytes (PMNs) are important mediators in acute inflammation • Neutrophils have **primary (azurophilic)** and **secondary (specific) granules:** – **Primary granules contain:** myeloperoxidase, phospholipase A2, lysozyme, acid hydrolases, elastase, defensins, and bactericidal permeability increasing protein (BPI) – **Secondary granules contain:** phospholipase A2, lysozyme, leukocyte alkaline phosphatase (LAP), collagenase, lactoferrin, vitamin B_{12}–binding proteins

► Neutrophil Margination and Extravasation

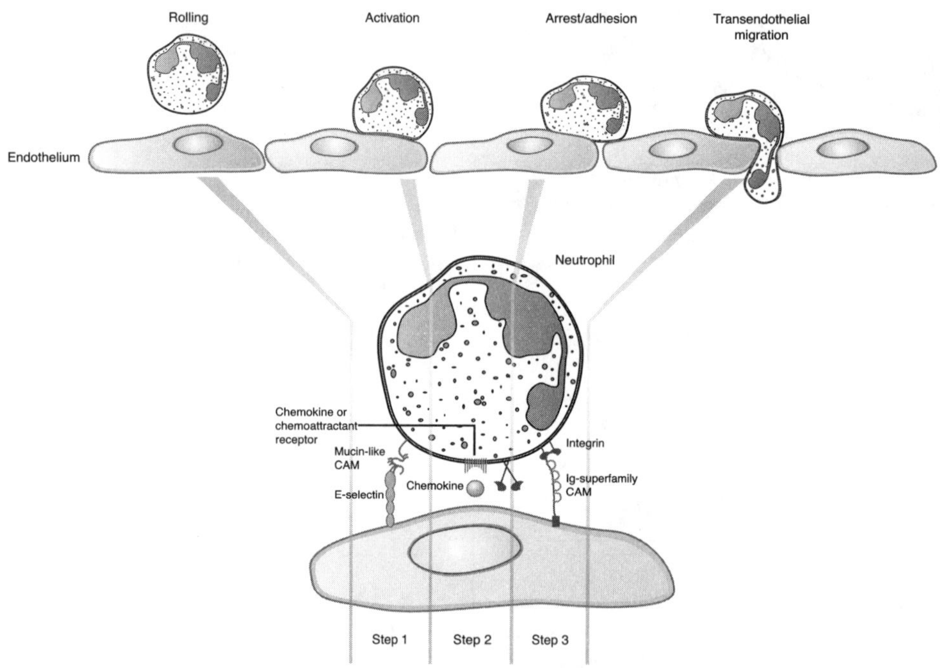

Neutrophil Margination and Adhesion

- At sites of inflammation, endothelial cells increase expression of **E-selectin** and **P-selectin**, allowing neutrophils to bind weakly.
- Then neutrophils are stimulated by chemokines to express their integrins.
- Tight adherence of the neutrophil to the endothelial cell allows migration through the basement membrane toward the inflammatory stimulus (chemotaxis).

► Neutrophil Migration/Chemotaxis

Chemoattractive Molecule	Origin
Chemokines (**IL-8**)	Tissue mast cells, platelets, neutrophils, monocytes, macrophages, eosinophils, basophils, lymphocytes
Complement split product **C5a**	Endothelial damage → activation Hageman factor → plasmin activation
Leukotriene B_4	Membrane phospholipids of macrophages, monocytes, neutrophils, mast cells → arachidonic acid cascade → lipoxygenase pathway
Formyl methionyl peptides	Released from **microorganisms**

► Other Chemical Mediators of Inflammation

Monoamine	Sources	Effects	Triggers for Release
Histamine	Basophils, platelets, and mast cells	Vasodilation and increased vascular permeability	• IgE-mediated mast cell reactions • Physical injury • Anaphylatoxins (C3a and C5a) • Cytokines (IL-1)
Serotonin	Platelets		Platelet aggregation
Enzyme	**Arachidonic Acid Product**	**Effects**	**Comments**
Cyclooxygenase	Thromboxane A_2	Vasoconstriction, platelet aggregation	Produced by platelets
	Prostacyclin (PGI_2)	**Vasodilation** and inhibits platelet aggregation	Produced by vascular endothelium
	PGE_2	Pain	—
	PGE_2, PGD_2, PGF_2	Vasodilation	—
Lipoxygenase	LTB_4	Neutrophil chemotaxis, **increased vascular permeability, vasoconstriction or vasodilation***	—
	LTC_4, LTD_4, LTE_4	**Bronchoconstriction, increased vascular permeability, vasoconstriction or vasodilation***	Slow-reacting substance of anaphylaxis

Kinin System

- Bradykinin—vasoactive peptide produced from kininogen by family of enzymes called kallikreins; degraded by different peptidases, including angiotensin-converting enzyme (ACE)
- Activated **Hageman factor (factor XII)** converts prekallikrein → kallikrein
- Kallikrein cleaves high molecular weight kininogen (HMWK) → **bradykinin** (produces increased vascular permeability, pain, vasodilation, bronchoconstriction)

***Can be tissue specific (e.g., vasoconstriction in kidneys and heart; vasodilation in skin and nasal mucosa)**

► Phagocytosis

- Several steps of phagocytosis: engulfment, fusion of the phagosome and lysosome, and digestion.
- Mechanisms of intracellular killing: NADPH oxidase-dependent, myeloperoxidase-dependent, and lysosome-dependent.
- **Opsonization** is the enhancement of phagocytosis with IgG and/or C3b.

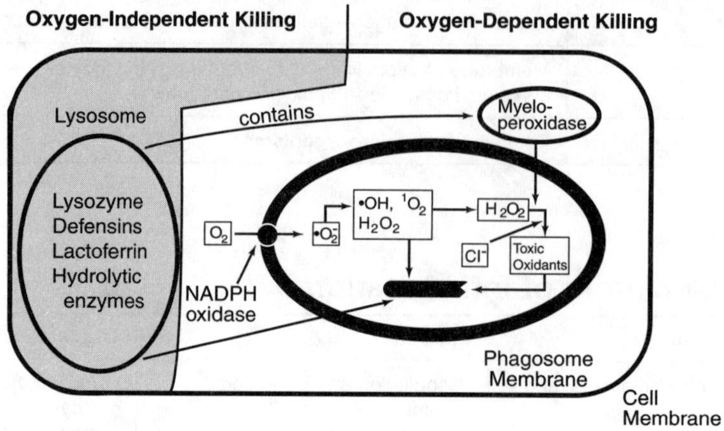

► Defects of Phagocytic Cells

Disease	Molecular Defect(s)	Symptoms
Chronic granulomatous disease (CGD)	Deficiency of **NADPH oxidase** (any one of four component proteins); failure to generate superoxide anion, other O_2 radicals	Recurrent infections with **catalase-positive** bacteria and fungi
Chédiak-Higashi syndrome	Granule structural defect	Recurrent infection with bacteria: chemotactic and degranulation defects; **absent NK** activity, **partial albinism**
Leukocyte adhesion deficiency	**Absence of CD18**—common β chain of the leukocyte integrins	Recurrent and chronic infections, failure to form pus, **does not reject umbilical cord** stump

► Complement Cascade

- The complement system is a set of interacting serum proteins that enhance inflammation (C3a, C4a, C5a) and opsonization (C3b) and cause lysis of particles (e.g., gram-negative bacteria) via C5b-9.
- The **alternative** pathway is initiated by **surfaces of pathogens**.
- The **classical** pathway is activated by **Ag/Ab complexes**.

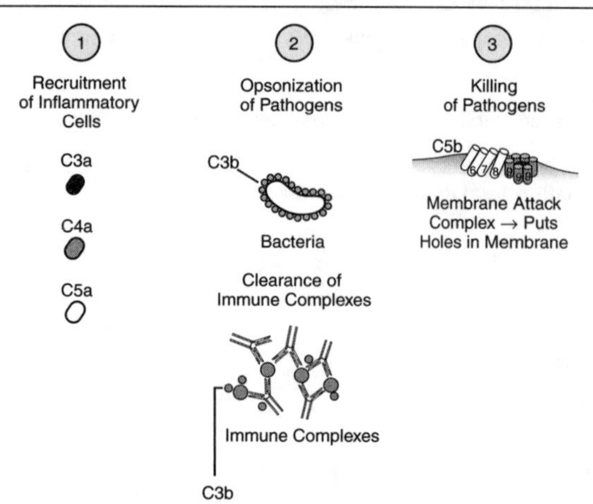

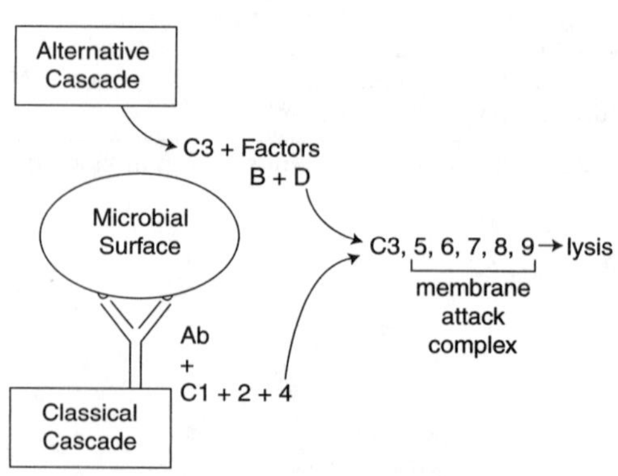

► Deficiencies of Complement or Its Regulation

Deficiencies in Complement Components	Deficiency	Signs/Diagnosis
Classical pathway	C1q, C1r, C1s, C2, C4	Marked increase in immune complex diseases, increased infections with pyogenic bacteria
Alternative pathway	Factor B, properdin	Increased neisserial infections
Both pathways	C3	Recurrent bacterial infections, immune complex disease
	C5, C6, C7, or **C8**	**Recurrent meningococcal and gonococcal infections**
Deficiencies in complement regulatory proteins	C1-INH (**hereditary angioedema**)	Serum depletion of C1, C2, C4 **Edema at mucosal surfaces**

► Summary of Acute Inflammation

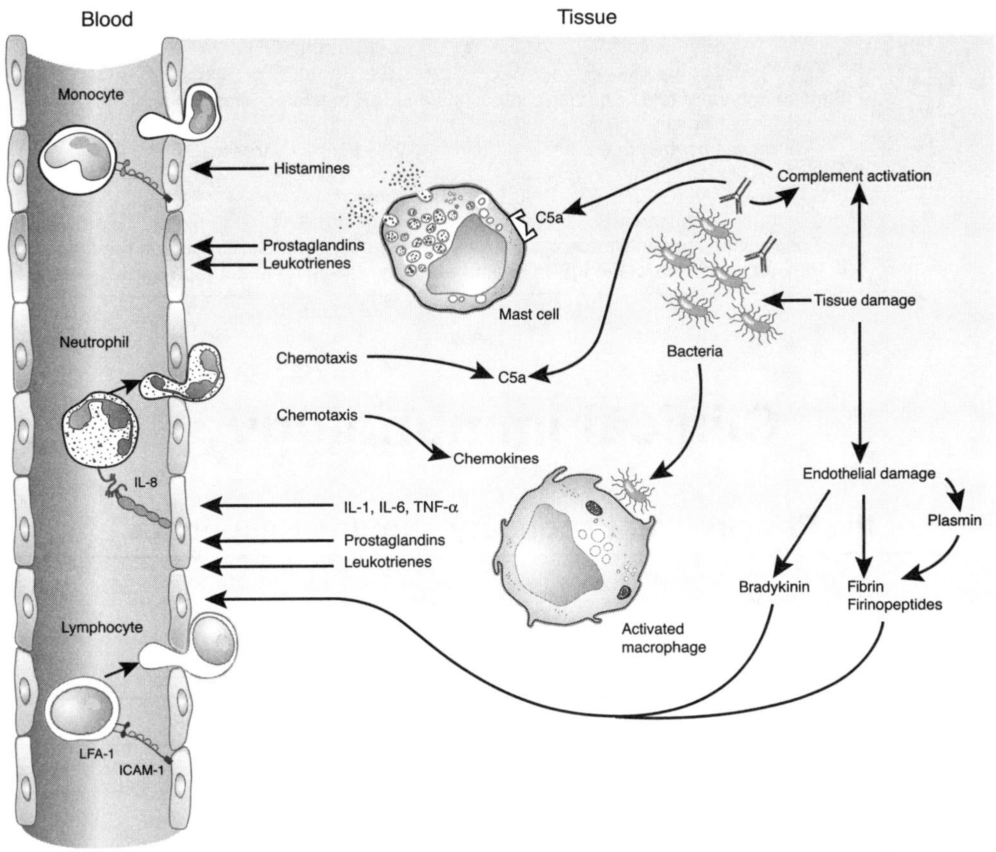

► Chronic Inflammation

<table>
<tr><th>Causes</th><th>Important Cell Types</th></tr>
<tr><td rowspan="8">• Following a bout of acute inflammation
• Persistent infections
• Infections with certain organisms (viruses, mycobacteria, parasites, fungi)
• Autoimmune diseases
• Response to foreign material</td><td>Macrophages</td></tr>
<tr><td>Derived from blood monocytes. During inflammation, macrophages are mainly recruited from the blood (circulating monocytes). Macrophages contain acid hydrolases, elastase, and collagenase, secrete monokines.
Chemotactic factors: C5a, MCP-1, MIP-1-α, PDGF, TGF-α
Tissue-based macrophages:
• Connective tissue (histiocyte)
• Lung (pulmonary alveolar macrophages)
• Liver (Kupffer cells)
• Bone (osteoclasts)
• Brain (microglia)
• Kidney (mesangial cells)</td></tr>
<tr><td>Lymphocytes (e.g., B cells, plasma cells)</td></tr>
<tr><td>• T cells
• Lymphocyte chemokine: lymphotaxin</td></tr>
<tr><td>Eosinophils</td></tr>
<tr><td>Play an important role in parasitic infections and IgE-mediated allergic reactions
• Eosinophilic chemokine: eotaxin
• Granules contain major basic protein, which is toxic to parasites</td></tr>
<tr><td>Basophils</td></tr>
<tr><td>• Tissue-based basophils are called mast cells, present in high numbers in the lung and skin
• Play an important role in IgE-mediated reactions (allergies and anaphylaxis), release histamine</td></tr>
</table>

Clinical Immunology

► Comparison of the Primary and Secondary Immune Responses

Feature	Primary Response	Secondary Response
Time lag after immunization	5–10 days	1–3 days
Peak response	Small	Large
Antibody isotype	IgM then IgG	Increasing IgG, IgA, or IgE
Antibody **affinity**	Variable to low	High (**affinity maturation**)
Inducing agent	All immunogens	**Protein antigens**
Immunization protocol	High dose of antigen (often with adjuvant)	Low dose of antigen (often without adjuvant)

▶ Types of Immunization Used in Medicine

Adjuvants increase immunogenicity nonspecifically. They are given with weak immunogens to enhance the response.

Type of Immunity	Acquired Through	Examples
Natural	Passive means	Placental IgG transport, colostrum
Natural	Active means	Recovery from infection
Artificial	Passive means	Immunoglobulins or immune cells given
Artificial	Active means	Vaccination

▶ Summary of Bacterial Vaccines

Organism	Vaccine	Vaccine Type
C. diphtheriae	DT**aP**	Toxoid
B. pertussis	DT**aP**	Toxoid
C. tetani	DT**aP**	Toxoid
H. influenzae	Hib	Capsular polysaccharide and protein
S. pneumoniae	PCV Pediatric	13 capsular serotypes and protein
	PPV Adult	23 capsular serotypes
N. meningitidis	MCV-4	4 capsular serotypes (Y, W-135, C, A) plus protein

▶ Summary of Viral Vaccines

Killed Vaccines	Live Viral Vaccines	Component Vaccines
Mnemonic: RIP-A (Rest In Peace Always—the killed viral vaccines): Rabies (killed human diploid cell vaccine) Influenza Polio (Salk) A Hepatitis	All but adenovirus are attenuated (**mnemonic: Mrr. V.Z. Mapsy**) Mumps Rotavirus Rubella Varicella – Zoster Measles Adenovirus (pathogenic [not attenuated] respiratory strains given in enteric coated capsules) Polio (Sabin) Small Pox Yellow Fever	Hepatitis B HPV (human papilloma virus)

► Defects of Humoral Immunity

Disease	Molecular Defect	Symptoms/Signs
Bruton X-linked hypogammaglobulinemia	Deficiency of a tyrosine kinase blocks B-cell maturation	Low immunoglobulin of all classes, **no circulating B cells**, **pre-B cells in bone marrow in normal numbers**, normal cell-mediated immunity
Selective IgA deficiency	Deficiency of IgA (most common)	Repeated **sinopulmonary and gastrointestinal infections**, ↑ atopic allergy
X-linked hyper-IgM syndrome	Deficiency of **CD40L** on activated T cells	**High serum titers of IgM without other isotypes** Normal B- and T-cell numbers, susceptibility to extracellular bacteria and opportunists
Common variable immunodeficiency	B-cell maturation defect and **hypogammaglobulinemia**	Both sexes affected, childhood onset, recurrent bacterial infections and increased susceptibility to *Giardia* Increased risk later in life to autoimmune disease, lymphoma, or gastric cancer

► Defects of T Cells and Severe Combined Immunodeficiencies

Category	Disease	Defect	Clinical Manifestation
Selective T-cell deficiency	**DiGeorge syndrome (velocardiofacial syndrome)**	Failure of formation of third and fourth pharyngeal pouches, **thymic aplasia**	Facial abnormalities, hypoparathyroidism, cardiac malformations, depression of T-cell numbers and absence of T-cell responses
	MHC class I deficiency	Failure of TAP 1 molecules to transport peptides to endoplasmic reticulum	**CD8+ T cells deficient**, CD4+ T cells normal, recurring viral infections, normal DTH, normal Ab production
	MHC class II deficiency	**Bare lymphocyte syndrome**	T cells present and responsive to nonspecific mitogens, no GVHD, **deficient in CD4+ T cells,** hypogammaglobulinemia; presents as SCID
Combined partial B- and T-cell deficiency	**Wiskott-Aldrich syndrome**	Defect in cytoskeletal glycoprotein, X-linked	Defective responses to bacterial polysaccharides and depressed IgM, gradual loss of humoral and cellular responses, **thrombocytopenia and eczema**
	Ataxia telangiectasia	Defect in kinase involved in the cell cycle	Ataxia (gait abnormalities), telangiectasia (capillary distortions in the eye), deficiency of IgA and IgE production
Complete functional B- and T-cell deficiency	Severe combined immunodeficiency (SCID)	Defects in common γ chain of IL-2 receptor (also present in receptors for IL-4, -7, -9, -15) X-linked	Chronic diarrhea; skin, mouth, and throat lesions; opportunistic (**fungal**) infections; low levels of circulating lymphocytes; cells unresponsive to mitogens
		Adenosine deaminase deficiency (results in toxic metabolic products in cells)	
		Defect in signal transduction from T-cell IL-2 receptors	

▶ Association Between Immunodeficiency Disease and Developmental Blocks

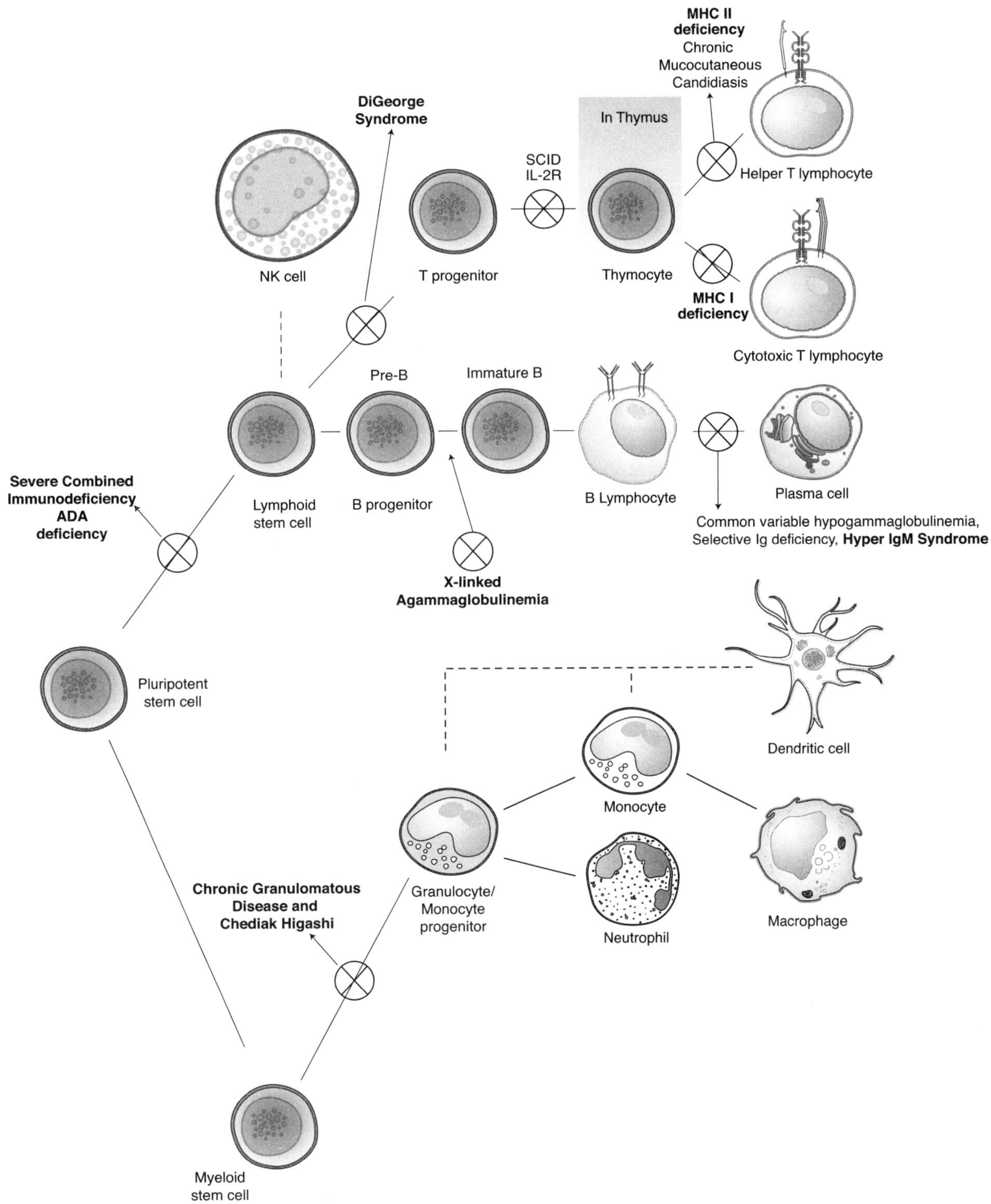

► Acquired Immunodeficiency Syndrome (AIDS)

Definition	When a patient is HIV-positive with CD4 count less than 200/mm^3 *or* HIV-positive with an AIDS-defining disease

Transmission	• Sexual contact: homosexual > heterosexual in U.S.
	  – Cofactors: herpes and syphilis
	• Parenteral transmission:
	  – Intravenous drug abuse
	  – Hemophiliacs
	  – Blood transfusions
	  – Accidental needle sticks in hospital workers
	• Vertical transmission (mother to child)

Pathogenesis	• Human immunodeficiency virus (HIV; an enveloped retrovirus containing reverse transcriptase)
	• HIV infects CD4+ cells (gp120 binds to CD4)
	  – CD4+ T cells (with CCR5 chemokine coreceptor)
	  – Macrophages (with CXCR4 chemokine coreceptor)
	• **Persons who are homozygous CCR5 defective cannot be infected**
	• Entry into cell by fusion requires gp41 and coreceptors

Diagnosis and Monitoring	• **Initial screening:** Serologic, ELISA • **Confirmation:** Serologic, Western blot • **Detection of virus in blood (evaluate viral load):** RT-PCR • **Detect HIV infection in newborns of HIV+ mother (provirus):** PCR* • **Early marker of infection:** p24 antigen • **Evaluate progression of disease:** CD4:CD8 T-cell ratio
Treatment	• Combination antiretroviral treatment • Reverse transcriptase inhibitors • Protease inhibitors • Prophylaxis for opportunistic infections based on CD4 count • Fusion inhibitors • Integrase inhibitors

*RT-PCR tests for circulating viral RNA and is used to monitor the efficacy of treatment. PCR detects integrated virus (provirus DNA). Viral load has been demonstrated to be the best prognostic indicator during infection.

► Opportunistic Infection and Common Sites of Infection in AIDS Patients

Opportunistic Infection	Common Sites of Infection
Pneumocystis jiroveci (carinii)	Lung (pneumonia), bone marrow, start prophylaxis at **< 200 CD4**
Histoplasma capsulatum	Lung, disseminated, start prophylaxis at **< 100 CD4** in endemic area
Toxoplasma gondii	CNS, start prophylaxis at **< 100 CD4**
Mycobacterium avium-intracellulare	Lung, gastrointestinal tract, disseminated, start prophylaxis at **< 50 CD4**
Cytomegalovirus	Lung, retina, adrenals, and gastrointestinal tract, start prophylaxis at **< 50 CD4**
Cryptosporidium parvum	Gastrointestinal tract, start prophylaxis at **< 50 CD4**
Cryptococcus neoformans	CNS (meningitis), start prophylaxis at **< 50 CD4**
Coccidioides immitis	Lung, disseminated
Giardia lamblia	Gastrointestinal tract
Herpes simplex virus	Esophagus and CNS (encephalitis)
Candida albicans	Oropharynx and esophagus
Aspergillus spp.	CNS, lungs, blood vessels
JC virus	CNS (progressive multifocal leukoencephalopathy)
Mycobacterium tuberculosis	Lung, disseminated

▶ Other Complications of AIDS

Hairy leukoplakia	Associated with Epstein-Barr virus (EBV)
Kaposi sarcoma	Associated with human herpes virus 8 (HHV8) Common sites: skin, GI tract, lymph nodes, and lungs
Non-Hodgkin lymphoma	Tend to be high-grade B-cell lymphomas Extranodal CNS lymphomas common
Miscellaneous	Cervical cancer HIV wasting syndrome AIDS nephropathy AIDS dementia complex

▶ HIV Therapies

Anti-HIV therapy usually involves three or more anti-retroviral agents including antimetabolite inhibitors of retroviral reverse transcriptase and viral protease. These aggressive drug combinations (highly active antiretroviral therapy, **HAART**) are typically initiated early after HIV infection and will often reduce viral load, preserve CD-4 counts, and limit opportunistic infections. Drug combinations also slow the development of resistance to drugs as opposed to monotherapy.

Drug	Mechanism of Action	Side Effects and Comments
	Nucleoside reverse transcriptase inhibitors (NRTIs)	
Abacavir (ABC) Didanosine (ddI) Emtricitabine (FTC) Lamivudine (3TC) Stavudine (d4T) Tenofovir (TDF) Zalcitabine (ddC) Zidovudine (ZDV, AZT)	Converted to nucleoside triphosphates, which **inhibit reverse transcriptase**, leading the inhibition of viral replication by chain termination	Dose-limiting pancreatitis (ddI) Dose-limiting peripheral neuropathy (ddC, ddI, d4T) Hypersensitivity reactions (ABC) Lactic acidosis (ddI, d4T) Fanconi syndrome (TDF) Dose-limiting BMS (ZDV) Minimal toxicity (FTC, 3TC) Least toxic and also used for hepatitis B (3TC)
	Non-nucleoside reverse transcriptase inhibitors (NNRTIs)	
Dela**vir**dine (DLV) Efa**vir**enz (EFV) Etra**vir**ine (ETR) Ne**vir**apine (NVP)	**Inhibit reverse transcriptase** noncompetitively	Rash (occasional Steven-Johnson syndrome) Adverse CNS effects (EFV) P450 interactions Increased transaminase levels (DLV, EFV)
	Protease inhibitors	
Ataza**navir** (ATV) Daru**navir** (DRV) Fosampre**navir** (FPV) Indi**navir** (IDV) Nelfi**navir** (NFV) Rito**navir** (RTV) Saqui**navir** (SQV) Lopi**navir** + Rito**navir** (LPV/r)	**Inhibits aspartate protease** (HIV-1 protease encoded by ***pol* gene**), blocking structural protein formation of the mature virion core	Inhibit CYP3A4 (especially ritonavir) Crystalluria (indinavir, maintain hydration) Elevated transaminases Lopinavir is only available in combination with ritonavir
	Fusion inhibitor	
Enfuvirtide	**Binds gp41** and **inhibits fusion** of HIV-1 to CD4+ cells	Local injection reactions (100% patients) Hypersensitivity reactions
	CCR5 antagonist	
Maraviroc (MVC)	**Blocks CCR5 receptor**, preventing HIV entry into target cells	Hepatotoxicity, orthostatic hypotension
	Integrase inhibitor	
Raltegravir (RAL)	**Inhibits integrase**, thus blocking viral integration	CPK elevation

► Hypersensitivity Reactions

Type	Antibody	Complement	Effector Cells	Examples
I (immediate)	**IgE**	No	**Basophil, mast cell**	Hay fever, atopic dermatitis, **insect venom sensitivity**, **anaphylaxis** to drugs, some food allergies, allergy to animals and animal products, **asthma**
II (cytotoxic)	IgG, IgM	Yes	PMN, macrophages, NK cells	Autoimmune or drug-induced hemolytic anemia, transfusion reactions, **HDNB**, hyperacute graft rejection, **Goodpasture disease**, **rheumatic fever**
II (noncytotoxic)	IgG	**No**	None	Myasthenia gravis, Graves disease, type 2 diabetes mellitus
III (immune complex)	IgG, IgM	Yes	PMN, macrophages	**SLE,** polyarteritis nodosa, poststreptococcal glomerulonephritis, Arthus reaction, serum sickness
IV (delayed, DTH)	None	No	CTL, TH1, macrophages	**Tuberculin test**, tuberculosis, leprosy, **RA**, Hashimoto thyroiditis, poison ivy (**contact dermatitis**), **GVHD**, IDDM

Definition of abbreviations: GVHD, graft-versus-host disease; HDNB, hemolytic disease of the newborn; IDDM, insulin-dependent diabetes mellitus; RA, rheumatoid arthritis; SLE, systemic lupus erythematosus.

► Important Autoimmune Diseases

Autoantibodies	Clinical Features	Comments
Systemic lupus erythematosus: chronic systemic autoimmune disease characterized by a loss of self-tolerance and production of autoantibodies		
Antinuclear antibody (ANA) (>95%): **Anti-dsDNA** (40–60%) **Anti-Sm** (20–30%)	• Hemolytic anemia, thrombocytopenia, leukopenia • Arthritis • Skin rashes (including classic malar rash) • Renal disease • Libman-Sacks endocarditis • Serositis • Neurologic symptoms	• Females >> Males (M:F = 1:9), peak age 20–45 years, African American > Caucasian • Mechanism of injury: type II and III hypersensitivity reactions • Treatment: steroids and other immunosuppressants
Sjögren syndrome: an autoimmune disease characterized by destruction of the lacrimal and salivary glands, resulting in the inability to produce saliva or tears		
Antiribonucleoprotein antibodies: Anti-SS-A (Ro) Anti-SS-B (La)	• Keratoconjuctivitis sicca (dry eyes) and corneal ulcers • Xerostomia (dry mouth) • Mikulicz syndrome: enlargement of the salivary and lacrimal glands	• Females > males; age range: 30–50 years • Often associated with rheumatoid arthritis and other autoimmune diseases (e.g., SLE) • Increased risk of developing lymphoma

(Continued)

► Important Autoimmune Diseases *(Cont'd.)*

Autoantibodies	Clinical Features	Comments
Scleroderma (progressive systemic sclerosis): characterized by fibroblast stimulation and deposition of collagen in the skin and internal organs; females > males; age range: 20–55 years; activation of fibroblasts by growth factors/cytokines leads to fibrosis		
Diffuse Scleroderma		
Anti-DNA topoisomerase I antibodies (Scl-70) (70%)	Widespread skin involvement Early involvement of the visceral organs • Esophagus—dysphagia • GI tract—malabsorption • Pulmonary fibrosis—dyspnea on exertion • Cardiac fibrosis—arrhythmias • Kidney fibrosis—renal insufficiency	Raynaud phenomenon is seen in almost all patients and often preceeds other symptoms. **Treatment:** vasodilators, ACE inhibitors, NSAIDs, steroids, d-penicillamine
Limited scleroderma (e.g., CREST syndrome)		
Anticentromere antibodies	• Skin involvement of the face and hands • Late involvement of visceral organs (relatively benign clinical course)	(**C**alcinosis, **R**aynaud phenomenon, **E**sophageal dysmotility, **S**clerodactyly, **T**elangiectasia)

Transplantation Immunology

► Grafts Used in Medicine

Grafts	Definition
Autologous (**autografts**)	Tissue is moved from one location to another in the same individual
Isograft	Transplants between genetically identical individuals (monozygotic twins)
Allograft	Transplants between genetically different members of the same species
Xenograft	Transplants between members of different species

► Graft Rejection Reactions

Type of Rejection	Time Taken	Cause
Hyperacute	Minutes to hours	Preformed anti-donor antibodies and complement (type II hypersensitivity)
Accelerated	Days	Reactivation of sensitized T cells
Acute	Days to weeks	Primary activation of T cells
Chronic	Months to years	Causes are unclear: antibodies, immune complexes, slow cellular reaction, recurrence of disease (type IV hypersensitivity)
Graft versus host	Weeks to months	Grafted bone marrow T cells attack host (type IV hypersensitivity)

Microbiology

Chapter 4

General Principles of Microbiology

► Comparison of Medically Important Microbial Groups

Characteristic	Viruses	Bacteria	Fungi	Parasites
Diameter	Minute (0.02–0.3 μ)	Small (0.3–2 μ)	3–10 μ	15–25 μ (trophozoites)
Cell type	**Acellular**—no nucleus	**Prokaryotic cells**	**Eukaryotic cells**	
	• DNA or RNA • 1 nucleocapsid, except in segmented or diploid viruses	• DNA and RNA • 1 chromosome • **No histones**	• DNA and RNA • More than one chromosome	
	Replicates in host cells	DNA replicates continuously	G and S phases	
		Exons, **no introns**	Introns and exons	
	Some have polycistronic mRNA and post-translational cleavage	**Mono- and polycistronic mRNA**	**Monocistronic RNA**	
	Uses host organelles; obligate intracellular parasites	**No membrane-bound organelles**	Mitochondria and other membrane-bound organelles	
	No ribosomes	**70S** ribosomes (30S+50S)	**80S** ribosomes (40S+60S)	
Replication	Make and assemble viral components	**Binary fission (asexual)**	Cytokinesis with mitosis/meiosis	
Cellular membrane	Some are enveloped, but no membrane function	Membranes have **no sterols, except *Mycoplasma***, which have cholesterol	**Ergosterol** is major sterol	Sterols, such as **cholesterol**
Cell wall	No cell wall	**Peptidoglycan**	Complex carbohydrate **cell wall: chitin**, glucans, or mannans	No cell wall

Note: Prions are infectious proteins (contain no nucleic acids). They are the agents of kuru, mad cow disease, etc.

Bacteriology

► Bacterial Growth Curve

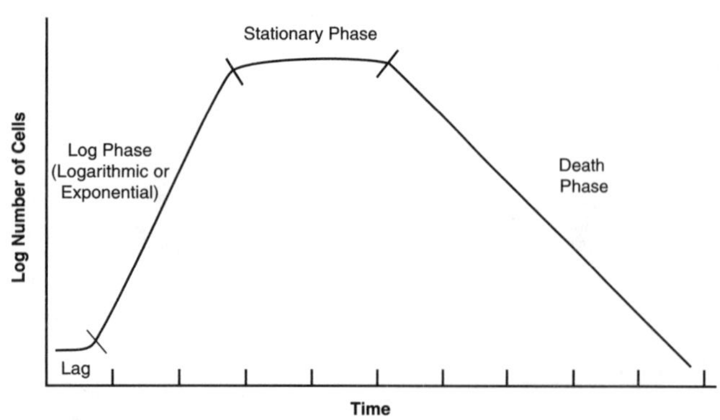

Lag Phase:
- Detoxifying medium
- Turning on enzymes to utilize medium

Log Phase:
- Rapid exponential growth
- Generation time—time it takes one cell to divide into two
- This is determined during log phase

Stationary Phase:
- Nutrients used up
- Toxic products begin to accumulate
- Number of new cells = the number of dying cells

Death Phase:
- Nutrients gone
- Toxic products kill cells
- Number of cells dying exceeds the number of cells dividing

► Features of Bacteria

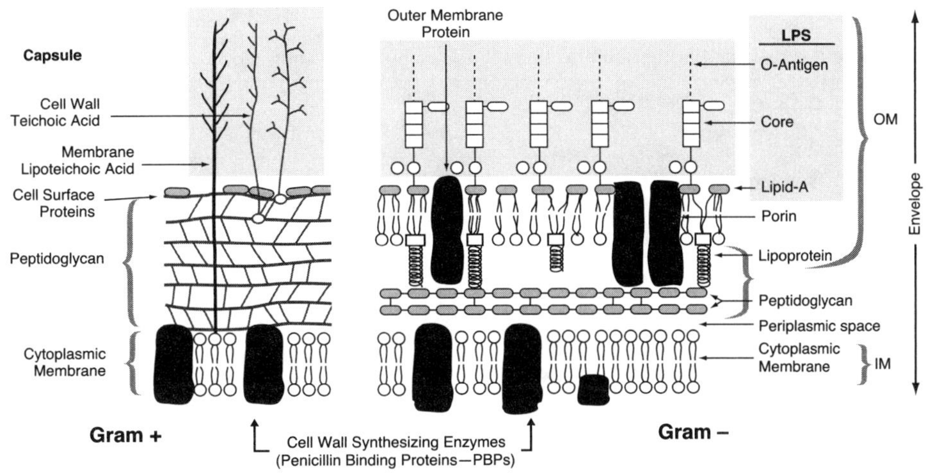

Envelope Structure	Gram ⊕ or ⊖	Chemical Composition	Function
Capsule (nonessential) = slime = glycocalyx	Both Gram ⊕ and Gram ⊖	**Polysaccharide gel** (except *B. anthracis*: poly-D-glutamate)	• **Antiphagocytic** • **Immunogenic** (except *S. pyogenes* and *N. meningitidis*, type B)
Outer membrane	**Gram** ⊖ only	Phospholipid/proteins LPS: • Lipid A • Polysaccharide	Hydrophobic membrane: • **LPS = endotoxin** • **Lipid A = toxic moiety** • PS = immunogenic portion
		Outer membrane proteins	Attachment, virulence, etc.
		Protein porins	Passive transport
Cell wall = peptidoglycan	Gram ⊕ (thick) Gram ⊖ (thin)	**Peptidoglycan**—open 3-D net of: • *N*-acetyl-glucosamine • *N*-acetyl-muramic acid • Amino acids (including DAP)	• Rigid support, cell shape, and protection from osmotic damage • Synthesis **inhibited by penicillins and cephalosporins** • **Confers Gram reaction**
	Gram ⊕ only	**Teichoic acids**	• Immunogenic, induces TNF-α, IL-1 • **Attachment**
	Acid-fast only	**Mycolic acids**	• Acid-fastness • **Resistance to drying and chemicals**
Periplasmic space	**Gram** ⊖ only	"Storage space" between the inner and outer membranes	• Enzymes to break down large molecules (β-lactamases) • Aids regulation of osmolarity
Cytoplasmic membrane = inner membrane = cell membrane = plasma membrane	Gram ⊕ Gram ⊖	Phospholipid bilayer with many embedded proteins	• Hydrophobic cell "sac" • Selective permeability and active transport • **Carrier for enzymes** for: – Oxidative metabolism – Phosphorylation – Phospholipid synthesis – DNA replication – Peptidoglycan cross linkage • **Penicillin binding proteins** (PBPs)

Definition of abbreviation: DAP, diaminopimelic acid; LPS, lipopolysaccharide.

► Normal Flora Organisms

Most infectious disease vignettes begin with the necessity to rule out the normal flora organisms that are cultured from the patient. Make sure you know those organisms that can confound a simple Gram-stain type of diagnosis, **e.g., notice in the oropharynx and vagina, normal flora organisms cannot be indistinguishable from pathogens by Gram stain alone!**

Site	Common or Medically Important Organisms	Less Common but Notable Organisms
Blood, internal organs	None, generally sterile	—
Cutaneous surfaces	*Staphylococcus epidermidis*	*Staphylococcus aureus, Corynebacteria* (diphtheroids), streptococci, anaerobes, e.g., peptostreptococci, *Candida* spp.
Nose	*Staphylococcus aureus*	*S. epidermidis,* diphtheroids, assorted streptococci
Oropharynx	**Viridans streptococci**, including *Streptococcus mutans*	Assorted streptococci, **nonpathogenic *Neisseria,* nontypeable *Haemophilus influenzae,*** *Candida albicans*
Gingival crevices	Anaerobes: *Bacteroides, Prevotella, Fusobacterium, Streptococcus, Actinomyces*	—
Stomach	None	—
Colon (microaerophilic/ anaerobic)	Adult: ***Bacteroides***/*Prevotella* (predominant organism), *Escherichia, Bifidobacterium*	*Eubacterium, Fusobacterium, Lactobacillus,* assorted gram-negative anaerobic rods *Enterococcus faecalis* and other streptococci
Vagina	**Lactobacillus**	Assorted streptococci, gram-negative rods, diphtheroids, yeasts, *Veillonella* (gram-negative diplococcus)

► Bacterial Toxins

Endotoxin

Endotoxin (lipopolysaccharide = LPS) is part of the gram-negative outer membrane. It is encoded on the chromosome.

- The toxic portion is lipid A. LPS is heat stable and not strongly immunogenic, so it cannot be converted to a toxoid.
- LPS activates macrophages, leading to release of TNF-α, IL-1, IL-6, and nitric oxide (NO). IL-1 is a major mediator of fever. Damage to the endothelium from bradykinin-induced vasodilation leads to shock. Coagulation (DIC) is mediated through the activation of Hageman factor. NO production causes hypotension, which contributes to shock.

Exotoxin

Exotoxins are protein toxins, generally quite toxic, and secreted by bacterial cells. They are encoded on plasmids or in lysogenic phage genomes.

- Exotoxins can be modified by chemicals or heat to produce a toxoid that still is immunogenic, but no longer toxic, so it can be used as a vaccine.
- Most are A-B (or two) component protein toxins. B component binds to specific cell receptors to facilitate the internalization of A (the active [toxic] component)

► Major Exotoxins

	Organism (Gram)	Toxin	Mode of Action	Role in Disease
Protein synthesis inhibitors	*Corynebacterium diphtheriae* (⊕)	**Diphtheria toxin**	• ADP ribosyl transferase **inactivates eEF-2** • *Targets:* **heart, nerves, epithelium**	Inhibits eukaryotic cell protein synthesis
	Pseudomonas aeruginosa (⊖)	**Exotoxin A**	• ADP ribosyl transferase **inactivates eEF-2** • *Target:* **liver**	Inhibits eukaryotic cell protein synthesis
	Shigella dysenteriae (⊖)	**Shiga toxin**	**Interferes with 60S ribosomal subunit**	• Inhibits protein synthesis in eukaryotic cells • Enterotoxic, cytotoxic, and neurotoxic
	Enterohemorrhagic *E. coli* (EHEC) (⊖)	**Verotoxin** (shiga-like)	**Interferes with 60S ribosomal subunit**	Inhibits protein synthesis in eukaryotic cells
Neurotoxins	*Clostridium tetani* (⊕)	**Tetanus toxin**	**Blocks release of glycine and GABA**	Inhibits neurotransmission in inhibitory synapses
	Clostridium botulinum (⊕)	**Botulinum toxin**	**Blocks release of acetylcholine**	Inhibits cholinergic synapses
Superantigens	***Staphylococcus aureus*** **(⊕)**	**TSST-1**	• Induces IL-1, IL-6, TNF-α, IFN-γ • Decreases liver clearance of LPS	Fever, increased susceptibility to LPS, rash, shock, capillary leakage
	Streptococcus pyogenes **(⊕)**	**Exotoxin A**, also called erythrogenic or pyrogenic toxin	**Similar to TSST-1**	Fever, increased susceptibility to LPS, rash, shock, capillary leakage, cardiotoxicity
cAMP inducers	Enterotoxigenic *Escherichia coli* (⊖)	Heat **labile toxin** (LT)	LT stimulates an adenylate cyclase by **ADP ribosylation of GTP-binding protein**	Both LT and ST promote secretion of fluid and electrolytes from intestinal epithelium
	Vibrio cholerae (⊖)	**Cholera toxin**	**Similar to *E. coli* LT**	Profuse, watery diarrhea
	Bacillus anthracis (⊕)	**Anthrax toxin (3 proteins** make 2 toxins)	• **EF = edema factor = adenylate cyclase** • **LF = lethal factor** • **PA = protective antigen (B component for both)**	• Decreases phagocytosis • Causes **edema, kills cells**
	Bordetella pertussis (⊖)	**Pertussis toxin**	**ADP ribosylates G_i,** the negative regulator of adenylate cyclase, leading to increased cAMP	• **Histamine sensitizing** • **Lymphocytosis promotion** (inhibits chemokine receptors) • **Islet activation**
Cytolysins	***Clostridium perfringens*** **(⊕)**	**Alpha toxin**	**Lecithinase**	• Damages cell membranes • **Myonecrosis**
	Staphylococcus aureus **(⊕)**	**Alpha toxin**	**Pore former**	Membrane becomes leaky

Definition of abbreviations: TSST-1, toxic shock syndrome toxin-1

▶ Important Pathogenic Factors and Diagnostic Enzymes

Factor	Function	Organisms
All **capsules**	**Antiphagocytic**	***S****treptococcus pneumoniae*, ***K****lebsiella pneumoniae*, ***H****aemophilus influenzae*, ***P****seudomonas aeruginosa*, ***N****eisseria meningitidis*, ***C****ryptococcus neoformans* (mnemonic: **s**ome **k**illers **h**ave **p**retty **n**ice **c**apsules) and many more
M protein	Antiphagocytic	Group A streptococci
A protein	Binds Fc of IgG to inhibit opsonization and phagocytosis	*Staphylococcus aureus*
Lipoteichoic acid	Attachment to host cells	All **gram-positive** bacteria
All **pili**	Attachment	Many gram-negatives
Pili of *N. gonorrhoeae*	**Antiphagocytic, antigenic variation**	*N. gonorrhoeae*
Hyaluronidase	Hydrolysis of ground substance	Group A streptococci
Collagenase	Hydrolysis of collagen	*Clostridium perfringens, Prevotella melaninogenica*
Urease	Increases pH of locale, contributes to kidney stones	***P****roteus,* ***U****reaplasma,* ***N****ocardia,* ***C****ryptococcus,* ***H****elicobacter* (mnemonic: **PUNCH**)
Kinases	Hydrolysis of fibrin	*Streptococcus, Staphylococcus*
Lecithinase	Destroys cell membranes	*Clostridium perfringens*
Heparinase	Thrombophlebitis	*Bacteroides*
Catalase	Destroys hydrogen peroxide **(major problem for CGD patients)**	• Most important: *Staphylococcus*, *Pseudomonas*, *Aspergillus*, *Candida*, Enterobacteriaceae • Most anaerobes lack catalase
IgA proteases	Destroy IgA, promote colonization of mucosal surfaces	*Neisseria, Haemophilus, Streptococcus pneumoniae*
Oxidase	Cytochrome c oxidase is the terminal electron acceptor	*Neisseria* and most gram-negatives, except the *Enterobacteriaceae*
Coagulase	Produces fibrin clot	***Staphylococcus aureus*** and *Yersinia pestis*

▶ Unusual Growth Requirements

Requirements in Culture	Organism
Factors **X and V**	***Haemophilus***
Cholesterol	*Mycoplasma*
High salt	*Staphylococcus aureus,* group D **enterococci** and ***Vibrio***
Cysteine	***Francisella, Legionella, Brucella,*** **and** ***Pasteurella*** (**mnemonic:** the 4 Sisters "ELLA" worship in the Cysteine Chapel)
High temperature (42° C)	***Campylobacter***
Lower than atmospheric oxygen pressure (microaerophilic); special CO_2 incubator	***Campylobacter*** and ***Helicobacter***

▶ Bacterial Genetics

Recombination	**Homologous**: The one-to-one exchange of linear extrachromosomal DNA for homologous alleles within the chromosome, using recombinase A **Site-specific**: The incorporation of extrachromosomal circles of DNA into another molecule of DNA using restriction endonucleases
Conjugation	The donation of chromosomal or plasmid genes from one bacterium to another through a conjugal bridge. • **F+ cells** have a fertility factor plasmid and serve as donors of plasmid DNA • **F− cells** do not have fertility factors and serve as the recipients of DNA in any cross. • **Hfr cells** have incorporated a fertility factor plasmid (now called episome) into their chromosome by site-specific recombination and serve as donors of chromosomal DNA • Conjugation is the most important means of transfer of drug resistance genes in gram-negative bacilli
Transduction	The delivery of bacterial genes from one bacterium to another via a virus vector. • **Generalized transduction**: Transfer of any genes from one bacterium to another via an accident in the assembly of a virus with a lytic life cycle. • **Specialized transduction**: The transfer of bacterial chromosomal genes located near the insertion site of a temperate phage from one bacterium to another via an accident of excision. • Transduction has been shown to be the means of transfer of drug resistance to methicillin (MRSA) and imipenem (*Pseudomonas*).
Transformation	The uptake and incorporation of free DNA from the environment by competent cells followed by homologous recombination. • Transformation is an important means of transfer of traits in bacteria that are naturally competent (*Streptococcus pneumoniae, Helicobacter, Neisseria,* and *Haemophilus influenzae*)
Lysogeny	The stable association of DNA molecules between a bacterium and a temperate phage. • It imparts the important traits: **C** = Cholera toxin, **O** = *Salmonella* O antigen, **B**= Botulinum toxin, **E** = Erythrogenic toxin of *Streptococcus pyogenes,* **D** = Diphtheria toxin, **S** = Shiga toxin. **Mnemonic: COBEDS:** when 2 people share a bed, someone gets a little bit pregnant (with phage). • Bacterial cells with stably integrated temperate phage DNA are said to have undergone **lysogenic conversion**.
Transposon	A mobile genetic element capable of movement within a cell. • They move by a variation of site-specific recombination and are responsible for the formation of multiple drug-resistance plasmids. • VRSA has arisen because *Enterococcus* donated a multi-drug resistance plasmid, produced by transposition, to MRSA.

Antibacterial Agents

▶ Mechanisms of Action of Antibacterial Agents

Mechanism of Action	Antibacterial Agents
Inhibition of bacterial cell-wall synthesis	Penicillins, cephalosporins, imipenem/meropenem, aztreonam, vancomycin
Inhibition of bacterial protein synthesis	Aminoglycosides, chloramphenicol, macrolides, tetracyclines, streptogramins, linezolid
Inhibition of DNA replication or transcription	Fluoroquinolones, rifampin
Inhibition of nucleic acid synthesis	Trimethoprim, flucytosine
Inhibition of folic acid synthesis	Sulfonamides, trimethoprim, pyrimethamine

► Cell Wall Synthesis Inhibitors

Class/Example	Mechanism of Action/Resistance	Spectrum	Toxicity/Notes
Penicillins			
Narrow spectrum, β-lactamase sensitive: penicillin G, penicillin V	**Mechanism:** inhibit cross-linking of peptidoglycan component of cell wall by transpeptidases; action mediated by binding of penicillin-binding proteins (PBPs) **Resistance:** production of β-lactamases, which cleave the β-lactam ring structure; change in PBPs; change in porins	Gram-positives Clostridia Syphilis	—
Very narrow spectrum, β-lactamase resistant: methicillin, nafcillin, oxacillin		Gram-positives, especially *S. aureus*	Resistant staph emerging "MRSA"
Broad spectrum, aminopenicillins, β-lactamase sensitive: ampicillin, amoxicillin		Gram-positives, enterococci, *H. influenzae* *L monocytogenes* *M. catarrhalis* *E. coli*	Activity may be augmented with penicillinase **β-lactamase inhibitors** (e.g., clavulanic acid, sulbactam, and tazobactam)
Extended spectrum, antipseudomonal, β-lactamase sensitive: mezlocillin, piperacillin, carbenicillin, ticarcillin, azlocillin		• Gram-negatives, including ***Pseudomonas*** • Gram-positives, including enterococci (mezlocillin and piperacillin)	—
Cephalosporins			
First generation: cefazolin, cephalexin	**Mechanism:** inhibition of cell wall formation similar to penicillins **Resistance:** same as penicillins	Gram-positives *Proteus mirabilis* *E. coli* *Klebsiella pneumoniae*	• Cross-allergenicity with penicillins occurs in 5% • Anaphylaxis, but not rash, a contraindication in penicillin-sensitive pt. • Disulfiram-like effects (cefotetan)
Second generation: cefotetan, cefoxitin, cefuroxime, cefaclor		Less gram-positive activity and more gram-negative activity than first generation • *B. fragilis* • *H. influenzae* • *M. catarrhalis* • *P. mirabilis* • *E. coli* • *K. pneumoniae* • *Neisseria, Enterobacter*	
Third generation: ceftazidime, cefoperazone, cefotaxime, ceftriaxone		Less gram-positive activity and more gram-negative activity than second generation • *Serratia* sp. • *Borrelia burgdorferi* • *H. influenzae* • *Neisseria* • *Enterobacter* Some have anti-*Pseudomonas* activity	• Most penetrate **blood-brain** barrier (not cefoperazone) • Reserved for serious infections • Disulfiram-like effects (cefoperazone)
Fourth generation: cefepime		More gram-negative activity while retaining first-generation gram-positive activity	More resistant to β- lactamases

(Continued)

► Cell Wall Synthesis Inhibitors *(Cont'd.)*

Class/Example	Mechanism of Action/Resistance	Spectrum	Toxicity/Notes
Carbapenems and Monobactams			
Carbapenems (meropenem, imipenem)	Similar mechanism to penicillins and cephalosporins	Gram-positives, gram-negative rods, anaerobes	• **Nephrotoxic** • GI distress • Rash • CNS toxicity • **Cilastatin administered concurrently** with imipenem increases the drug's half-life and reduces nephrotoxicity • Beta-lactamase resistant
Monobactams (aztreonam)		Gram-negative rods	• GI distress with superinfection, vertigo, headache • Synergistic with aminoglycosides • Beta-lactamase resistant
Non-Beta Lactam Cell Wall Synthesis Inhibitors			
Vancomycin	Binds cell wall precursors (D-ala-D-ala muramyl pentapeptide), preventing polymerization, peptidoglycan elongation	Drug resistant gram-positives, e.g., MRSA sepsis (IV) or *C. difficile* (oral [not absorbed from lumen])	• Chills, fever, ototoxicity, nephrotoxicity • Flushing or **"red man syndrome"** upon rapid infusion • Resistant strains (VRSA, VRE) emerging

Definition of abbreviations: VRE, vancomycin-resistant enterococcus; VRSA, vancomycin-resistant *Staphylococcus aureus.*

► Summary of Mechanisms of Protein Synthesis Inhibition

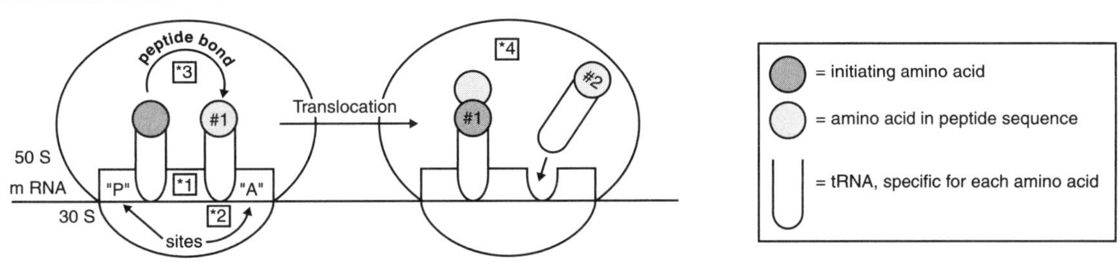

Event	Antibiotics and Binding Sites	Mechanism
1. Formation of initiation complex	Aminoglycosides (30S) Linezolid (50S)	Interfere with initiation codon functions—block association of 50S ribosomal subunit with mRNA-30S (bacteriostatic); misreading of code—incorporation of wrong amino acid (bactericidal)
2. Amino-acid incorporation	Tetracyclines (30S) Dalfopristin/quinupristin (50S)	Block the attachment of aminoacyl tRNA to acceptor site (bacteriostatic)
3. Formation of peptide bond	Chloramphenicol (50S)	Inhibit the activity of peptidyltransferase (bacteriostatic)
4. Translocation	Macrolides and clindamycin (50S)	Inhibit translocation of peptidyl tRNA from acceptor to donor site (bacteriostatic)

► Protein Synthesis Inhibitors

Drug/Class	Site of Inhibition	Spectrum	Mechanisms of Resistance	Toxicities	Notes
Chloramphenicol	50S	Wide spectrum, including: • *H. influenzae* • *N. meningitidis* • *Bacteroides* • *Rickettsia* • *Salmonella*	Plasmid-mediated acetyltransferases that inactivate the drug	• **"Gray baby" syndrome** (↓ glucuronyl transferase in neonates) • **Aplastic anemia**/bone marrow suppression • GI irritation	• Toxicity limits clinical use • Reserved for severe *Salmonella* and bacterial meningitis in β-lactam–sensitive patients
Tetracyclines: • tetracycline • doxycycline • minocycline	30S	Gram ⊕ and Gram ⊖: • *Rickettsia* • *Chlamydia* • *Mycoplasma* • *H. pylori* • *Brucella* • *Vibrio*	Plasmid-mediated efflux pumps and reduced uptake via transport systems	• GI irritation • **Tooth enamel dysplasia** • **Bone growth irregularities** • Hepatotoxicity • **Photosensitivity** • Vestibular toxicity	• **Fanconi syndrome** with expired tetracycline • Oral absorption limited by multivalent cations
Macrolides: • erythromycin, • azithromycin • clarithromycin	50S	Gram ⊕, some Gram ⊖: • *Chlamydia* • *Mycoplasma* • *Ureaplasma* • *Legionella* • *Campylobacter*	Methylation of binding site on 50S; increased efflux from multidrug exporters	• **GI irritation** • Cholestasis • Hepatitis • Skin rashes • ↓ CYP3A4 (except azithromycin)	Useful in atypical pneumonia
Ketolides • Telithromycin	50S	Similar spectrum to macrolides	Many macrolide-resistant strains are susceptible to ketolides	• Severe hepatotoxicity • Visual disturbances • Fainting	Its use is limited because of toxicity
Clindamycin	50S	Narrow spectrum: Gram ⊕, anaerobes	Methylation of binding site on 50S	• GI irritation • Skin rash • ***C. difficile* superinfection**	—
Aminoglycosides: • gentamicin • neomycin • tobramycin • streptomycin	30S	Gram ⊖ rods, aerobic only	Plasmid-mediated **group transferases**	Ototoxicity, nephrotoxicity	Neomycin for bowel prep (stays in bowel lumen)
Oxazolidinones: • linezolid	50S	Gram ⊕ cocci	Resistance rare	• Thrombocytopenia, neutropenia, esp. in immunocompromised • MAO inhibition (dietary and drug restrictions)	No cross-resistance with other protein synthesis inhibitors, so often reserved for resistant infections

▶ Folic Acid Synthesis Inhibitors

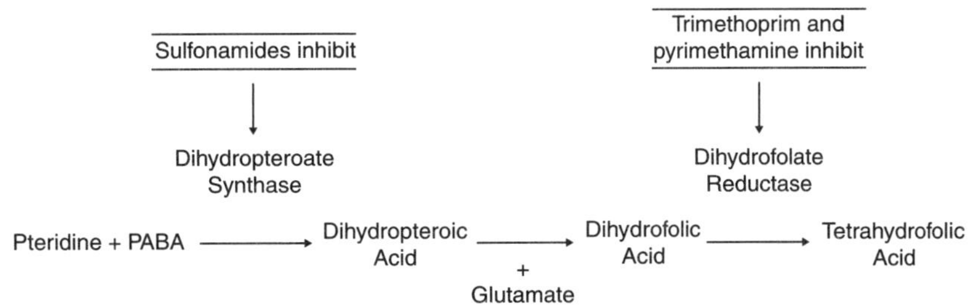

Class/Drug	Mechanism of Action	Spectrum	Mechanism of Resistance	Toxicity	Notes
Sulfonamides	PABA antimetabolite inhibits bacterial dihydropteroate synthase, thus curbing folate synthesis	Gram ⊖, gram ⊕, *Chlamydia*, *Nocardia*	Decreased accumulation of drugs, decreased affinity of drug for **dihydropteroate synthase**	• Hypersensitivity • Hemolytic anemia in G6PD-deficient • Nephrotoxicity • Kernicterus in newborns	Combined with trimethoprim for increased efficacy
Trimethoprim	Inhibits bacterial dihydrofolate reductase, thus inhibiting folate synthesis	*H. influenzae* *M. catarrhalis*	Production of bacterial **dihydrofolate reductase** with decreased affinity for drug	• Megaloblastic anemia • Leukopenia • Granulocytopenia	• Adverse effects may be reduced by concurrent **folinic acid** • Good for UTIs because it is excreted in urine unchanged

▶ DNA Replication Inhibitors

Class/Drug	Mechanism of Action	Spectrum	Mechanism of Resistance	Toxicity	Notes
Fluoroquinolones: • cipro**floxacin** • o**floxacin** • levo**floxacin** • moxi**floxacin**	Interfere with bacterial DNA topoisomerase II and IV (DNA gyrase), resulting in inhibition of DNA synthesis	Gram ⊖ rods, *Neisseria*, occasional gram ⊕	• Decreased intracellular drug concentrations through efflux pumps and altered porins • Alteration of drug's binding site	• **GI distress** • Skin rash • Superinfection • Tendonitis and tendon rupture	Contraindicated in pregnancy due to cartilage formation abnormalities in animal studies

▶ Miscellaneous

Class/Drug	Mechanism of Action	Spectrum	Mechanism of Resistance	Toxicity	Notes
Metronidazole	When reduced, interferes with nucleic acid synthesis (bactericidal)	Anaerobes (except *Actinomyces*)	Rare plasma-mediated resistance	• GI distress • Disulfiram-like reaction with alcohol • Peripheral neuropathy, ataxia	• Strong metallic taste • DOC in pseudomembranous colitis

Definition of abbreviations: DOC, drug of choice; G6PD, glucose-6-phosphate dehydrogenase; PABA, para-aminobenzoic acid; UTI, urinary tract Infection.

Parasites

► Obligate Intracellular Parasites

- Cannot be cultured on inert media. Intracellular organisms (both obligate and facultative) are protected from antibody and complement. Intracellular pathogens tend to elicit cell-mediated immune responses, so end pathologic lesion is frequently a granuloma
- **All rickettsiae, chlamydiae, *Mycobacterium leprae***
- **All viruses**
- ***Plasmodium, Toxoplasma gondii, Babesia***, *Leishmania, Trypanosoma cruzi* (amastigotes in cardiac muscle)

► Facultative Intracellular Parasites

Live inside phagocytic cells in the body, but can be cultured on inert media

- *Francisella tularensis*
- ***Listeria monocytogenes***
- ***Mycobacterium tuberculosis***
- *Brucella* species
- Nontuberculous mycobacteria
- *Salmonella typhi*
- *Legionella pneumophila*
- *Yersinia pestis*
- *Nocardia*
- *Borrelia burgdorferi*
- ***Histoplasma capsulatum***

► Protozoans

Common Name	Amebae	Flagellates	Apicomplexa (Intracellular)
Important genera	***Entamoeba*** *Naegleria* *Acanthamoeba*	LUMINAL (GUT, UG) ***Trichomonas*** ***Giardia*** HEMOFLAGELLATES *Leishmania* *Trypanosoma*	BLOOD/TISSUE ***Plasmodium*** ***Toxoplasma*** *Babesia* INTESTINAL ***Cryptosporidium*** *Isospora*

▶ Protozoan Parasites

Species	Disease/Organs Most Affected	Form/Transmission	Diagnosis
Entamoeba histolytica	• **Amebiasis:** dysentery • **Inverted, flask-shaped lesions** in large intestine with extension to peritoneum and liver, lungs, brain, and heart • Blood and pus in stool • Liver abscesses	• Cysts • Fecal-oral transmission: water, fresh fruits, and vegetables • Travel to tropics	• Trophozoites or cysts (with 4 nuclei) in stool 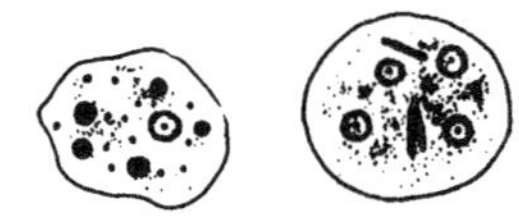 • Nuclei have sharp central karyosome and fine chromatin "spokes" 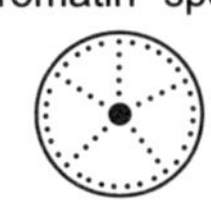 • Serology
Giardia lamblia	**Giardiasis:** Ventral sucking disk attaches to lining of duodenal wall, causing a **fatty**, foul-smelling diarrhea (diarrhea → ***malabsorption*** in duodenum, jejunum)	• Cysts • Fecal (human, beaver, muskrat, etc.), oral transmission: water, food, day care, oral-anal sex • Campers and hikers	• Trophozoites or cysts in stool or fecal antigen test (replaces "string" test) 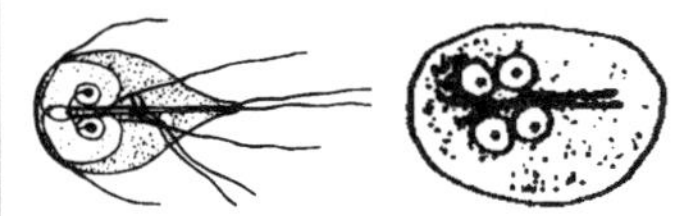 • "Falling leaf" motility
***Cryptosporidium* spp.**	Cryptosporidiosis: transient diarrhea in healthy; severe in immunocompromised hosts	• Cysts • Undercooked meat, water; not killed by chlorination	**Acid fast oocysts** in stool: biopsy shows dots (cysts) in intestinal glands 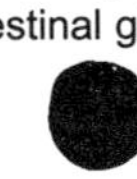
Trichomonas vaginalis (urogenital)	Trichomoniasis: frothy green, unpleasant smelling vaginal discharge, itching, burning vaginitis	• Trophozoites • **Sexual**	Motile trophozoites in methylene blue wet mount 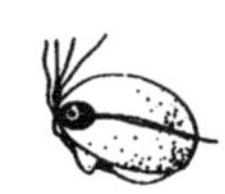

▶ Free-Living Amebae That Occasionally Infect Humans

Species	Disease/Locale	Form/Transmission	Diagnosis
Naegleria	**Primary amebic meningoencephalitis** (PAM): severe prefrontal headache, nausea, high fever, often an altered sense of smell; often fatal	• Free-living amebae picked up while swimming or **diving in very warm fresh water** • Penetrates cribriform plate	• Motile trophozoites in CSF • Culture on plates seeded with gram ⊖ bacteria; amebae will leave trails
Acanthamoeba	**Keratitis; GAE** in immunocompromised patients; insidious onset but progressive to death	• Free-living amebae in contaminated **contact lens solution (airborne cysts)** • Not certain for GAE; inhalation or contact with contaminated soil or water	• Star-shaped cysts on biopsy; rarely seen in CSF • Culture as above

Definition of abbreviations: CSF, cerebrospinal fluid; GAE, granulomatous amaebic encephalitis.

► *Plasmodium* Life Cycle

Each *Plasmodium* has two distinct hosts:

- A vertebrate, such as the human (intermediate host), where asexual phase (schizogony) takes place in the liver and red blood cells
- An arthropod (definitive) host (*Anopheles* mosquito), where gametogony (sexual phase) and sporogony take place

Disease is caused by a variety of mechanisms, including metabolism of hemoglobin and lysis of infected cells, leading to anemia and to agglutination of the infected RBCs. Paroxysms (chills, fever spike, and malarial rigors) occur when the infected RBCs are lysed, liberating a new crop of merozoites.

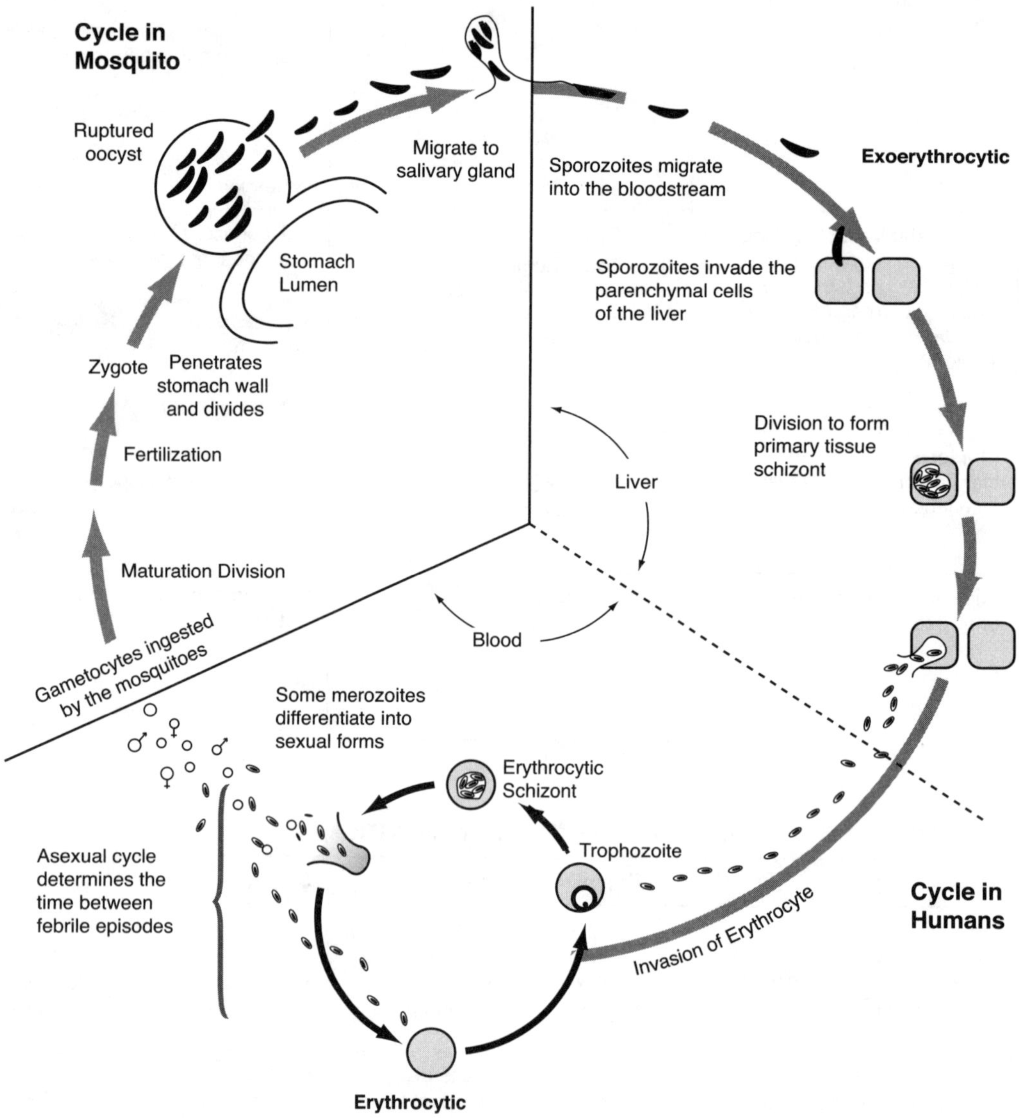

Definition of abbreviation: RBCs, red blood cells.

► *Plasmodium* Species

Species	Disease	Important Features	Blood Smears	Liver Stages
Plasmodium vivax	Benign tertian	48-hour fever spikes	Enlarged host cells; ameboid trophozoites	Persistent hypnozoites Relapse*
Plasmodium ovale	Benign tertian	48-hour fever spikes	Oval, jagged, infected RBCs	Persistent hypnozoites Relapse
Plasmodium malariae	Quartan or malarial	72-hour fever spikes; recrudescence*	Bar and band forms; rosette schizonts	No persistent stage*
Plasmodium falciparum	Malignant tertian	Irregular fever spikes; causes cerebral malaria; most dangerous	Multiple ring forms crescent-shaped gametes	No persistent stage*

Definition of abbreviations: PO, by mouth; RBCs, red blood cells.

*Recrudescence is a recurrence of symptoms from low levels of organisms remaining in **red** cells. Relapse is an exacerbation from liver stages (hypnozoites).

†Use quinine sulfate plus pyrimethamine-sulfadoxine.

► Antimalarial Drugs

1. Suppressive (to avoid infection)
2. Therapeutic (eliminate erythrocytic)
3. Radical cure (eliminate exoerythrocytic)
4. Gametocidal (destruction of gametocytes)

Successful treatment is accomplished with chloroquine followed by primaquine. Chloroquine therapy is suppressive, therapeutic, and gametocidal, whereas primaquine eliminates the exoerythrocytic form.

Chloroquine-Sensitive Malaria	
P. falciparum	Chloroquine
P. malariae	Chloroquine
P. vivax	Chloroquine plus primaquine
P. ovale	Chloroquine plus primaquine
Chloroquine-Resistant Malaria	
Prophylaxis:	mefloquine; backup drugs: doxycycline, atovaquone-proguanil
Treatment:	quinine ± either doxycycline, clindamycin, or pyrimethamine

► Adverse Effects of Antimalarial Drugs

Drug	Side Effects	Contraindications and Cautions
Chloroquine, hydroxychloroquine	GI distress, pruritus, headache, dizziness, hemolysis, retinopathy	Avoid in psoriasis
Mefloquine	NVD, dizziness, syncope, extrasystoles, CNS effects (rare)	Avoid in seizures, psychiatric disorders, and in cardiac conduction defects
Primaquine	GI distress, headache, dizziness, neutropenia, hemolysis	Avoid in pregnancy, G6PD deficiency, and autoimmune disorders
Quinine	GI distress, cinchonism, CNS effects, hemolysis, hematotoxicity	Avoid in pregnancy

Definition of abbreviations: CNS, central nervous system; GI, gastrointestinal; G6PD, glucose-6-phosphate dehydrogenase; NVD, nausea, vomiting, diarrhea.

▶ Hemoflagellates

Hemoflagellates (Trypanosomes and *Leishmania*) infect blood and tissues. They are found in:

- Human blood as **trypomastigotes** with flagellum and an undulating membrane.
- Intracellular as **amastigotes (oval cells having neither the flagellum nor undulating membrane)**. *Leishmania* spp. have only amastigotes in the human.

Trypomastigote	Amastigote
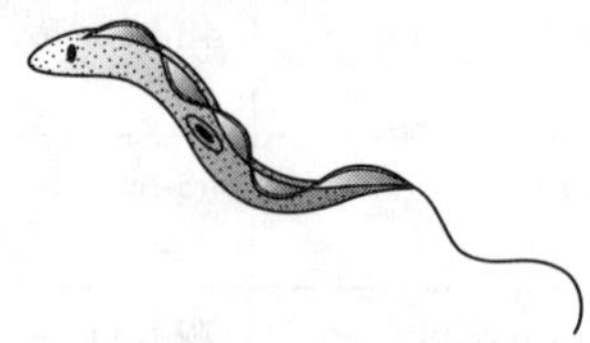	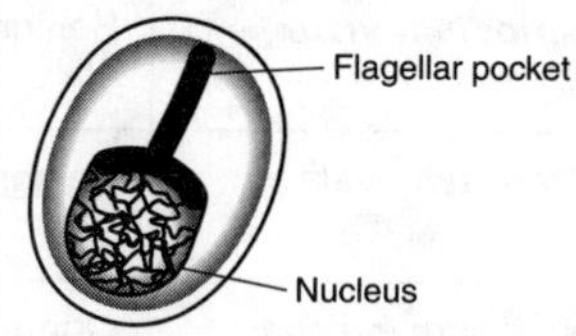

Species	Disease	Vector/Form/ Transmission	Diagnosis
Trypanosoma cruzi*	• **Chagas disease** (American trypanosomiasis) • Latin America • Swelling around eye (**Romaña's sign**): common early sign • Cardiac muscle (dilated cardiomyopathy), megaesophagus, megacolon	**Reduviid bug (kissing or cone bug)** passes trypomastigote **in feces**	Blood films, **trypomastigotes**
Trypanosoma brucei gambiense ***Trypanosoma b. rhodesiense***	• **African sleeping sickness** (African trypanosomiasis) • **Antigenic variation**	Trypomastigote in saliva of **tsetse fly**	• **Trypomastigotes in blood films**, CSF • High immunoglobulin levels in CSF
Leishmania donovani† complex	• **Visceral leishmaniasis** • Kala-azar	**Sandfly** bite	**Amastigotes in macrophages** in bone marrow, liver, spleen
Leishmania (about 15 different species)	Cutaneous leishmaniasis (Oriental sore, etc.)	**Sandfly** bite	**Amastigotes in macrophages** in cutaneous lesions
Leishmania braziliensis complex	Mucocutaneous leishmaniasis	**Sandfly** bite	Same

Definition of abbreviations: CSF, cerebrospinal fluid.

**T. cruzi*: An estimated 0.5 million Americans are infected, creating some risk of transfusion transmission in the United States. In babies, acute infections are often serious and involve the CNS. In older children and adults, mild acute infections may become chronic with the risk of development of cardiomyopathy and heart failure.

† All *Leishmania*: intracellular, sandfly vector, stibogluconate

▶ Miscellaneous Apicomplexa Infecting Blood or Tissues

Species	Disease/Locale of Origin	Transmission	Diagnosis
Babesia (primarily a disease of cattle) Humans: *Babesia microti*, WA1 and MO1 strains	Babesiosis (hemolytic, **malaria-like**) Same range as Lyme: N.E., N. Central, California, and N.W. United States	• ***Ixodes* tick** • Coinfections with ***Borrelia*** and *Ehrlichia*	Giemsa stain of blood smear
Toxoplasma gondii	• Most common parasitic disease • Infections **after birth are most commonly asymptomatic** or mild; may mimic mononucleosis • Produces **severe disease in AIDS** or other immunocompromised **(ring-enhancing lesions in brain)** • **Primary maternal infection during pregnancy may infect fetus:** – **Severe** congenital infections (intracerebral calcifications, chorioretinitis, hydro- or microcephaly, seizures) **if *Toxoplasma* crosses the placenta early** – **Later term congenital infection** may produce **progressive blindness**	**Cat** is **essential definitive** host; many other animals are intermediate hosts Mode: • Raw meat in U.S.; pork is #1 • Contact with cat feces	Serology**:** High IgM or rising IgM acute infection

▶ Major Protozoal Infections and Drugs of Choice

Infection	Drug of Choice	Comments
Amebiasis	Metronidazole	Diloxanide for noninvasive intestinal amebiasis
Giardiasis	Metronidazole or furazolidone	—
Trichomoniasis	Metronidazole	Treat both partners
Toxoplasmosis	Pyrimethamine and sulfadiazine	TMP-SMX is also prophylactic against *Pneumocystis jiroveci* in AIDS
Leishmaniasis	Stibogluconate	—
Trypanosomiasis	• Nifurtimox (Chagas disease) • Arsenicals, pentamidine, suramin (African sleeping sickness)	—

▶ Metazoans: Worms*

Phylum	Flatworms (Platyhelminthes)		Roundworms (Nemathelminthes)
Class (common name)	**Trematodes** (flukes)	**Cestodes** (tapeworms)	**Nematodes**† (roundworms)
Genera	*Fasciola* *Fasciolopsis* *Paragonimus* *Clonorchis* ***Schistosoma***	***Diphyllobothrium*** *Hymenolepis* *Taenia* *Echinococcus*	***Necator*** ***Enterobius*** (W)*uchereria/Brugia* ***Ascaris*** and ***Ancylostoma*** *Toxocara, Trichuris,* and *Trichinella* *Onchocerca* *Dracunculus* Eyeworm (*Loa loa*) *Strongyloides*

*Metazoans also include the Arthropoda, which serve mainly as intermediate hosts (the crustaceans) or as vectors of disease (the Arachnida and Insecta).

†Nematodes **mnemonic** (turn the "W" upside down)

► Trematode (Fluke) Diseases

Trematodes:

- Are commonly called flukes, which are generally flat and fleshy, leaf-shaped worms
- Are hermaphroditic, except for *Schistosoma*, which has separate males and females
- Have complicated life cycles occurring in two or more hosts
- Have operculated eggs (except for *Schistosoma*)
- **The first intermediate hosts are snails**

Organism	Common Name	Acquisition	Progression in Humans	Important Ova
Schistosoma mansoni ***S. japonicum***	**Intestinal schistosomiasis**	Contact with water; skin penetration	Skin penetration (itching) → mature in veins of mesentery → eggs cause granulomas in liver (**portal hypertension** and liver fibrosis in chronic cases)	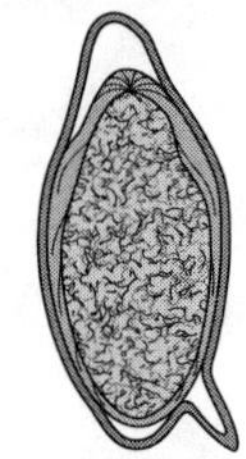 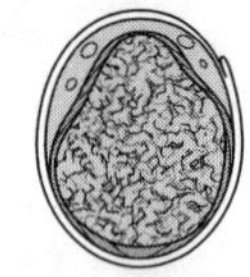
Schistosoma haematobium	**Vesicular schistosomiasis**	Contact with water; skin penetration	Skin penetration (itching) → mature in bladder veins; chronic infection has high association with **bladder carcinoma in Egypt and Africa**	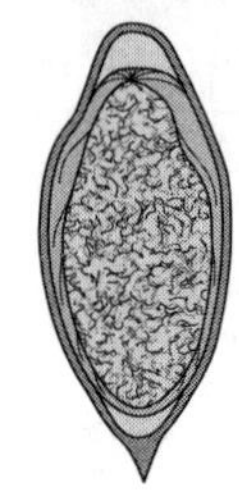
Nonhuman schistosomes	**Swimmer's itch**	Contact with water; skin penetration (Great Lakes)	Penetrate skin, producing **dermatitis** without further development in humans; itching is most intense at 2 to 3 days	—
Clonorchis sinensis	**Chinese liver fluke**	Raw fish ingestion	Inflammation of **biliary tract**, pigmented gallstones, **cholangiocarcinoma**	Operculated eggs
Paragonimus westermani	**Lung fluke**	Raw crabs, crayfish	**Hemoptysis**, secondary bacterial infection of lung	Operculated eggs

► Gastrointestinal Cestodes (Tapeworms)

- Consist of three basic portions: the head or scolex; a "neck" section, which produces the proglottids; and the segments or proglottids, which mature as they move away from the scolex
- Are diagnosed by finding eggs or proglottids in the feces
- Have complex life cycles involving extraintestinal larval forms in intermediate hosts; when humans are intermediate host, these infections are generally more serious than intestinal infections with adult tapeworms

Cestode (Common Name)	Form/ Transmission	Human Host Type	Disease/Organ Involvement/ Symptoms (Sx)	Diagnosis
***Taenia solium* (pork tapeworm)** IH: swine; rare: humans DH: humans,developing and Slavic countries	Water, vegetation, food contaminated with **eggs** Autoinfection	IH	**Cysticercosis**/eggs → larva develop in brain, eye, heart, lung, etc. **Epilepsy** with onset after age 20	Biopsy
	Rare/raw pork containing the **cysticerci** ingested by humans	DH	• **Intestinal tapeworm** • Sx: same as for *Taenia saginata*	**Proglottids** or **eggs** in feces
***Diphyllobothrium latum* (fish tapeworm)** 2 IHs: crustaceans → fish; rare: humans DH: humans/mammals; cool lake regions	Drinking pond water containing copepods (crustaceans) carrying the **larval** forms or frog/snake poultices	IH	**Sparganosis**/larvae penetrate intestinal wall and encyst	Biopsy
	Rare, raw pickled fish containing a **sparganum**	DH	**Intestinal tapeworm** (up to 10 meters)/small intestine, **megaloblastic anemia**	Proglottids or eggs in feces
Echinococcus granulosus IH: herbivores; rare: humans DH: carnivores in sheep-raising areas	Ingestion of eggs	IH	**Hydatid cyst disease**; liver and lung, where cysts containing brood capsules develop	Imaging, serology

Definition of abbreviations: IH, intermediate host; DH, definitive host.

► Roundworms (Nematodes)

Roundworms are transmitted by:

- Ingestion of eggs (*Enterobius*, *Ascaris*, or *Trichuris*)
- Direct invasion of skin by larval forms (*Necator*, *Ancylostoma*, or *Strongyloides*)
- Ingestion of meat containing larvae (*Trichinella*)
- Infection involving insects transmitting the larvae with bites (*Wuchereria*, *Loa loa*, *Mansonella*, *Onchocerca*, and *Dracunculus*)

► Roundworms (Nematodes) Transmitted By Eggs

Species	Disease/Organs Most Affected	Form/Transmission	Diagnosis
Enterobius vermicularis (Most frequent helminth parasite in U.S.)	**Pinworms**, large intestine, perianal itching	• **Eggs**/person to person • **Autoinfection**	• **Scotch tape swab** of perianal area • Ova have flattened side with larvae inside 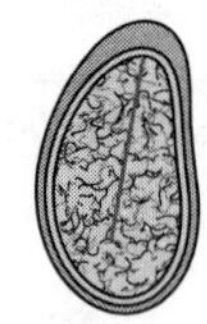
Trichuris trichiura	**Whipworm** cecum, appendicitis, and rectal prolapse	**Eggs** ingested	**Barrel-shaped eggs with bipolar plugs** in stools 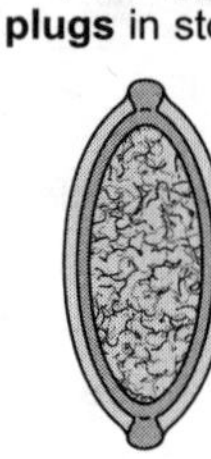
Ascaris lumbricoides (Most common helminth worldwide; largest roundworm)	**Ascariasis** Ingest egg → larvae migrate through lungs (cough) and mature in small intestine; may obstruct intestine or bile duct	**Eggs** ingested	**Bile stained, knobby eggs** 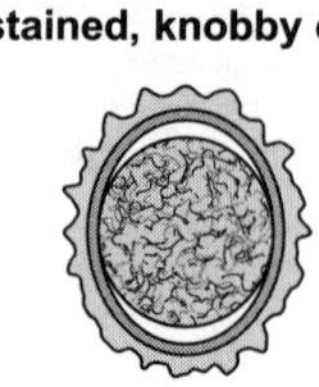 Adult 35 to 40 cm
Toxocara canis or cati (Dog/cat ascarids)	**Visceral larva migrans** Larvae wander aimlessly until they die, cause inflammation	**Eggs** ingested/from handling puppies or from eating dirt in yard (pica)	Clinical findings and serology

▶ Roundworms (Nematodes) Transmitted by Larvae

Species	Disease/Organs	Form/Transmission	Diagnosis
Necator americanus (New World hookworm)	**Hookworm** infection Lung migration → pneumonitis Bloodsucking → anemia	Filariform **larva penetrates intact skin of bare feet**	Fecal larvae (up to 13 mm) and ova: oval, transparent with 2–8 cell-stage visible inside Fecal occult blood may be present
Ancylostoma braziliense ***Ancylostoma caninum*** (dog and cat hookworms)	**Cutaneous larva migrans**/ intense skin itching, snake-like tracks	Filariform larva penetrates intact skin but cannot mature in humans	Usually a presumptive diagnosis; exposure
Strongyloides stercoralis	**Threadworm** strongyloidiasis: *Early:* pneumonitis, abdominal pain, diarrhea *Later:* malabsorption, ulcers, bloody stools	Filariform **larva penetrates intact skin; autoinfection** leads to indefinite infections unless treated	Larvae in stool, serology
Trichinella spiralis	Trichinosis: larvae encyst in muscle → pain	**Viable encysted larvae in meat** are consumed: wildgame meat	Muscle biopsy; clinical findings: **fever, myalgia, splinter hemorrhages, eosinophilia**

▶ Filarial Nematodes

Species	Disease	Transmission/Vector	Diagnosis
Wuchereria bancrofti; Brugia malayi	Elephantiasis	Mosquito	Microfilariae in blood, eosinophilia
Loa loa (African eye worm)	Pruritus, calabar swellings	Chrysops, mango flies	Microfilariae in blood, eosinophilia
Onchocerca volvulus	River blindness, itchy "leopard" rash	Blackflies	Skin snips from calabar swellings
Dracunculus medinensis (Guinea worm, fiery serpent)	Creeping eruptions, ulcerations, rash	Drinking water with infected copepods	Increased IgE; worm eruption from skin

▶ Drugs for Helminthic Infections

Most intestinal nematodes (worms)	• Mebendazole (↓ glucose uptake and ↓ microtubular structure) • Pyrantel pamoate (NM agonist → spastic paralysis)
Most cestodes (tapeworms) and trematodes (flukes)	• Praziquantel (↑ Ca^{2+} influx, ↑ vacuolization)

Virology

▶ Viral Structure and Morphology

The Basic Virion	Viral Structure
DNA or RNA + Structural proteins = Nucleocapsid (naked capsid virus) Nucleocapsid + Host membrane with viral specified glycoproteins* = Enveloped virus *critical for infectiousness of viral progeny	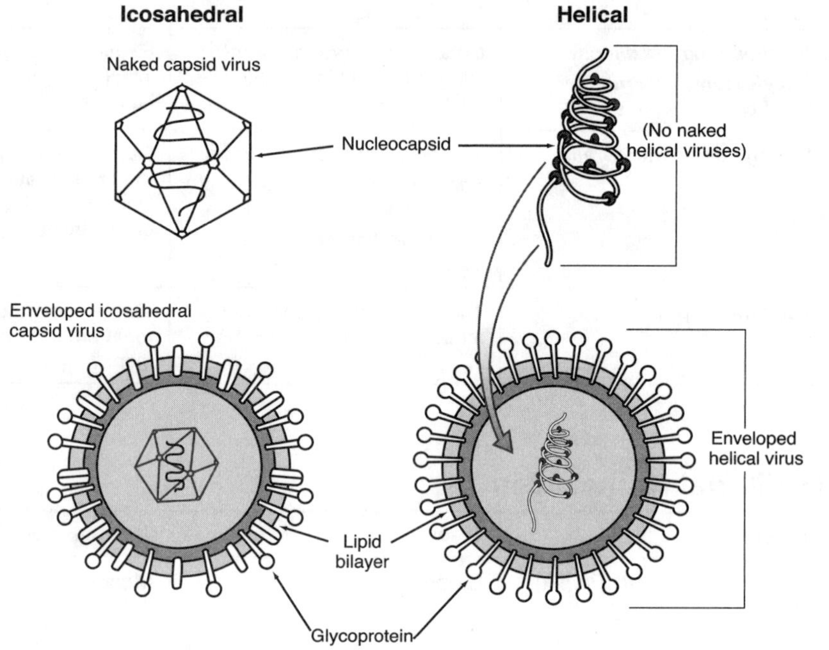

▶ DNA Viruses

General Comments About DNA Viruses:

- All are double-stranded except Parvo
- All are icosahedral except Pox, which are brick-shaped complex
- All replicate in the nucleus except Pox

Virus Family	DNA Type	Polymerase	Envelope	Area of Replication	Major Viruses
Parvovirus	**ssDNA**	No	**Naked**	Nucleus	**B19**
Papilloma	dsDNA Circular	No	**Naked**	Nucleus	Papilloma
Polyomavirus	dsDNA Circular	No	**Naked**	Nucleus	Polyoma
Adenovirus	dsDNA Linear	No	**Naked**	Nucleus	Adenovirus
Hepadnavirus	Partially dsDNA Circular	**Yes**	Enveloped	Nucleus via RNA intermediate	HBV
Herpesvirus	dsDNA Linear	No	Enveloped **Nuclear**	Nucleus, assembled in nucleus	**HSV, VZV, EBV, CMV** HHV-6, HHV-8
Poxvirus	dsDNA Linear	**Yes**	Enveloped	**Cytoplasm**	Variola, vaccinia Molluscum contagiosum

Definition of abbreviations: CMV, cytomegalovirus; ds, double-stranded; EBV, Epstein-Barr virus; HBV, hepatitis B virus; HSV, herpes simplex virus; ss, single-stranded; VZV, varicella-zoster virus.

Note: Viruses are listed from top to bottom in order of increasing size. If you know them in this order, then you can remember that the smallest 4 are naked (wearing more clothing makes you larger).

Mnemonic: Pardon **P**a**P**a **A**s **He H**as **Pox**

Mnemonic: **Naked viruses PAPP** (you need to be naked for a Pap smear)

▶ RNA Viruses

General Comments About RNA Viruses:

- All are single-stranded except Reo
- Most are enveloped. Only naked ones are **H**epe, **C**alici, **P**ico, and **R**eo (**Mnemonic: H**elp! **CPR!**)
- Some are segmented; **Mnemonic: ROBA: R**eo, **O**rthomyxo, **B**unya, and **A**rena – ROBA sounds like ROBOT
- Positive sense RNA = (+)RNA (can be used itself as mRNA)
- Negative sense RNA = (–)RNA
  - Complementary to mRNA
  - Cannot be used as mRNA
  - Requires virion-associated, RNA-dependent RNA polymerase (as part of mature virus)
- Others that carry a polymerase are Reo, Arena, and Retro

▶ Double-Stranded RNA Viruses: Reoviridae

	RNA Structure	Polymerase	Envelope	Shape	Major viruses
Reovirus	• Linear dsRNA • **10–11 segments**	Yes	**Naked**	• Icosahedral • **Double shelled**	• Reovirus • **Rotavirus**

▶ Positive-Sense RNA Viruses

Family	RNA Structure	Polymerase	Envelope	Shape	Area of Replication	Major Viruses
Calicivirus	• ss⊕RNA, linear • Nonsegmented	No	**Naked**	Icosahedral	Cytoplasm	• Norwalk • Norolike
Hepevirus	• ss⊕RNA, linear • Nonsegmented	No	**Naked**	Icosahedral	Cytoplasm	Hepatitis E
Picornavirus	• ss⊕RNA, linear • Nonsegmented	No	**Naked**	Icosahedral	Cytoplasm	• Polio, ECHO, Entero • Rhino, coxsackie • Hepatitis A
Flavivirus	• ss⊕RNA, linear • Nonsegmented	No	Enveloped	Icosahedral	Cytoplasm	Yellow fever, dengue, SLE, hepatitis C, **West Nile virus**
Togavirus	• ss⊕RNA, linear • Nonsegmented	No	Enveloped	Icosahedral	Cytoplasm	Rubella WEE, EEE, VEE
Coronavirus	• ss⊕RNA, linear • Nonsegmented	No	Enveloped	**Helical**	Cytoplasm	Coronaviruses **SARS agent**
Retrovirus	• **Diploid** • ss⊕RNA, linear • Nonsegmented	**RNA-dependent DNA polymerase**	Enveloped	Icosahedral or truncated conical	**Nucleus**	HIV HTLV Sarcoma

Definition of abbreviations: EEE, eastern equine encephalitis; HIV, human immunodeficiency virus; HTLV, human T-cell lymphocytotropic virus; VEE, Venezuelan equine encephalitis; WEE, Western equine encephalitis.

Mnemonic: Again from smallest (top) to largest (bottom): **C**all **H**enry, **P**ico, and **Flo T**o **C**ome **R**ightaway
Mnemonic: Picornaviruses: **PEE Co Rn A** viruses (**P**olio, **E**ntero, **E**cho, **C**oxsackie, **R**hino, Hep **A**)

► Negative-Sense RNA Viruses

Virus	RNA	Polymerase	Envelope	Shape	Area Where Multiplies	Major Viruses
Paramyxovirus	• ss⊖RNA, linear • Nonsegmented	Yes	Yes	Helical	Cytoplasm	Mumps, measles RSV, parainfluenza
Rhabdovirus	• ss⊖RNA, linear • Nonsegmented	Yes	Yes	**Bullet-shaped**, helical	Cytoplasm	Rabies, VSV
Filovirus	• ss⊖RNA, linear • Nonsegmented	Yes	Yes	Helical	Cytoplasm	Marburg, Ebola
Orthomyxovirus	• ss⊖RNA, linear • **8 segments**	Yes	Yes	Helical	**Cytoplasm and nucleus**	Influenza
Bunyavirus	• ss⊖RNA, linear to circular • 3 segments, ambisense	Yes	Yes	Helical	Cytoplasm	California and LaCrosse encephalitis, Hantavirus
Arenavirus	• ss⊖RNA, circular, • 2 segments: 1 ⊖ sense, 1 ambisense	Yes	Yes	Helical	Cytoplasm	Lymphocytic choriomeningitis virus, Lassa fever

Definition of abbreviations: ds, double-stranded; RSV, respiratory syncytial virus; ss, single-stranded; VSV, vesicular stomatitis virus.

Mnemonic (in order of increasing size): **P**ain **R**esults **F**rom **O**ur **B**unions **A**lways (Pain is a negative thing!)
Or, to remind you of life-cycle: **B**ring **A** **P**olymerase **O**r **F**ail **R**eplication

► Viral Genetics

Phenotypic mixing	• Related viruses coinfect cell (virus A and virus B) • Resulting proteins on the surface are a mixture capsid of AB around nucleic acid of either A or B
Phenotypic masking	• Related viruses coinfect cell (virus A and virus B) • Capsid of proteins of virus A form around nucleic acid of B
Complementation	• Two related defective viruses infect the same cell; if they are defective in different genes, viral progeny (still with mutated DNA) will be formed • If they are defective in the same gene, no progeny will be formed • Coinfection of hepatitis B and D is a clinical example of complementation where HBV supplies the needed surface antigen for hepatitis D
Genetic reassortment (genetic shift)	• Two different strains of a segmented RNA virus infect the same cell. • Major new genetic combinations are produced through "shuffling," resulting in stable and dramatic changes • This results in **pandemics** of disease
Genetic drift	• Minor antigenic changes from mutation • Occurs in many viruses, particularly RNA types • Most noted in HIV and influenza
Viral vectors	• Recombinant viruses are produced that have combinations of human replacement genes with the defective viral nucleic acid

▶ Antiviral Agents

As viruses rely on host machinery to produce viral products, selectivity must be achieved by targeting minute differences in viral enzymes. This may be accomplished at any stage in the viral "life cycle" including adsorption, penetration, nucleic acid synthesis, late protein synthesis, protein processing, viral product packaging, and viral release.

Class/Agent	Mechanism of Action	Spectrum/Clinical Applications	Mechanism(s) of Resistance	Toxicity/Notes
ANTIHERPETICS				
Acyclovir Famciclovir Valacyclovir	**Inhibit viral DNA polymerases** Activated by viral thymidine kinase (TK); • Famciclovir is oral prodrug converted to penciclovir • Valacyclovir is oral prodrug of acyclovir • Mechanism of penciclovir same as acyclovir	HSV, VZV (esp. famciclovir, valacyclovir)	Decreased activity or loss of thymidine kinase/DNA polymerase	• Fairly well-tolerated (esp. oral), some nausea/vomiting • IV use associated with seizure, delirium, crystalluria (maintain hydration) • Famciclovir and valacyclovir have much greater oral bioavailability and longer $t_{1/2}$ than acyclovir
Ganciclovir	Similar to acyclovir	CMV (e.g., CMV retinitis), HSV, VZV	Similar to acyclovir	Dose-limiting leukopenia, thrombocytopenia; crystalluria (maintain hydration)
Foscarnet	**Inhibits DNA and RNA polymerases**; does not require activation by kinases (may be effective in acyclovir-, ganciclovir-resistant strains)	• CMV retinitis in AIDS patients • Acyclovir-resistant mucocutaneous HSV in immuno-compromised patients		• Dose limiting nephrotoxicity • Electrolyte imbalance (can lead to seizures)
ANTI-INFLUENZA DRUGS				
Amantadine Rimantadine	Block viral penetration/ uncoating of influenza A virus via interaction with viral M2 protein	• Influenza A (prophylaxis) • Amantadine also used in Parkinson disease to stimulate dopamine release	Current isolates are resistant Resistance due to mutations in M2 protein (no cross resistance to neuraminidase inhibitors)	• Ataxia • Increased seizure activity • Dizziness & hypotension • Rimantadine better tolerated in elderly
Oseltamivir Zanamivir	**Inhibit neuraminidases** made by influenza A and B (enzymes that promote virion release and prevent clumping of these virions), decreasing viral spread	Prophylaxis, but may ↓ duration of flu symptoms by 2-3 days	Mutations to viral neuraminidase	Oseltamivir: oral prodrug; GI discomfort Zanamivir: inhalational drug; cough, bronchospasm in asthmatics
Ribavirin	Inhibits viral RNA synthesis by altering the nucleotide pools and normal messenger RNA formation	Influenza A & B, Parainfluenza, RSV, paramyxoviruses HCV (combined with α–interferon), HIV	Unknown	Dose-dependent hemolytic anemia

(Continued)

► Antiviral Agents *(Cont'd.)*

Class/Agent	Mechanism of Action	Spectrum/Clinical Applications	Mechanism(s) of Resistance	Toxicity/Notes
HIV THERAPY: For details on HIV therapy, see Ch. 4, General Principles of Immunology				
Interferons[†]	Interferons are a class of related proteins with antiviral, antiproliferative, and immune regulating activity. They induce the synthesis of a number of antiviral proteins (e.g., RNAse and a protein kinase) that protect the cell against subsequent challenges by a variety of viruses.	• Hepatitis B & C • Kaposi sarcoma • Leukemias • Malignant melanoma	Anti-interferon antibodies are seen with prolonged use	• Interferons can cause influenza-like symptoms, especially in the first week of therapy • Bone marrow suppression • Profound fatigue, myalgia, weight loss, and increased susceptibility to bacterial infections • Depression is seen in up to 20% of patients

Definition of abbreviations: CMV, cytomegalovirus; HCV, hepatitis C virus; HSV, herpes simplex virus; RSV, respiratory syncytial virus; VZV, varicella zoster virus.

†For more information on interferons and other immunosuppressants, see Chapter 4, General Principles of Immunology

Mycology

► Mycology: Overview

Fungi are eukaryotic organisms with complex carbohydrate cell walls (the reason they frequently calcify in chronic infections) and ergosterol as their major membrane sterol (which is targeted with nystatin and the imidazoles). Morphologic and geographic clues are very important in determining the identity of the organism.

Fungi come in two basic forms	• **Hyphae**—filamentous forms may either have cross walls (septate) or lack them (aseptate) • **Yeasts**—single-celled oval/round forms • **Dimorphic fungi**—may convert from hyphal to yeast forms (key examples: *Histoplasma*, *Blastomyces*, *Coccidioides*, and *Sporothrix*). **Mnemonic: H**eat **C**hanges **B**ody **S**hape: yeast in the heat, mold in the cold
Pseudohyphae	• Hyphae formed by budding off yeasts; formed by ***Candida albicans***; the basis of the germ tube test for diagnosis of invasive *C. albicans*
Spores are used for reproduction and dissemination	• **Conidia**—asexual spores form off hyphae • **Blastoconidia**—asexual spores like buds on yeasts • **Arthroconidia**—asexual spores formed with joints between • **Spherules** with **endospores**—sexual spores in tissues (*Coccidioides*)

► Nonsystemic Fungal Infections

Organism	Disease	Notes
Malassezia furfur 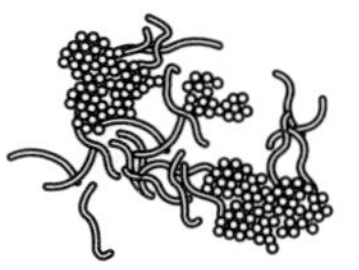	**Pityriasis** or **tinea versicolor**	• Superficial infection of keratinized cells • **Hypopigmented spots on the chest/back** (blotchy suntan) • KOH mount of skin scales: "spaghetti and meatballs," yeast clusters and short, curved septate hyphae • Treatment is topical selenium sulfide; recurs.
	Fungemia	• In **premature infants**
Candida albicans, *Candida* spp.	**Cutaneous or mucocutaneous candidiasis**	• Causes oral thrush and vulvovaginitis in immunocompetent individuals • Source of opportunistic infections in hospitalized and immunocompromised (*see* Opportunistic Mycoses) 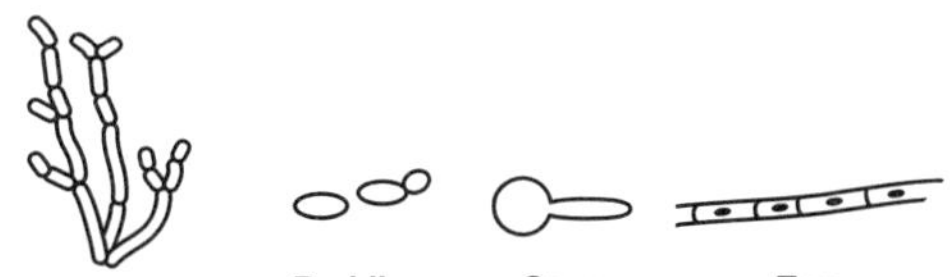
Trichophyton, Microsporum, Epidermophyton 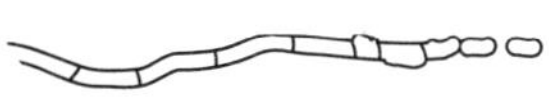	**Tinea** (capitis, barbae, corporis, cruris, pedis)	• Infects **skin, hair, and nails** • **Monomorphic** filamentous fungi • KOH mount shows **arthroconidia, hyphae** • **Pruritic lesions with serpiginous borders and central clearing**
Sporothrix schenckii 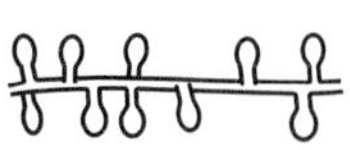 Hyphae with sleeves 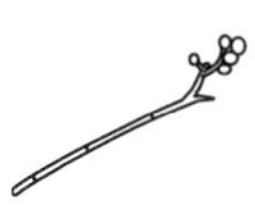 or rosettes of conidia	• **Sporotrichosis (rose gardener's disease)** • **Pulmonary sporotrichosis** (in alcoholics/homeless)	Dimorphic fungus: • Environmental form: hyphae with rosettes and sleeves of conidia • Tissue form: cigar-shaped yeast

► Systemic Fungal Infections

Organism	Disease	Notes
		General Comments
Histoplasma ***Coccidioides*** ***Blastomyces***	• Acute pulmonary (asymptomatic or self-resolving in about 95% of the cases) • Chronic pulmonary • Disseminated infections	**Diagnosis:** • Sputum cytology (calcofluor white staining helpful) • **Sputum cultures** on blood agar and **special fungal media** (inhibitory mold agar, Sabouraud's agar) • **Peripheral blood cultures are useful for *Histoplasma* because it circulates in RES cells**
		Specific Organisms
Histoplasma capsulatum 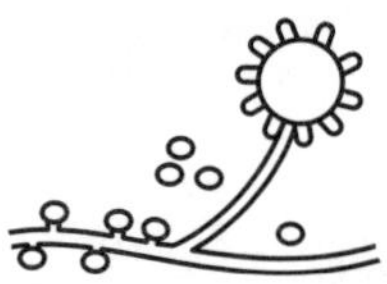	Fungus flu (a pneumonia) • Asymptomatic or flu-like • **Hepatosplenomegaly** may be present • May **disseminate in AIDS patient** 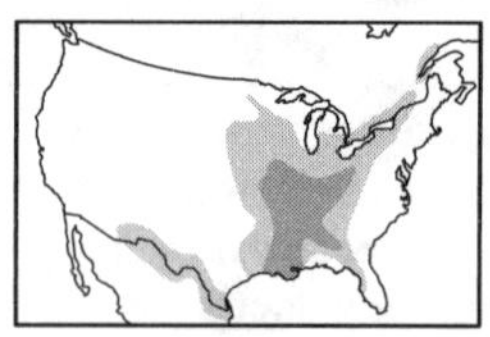	**Dimorphic fungus:** • **Environmental form: hyphae** with **microconidia** and **tuberculate macroconidia** – Endemic region: **Eastern Great Lakes, Ohio, Mississippi,** and **Missouri River beds** – Found in **soil (dust) enriched with bird or bat feces** (caves, chicken coops) • **Tissue form: small intracellular yeasts** with narrow neck on bud; **no capsule** • **Facultative intracellular parasite** found in **RES cells** (tiny; can get 30 or so in a human cell)
Coccidioides immitis 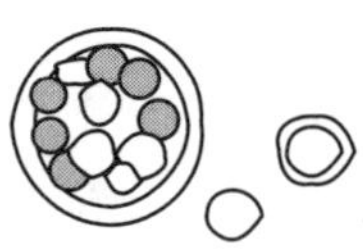 (endospores/spherules) 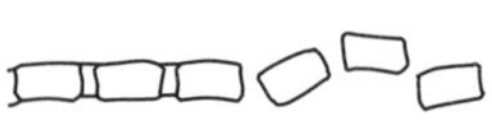 (arthroconidia)	Coccidioidomycosis (San Joaquin Valley fever) 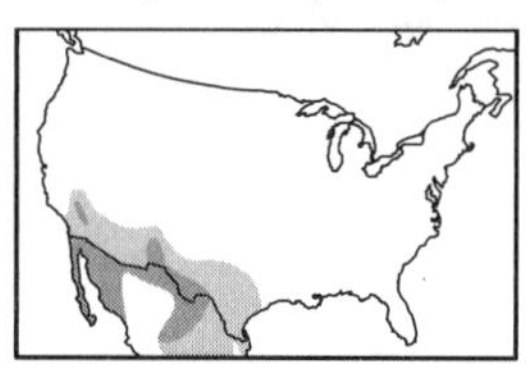	• Dimorphic fungus • Asymptomatic to **self-resolving pneumonia** • Desert bumps (erythema nodosum) • **Pulmonary lesions may calcify** • **May disseminate in AIDS and immunocompromised** (meningitis, mucocutaneous lesions) • Has a tendency to **disseminate in third trimester of pregnancy**
Blastomyces dermatitidis 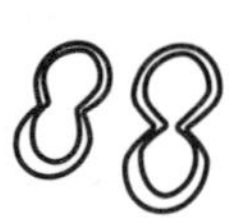	Blastomycosis 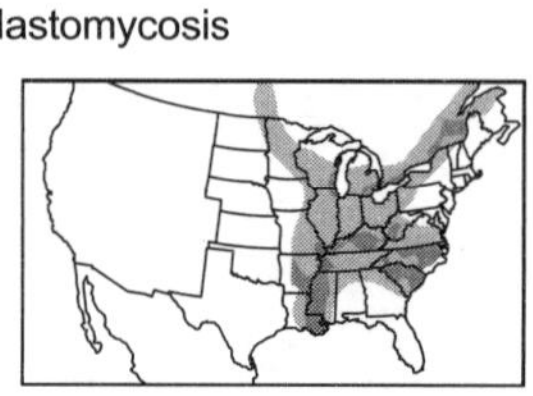	• Dimorphic fungus • Environmental form: hyphae with conidia • Tissue form: broad-based budding yeast • Pulmonary disease • Disseminated disease

Definition of abbreviations: RES, reticuloendothelial.

► Opportunistic Fungi

Aspergillus fumigatus 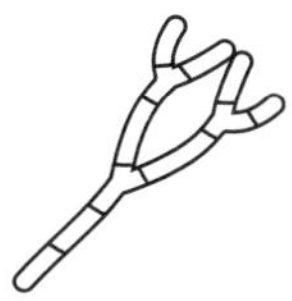	• **Allergic bronchopulmonary aspergillosis**/asthma, cystic fibrosis • **Fungus ball:** free in preformed lung cavities • **Invasive aspergillosis**/severe neutropenia, CGD, CF, burns – Invades tissues, causing infarcts and hemorrhage – Nasal colonization →**pneumonia or meningitis** – **Cellulitis**/in burn patients; may also disseminate	• **Dichotomously branching** • **Generally acute angles** • **Septate** • Compost pits, moldy marijuana • May cause disease in immunocompromised patients **Treatment:** itraconazole, amphotericin B; depends on severity of infection
Candida albicans (and other spp. of *Candida*)	• Involvement of the oral cavity and digestive tract • Septicemia, endocarditis in IV drug abusers • Mucocutaneous candidiasis	**Diagnosis:** • KOH: pseudohyphae, true hyphae, budding yeasts • Septicemia: culture lab identification: biochemical tests/formation of germ tubes **Treatment:** • Topical imidazoles or oral imidazoles; nystatin • Disseminated: amphotericin B or fluconazole
Cryptococcus neoformans 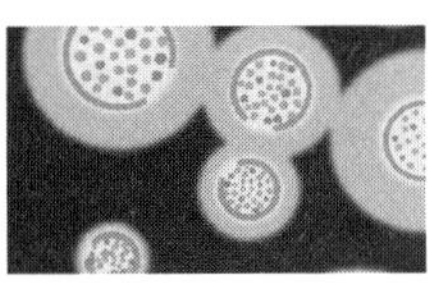	• **Meningitis/Hodgkin, AIDS (the dominant meningitis)** • **Acute pulmonary** (usually asymptomatic)/**pigeon breeders**	• **Encapsulated yeast (monomorphic)** • **Environmental source:** Soil enriched with pigeon droppings • **Diagnosis of meningitis: CSF** – Detect capsular antigen in CSF (by latex particle agglutination or counter immunoelectrophoresis) – **India ink mount** (misses 50%) of CSF sediment to find budding yeasts with capsular "halos" – Cultures (urease ⊕ yeast) • **Treatment:** amphotericin B plus flucytosine until afebrile and culture ⊖, then fluconazole
Mucor, Rhizopus, Absidia (Zygomycophyta family) 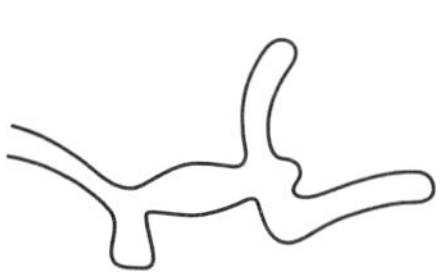	**Rhinocerebral infection** (mucormycosis) caused by *Mucor* (or other Zygomycophyta)	• Nonseptate, filamentous fungi • Characterized by paranasal swelling, necrotic tissues, hemorrhagic exudates from nose and eyes, mental lethargy • Occurs in **ketoacidotic diabetic patients** and **leukemic patients** • These fungi penetrate without respect to anatomic barriers, progressing rapidly from sinuses into brain tissue • **Diagnosis:** KOH of tissue; broad, ribbon-like nonseptate hyphae with about 90° angles on branches • **Treatment:** débride necrotic tissue and start amphotericin B fast; high fatality rate because of rapid growth and invasion
Pneumocystis jiroveci (formerly *carinii*) 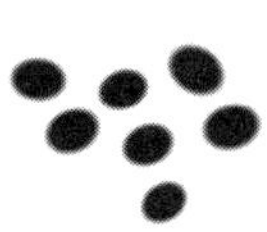	Pneumonia in AIDS patients, malnourished babies, premature neonates, other immunocompromised	• An exudate with foamy or **honeycomb appearance on H & E stain** • **Patchy infiltrative (ground-glass appearance) on x-ray** • **Diagnosis: silver-staining cysts** in bronchial alveolar lavage fluids or biopsy • Treatment: trimethoprim/sulfamethoxazole, pentamidine

Definition of abbreviations: CF, cystic fibrosis; CSF, cerebrospinal fluid; CGD, chronic granulomatous disease; KOH, potassium hydroxide.

► Antifungal Agents

Because fungi are eukaryotic, finding selectively toxic antifungal agents is difficult. Consequently, treating fungal infections poses a clinical challenge, especially in immunocompromised patients. Fungal cell membranes contain **ergosterol**, a sterol not found in mammalian tissue. Thus, this difference provides the basis for most systemically administered antifungal agents.

Class/Agent	Mechanism of Action	Spectrum/Clinical Use	Mechanism(s) of Resistance	Toxicity/Notes
Agents for Systemic Infections				
Amphotericin B	Binds ergosterol, causing formation of artificial pores, thus altering membrane permeability, killing the cell	Widest antifungal spectrum: *Aspergillus* *Coccidioides* *Blastomyces* *Candida albicans* *Cryptococcus* *Histoplasma* *Mucor* *Sporothrix schenckii*	Very uncommon; ↓ or structurally altered ergosterol	• Fever and chills ("cytokine storm") • **Nephrotoxicity** limits dosing (cumulative over lifetime) • Reversible anemia (secondary to ↓ erythropoietin) • Arrhythmias • IV only
Flucytosine	Permease allows entry, deaminated to 5-FU, then converted to 5-FdUMP (thymidylate synthase inhibitor)	Narrow spectrum: *Cryptococcus* *Candida albicans* (systemic)	Rapid if used as a single agent; ↓ activity of fungal permeases and deaminases	• Reversible **bone marrow suppression** • Alopecia • Typically **combined with amphotericin B** or fluconazole
Azoles: fluconazole, itraconazole, voriconazole, ketoconazole	Inhibit synthesis of ergosterol, leading to altered membrane permeability	Varies: *Candida* *Coccidioides* *Cryptococcus* *Aspergillus* *Histoplasma*	↓ sensitivity of target enzymes	• Vomiting and diarrhea • Skin rash • Hepatotoxicity (rare) • **Gynecomastia** • ↓ P450
Echinocandin/ caspofungin	Inhibits synthesis of β-1,2 glycan, a component of fungal cell walls	*Candida* *Aspergillus*	—	• Not very toxic • Headache • Infusion-related reactions
Systemic Agents for Superficial Infections				
Griseofulvin	• Uptake by energy-dependent transport • Interferes with microtubule formation in dermatophytes • May inhibit polymerization of nucleic acids	• Dermatophytes of the hair and scalp • Accumulates in keratin	↓ in transport/uptake	• Confusion and vertigo • Headache • Blurred vision • Nausea/vomiting • ↑ P450 • GI irritation • **Disulfiram-like reaction** with ethanol
Terbinafine	Inhibits squalene epoxidase (for sterol biosynthesis)	Accumulates in keratin, used in onychomycosis		• GI irritation • Rash • Headache • Taste disturbance
Azoles (*see* above)	—	—	—	—
Topical Antifungals†				
Nystatin	Disrupts membrane by binding ergosterol	*Candida*, especially in oral candidiasis (thrush)	Same as amphotericin B	• Contact dermatitis • Stevens-Johnson syndrome

†Topical azoles, such as miconazole and clotrimazole are also widely used.

Embryology

Chapter 5

General Principles of Embyrology

General Principles of Embryology

► Early Embryology

Week 1

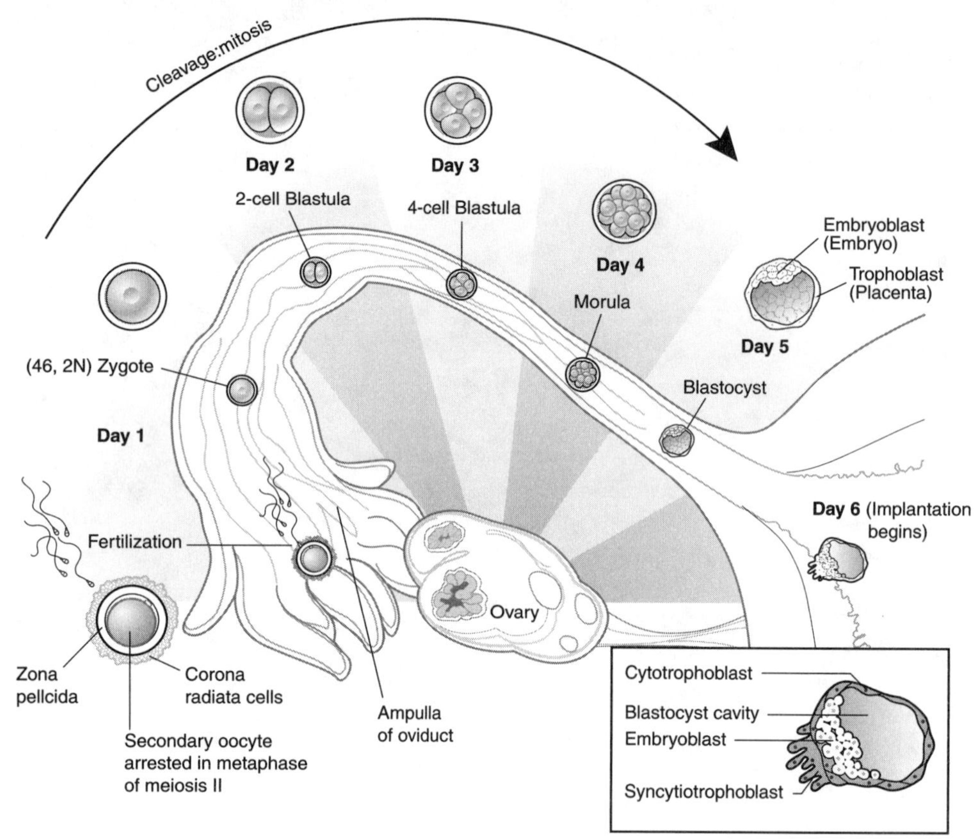

Fertilization occurs in the **ampulla of the uterine tube** when the male and female pronuclei fuse to form a **zygote**. At fertilization, the secondary oocyte rapidly completes meiosis II.

During the first 4 to 5 days of the first week, the zygote undergoes rapid mitotic division (**cleavage**) in the oviduct to form a **blastula**, consisting of increasingly smaller **blastomeres**. This becomes the **morula** (32-cell stage).

A **blastocyst** forms as fluid develops in the morula. The blastocyst consists of an inner cell mass known as the **embryoblast**, and the outer cell mass known as the **trophoblast** becomes the placenta.

At the end of the first week, the trophoblast differentiates into the **cytotrophoblast** and **syncytiotrophoblast** and then implantation begins. Implantation usually occurs in the **posterior superior wall** of the uterus.

Clinical Correlation: Ectopic Pregnancy	
Tubal	The **most common form** of ectopic pregnancy Usually occurs when the blastocyst **implants within the ampulla** of the uterine tube because of delayed transport **Risk factors:** endometriosis, pelvic inflammatory disease (PID), tubular pelvic surgery, or exposure to diethylstilbestrol (DES) **Clinical signs:** abnormal or brisk uterine bleeding, sudden onset of abdominal pain that may be confused with appendicitis, missed menstrual period (e.g., LMP 60 days ago), positive human chorionic gonadotropin (hCG) test, culdocentesis showing intraperitoneal blood, positive sonogram
Abdominal	Most commonly occurs in the **rectouterine pouch** (pouch of Douglas)

(Continued)

▶ Early Embryology *(Cont'd.)*

Week 2

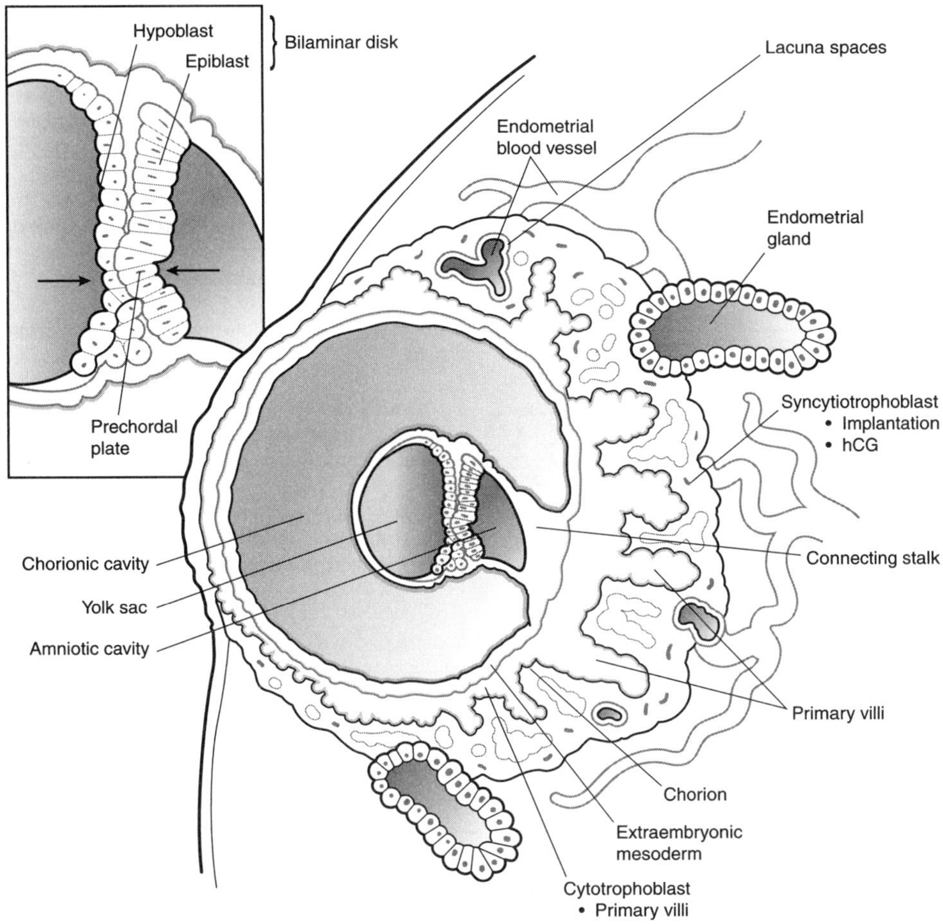

The embryoblast differentiates into the **epiblast** and **hypoblast**, forming a **bilaminar embryonic disk**.

The epiblast forms the **amniotic cavity**, and hypoblast cells migrate from the **primary yolk sac**.

The **prechordal plate**, formed from fusion of epiblast and hypoblast cells, is the site of the future **mouth**.

Extraembryonic mesoderm is derived from the epiblast. **Extraembryonic somatic mesoderm** lines the cytotrophoblast, forms the connecting stalk, and covers the amnion. **Extraembryonic visceral mesoderm** covers the yolk sac.

The connecting stalk suspends the conceptus within the chorionic cavity. The wall of the chorionic cavity is called the **chorion**, consisting of extraembryonic somatic mesoderm, the cytotrophoblast, and the syncytiotrophoblast.

Clinical Correlation

Human chorionic gonadotropin (hCG) is a glycoprotein produced by the syncytiotrophoblast. It stimulates progesterone production by the corpus luteum. hCG can be assayed in maternal blood or urine and is the basis for early pregnancy testing. hCG is detectable throughout pregnancy. **Low hCG** levels may predict a spontaneous abortion or ectopic pregnancy. **High hCG** levels may predict a multiple pregnancy, hydatidiform mole, or gestational trophoblastic disease.

(Continued)

▶ Early Embryology *(Cont'd.)*

Weeks 3 Through 8

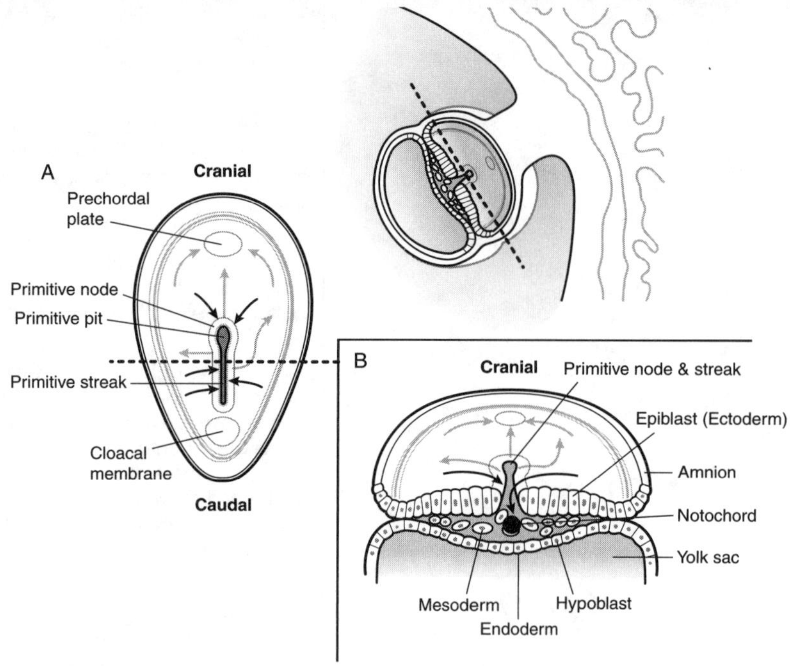

Third week: gastrulation and early development of nervous and cardiovascular systems; corresponds to first missed period

Gastrulation—a process that produces the three primary germ layers: **ectoderm, mesoderm**, and **endoderm**; begins with the formation of the **primitive streak** within the epiblast

Ectoderm → **neuroectoderm** and **neural crest** cells

Mesoderm → **paraxial mesoderm** (35 pairs of somites), **intermediate mesoderm**, and **lateral mesoderm**

All major organ systems begin to develop during the **embryonic period (Weeks 3–8)**. By the end of this period, the embryo begins to look human.

Clinical Correlation

Sacrococcygeal teratoma: a tumor that arises from remnants of the primitive streak; often contains various types of tissue (bone, nerve, hair, etc.).

Chordoma: a tumor that arises from remnants of the notochord, found either intracranially or in the sacral region

Caudal dysplasia (sirenomelia): a constellation of syndromes ranging from minor lesions of the lower vertebrae to complete fusion of lower limbs. Occurs as a result of abnormal gastrulation, in which migration of mesoderm is disturbed. Associated with VATER (vertebral defects, anal atresia, tracheoesophageal fistula, and renal defects) or VACTERL (vertebral defects, anal atresia, cardiovascular defects, tracheoesophageal fistula, renal defects, and upper limb defects)

Hydatidiform mole: results from the partial or complete replacement of the trophoblast by dilated villi

- **In a complete mole, there is no embryo;** a haploid sperm fertilizes a blighted ovum and reduplicates so that the karyotype is 46,XX, with all chromosomes of paternal origin. In a **partial mole**, there is a haploid set of maternal chromosomes and usually two sets of paternal chromosomes so that the typical karyotype is 69,XXY.
- **Molar pregnancies have high levels of hCG, and 20% develop into a malignant trophoblastic disease, including choriocarcinoma.**

▶ Germ-Layer Derivatives

Ectoderm	
Surface ectoderm	Epidermis, hair, nails, inner and external ear, tooth enamel, lens of eye, anterior pituitary (from Rathke pouch), major salivary, sweat, and mammary glands; epithelial lining of nasal and oral cavities and ear
Neuroectoderm	CNS (brain and spinal cord), retina and optic nerve, pineal gland, neurohypophysis, astrocytes, oligodendrocytes, ependymal cells
Neural crest	Adrenal medulla, ganglia (sensory, autonomic), melanocytes, Schwann cells, meninges (pia, arachnoid), pharyngeal arch cartilage, bones of the skull, odontoblasts, parafollicular (C) cells, laryngeal cartilage, aorticopulmonary septum, endocardial cushions (abnormal development can lead to many congenital defects)
Mesoderm	Muscle (smooth, cardiac, skeletal), connective tissue, serous membranes, bone and cartilage, blood and blood vessels, lymphatics, cardiovascular organs, adrenal cortex, gonads and internal reproductive organs, spleen, kidney and ureter, dura mater
Endoderm	Epithelial parts: GI tract, tonsils, thymus, pharynx, larynx, trachea, bronchi, lungs, urinary bladder, urethra, tympanic cavity, auditory tube and other pharyngeal pouches Parenchyma: liver, pancreas, tonsils, thyroid, parathyroids, glands of GI tract, submandibular and sublingual glands

▶ Placenta

The placenta permits exchange of nutrients and waste products between maternal and fetal circulations.

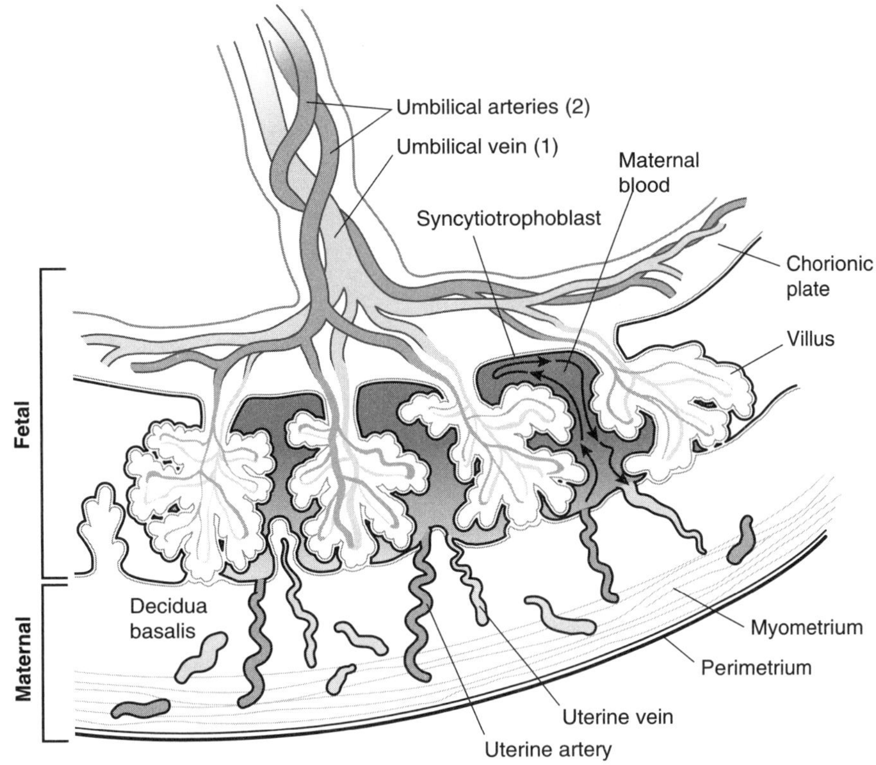

Fetal component	Chorionic plate and villi **Syncytiotrophoblast:** outer layer of chorionic villi; secretes hCG **Cytotrophoblast:** inner layer of chorionic villi
Maternal component	**Decidua basalis:** Maternal blood vessels from the decidua conduct blood into the intervillous spaces of the placenta, where floating villi are present
Placental barrier	The syncytiotrophoblast, cytotrophoblast, basement membrane, fetal capillary endothelium separate the maternal and fetal blood
Umbilical cord	1 **umbilical vein** supplies **oxygenated** blood from the placenta to the fetus 2 **umbilical arteries** carries **deoxygenated** blood back from the fetus to the placenta **Urachus**: Removes nitrogenous waste from the fetal bladder

▶ Twinning

The type of twinning depends on the point in time in which cleavage occurs. If the twinning occurs very early on (before the chorion forms), two separate chorions will form (dichorionic). All other possible types of twins are monochorionic because the chorion has already formed. Fraternal twins are **dizygotic** and identical twins are **monozygotic**.

Placental morphology	Time of cleavage	Type of twin
Dichorionic diamniotic	Very early (Days 1–3)	Fraternal or identical
Monochorionic diamniotic	Early (Days 4–8)	Identical
Monochorionic monoamniotic	Later (Days 8–13): identical Even later (Days 13–15): conjoined	Identical, conjoined

► Teratogens

ACE inhibitors; ARBS	Renal damage
Aminoglycosides	CN VIII toxicity
Androgens	Masculinization of female fetus
Anticonvulsants	Neural tube defects (carbamazepine, valproic acid), phenytoin (fetal hydantoin syndrome); multiple congenital defects
Antithyroid drugs	Congenital goiter, hypothyroidism
Diethylstilbestrol (DES)	Vaginal clear cell adenocarcinoma; vaginal adenosis
Ethanol	Fetal alcohol syndrome (e.g., growth retardation, facial abnormalities, microcephaly, cardiac defects)
Folate antagonists	Multiple congenital anomalies
Lithium	Ebstein anomaly
Radiation	Multiple abnormalities
Tetracyclines	Discoloration of teeth
Thalidomide	Phocomelia (limb reduction defects)
Warfarin	Bone and cartilage abnormalities, hemorrhage, etc.
Vitamin A excess; vitamin A derivatives	Multiple abnormalities, e.g., cleft palate, cardiac abnormalities, mental retardation

Physiology

Chapter 6

► Physiologic Terminology

Equilibrium	Equilibrium occurs when the balance of opposing forces has reached the **lowest free energy state**, and as a result, a given variable has reached a constant value.
Steady state	Steady state is a condition in which a variable is maintained within narrow limits by regulating an opposing activity. This process requires energy.
Negative feedback	This is a common system that acts to oppose changes in the internal environment. Negative feedback systems promote stability and act to restore steady-state function after a perturbation.
Positive feedback	This is a less common system (also called a vicious cycle) that acts to magnify a change in the internal environment; the initial change in a system is increased as a result of feedback activity. In a viable organism, any positive feedback system is ultimately overridden by one or more negative feedback systems.

Negative Feedback Example

Follicular Phase

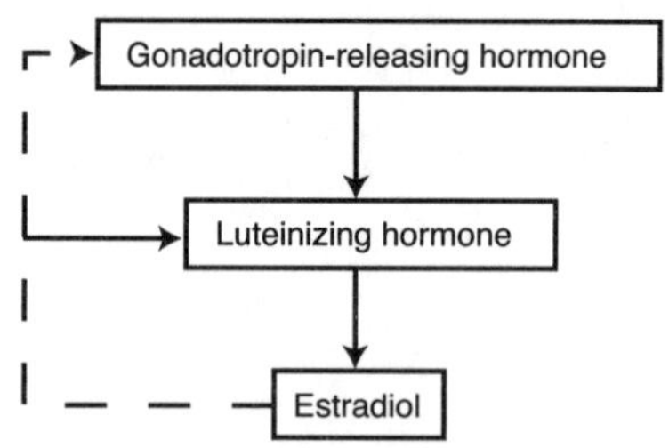

Positive Feedback Example

Pre-ovulatory Phase

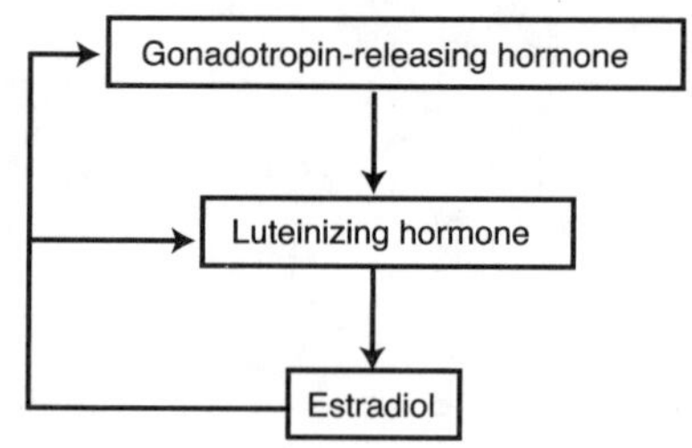

The figures above show the negative feedback relationship between estrogens and the gonadotropins that dominates during the follicular phase, which transforms into a positive feedback relationship, producing the LH surge prior to ovulation. Solid arrows show direct relationships (stimulation) and dashed arrows show inverse relationships (inhibition).

► Transport

Type of Transport	Energy Source	Example	Other Characteristics	Clinical Correlation
Simple diffusion	Passive	Pulmonary gases	—	Pulmonary edema decreases diffusion
Carrier-mediated or facilitated diffusion	Passive	Glucose uptake by muscle	• Insulin controls carrier population • Chemical specificity	Insulin-dependent glucose uptake impaired in diabetes mellitus
Primary active transport	Direct use of ATP	Na^+/K^+-ATPase Ca^{2+}-ATPase	Antiport (countertransport) Regulates cellular Ca^{2+}	Inhibition by cardiac glycosides Deficiency causes neuromuscular disorders
Secondary active transport	Electrochemical gradient for sodium is most common driving force	Na^+-glucose in kidney Na^+-H^+ exchange	Symport (cotransport) Antiport (countertransport)	Osmotic diuresis results when transporters saturated Renal tubular acidosis

Key Points

- Passive processes are directly related to concentration gradients.
- Active processes create or increase a concentration gradient and thus depend upon metabolic energy.
- Both carrier-mediated facilitated diffusion and active transport can be saturated; maximum transport rate depends on population and activity of transport molecules.
- Primary active transport proteins have an ATPase as part of their structure.
- Most secondary active transport depends upon the electrochemical gradient of sodium ions, which in turn depends on the activity of the primary active transporter, sodium-potassium ATPase.

▶ Diffusion Kinetics

Simple diffusion

The rate is estimated by **Fick's law of diffusion**: $J = -DA(\Delta C/\Delta X)$

J = net flux, D = diffusion coefficient, A = surface area, ΔC = concentration or pressure gradient, ΔX = diffusion distance

Changes in surface area or diffusion distance are most important in disease states (e.g., the decrease in surface area caused by destruction of alveoli in emphysema or the decreased diffusion of oxygen during pulmonary edema related to increased diffusion distance).

Carrier-mediated transport

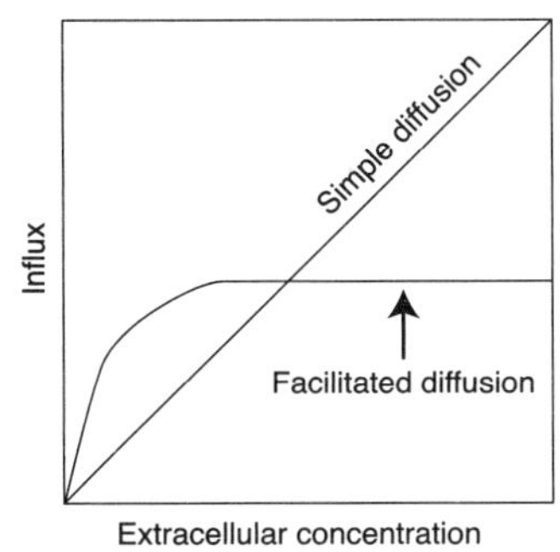

Assumption: intracellular concentration is negligible

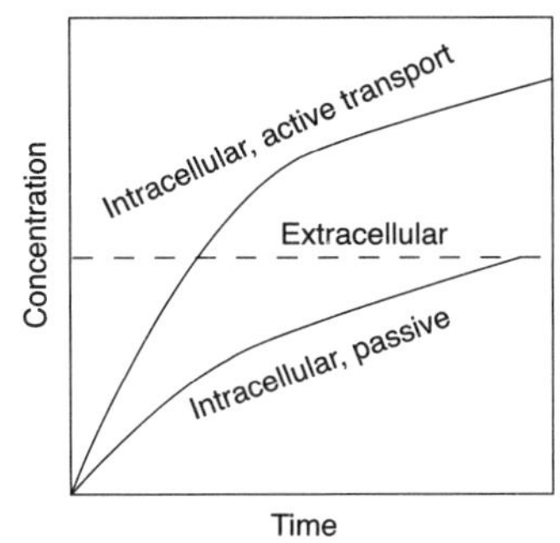

Assumption: extracellular concentration does not change

Facilitated diffusion increases transport rate above that capable with **simple diffusion**, but has saturation kinetics (*left*).

Active transport can produce a concentration gradient, and **passive processes** will lead to an equilibrium state (*right*).

▶ Fluid Volume Compartments and Distribution

	% of Body Weight	Fraction of TBW	Markers Used to Measure Volume	Primary Cations	Primary Anions
Total body water (TBW)	60	1.0	Tritiated H_2O D_2O, antipyrine	—	—
Intracellular fluid volume (ICF)	40	⅔	TBW – ECF*	K^+	Organic phosphates; protein
Extracellular fluid volume (ECF)	20	⅓	Inulin Mannitol	Na^+	Cl^- HCO_3^-
Plasma	5	1/12 (¼ of ECF)	RISA Evans blue	Na^+	Cl^- HCO_3^- Plasma proteins
Interstitial fluid	15	¼ (¾ of ECF)	ECF-plasma volume*	Na^+	Cl^- HCO_3^-

Principles of Fluid Distribution

1. Osmolarity of the ICF and ECF are equal.
2. Intracellular volume changes only when extracellular osmolarity changes.
3. All substances enter or leave the body by passing through the extracellular compartment.

Measurement of Fluid Volumes

$$\text{Volume} = \frac{\text{Mass}}{\text{Concentration}}$$

Example: 100 mg of inulin is infused. After equilibration, its concentration = 0.01 mg/mL. What is patient's ECF volume?

Answer: ECF = 100 mg/0.01 mg/mL = 10,000 mL, or 10 L

Osmolarity and Mass

1. Plasma osmolarity in mOsm/L can be quickly estimated as twice the plasma sodium concentration in mmol/L. More rigorously, plasma osmolarity (mOsm/L) = (2 × serum sodium [mEq/L]) + (BUN [mg/dL]/2.8) + (glucose [mg/dL]/18).
2. Mass of solutes in the TBW, ICF, or ECF in mOsm is calculated by the relevant volume multiplied by the osmolarity.

Definition of abbreviation: RISA, radio-iodinated serum albumin.
*Indirect measurement

► Summary of Volume and Osmolarity Changes of Body Fluids

Body osmolarity and intracellular and extracellular fluid volumes change in clinically relevant situations. The **Darrow-Yannet diagram** *(right)* represents this information. The *y*-axis is solute concentration or osmolarity. The *x*-axis is the volume of ICF and ECF. The *solid line* represents the control state, and the *dashed line* represents changes in volume or osmolarity. In this example, osmolarity ↓, ICF volume ↑, and ECF volume ↓.

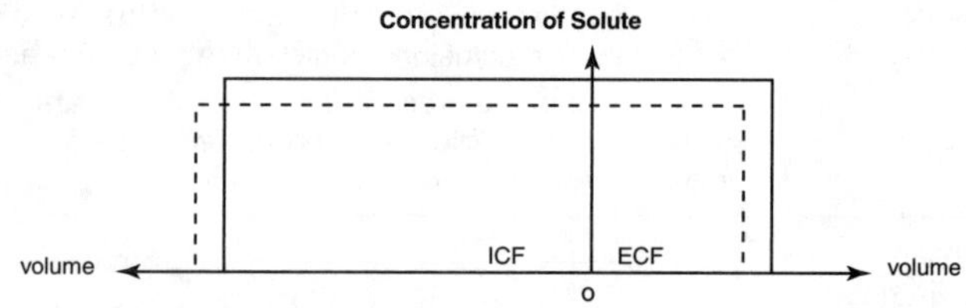

Type	Examples	ECF Volume	Body Osmolarity	ICF Volume	D-Y Diagram
Isosmotic volume contraction (loss of isotonic fluid)	Diarrhea, hemorrhage, vomiting	↓	No change	No change	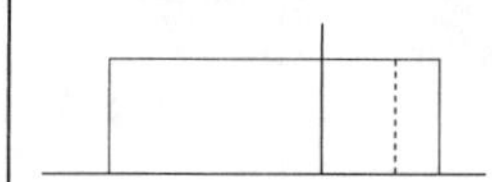
Isosmotic volume expansion (gain of isotonic fluid)	Isotonic saline infusion	↑	No change	No change	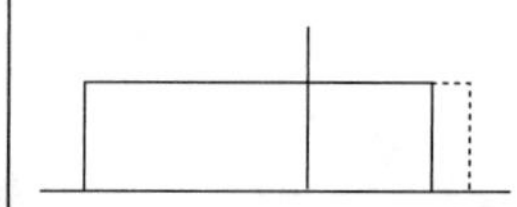
Hyperosmotic volume contraction (loss of water)	Dehydration, diabetes insipidus	↓	↑	↓	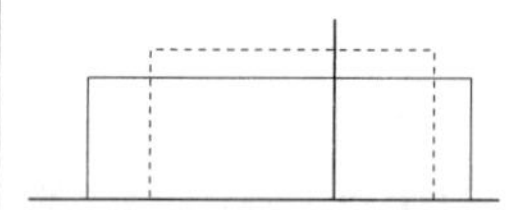
Hyperosmotic volume expansion (gain of NaCl)	Excessive NaCl intake, hypertonic mannitol, chronic aldosterone excess	↑	↑	↓	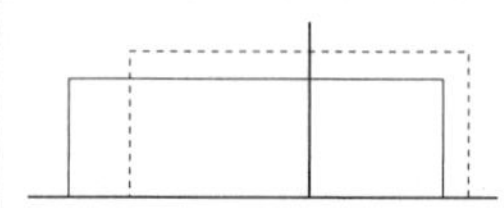
Hyposmotic volume contraction (loss of NaCl)	Adrenal insufficiency	↓	↓	↑	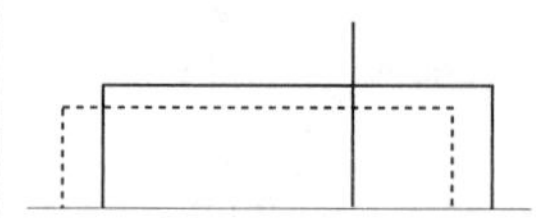
Hyposmotic volume expansion (gain of water)	SIADH, water intoxication	↑	↓	↑	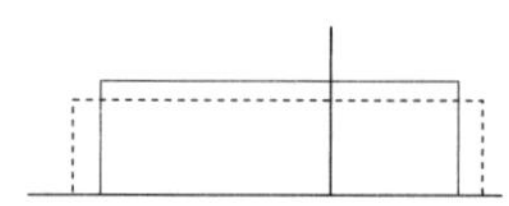

Definiton of abbreviation: SIADH, syndrome of inappropriate antidiuretic hormone.

▶ Membrane Potentials

Equilibrium potential

Amount of voltage needed to balance the chemical force due to its concentration gradient

The **Nernst equation** can determine this. For a monovalent cation:

$$E_x = \frac{60\text{ mV}}{Z}\log_{10}\frac{[X]_o}{[X]_i}$$; E_x = equilibrium potential, [X] = ion concentration (out and in), Z = charge

(Na^+ = 1, Cl^- = –1, Ca^{2+} = 2)

Resting membrane (RM) potential

- RM is the potential difference across a cell membrane in millivolts (mV); –70 mV is typical.
- RM occurs because of an **unequal distribution of ions** between the ICF and ECF and the **selective permeability** of the membrane to ions. **Proteins (anions)** in cells that do not diffuse help establish the electrical potential across the membrane.
- The relative effect of an ion on the membrane potential is in proportion to the conductance or permeability of that ion. The **greater the conductance**, the closer the membrane will approach the **equilibrium potential** of that ion.
- The resting potential of cells is negative inside. **Hyperpolarization** occurs when the membrane potential becomes more negative. **Depolarization** occurs when the membrane potential becomes less negative or even positive.

Chord conductance equation

$$E_m = (g_K/\Sigma g \times E_K) + (g_{Na}/\Sigma g \times E_{Na}) + (g_{Cl}/\Sigma g \times E_{Cl})$$

E_m = membrane potential in mV; g = conductance of individual ion; Σg = total conductance of cell membrane; E = equilibrium potential of individual ion from Nernst equation

- Used to calculate membrane potential; useful to evaluate effects of ion conductance and concentrations; explains action potential, synaptic potentials, and electrolyte disorders

Properties of ions in a typical neuron

Ion	Extracellular (mM)	Intracellular (mM)	Equilibrium Potential (mV)	Conductance
Na^+	150.0	15.0	+60	Very low
K^+	5.5	150.0	–90	High
Cl^-	125.0	9.0	–70	High

- Because potassium and chloride have a high conductance, their equilibrium potentials dominate the membrane potential, so the inside of the cell is negative.
- Changes in EC K^+ can produce large changes in the membrane potential:

↑ EC K^+ → depolarization; ↓ EC K^+ → hyperpolarization.

- Changes in EC Na^+ have little effect on membrane potential, but an increase in Na^+ conductance → depolarization.

Definition of abbreviation: EC, extracellular.

► Action Potential

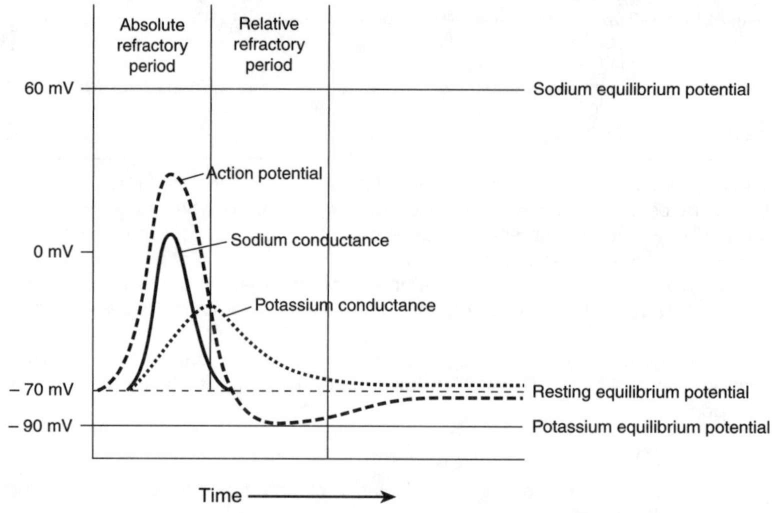

The action potentials (AP) of excitable cells involve the opening and closing of voltage-gated channels for sodium, potassium, and in some cells, calcium. The figure above shows a neuronal AP. The opening of a channel increases conductance.
Steps are shown below.

- Inward currents depolarize the membrane potential to **threshold**.
- **Voltage-gated Na^+ channels open**, causing an **inward Na^+ current**. The membrane potential approaches the Na^+ equilibrium potential. These channels can be blocked by **tetrodotoxin**.
- These Na^+ channels close rapidly **(inactivation)**, even though the membrane is still depolarized.
- Depolarization slowly opens K^+ channels, **increasing K^+ conductance (outward current)**, leading to **repolarization**.
- **Absolute refractory period:** An AP cannot be elicited because Na^+ channels are closed.
- **Relative refractory period:** Only a greater than normal stimulus can produce an AP because the K^+ conductance is still higher than at rest.
- The **Na^+-K^+ pump** restores ion concentrations. It is **electrogenic** (3 Na^+ pumped out for every 2 K^+ pumped in).

Clinical Correlations

Calcium has a low resting conductance and does not contribute to the resting potential. It has a very positive equilibrium potential, so when conductance increases (e.g., cardiac and smooth muscle cells), **depolarization** occurs. Calcium concentration affects the action potentials and force of contraction of **cardiac and smooth muscle**.

Hypercalcemia stabilizes excitable membranes, leading to flaccid paralysis of skeletal muscle. **Hypocalcemia** destabilizes membranes, leading to spontaneous action potentials and spasms.

Abnormal increases and decreases of **extracellular potassium** have severe consequences for cardiac conduction and rhythm.

Renal and gastrointestinal disorders are likely to cause abnormalities of electrolytes and alteration of resting potentials and action potentials.

Pathology

Chapter 7

Cellular Injury and Adaptation

Changing conditions in the cell's environment can produce changes from adaptation to injury or even cell death. The cellular response to injury depends on the *type, duration*, and *severity* of injury, the *type of cell* injured, *metabolic state*, and *ability to adapt*.

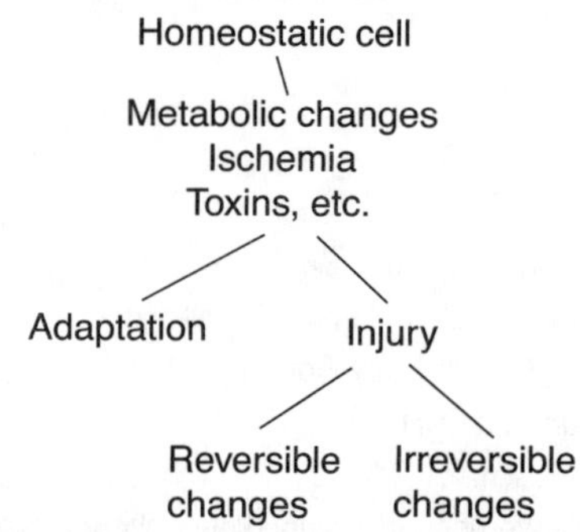

Causes	Examples
Hypoxia (most common)	• Ischemia (e.g., arteriosclerosis, thromboembolus) • Cardiopulmonary failure • Severe anemia
Infections	Viruses, bacteria, parasites, rickettsiae, fungi, prions
Immunologic reactions	• Hypersensitivity reactions • Autoimmune
Congenital/metabolic disorders	• Inborn errors of metabolism (e.g., phenylketonuria, galactosemia, glycogen storage diseases)
Chemical injury	• Drugs (e.g., therapeutic, drugs of abuse) • Poisons • Pollution • Occupational exposure (e.g., CCl_4, CO, asbestos)
Physical injury	Trauma, burns, frostbite, radiation
Nutritional or vitamin imbalance	• Inadequate calorie/protein intake (e.g., marasmus, kwashiorkor, anorexia nervosa) • Excess caloric intake (e.g., obesity, atherosclerosis) • Vitamin deficiencies • Hypervitaminosis

Important Mechanisms of Cell Injury

- Oxygen-free radicals (superoxide [$O_2^{\cdot -}$], hydroxyl radical [OH·], hydrogen peroxide [H_2O_2]) damage DNA, proteins, lipid membranes, and circulating lipids (LDL) by peroxidation
- Decreased oxidative phosphorylation
- ATP depletion
- Increased cell-membrane permeability
- Influx of calcium—activates a wide spectrum of enzymes: proteases, ATPases, phospholipases, endonucleases
- Mitochondrial dysfunction, formation of mitochondrial permeability transition (MPT) channels
- Release of cytochrome c is a trigger for apoptosis

Protective Factors Against Free Radicals

1. *Antioxidants*—vitamins A, E, and C
2. *Superoxide dismutase*—superoxide → hydrogen peroxide
3. *Glutathione peroxidase*—hydroxyl ions or hydrogen peroxide → water
4. *Catalase*—hydrogen peroxide → oxygen and water

▶ Direct and Indirect Results of Reversible Cell Injury

Direct Result	Consequences	Pathophysiologic Correlates
Decreased synthesis of ATP by oxidative phosphorylation	Decreased function of Na^+/K^+ ATPase → influx of Na^+ and water, efflux of K^+, and swelling of the ER	Cellular swelling (hydropic swelling), swelling of endoplasmic reticulum, membrane blebs, myelin figures
Increased glycolysis → glycogen depletion	Increased lactic acid production → decreased intracellular pH	Tissue acidosis
Ribosomes detach from rough ER	Decreased protein synthesis	Lipid deposition (fatty change)

▶ As the Degree of Cellular Injury Worsens . . .

Severe plasma membrane damage	Massive influx of calcium, efflux of intracellular enzymes and proteins into the circulation	Markers of cellular damage detectable in serum (LDH, CK, ALT, AST, troponin, etc.)
Calcium influx into mitochondria	Irreparable damage to oxidative phosphorylation	Mitochondrial densities
Lysosomal contents leak out	Lysosomal hydrolases are activated intracellularly	Autolysis, heterolysis, nuclear changes (pyknosis, karyorrhexis, karyolysis)

▶ Irreversible Injury and Cell Death

Morphologic Pattern	Characteristics
Coagulative necrosis	**Most common** (e.g., heart, liver, kidney) Proteins denatured, nucleus is lost, but cellular shape is maintained
Liquefactive necrosis	**Abscesses**, **brain infarcts**, pancreatic necrosis Cellular destruction by hydrolytic enzymes
Caseous necrosis	Seen in **tuberculosis** Combination of coagulation and liquefaction necrosis → soft, friable, and "cottage-cheese–like" appearance
Fat necrosis	Caused by the action of lipases on fatty tissue (e.g., with **pancreatic damage**) Chalky white appearance
Fibrinoid necrosis	Eosinophilic homogeneous appearance—resembles fibrin
Gangrenous necrosis	*Common sites:* lower limbs, gallbladder, GI tract, and testes Dry gangrene—coagulative necrosis Wet gangrene—liquefactive necrosis
Apoptosis	A specialized form of **programmed cell death**, an active process under genetic control Often affects only single cells or small groups of cells Mediated by a cascade of **caspases** (digest nuclear and cytoskeletal proteins and activate endonucleases)

Myocardial ischemia is a good example of cellular injury and death.

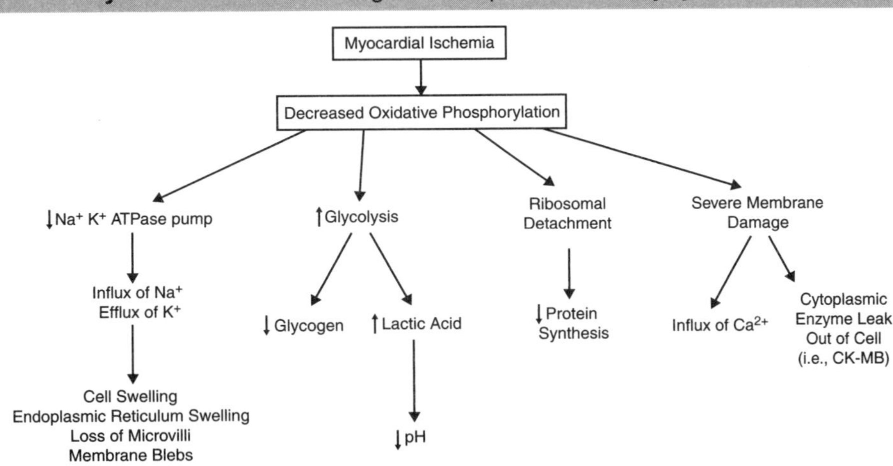

► Apoptosis

Morphology	Stimuli for Apoptosis	Genetic Regulation	Physiologic Examples	Pathologic Examples
• Cells shrink, cytoplasm is dense and eosinophilic • Nuclear chromatin condenses, then fragments • Cell membrane blebs • Cell fragments (apoptotic bodies) are phagocytized by adjacent cells or macrophages • **Lack of inflammatory response**	• Cell injury and DNA damage • Lack of hormones, cytokines, or growth factors • Receptor-ligand signals: – **Fas** binding to Fas ligand – Tumor necrosis factor (**TNF**) binding to TNF receptor 1 (TNFR1)	• ***bcl-2*** (inhibits apoptosis) • ***p-53*** (stimulates apoptosis)	• Embryogenesis—organogenesis and development • Hormone-dependent apoptosis (menstrual cycle) • Selective death of lymphocytes in thymus	• Viral hepatitis (Councilman body) • Graft versus host disease • Cystic fibrosis (CF)—duct obstruction and pancreatic atrophy

► Adaptive Cellular Responses to Injury (Potentially Reversible)

Types	Definitions	Causes
Atrophy	**Decrease in cell size and functional ability.** Cells shrink; lipofuscin granules can be seen microscopically. EM—autophagosomes	• Deceased workload/disuse • Ischemia • Lack of hormonal or neural stimulation • Malnutrition • Aging
Hypertrophy	**An increase in cell size and functional ability** mediated by growth factors, cytokines, and other trophic stimuli, leading to increased expression of genes and increased protein synthesis. May coexist with hyperplasia.	• Increased mechanical demand, e.g., striated muscle of weight lifters, cardiac muscle in hypertension • Increased endocrine stimulation, e.g., puberty, pregnancy, lactation
Hyperplasia	**An increase in the number of cells** in a tissue or organ, mediated by growth factors, cytokines, and other trophic stimuli. Increased expression of growth-promoting genes (proto-oncogenes), increased DNA synthesis, and cell division	**Physiologic causes:** • Compensatory (e.g., after partial hepatectomy) • Hormonal stimulation (e.g., breast development at puberty) • Antigenic stimulation (e.g., lymphoid hyperplasia) **Pathologic causes:** • Endometrial hyperplasia • Prostatic hyperplasia of aging
Metaplasia	**A reversible change of one cell type to another**	Irritation
Dysplasia	**An abnormal proliferation of cells** characterized by changes in cell size, shape, and loss of cellular organization; premalignant, e.g., cervical dysplasia	Similar to stimuli that produce cancer (e.g., HPV, esophageal reflux)

Regeneration and Repair

Wound healing involves **regeneration** of cells in a damaged tissue, along with repair of the connective tissue matrix.

▶ Capacity of Cells to Regenerate

Cell Type	Properties	Examples
Labile	Regenerate throughout life	Skin and mucosal lining cells Hematopoietic cells Stem cells
Stable	Replicate at a low level throughout life Have the capacity to divide if stimulated by some initiating event	Hepatocytes Proximal tubule cells Endothelium
Permanent	Cannot replicate	Neurons and cardiac muscle

Growth Factors and Cytokines Involved in Growth Repair

- Transforming growth factor α (TGF-α)
- Platelet-derived growth factor (PDGF)
- Fibroblast growth factor (FGF)
- Vascular endothelial growth factor (VEGF)
- Epidermal growth factor (EGF)
- Tumor necrosis factor α (TNF-α) and IL-1

▶ Connective Tissue Components

Collagen production requires vitamin C (wound healing impaired in scurvy) and copper. Different types of collagen are found in different body sites.

- Type I collagen is the most common form.
- Type II collagen is found in cartilage.
- Type III collagen is an immature form found in granulation tissue.
- Type IV collage is found in basement membranes.

Other extracellular matrix components include:

- adhesion molecules
- proteoglycans
- glycosaminoglycans

▶ Wound Healing

Primary Union (healing by first intention)

Occurs with clean wounds when there has been little tissue damage and wound edges are closely approximated, e.g., a surgical incision

Secondary Union (healing by second intention)

Occurs in wounds that have large tissue defects (the two skin edges are not in contact):

- Granulation tissue fills in the defects
- Often accompanied by significant wound contraction; may produce large residual scar

Keloids

Occur as result of excessive scar collagen deposition/hypertrophy, especially in dark-skinned people

Connective Tissue Diseases

Scurvy

Vitamin C deficiency first affecting collagen with highest hydroxyproline content, such as that found in blood vessels. Thus, an early symptom is bleeding gums.

Ehlers-Danlos (ED) Syndrome

Defect in collagen synthesis or structure. There are many types. ED type IV is a defect in type III collagen.

Osteogenesis Imperfecta

Defect in collagen type I

Staining Methods

Stain	Cell Type/Component
Hematoxylin (stains blue to purple)	Nuclei, nucleoli, bacteria, calcium
Eosin (stains pink to red)	Cytoplasm, collagen, fibrin, RBCs, thyroid colloid
Prussian blue	Iron
Congo red	Amyloid
Periodic acid-Schiff (PAS)	Glycogen, mucin, mucoprotein, glycoprotein, as well as fungi
Gram stain	Microorganisms
Trichrome	Collagen
Reticulin	Reticular fibers in loose connective tissue
Immunohistochemical (antibody) stains:	
• Cytokeratin	• Epithelial cells
• Vimentin	• Connective tissue
• Desmin	• Muscle
• Prostate-specific antigen (PSA)	• Prostate
• S-100, neuron specific enolase, neurofilament	• Neurons, neuronally derived, neural crest–derived growths
• GFAP	• Glial cells (including astrocytes)
• Tartrate-resistant acid phosphatase (TRAP)	• Hairy cell leukemia
• Bombesin	• Small cell lung cancer, carotid body tumor

Definition of abbreviations: GFAP, glial fibrillary acidic protein.

Amyloidosis

An accumulation of various insoluble fibrillar in various tissues. It stains with **Congo red** and shows **apple-green birefringence** with polarized light.

Disease	Major Fibril Protein	Precursor Protein
Primary amyloidosis (e.g., plasma cell disorders)	AL	Kappa or lambda chains
Secondary amyloidosis (e.g., neoplasia, rheumatoid arthritis, SLE, TB, Crohn disease, osteomyelitis, familial Mediterranean fever)	AA	Serum amyloid associated (SAA)
Renal hemodialysis	$A\beta_2M$	β_2 microglobin
Senile cerebral amyloidosis	Aβ	β-amyloid precursor protein
Cardiac amyloidosis	ATTR	Transthyretin
Medullary carcinoma of thyroid	A Cal	Calcitonin
Type 2 diabetes, pancreatic islet-cell tumors	A Amylin	Amylin

Definition of abbreviations: ATTR, amyloid transthyretin; SLE, systemic lupus erythematosus; TB, tuberculosis.

Neoplasia

Carcinogenesis is a multistep process involving multiple genetic changes from inherited germ-line mutations or acquired mutations, leading to monoclonal expansion of a mutated cell.

Progression of epithelial cancer: normal epithelium → atypical hyperplasia → dysplasia → carcinoma in situ → invasion, metastasis (collagenases, hydrolases aid in penetration of barriers, such as basement membrane)

► Basic Terms

Anaplasia	Loss of cell differentiation and tissue organization
Atypical hyperplasia	Increased cell number with morphologic abnormalities
Carcinoma	Malignant tumor of epithelium
Carcinoma in situ	Malignant tumor of epithelium that does not penetrate basement membrane to underlying tissue
Desmoplasia	Excessive fibrous tissue formation in tumor stroma
Dysplasia	Abnormal atypical cellular proliferation
Metaplasia	Replacement of one type of adult cell or tissue by another (within the same germ cell line) that is not normally present in that site
Metastasis	Secondary, discontinuous malignant growth (spread), such as a lung metastasis of a colon carcinoma
Sarcoma	A mesenchymal (nonepithelial) malignant tumor

► Selected Risk Factors for Cancer

Geographic/Racial	Stomach cancer (Japan); hepatocellular carcinoma (Asia)
Occupational/Environmental exposures	**Aflatoxin:** hepatocellular carcinoma **Alkylating agents:** leukemia, lymphoma, other cancers **Aromatic "–amines" and "azo–" dyes:** hepatocellular carcinoma **Arsenic:** squamous cell carcinomas of skin and lung, angiosarcoma of liver **Asbestos:** bronchogenic carcinoma, mesothelioma **Benzene:** leukemia **Chromium and nickel:** bronchogenic carcinoma **Cigarette smoke:** multiple malignancies **CCl_4:** fatty change and centrilobular necrosis of the liver **Ionizing radiation:** thyroid cancer, leukemia **Naphthylamine:** bladder cancer **Nitrosamines:** gastric cancer **Polycyclic aromatic hydrocarbons:** bronchogenic carcinoma **Ultraviolet exposure:** skin cancers **Vinyl chloride:** angiosarcoma of liver
Age	Increases risk of most cancers (exceptions: Wilms, etc.)
Hereditary predisposition	Familial retinoblastoma; multiple endocrine neoplasia, familial polyposis coli
Acquired risk factors	Cervical dysplasia, endometrial hyperplasia, cirrhosis, ulcerative colitis, chronic atrophic gastritis

▶ Mechanisms of Carcinogenesis

There are many proposed mechanisms of carcinogenesis. The most important mutations involve growth-promoting genes (proto-oncogenes), growth-inhibiting tumor suppressor genes, and genes regulating apoptosis.

Clinically Important Oncogenes

Proto-oncogenes are normal cellular genes involved with growth and cellular differentiation. **Oncogenes** are derived from proto-oncogenes by changing the gene sequence (resulting in a new gene product, oncoprotein) or a loss of gene regulation → overexpression of the normal gene product. Oncogenes lack regulatory control and are overexpressed → unregulated cellular proliferation.

Oncogene	Tumor	Gene Product	Mechanism of Activation
		Growth factor	
hst-1/int-2	Cancer of the stomach, breast, bladder, and melanoma	Fibroblast growth factor	Overexpression
sis	Astrocytoma	Platelet-derived growth factor	Overexpression
		Growth factor receptor	
erb-B1	SCC of lung	Epidermal growth factor receptor	Overexpression
erb-B2	Breast, ovary, lung	Epidermal growth factor receptor	Amplification
erb-B3	Breast	Epidermal growth factor receptor	Overexpression
ret	MEN II and III, familial thyroid (medullary) cancer	Glial neurotrophic factor receptor	Point mutation
		Signal transduction proteins	
abl	CML, ALL	*bcr-abl* fusion protein with tyrosine kinase activity	Translocation t(9;22)
Ki-ras	Lung, pancreas, and colon	GTP-binding protein	Point mutation
c-myc	Burkitt lymphoma	Nuclear regulatory protein	Translocation t(8;14)
L-myc	Small cell lung carcinoma	Nuclear regulatory protein	Amplification
N-myc	Neuroblastoma	Nuclear regulatory protein	Amplification
		Cell-cycle regulatory proteins	
bcl-1	Mantle cell lymphoma	Cyclin D_1 protein	Translocation t(11;14)
CDK4	Melanoma, glioblastoma multiforme	Cyclin-dependent kinase	Amplification
c-kit	Gastrointestinal stromal tumor (GIST)	KIT (also called CD117) is a stem cell factor receptor, a receptor tyrosine kinase	Overexpression or mutation

Definition of abbreviations: ALL, acute lymphocytic leukemia; CML, chronic myelogenous leukemia; MEN, multiple endocrine neoplasia; SCC, squamous cell carcinoma.

(Continued)

▶ Mechanisms of Carcinogenesis *(Cont'd.)*

Inactivation of Tumor Suppressor Genes

Tumor suppressor genes encode proteins that regulate and suppress cell proliferation by inhibiting progression through the cell cycle. Inactivation of these genes → uncontrolled cellular proliferation.

Gene	Chromosome	Tumors
VHL	3p25	Von Hippel-Lindau disease, renal cell carcinoma
WT-1	11p13	Wilms tumor
WT-2	11p15	Wilms tumor
Rb	13q14	Retinoblastoma, osteosarcoma
p53	17p13.1	Lung, breast, colon, etc.
BRCA-1	17q12-21	Hereditary breast and ovary cancers
BRCA-2	13q12-13	Hereditary breast cancer
APC	5q21	Adenomatous polyps and colon cancer
DCC	18q21	Colon cancer
NF-1	17q11.2	Neurofibromas
NF-2	22q12	Acoustic neuromas, meningiomas
p16	9p	Melanoma
DPC4	18q21	Pancreatic cancer

Failure of Apoptosis Is Another Cause of Cancer

bcl-2

- **Prevents apoptosis**
- Overexpressed in follicular lymphomas t(14:18) (chromosome 14 [immunoglobulin heavy chain gene]; chromosome 18 [*bcl-2*])

bax, bad, bcl-xS, bid

- **Promote apoptosis**
- ***p53*** promotes apoptosis in mutated cells by stimulating *bax* synthesis; inactivation → failure of apoptosis

c-myc

- Promotes cellular proliferation
- When associated with *p53* → promotes apoptosis; when associated with *bcl-2* → inhibits apoptosis

▶ Oncogenic Viruses

Specific virus	Human T-cell leukemia virus (HTLV-1)*	Hepatitis B (HBV) Hepatitis C (HCV)*	Epstein-Barr	Human papilloma virus (types 16, 18 in genital sites)	Human herpesvirus 8 (HHV-8)
Associated disease	Adult T-cell leukemia/ lymphoma	Hepatocellular carcinoma	Burkitt lymphoma, B-cell lymphoma, nasopharyngeal carcinoma	Cervical, vulvar, vaginal, penile, and anal carcinoma; some head and neck cancers	Kaposi sarcoma

*RNA oncogenic viruses (all other are DNA).

► Serum Tumor Markers

These are usually normal cellular components that are increased in neoplasms but may also be elevated in non-neoplastic conditions. Can be used for screening, monitoring of treatment efficacy, and detecting recurrence.

Marker	Associated Cancers
α-fetoprotein (AFP)	Hepatocellular carcinoma, nonseminomatous testicular germ-cell tumors
β-human chorionic gonadotropin (hCG)	Trophoblastic tumors, choriocarcinoma
Calcitonin	Medullary carcinoma of the thyroid
Carcinoembryonic antigen (CEA)	Carcinomas of the lung, pancreas, stomach, breast, colon
CA-125	Ovarian epithelial carcinoma
CA19-9	Pancreatic adenocarcinoma
Placental alkaline phosphatase	Seminoma
Prostatic acid phosphatase	Prostate cancer
Prostate-specific antigen (PSA)	Prostate cancer
S-100	Melanoma, neural-derived tumors, astrocytoma

► Paraneoplastic Syndromes

Syndrome	Neoplasm	Mechanism
Carcinoid syndrome	Carcinoid tumor (metastatic, bronchial, ovarian)	Serotonin, bradykinin
Cushing syndrome	Small cell carcinoma of the lung, neural tumors	ACTH, ACTH-like peptide
Hypercalcemia	Squamous cell carcinoma of the lung; breast, renal, and ovarian carcinomas	PTH-related peptide, TGF-α, TNF, IL-1
Lambert-Eaton myasthenic syndrome	Small cell carcinoma of the lung	Antibodies against presynaptic voltage-gated Ca^{2+} channels at the neuromuscular junction
Polycythemia	Renal cell carcinoma, hepatocellular carcinoma, cerebellar hemangioblastoma	Erythropoietin
SIADH	Small cell carcinoma of the lung; intracranial neoplasms	ADH

Definition of abbreviations: ACTH, adrenocorticotropic hormone; IL, interleukin; TGF, transforming growth factor; TNF, tumor necrosis factor; PTH, parathyroid hormone; SIADH, syndrome of inappropriate antidiuretic hormone

▶ Grading and Staging

Grade	• An estimate of the cytologic malignancy of a tumor, including the degree of anaplasia and number of mitoses. • Nuclear size, chromatin content, nucleoli, and nuclear-to-cytoplasmic ratio are all used.
Stage	• The clinical estimate of the extent of spread of a malignant tumor. Low stage means a localized tumor. Stage rises as tumors spread locally then metastasize. • **TNM** is typically used; **T** = size of **t**umor; **N** = **n**ode involvement; **M** = **m**etastases

▶ Cancer Incidence and Mortality

Incidence	**Males**	**Females**
	Prostate: 29%	Breast: 30%
	Lung and bronchus: 14%	Lung and bronchus: 14%
	Colon and rectum: 9%	Colon and rectum: 9%
Mortality	**Males**	**Females**
	Lung and bronchus: 28%	Lung and bronchus: 26%
	Prostate: 11%	Breast: 15%
	Colon and rectum: 8%	Colon and rectum: 9%

Section II

Organ Systems

The Nervous System

Chapter 1

Development of the Nervous System

Neurulation

- **Neurulation** begins in the third week of fetal development.
- The **notochord** induces the overlying ectoderm to form the neural plate.
- By end of the third week, **neural folds** grow over midline and fuse to form **neural tube**.
- During closure, **neural crest** cells form from neuroectoderm.

- **Neural tube** → brain and spinal cord (plus lower motoneurons, preganglionic neurons)
- Brain stem and spinal cord have an **alar** plate (**sensory**) and a **basal** plate (**motor**); plates are separated by the **sulcus limitans**.
- **Neural tube** → 3 primary vesicles → 5 primary vesicles

- **Neural crest** → sensory and postganglionic neurons

- **Peripheral NS (PNS):** cranial nerves (12 pairs) and spinal nerves (31 pairs)

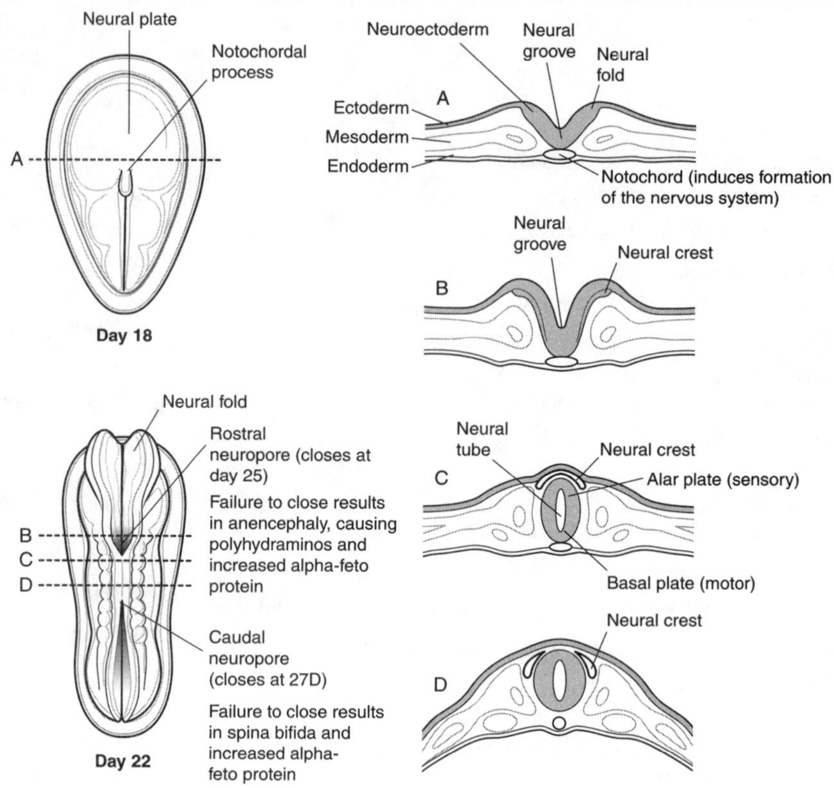

► Central Nervous System Development

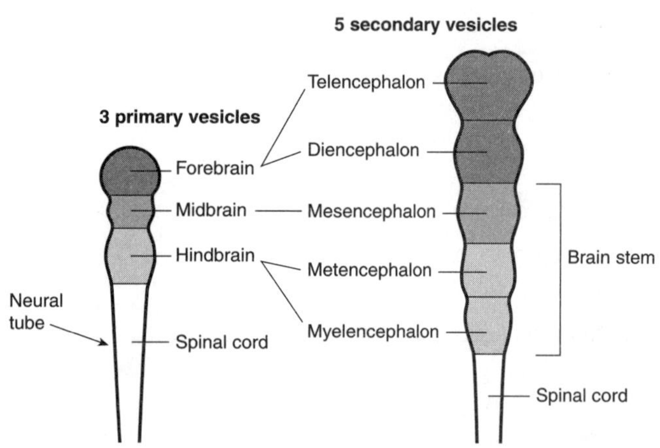

Adult Derivatives		
Structures		Ventricles
Telencephalon	Cerebral hemispheres, most of basal ganglia	Lateral ventricle
Diencephalon	Thalamus, hypothalamus, subthalamus, epithalamus (pineal gland), retina	Third ventricle
Mesencephalon	Midbrain	Cerebral aqueduct
Metencephalon	Pons, cerebellum	Fourth ventricle
Myelencephalon	Medulla	

► Congenital Malformations of the Nervous System

Condition	Types	Description
Anencephaly	—	Failure of **anterior neuropore** to close Brain does not develop Incompatible with life Increased AFP
Spina bifida	Failure of **posterior neuropore** to close	
	Spina bifida occulta **(Figure A)**	Mildest form **Vertebrae** fail to form around spinal cord **No** increase in **AFP** Asymptomatic
	Spina bifida with meningocele **(Figure B)**	**Meninges** protrude through vertebral defect Increase in AFP
	Spina bifida with meningomyelocele **(Figure C)**	**Meninges** and **spinal cord** protrude through vertebral defect Increase in AFP
	Spina bifida with myeloschisis **(Figure D)**	Most severe **Spinal cord** can be seen **externally** Increase in AFP

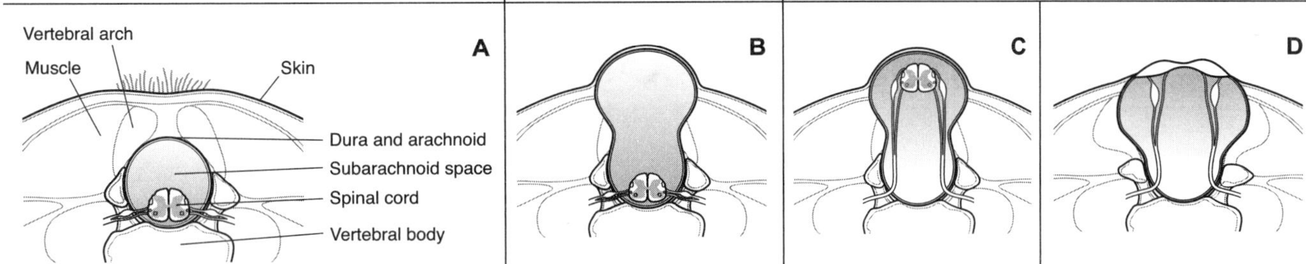

Condition	Types	Description
Arnold-Chiari malformation	Type I	Most common Mostly **asymptomatic** Downward displacement of cerebellar tonsils through foramen magnum
	Type II	More often **symptomatic** Downward displacement of **cerebellar vermis** and **medulla** through foramen magnum Compression of IV ventricle → obstructive **hydrocephaly** Frequent lumbar **meningomyelocele** Frequent association with **syringomyelia**
Dandy-Walker malformation		Failure of foramina of Luschka and Magendie to open → **dilation of IV ventricle** Agenesis of cerebellar vermis and splenium of the corpus callosum
Hydrocephalus		Most often caused by stenosis of cerebral aqueduct CSF accumulates in ventricles and subarachnoid space Increased head circumference
Holoprosencephaly		Incomplete separation of cerebral hemispheres One ventricle in telencephalon Seen in trisomy 13 (Patau)

Definition of abbreviation: AFP, α-fetoprotein.

Peripheral Nervous System

▶ Autonomic and Somatic Nervous Systems

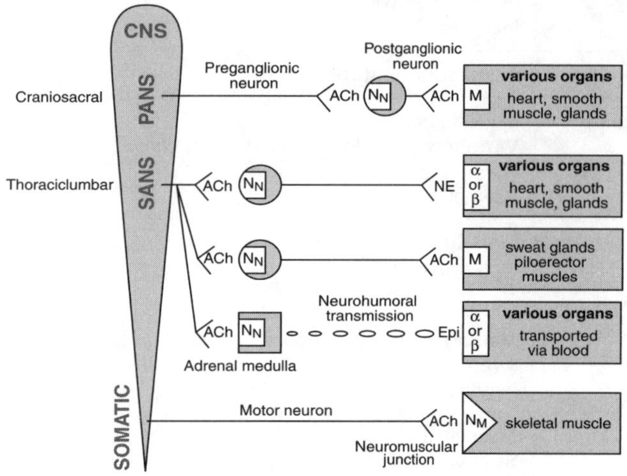

- **Somatic NS:** 1 neuron (from spinal cord → effector organ)
- **Autonomic NS:** 2 neurons (from spinal cord → effector organ)
  - **Preganglionic** neuron: cell body in CNS
  - **Postganglionic** neuron: cell body in ganglia in PNS
  - **Parasympathetic:** long preganglionic, short postganglionic
  - **Sympathetic:** short preganglionic, long postganglionic (except adrenal medulla)

Definition of abbreviations: N_N, neuronal nicotinic receptor; N_M, muscle nicotinic receptor; NE, norepinephrine; M, muscarinic receptor; ACh, acetylcholine.

Note: Arrows indicate lesion sites that result in Horner syndrome.

▶ Parasympathetic Nervous System

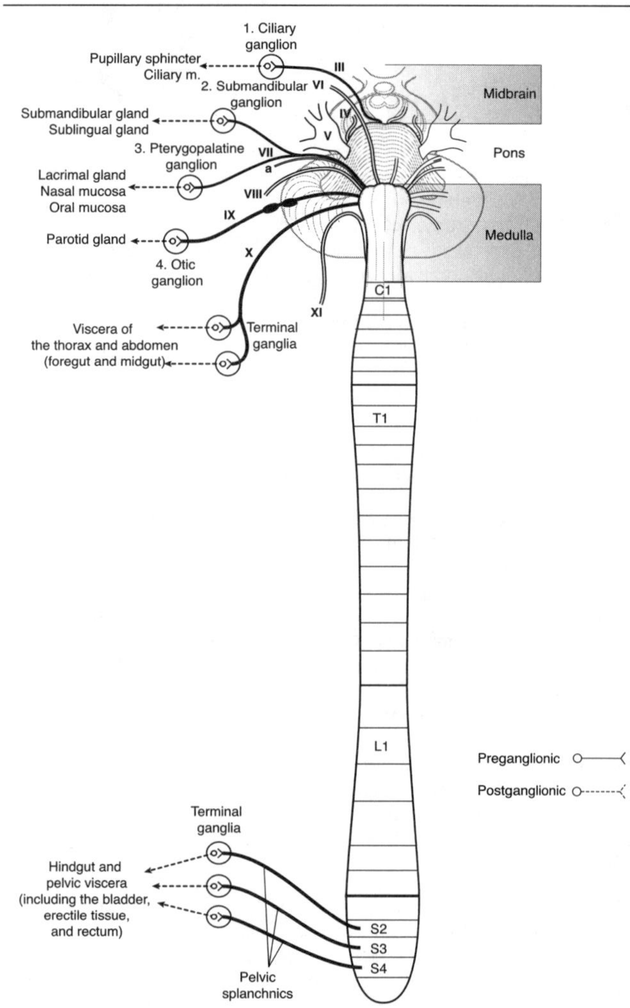

▶ Sympathetic Nervous System

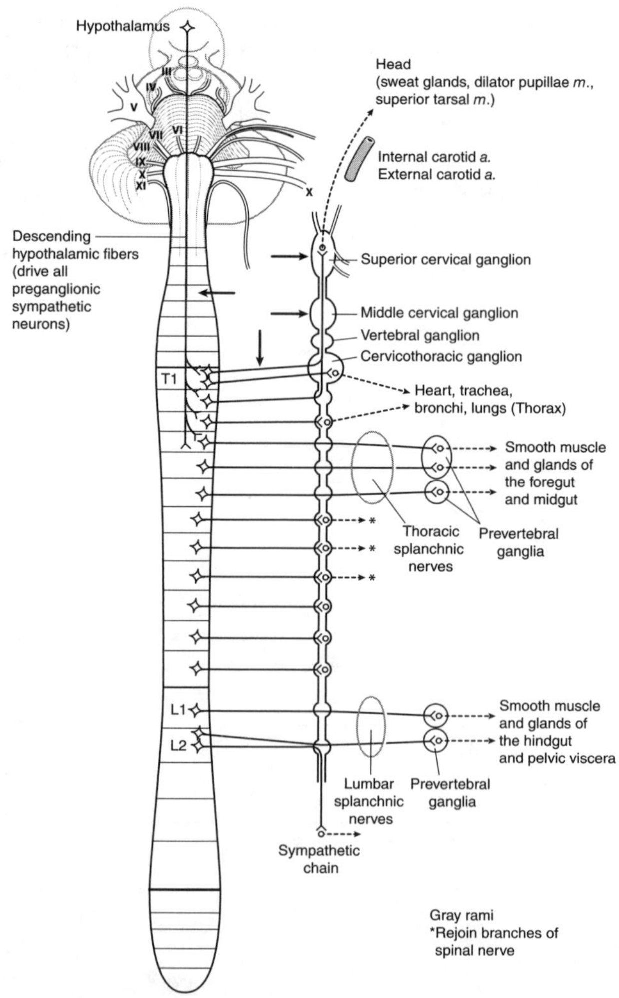

Note: Arrows indicate lesion sites that result in Horner syndrome.

▶ Parasympathetic = Craniosacral Outflow

Origin	Site of Synapse	Innervation
Cranial nerves III, VII, IX	4 cranial ganglia (ciliary, submandibular, pterygopalatine, otic)	Glands and smooth muscle of the **head**
Cranial nerve X	Terminal ganglia (in or near the walls of viscera)	Viscera of the neck, **thorax**, **foregut**, and **midgut**
Pelvic splanchnic nerves (S2, S3, S4)	Terminal ganglia (in or near the walls of viscera)	**Hindgut** and **pelvic viscera** (including bladder, rectum, and erectile tissue)

▶ Sympathetic = Thoracolumbar Outflow

Origin	Site of Synapse	Innervation
Spinal cord levels T1–L2	Sympathetic chain ganglia (paravertebral ganglia)	Smooth and cardiac muscle and glands of **body wall** and **limbs**; head and **thoracic viscera**
Thoracic splanchnic nerves T5–T12	Prevertebral ganglia (collateral; e.g., celiac, aorticorenal superior mesenteric ganglia)	Smooth muscle and glands of the **foregut** and **midgut**
Lumbar splanchnic nerves L1, L2	Prevertebral ganglia (collateral; e.g., inferior mesenteric and pelvic ganglia)	Smooth muscle and glands of the **pelvic viscera** and **hindgut**

▶ Autonomic Effects on Organ Systems

As a general rule, the **sympathetic autonomic nervous system (SANS)** mediates **"fight or flight"** responses, such as increasing heart rate and contractility, dilating airways and pupils, inhibiting GI and GU functions, and directing blood flow away from skin and GI tract and toward skeletal muscles. In contrast, the **parasympathetic autonomic nervous system (PANS)** causes the body to **"rest and digest,"** reducing heart rate and contractility, contracting airways and pupils, inducing secretion from lacrimal and salivary glands, and promoting GI and GU motility. Blood vessels are solely innervated by SANS nerve fibers.

	Sympathetic "Fight or Flight"		Parasympathetic "Rest and Digest"	
Organ	**Action**	**Receptor**	**Action**	**Receptor**
	Cardiovascular			
Heart				
SA node	↑ heart rate	β_1, (β_2)	↓ heart rate	M_2
Atria	↑ contractility		↓ contractility	
AV node	↑ conduction velocity and automaticity[1]		↓ conduction velocity and automaticity[1]	
Ventricles	↑ contractility		↓ contractility (slight)	
Arterioles[2]	Contract: ↑ resistance	α_1	—	$(M_3)^3$
Veins	Contract: ↑ venous pressure	α_1	—	—
Kidney	Renin release	β_1	—	—
	Respiratory			
Bronchiolar smooth muscle	Relax: ↓ resistance	β_2	Contract: ↑ resistance	M_3

(Continued)

[1]When acting as a pacemaker; otherwise, the SA node suppresses automaticity in these cells

[2]β_2 receptors that mediate relaxation and decrease resistance are also present on coronary arteries and arterioles. Low doses of epinephrine (or β_2 agonists) act selectively on β_2 receptors and can decrease systemic vascular resistance, but increased sympathetic tone increases systemic vascular resistance because vasoconstriction dominates.

[3]M_3 receptors are on vascular endothelium (not smooth muscle, like the adrenergic receptors) and cause vasodilation via nitric oxide (NO) generation; this has little physiologic significance because vasculature is not innervated by PANS, but is more important with muscarinic agonist administration.

▶ Autonomic Effects on Organ Systems (*Cont'd.*)

	Sympathetic "Fight or Flight"		Parasympathetic "Rest and Digest"	
Organ	**Action**	**Receptor**	**Action**	**Receptor**
Gastrointestinal				
GI smooth muscle				
Walls	↓ GI motility	α_2,[4] β_2	↑ GI motility	M_3
Sphincters	Contracts	α_1	Relaxes	M_3
Glandular secretion	—	—	Increases	M_3
Liver	Gluconeogenesis	β_2, α	—	—
	Glycogenolysis	β_2, α	—	—
Fat cells	Lipolysis	β_3	—	—
Genitourinary				
Bladder				
Walls	Relaxes	β_2	Contracts	M_3
Sphincters	Contracts	α_1	Relaxes	M_3
Uterus, pregnant	Relaxes	β_2	—	—
	Contracts	α	Contracts	M_3
Penis, seminal vesicles	Ejaculation	α	Erection	M
Skin				
Sweat glands	Secretion	M,[5] α[6]	—	—
Eye				
Radial dilator muscle	Contracts (dilates pupil)	α_1	—	—
Pupillary sphincter muscle	—	—	Contracts (constricts pupil)	M_3
Ciliary muscle	Relaxes—far vision	β	Contracts—near vision	M_3

[4] Probably via inhibition of cholinergic nerve terminals

[5] Generalized

[6] Localized (e.g., palms of hands)

► Cholinergic Transmission

Acetylcholine (ACh) is synthesized from acetate and choline in synaptic nerve terminals via **choline acetyltransferase (ChAT)** and stored in synaptic vesicles and released by Ca^{2+} influx upon depolarization. The **uptake of choline** into the nerve terminal is the **rate-limiting step** of ACh synthesis and can be blocked by **hemicholinium**. ACh then binds to postsynaptic receptors to elicit somatic (N_M) or autonomic (N_N and M) effects. Signal termination occurs by degradation of ACh by **acetylcholinesterase (AChE)**.

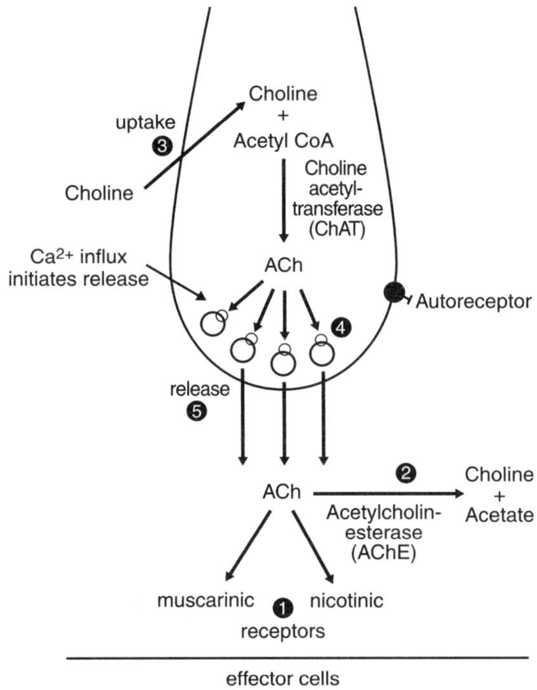

Receptor	Signal	Function
N_M	Cation channel	Stimulates skeletal muscle contraction (somatic)
N_N	Cation channel	Stimulates autonomic ganglia and adrenal medulla
M_1	↑ IP_3, DAG (G_q)	↑ gastric acid secretion from parietal cells; CNS and PNS effects
M_2	↓ cAMP (G_i)	↓ heart rate and contractility
M_3	↑ IP_3, DAG (G_q)	↑ smooth muscle contraction (e.g., GI, GU, bronchial, pupillary constriction); ↑ secretions; vascular endothelium (dilation via NO)

Definition of abbreviations: DAG, diacylglycerol; GI, gastrointestinal; GU, genitourinary; IP_3, inositol triphosphate.
Note: The numbers in the figure correspond to the numbers in the table below.

► Cholinergic Pharmacology

Mechanism of Action	Agent	Clinical Uses	Other Notes and Toxicity
❶ ACh receptor			
Nicotinic (N_M) agonist/antagonists (skeletal muscle)	(*See* neuromuscular blockers, page 427.)		
Nicotinic (N_N) antagonists (ganglion blockers)	Hexamethonium Mecamylamine	Rarely used due to toxicities	Blocks both SANS and PANS; effectively reduces predominant tone (*see table below*)
Cholinergic agonists M = muscarinic N = nicotinic B = both	Bethanechol (M)	Ileus (postop/neurogenic) Urinary retention	Heart block, cardiac arrest Syncope
	Methacholine (M)	Diagnosis of bronchial hyperreactivity in asthma	Partially sensitive to cholinesterase (others listed here are resistant)
	Pilocarpine (M)	Glaucoma (topical) Xerostomia	—
	Carbachol (B)	Glaucoma (topical)	—
	Nicotine (N)	Smoking deterrence	—

(Continued)

► Cholinergic Pharmacology (*Cont'd.*)

Mechanism of Action	Agent	Clinical Uses	Other Notes and Toxicity
Muscarinic antagonists Class known as "Belladonna" alkaloids (meaning "beautiful lady") from their origin from *Atropa belladonna*, which was used to dilate pupils (believed to make women look more attractive). Other drugs with anti-muscarinic effects: • Antihistamines • Tricyclics • Antipsychotics • Quinidine • Amantadine • Meperidine	Atropine	Counteracts cholinergic toxicity Antidiarrheal Mydriatic agent for eye exams Reversal of sinus bradycardia and heart block	Mydriasis and cycloplegia ***(blind as a bat)*** Decreased secretions ***(dry as a bone)*** Vasodilation ***(red as a beet)*** Delirium and hallucinations ***(mad as a hatter)*** Hyperthermia Tachycardia Urinary retention and constipation Sedation, amnesia
	Homatropine Cyclopentolate Tropicamide	Ophthalmology (topical), for mydriasis	—
	Ipratropium	Asthma and COPD	Localized effect because is a quaternary amine; few antimuscarinic side effects
	Scopolamine	Motion-sickness Antiemetic	(*See side effects for atropine.*)
	Benztropine Trihexyphenidyl Biperiden	Parkinsonism Acute extrapyramidal symptoms from neuroleptics	
	Glycopyrrolate Dicyclomine	Reduces hypermotility in GI and GU tracts	
❷ Metabolism of ACh (AChE inhibitors)			
Short-acting:	Edrophonium	Diagnosis of myasthenia gravis	Seizures
Tertiary amines:	Physostigmine	Glaucoma Reversal of anticholinergic toxicity	Carbamylating inhibitor Seizures
Quaternary amines:	Neostigmine Pyridostigmine Ambenonium	Ileus, urinary retention Myasthenia gravis Reversal of nondepolarizing neuromuscular blockers	Carbamylating inhibitors
Lipid-soluble:	Donepezil Tacrine Rivastigmine Galantamine	Alzheimer disease	Hepatotoxicity GI bleeding

(Continued)

► Cholinergic Pharmacology (*Cont'd.*)

Mechanism of Action	Agent	Clinical Uses	Other Notes and Toxicity
Organophosphates:	Echothiophate	Glaucoma	
• Long-acting and irreversible	Malathion Parathion	Insecticide	**Mnemonic: DUMBBELSS** **D**iarrhea **U**rination **M**iosis **B**radycardia **B**ronchoconstriction **E**xcitation (CNS and muscle) **L**acrimation **S**alivation **S**weating Acute treatment with **atropine** and **pralidoxime (2-PAM)** to regenerate AChE before aging occurs
• Causes time-dependent **aging**, which permanently inactivates AChE	Sarin VX	Nerve agents (chemical warfare)	
❸ Reuptake inhibitors	Hemicholinium	Only used in research settings	Blocks choline reuptake, slowing ACh synthesis
❹ Vesicular transport inhibitors	Vesamicol	Only used in research settings	Blocks ACh uptake into vesicles, preventing storage and leading to ACh depletion
❺ Vesicle release inhibitors	Botulinum toxin	Blepharospasm Strabismus/Hyperhydrosis Cervical dystonia Cosmetic (removes wrinkles)	Prevents fusion of cholinergic vesicles to membrane, thereby inhibiting ACh release

Definition of abbreviations: ACh, acetylcholine; AChE, acetylcholinesterase; ChAT, choline acetyltransferase; COPD, chronic obstructive pulmonary disorder.

► Predominant Tone and the Effect of Ganglionic Blockers

The effects of ganglionic blockers can be easily predicted if you know the predominant autonomic tone to a particular effector organ. The effect of the blockade will be the opposite of what the predominant tone causes. In general, the predominant tone to blood vessels and sweat glands is sympathetic, and most everything else is parasympathetic.

Site	Predominant Tone	Effect of Ganglionic Blockade
Arterioles	Sympathetic	Dilation (↓ blood pressure)
Veins	Sympathetic	Dilation (↓ venous return)
Heart	Parasympathetic	↑ heart rate
GI tract	Parasympathetic	↓ motility and secretions
Eye	Parasympathetic	Pupillary dilation, focus to far vision
Urinary bladder	Parasympathetic	Urinary retention
Salivary glands	Parasympathetic	Dry mouth
Sweat glands	Sympathetic (cholinergic)	Anhidrosis

► Adrenergic Transmission

Norepinephrine (NE), **epinephrine (EPI)**, and dopamine are part of the **catecholamine** family, which are synthesized from **tyrosine**. The first step of the synthetic pathway is carried out by **tyrosine hydroxylase**; it is also the **rate-limiting** step. NE levels inside the presynaptic terminal may also be regulated by metabolism by **monoamine oxidase (MAO)**. Once released, NE binds to various adrenergic receptors to transmit its signal. NE primarily binds α_1, α_2, and β_1 receptors, whereas EPI (released by the adrenal medulla) binds α_1, α_2, β_1, and β_2 receptors. **Reuptake** (especially uptake-1) and diffusion are most important in the termination of action of NE (and DA). Metabolism occurs via **catechol-*O*-methyltransferase ([COMT]** extracellular) and **MAO** (intracellular). Metabolites such as **metanephrine**, **normetanephrine**, **vanillylmandelic acid (VMA)** can be measured in the urine and are used in the diagnosis of diseases such as pheochromocytoma.

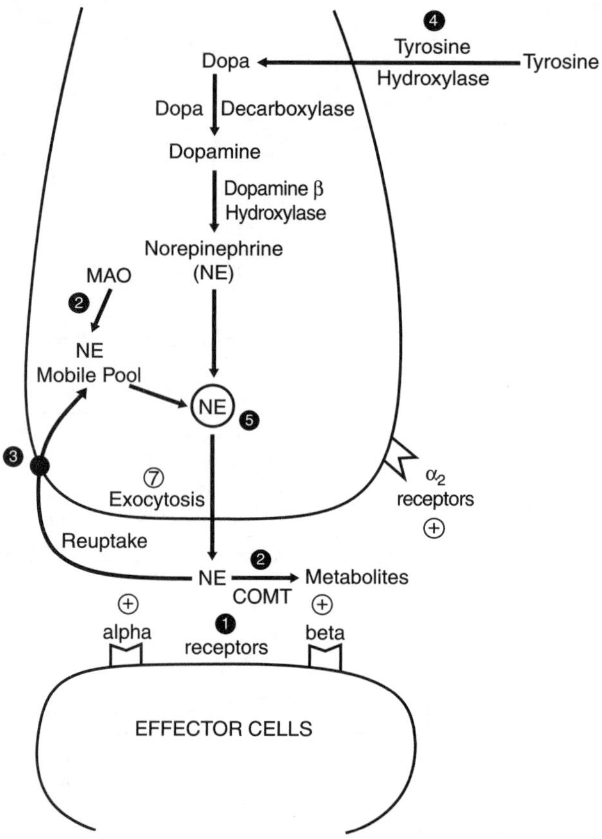

Receptor	Signal	Function
α_1	↑ IP_3, DAG (G_q)	↑ smooth muscle contraction (in vascular walls, radial dilator muscle [eye], and GI and bladder sphincters); ↑ glycogenolysis in liver
α_2	↓ cAMP (G_i)	Inhibits neurotransmitter release; inhibits insulin release and lipolysis
β_1	↑ cAMP (G_s)	↑ heart rate and contractility; ↑ AV conduction velocity; ↑ renin secretion
β_2		↑ smooth muscle relaxation (in vascular, bronchial, GI, and bladder walls); ↑ glycogenolysis in liver, ↑ insulin release
β_3		↑ lipolysis from adipose tissues

Mnemonic: You can get an adrenaline rush from a **QISSS** ($G_qG_iG_sG_sG_s$).

Definition of abbreviations: DAG, diacylglycerol; GI, gastrointestinal; GU, genitourinary; IP_3, inositol triphosphate.

Note: The numbers in the figure correspond to the numbers in the following table.

► Adrenergic Pharmacology

Mechanism of Action	Agent	Clinical Uses	Other Notes and Toxicity
❶ Adrenergic receptor			
α-adrenergic agonists	α_1: Phenylephrine	Nasal congestion Vasoconstriction Mydriasis (topical)	—
	α_1: Methoxamine	Paroxysmal supraventricular tachycardia	Bradycardia (vagal reflex)
	α_2: Clonidine Methyldopa	Hypertension	Decreases sympathetic outflow Methyldopa: prodrug converted to methylnorepinephrine
α-adrenergic antagonists	**Nonselective:** Phentolamine	Pheochromocytoma	**Reversible**, competitive inhibitor Postural hypotension, reflex tachycardia
	Nonselective: Phenoxybenzamine	Pheochromocytoma	**Irreversible** inhibitor Postural hypotension, reflex tachycardia
	α_1: Prazosin Doxazosin Terazosin Tamsulosin	Hypertension Benign prostatic hypertrophy	Postural hypotension on first dose
	α_2: Yohimbine	Impotence Postural hypotension	Clinical use limited
	α_2: Mirtazapine	Depression	May also block 5HT receptors
β-adrenergic agonists	$\beta_1 = \beta_2$: Isoproterenol	Bronchospasm Heart block and bradyarrhythmias	Clinical use limited ↓ BP, ↑ HR Arrhythmias
	$\beta_1 > \beta_2$: Dobutamine	Acute heart failure	—
	β_2: Albuterol Terbutaline Metaproterenol Salmeterol	Asthma	Tachycardia, skeletal muscle tremor Pulmonary delivery to minimize side effects Salmeterol is long-acting Suppress premature labor (terbutaline)
β-adrenergic antagonists	β_1: Acebutolol Atenolol Esmolol Metoprolol	Hypertension Angina Chronic heart failure (carvedilol, metoprolol) Arrhythmia Glaucoma (timolol) Migraine, tremor, thyrotoxicosis (propanolol)	Sedation Decreases libido Bradycardia β_1 selectivity safer in asthma, diabetes, and vascular diseases Pindolol and acebutolol have **intrinsic sympathomimetic activity** (useful in asthmatics); should not be used in patients with recent MI
	Nonselective: Pindolol Propranolol Nadolol Timolol		
	α and β: Labetalol Carvedilol	CHF (carvedilol) Hypertension (labetalol)	Similar to above Liver damage (labetalol)

Definition of abbreviation: CHF, congestive heart failure.

(Continued)

► Adrenergic Pharmacology (*Cont'd.*)

Mechanism of Action	Agent	Clinical Uses	Other Notes and Toxicity
❷ Metabolism			
MAO inhibitors MAO-A: mainly liver but Anywhere MAO-B: mainly in Brain	Phenelzine Tranylcypromine	Depression	Nonselective MAO-A/B inhibitors Tyramine (red wine, cheese) ingestion → hypertensive crisis Insomnia Postural hypotension MAO-AIs: moclobemide (reversible), clorgyline available in Europe
	Selegiline Rasagiline	Parkinson disease	Selective MAO-B inhibitor
COMT inhibitors	Entacapone Tolcapone	Parkinson disease	—
❸ Reuptake inhibitors	Cocaine	Local anesthesia Abuse	Inhibits monoamine reuptake Addiction
Tricyclic antidepressants	Amitriptyline Imipramine Desipramine Nortriptyline	Depression	Inhibits monoamine reuptake Sedation Postural hypotension Tachycardia Atropine-like effects
❹ Synthesis inhibitors	α-Methyltyrosine (metyrosine)	Hypertension	Inhibits tyrosine hydroxylase Only for hypertension associated with pheochromocytoma
❺ Drugs affecting release			
Adrenergic neuron blockers	Reserpine	Hypertension	Inhibits monoamine vesicular uptake, leading to neurotransmitter depletion Sedation, depression
	Guanethidine	Hypertension	Inhibits NE release from sympathetic nerve endings Requires neuronal uptake to work, so interferes with other drugs that require uptake carrier (e.g., cocaine, amphetamine, cyclic antidepressants)
Indirect-acting sympathomimetics	Amphetamine Methylphenidate	Narcolepsy and ADHD	Displaces NE from mobile pool Addiction Restlessness and rebound fatigue
	Ephedrine Pseudoephedrine	For vasoconstriction	Displaces NE from mobile pool Pseudoephedrine: OTC for nasal congestion

Definition of abbreviations: ADHD, attention deficit and hyperactivity disorder; COMT, catechol-O-methyltransferase; MAO, monoamine oxidase; NE, norepinephrine; OTC, over the counter.

Meninges, Ventricular System, and Venous Drainage

▶ Meninges and Meningeal Spaces

The meninges consist of three connective tissue membranes that surround the brain and spinal cord. Meningeal spaces are spaces or potential spaces adjacent to the meninges.

Meninges	Meningeal Space	Anatomic Description	Clinical Correlate
	Epidural space	Tight potential space between dura and skull Contains **middle meningeal artery**	**Epidural hematoma** Temporal bone fracture → rupture of **middle meningeal artery** **Lens-shaped biconvex** hematoma
Dura		Tough outer layer; dense connective tissue	
	Subdural space	Contains **bridging veins**	**Subdural hematoma** Rupture of bridging veins **Crescent-shaped** hematoma
Arachnoid		Delicate, nonvascular connective tissue	
	Subarachnoid space	Contains **CSF** Ends at S2 vertebra	**Subarachnoid hemorrhage** **"Worst headache of my life"** Often caused by **berry aneurysms** **Lumbar puncture** between L4, L5 discs
Pia		Thin, highly vascular connective tissue Adheres to brain and spinal cord	

▶ Meningitis (infection of the meninges, especially the pia and arachnoid)

Acute purulent (bacterial) meningitis	• **Headache, fever, nuchal rigidity**, obtundation; coma may occur • Meninges opaque; neutrophilic exudate present • Sequelae: hydrocephalus, herniation, cranial nerve impairment
Acute aseptic (viral) meningitis	• Leptomeningeal inflammation (lymphomonocytic infiltrates) due to viruses (Enterovirus most frequent) • Fever, signs of meningeal irritation, depressed consciousness, but low mortality
Mycobacterial meningoencephalitis	• Can be caused by *Mycobacterium tuberculosis* or atypical mycobacteria • Usually involves the **basal surface** of the brain with tuberculomas within the brain and dura mater • Frequent in AIDS patients, particularly by *Mycobacterium avium-intracellulare* (MAI)
Fungal meningoencephalitis	• *Candida, Aspergillus, Cryptococcus*, and *Mucor* species most frequent agents • *Aspergillus* and *Mucor* attack blood vessels → vasculitis, rupture of blood vessels, and hemorrhage • *Cryptococcus* causes diffuse meningoencephalitis

▶ Organisms Causing Bacterial Meningitis by Age Group

Neonates	Infants/Children	Adolescents/Young Adults	Elderly
Group B streptococci ***Escherichia coli*** *Listeria monocytogenes*	***Haemophilus influenzae* B** (if not vaccinated) *Streptococcus pneumoniae* *Neisseria meningitidis*	***Neisseria meningitidis***	***Streptococcus pneumoniae*** *Listeria monocytogenes*

▶ CSF Parameters in Meningitis

Condition	Cells/μl	Glucose (mg/dL)	Proteins (mg/dL)	Pressure (mm H_2O)
Normal values	<5 lymphocytes	45–85 (50–70% of blood glucose)	15–45	70–180
Purulent (bacterial)	Up to 90,000 neutrophils	Decreased (<45)	Increased (>50)	Markedly elevated
Aseptic (viral)	100–1,000 most lymphocytes	Normal	Increased (>50)	Slightly elevated
Granulomatous (mycobacterial/fungal)	100–1,000 most lymphocytes	Decreased (<45)	Increased (>50)	Moderately elevated

▶ Viral Encephalitis

Pathology: perivascular cuffs, microglial nodules, neuron loss, and neuronophagia
Clinical: fever, headache, mental status changes, often progressing to coma

Arthropod-Borne	Herpes Simplex	Rabies	HIV
St. Louis, California, Eastern equine, Western equine, Venezuelan	Characteristic **hemorrhagic necrosis of temporal lobes**	**Negri bodies** in hippocampal and Purkinje neurons of the cerebellum	**Microglial nodules, multinucleated giant cells**

▶ Ventricular System and Venous Drainage

The brain and spinal cord float within a protective bath of cerebrospinal fluid (CSF), which is produced by the lining of the ventricles, the choroid plexus. CSF circulation begins in the ventricles and then enters the subarachnoid space to surround the brain and spinal cord.

Ventricles and CSF Circulation

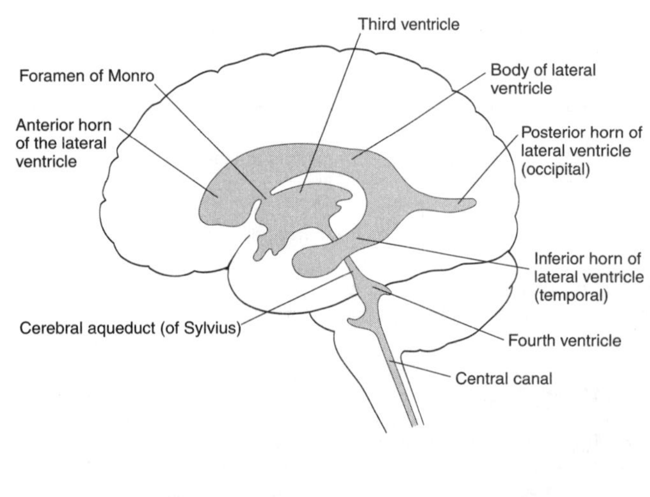

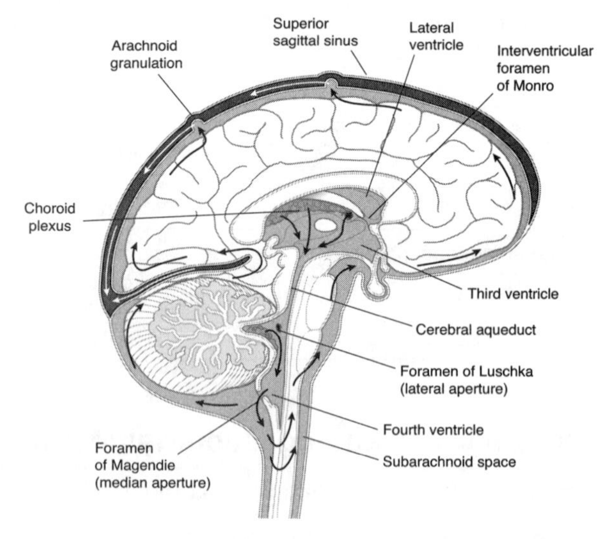

Lateral ventricles $\xrightarrow{A}$ third ventricle $\xrightarrow{B}$ fourth ventricle → subarachnoid space (via foramina of Luschka and foramen of Magendie)
(**A**, interventricular foramen of Monro; **B**, cerebral aqueduct.)

(Continued)

▶ Ventricular System and Venous Drainage (*Cont'd.*)

CSF Production and Barriers

Choroid plexus—contains **ependymal cells** and is found in the lateral, third, and fourth ventricles. **Secretes CSF.** Tight junctions form **blood-CSF barrier**.

Blood-brain barrier—formed by capillary endothelium with tight junctions; astrocyte foot processes contribute.

Once CSF is in the subarachnoid space, it goes up over convexity of the brain and enters the venous circulation by passing through **arachnoid granulations** into the **superior sagittal sinus**.

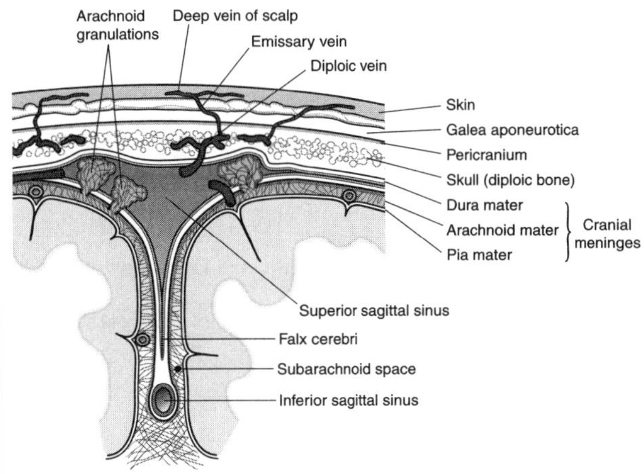

Sinuses

Superior sagittal sinus (in superior margin of falx cerebri)—drains into two **transverse sinuses**. Each of these drains blood from the **confluence of sinuses** into **sigmoid sinuses**. Each sigmoid sinus exits the skull (via **jugular foramen**) as the **internal jugular veins**.

Inferior sagittal sinus (in inferior margin of falx cerebri)— terminates by joining with the great cerebral vein of Galen to form the **straight sinus** at the falx cerebri and tentorium cerebelli junction. This drains into the confluence of sinuses.

Cavernous sinus—a plexus of veins on either side of the **sella turcica**. Surrounds internal carotid artery and cranial nerves III, IV, V, and VI. It drains into the transverse sinus (via the **superior petrosal sinus**) and the internal jugular vein (via the **inferior petrosal sinus**).

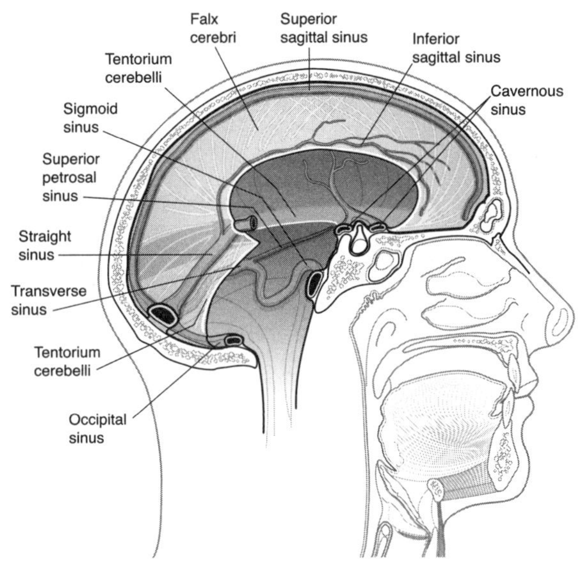

▶ Hydrocephalus

Excess Volume or Pressure of CSF, Leading to Dilated Ventricles

Noncommunicating	**Obstruction of flow within ventricles**; most commonly occurs at narrow points, e.g., foramen of Monro, cerebral aqueduct, fourth ventricle
Communicating	**Impaired CSF reabsorption** in arachnoid granulations or obstruction of flow in subarachnoid space
Normal pressure	CSF is not absorbed by arachnoid villi (a form of communicating hydrocephalus). CSF pressure is usually normal. Ventricles chronically dilated. Produces **triad** of **dementia, ataxic gait,** and **urinary incontinence**.
Hydrocephalus ex vacuo	Descriptive term referring to excess CSF in regions where brain tissue is lost due to atrophy, stroke, surgery, trauma, etc.

Neurohistology and Pathologic Correlates

► Cell Types of the Nervous System

Neurons	Glia (non-neuronal cells of the nervous system)
Composed of: • **Dendrites:** receive info and transmit to the cell body • **Cell body:** contains organelles • **Axon:** transmits electrical impulse down to the nerve terminals • **Nerve terminals:** contain synaptic vesicles and release neurotransmitter into the synapse	• **Oligodendrocytes:** form **myelin** in the **CNS** (one cell myelinates many axons) • **Astrocytes:** control microenvironment of neurons and help maintain the blood/brain barrier with foot processes • **Schwann cells:** form **myelin** in the **PNS** (one cell myelinates one internode) • **Ependymal cells:** ciliated neurons that line the ventricles and central canal of the spinal cord • **Microglia:** are **phagocytic** and are part of the **mononuclear phagocyte system**

► Disorders of Myelination

Demyelinating diseases are acquired conditions involving selective damage to myelin. Other diseases (e.g., infectious, metabolic, inherited) can also affect myelin and are generally called **leukodystrophies**.

Disease	Symptoms	Notes
Multiple sclerosis (MS)	**Symptoms separated in space and time** Vision loss (**optic neuritis**) **Internuclear ophthalmoplegia** (MLF degeneration) Motor and sensory deficits Vertigo Neuropsychiatric	Occurs twice as often in **women** Onset often in **third or fourth decade** Higher prevalence in **temperate zones** **Relapsing–remitting course** is most common Well-circumscribed **demyelinated plaques** often in periventricular areas Chronic inflammation; axons initially preserved Type IV hypersensitivity Increased IgG **(oligoclonal bands)** in CSF **Treatment:** high-dose steroids, interferon-beta, glatiramer (Copaxone®), natalizumab
Metachromatic leukodystrophy	Varied neurologic and psychiatric symptoms	**Arylsulfatase A deficiency**
Progressive multifocal leukoencephalopathy (PML)	Varied neurologic symptoms, dementia	Caused by **JC virus** Affects **immunocompromised, especially AIDS** Demyelination, astrogliosis, lymphohistiocytosis
Central pontine myelinolysis (CPM)	**Pseudobulbar palsy** **Spastic quadriparesis** Mental changes May produce the "locked-in" syndrome Often fatal	Focal demyelination of central area of basis pontis (affects corticospinal, corticobulbar tracts) Seen in **severely malnourished, alcoholics, liver disease** Probably **caused by overly aggressive correction of hyponatremia**
Guillain-Barré syndrome	Acute symmetric ascending inflammatory neuropathy **Weakness begins in lower limbs and ascends; respiratory failure can occur** in severe cases Autonomic dysfunction may be prominent Cranial nerve involvement is common Sensory loss, pain, and paresthesias occur **Reflexes invariably decreased or absent**	Two-thirds of patients have **history of respiratory or GI illness 1–3 weeks prior to onset**, 30% post *Campylobacter* Elevated CSF protein with normal cell count **(albuminocytologic dissociation)**
Charcot-Marie-Tooth disease	Slowly progressing weakness in distal limbs; usually lower extremities before upper extremities Abnormal proprioception/vibration sensation	Most common inherited neurologic disorder Onset usually in 1st two decades of life Different constellation of symptoms can occur, demyelination or axonal disease

(Continued)

▶ Disorders of Myelination (*Cont'd.*)

Acute disseminated (postinfectious) encephalomyelitis	Symptoms can be similar to MS, but is associated with constitutional symptoms, mental status changes, seizures, and fewer dorsal column abnormalities	Nonvasculitic inflammatory demyelinating disease History of preceding infectious illness or immunization Most often in prepubertal children

Definition of abbreviation: MLF, medial longitudinal fasciculus.

▶ Tumors of the CNS and PNS

One half of brain and spinal cord tumors are metastatic. Some differences between primary and metastatic tumors are listed below:

Primary	Metastatic
Poorly circumscribed	Well circumscribed
Usually single	Often multiple
Location varies by specific type	Usually located at the junction between gray and white matter

▶ Primary Tumors

Tumor	Features	Pathology
Glioblastoma multiforme (grade IV astrocytoma)	• **Most common primary brain tumor** • **Highly malignant** • Usually lethal in 8–12 months	• Can cross the midline via the corpus callosum ("**butterfly glioma**") • Areas of necrosis surrounded by rows of neoplastic cells (**pseudopalisading necrosis**)
Pilocytic astrocytoma (grade 1)	• Tumor of children and young adults • Usually in **posterior fossa in children**	• **Rosenthal fibers** • Immunostaining with **GFAP**
Oligodendroglioma	• Slow growing • Long survival (average 5–10 years)	**"Fried-egg" appearance**—perinuclear halo
Ependymoma	• Ependymal origin • Can arise in IV ventricle and lead to **hydrocephalus**	Rosettes and pseudorosettes
Medulloblastoma	• Highly malignant cerebellar tumor • A type of primitive neuroectodermal tumors (PNET)	Blue, small, round cells with Homer-Wright pseudorosettes
Meningioma	• Second most common primary brain tumor • Dural convexities; parasagittal region	• Attaches to the dura, compresses underlying brain without invasion • Microscopic—**psammoma bodies**
Schwannoma	• Third most common primary brain tumor • Most frequent location: **CN VIII at cerebellopontine angle** • **Hearing loss, tinnitus** • Good prognosis after surgical resection	• Antoni A (hypercellular) and B (hypocellular) areas • **Bilateral acoustic schwannomas—pathognomonic for neurofibromatosis type 2**
Retinoblastoma	• Sporadic—unilateral • **Familial—bilateral; associated with osteosarcoma**	Small, round, blue cells; may have rosettes
Craniopharyngioma	• Derived from odontogenic epithelium (remnants of **Rathke pouch**) • Usually children and young adults • Often calcified • Symptoms due to encroachment on pituitary stalk or optic chiasm • Benign but may recur	Histology resembles **adamantinoma** (most common tumor of tooth)

Definition of abbreviation: GFAP, glial fibrillary acidic protein.

Spinal Cord

The spinal cord is divided internally into 31 segments that give rise to **31 pairs of spinal nerves** (from rostral to caudal): **8 cervical**, **12 thoracic**, **5 lumbar**, **5 sacral**, and **1 coccygeal**. Each segment is divided into an inner butterfly-like gray matter containing neuronal cell bodies and a surrounding area of white matter. The ventral horn contains alpha and gamma motoneurons; the intermediate horn contains preganglionic neurons and Clarke's nucleus; and the dorsal horn contains sensory neurons. The outer covering of the spinal cord is the white matter containing ascending and descending axons that form tracts located within funiculi.

► General Spinal Cord Features

Conus medullaris	Caudal end of the spinal cord (S3–S5). In adult, ends at the L2 vertebra
Cauda equina	Nerve roots of the lumbar, sacral, and coccygeal spinal nerves
Filum terminale	Slender pial extension that tethers the spinal cord to the bottom of the vertebral column
Doral root ganglia	Cell bodies of primary sensory neurons
Dorsal and ventral roots	Each segment has a pair
Dorsal	**In (sensory)**
Ventral	**Out (motor)**
Spinal nerve	Formed from dorsal and ventral roots (mixed nerve)
Cervical enlargement	(C4–T1) → branchial plexus → upper limbs
Lumbar enlargement	(L2–S3) → lumbar and sacral plexuses → lower limbs

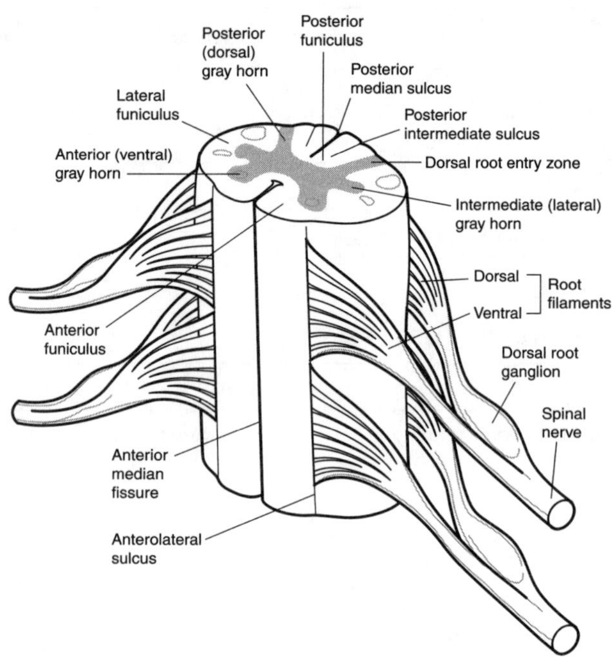

The following figure shows additional features of the spinal cord, such as the gray and white communicating rami, which are part of the autonomic nervous system.

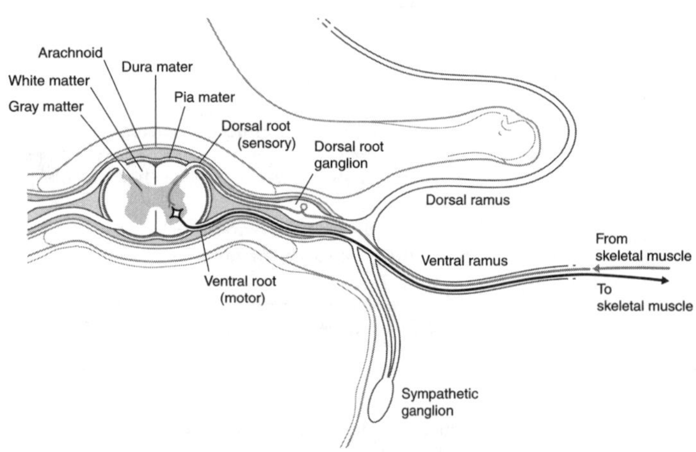

Communicating Rami

Gray communicating rami contain **unmyelinated postganglionic sympathetic** fibers at all levels of spinal cord.

White communicating rami contain **myelinated preganglionic sympathetic** fibers from T1–L3.

Gray Matter

Dorsal horn: sensory comes in

Intermediate zone: has preganglionic nerve cell bodies; Clarke's column (C8–L3)

Ventral horn: has alpha and gamma motoneuron cell bodies; motor goes out

White Matter

Tract: a collection of axons with the same origin, function, and termination; are named by stating site of origin followed by site of termination, e.g., corticospinal (cortex → spinal cord)
Fasciculi: bundle of axons
Funiculi: a region of white matter (dorsal, lateral, ventral) that may have functionally different fasciculi

► Descending Pathways

The most essential descending pathway is that which mediates voluntary skilled motor activity. This is formed by the **upper motor neuron (UMN; corticospinal tract)** and the **lower motor neuron (LMN)**.

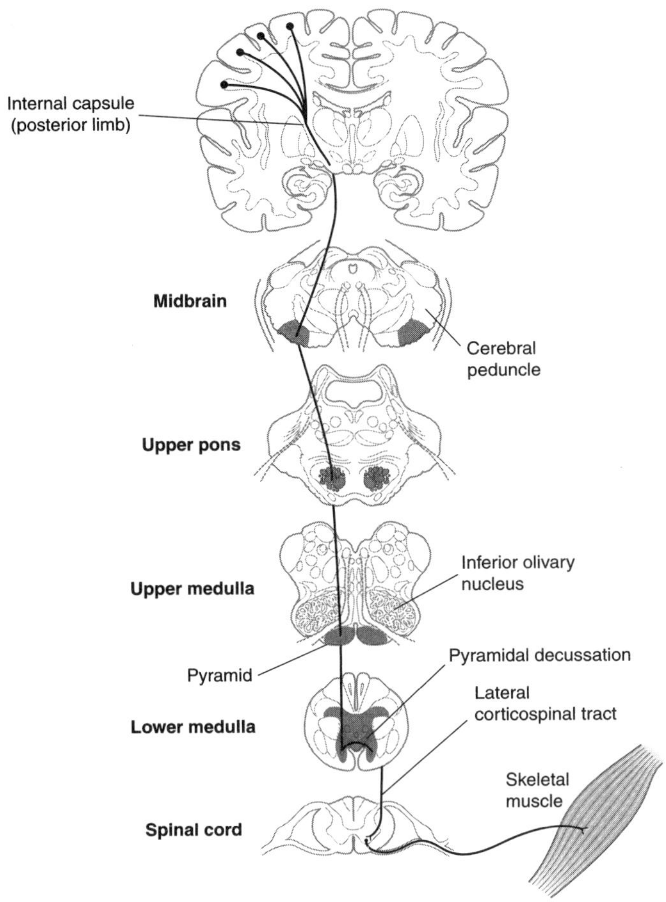

Voluntary Motor System

Function: voluntary refined movements of distal extremities

Components:

1. **Upper motor neuron (UMN):** cortex → ventral horn
2. **Lower motor neuron (LMN):** ventral horn → skeletal muscle

Lateral Corticospinal Tract

Cortex (primary motor, premotor, primary sensory)
↓
Posterior limb of **internal capsule**
↓
Crus cerebri (midbrain)
↓
Base of **pons**
↓
Pyramids (medulla)
↓
Pyramidal decussation (80–90% cross)
↓
Lateral corticospinal tract (spinal cord)
↓
Ventral horn (spinal cord): **synapse**

Note: The 10–20% of fibers that do not cross descend as the anterior corticospinal tract.

► Upper versus Lower Motor Neuron Lesions

Clinical Signs	Upper Motor Neuron	Lower Motor Neuron
Paralysis	Spastic	Flaccid
Muscle tone	Hypertonia	Hypotonia
Muscle bulk	Disuse atrophy	Atrophy, fasciculations
Deep tendon reflexes	Hyperreflexia	Hyporeflexia
Pathologic reflexes	Babinski	None
Area of body involved:		
Size:	Large	Small
Side:	Contralateral if above decussation; ipsilateral if below decussation	Ipsilateral

► Commonly Tested Muscle Stretch Reflexes

The **deep tendon (stretch, myotatic) reflex** is monosynaptic and ipsilateral. The **afferent limb** consists of a **muscle spindle receptor, Ia sensory neuron,** and **efferent limb (lower motor neuron)**. These reflexes are useful in the clinical exam.

Reflex	Cord Segment Involved	Muscle Tested
Knee (patellar)	L2–L4	Quadriceps
Ankle	S1	Gastrocnemius
Biceps	C5–C6	Biceps
Triceps	C7–C8	Triceps
Forearm	C5–C6	Brachioradialis

► Ascending Pathways

The two most important ascending pathways use a three-neuron system to convey sensory information to the cortex. Key general features are listed below.

Pathway	Function	Overview
Dorsal column–medial lemniscus	Discriminative touch, conscious proprioception, vibration, pressure	**3 neuron system:** 1° neuron: cell body in **DRG** 2° neuron: **decussates** 3° neuron: **thalamus (VPL)** → **cortex**
Anterolateral (spinothalamic)	Pain and temperature	

Definition of abbreviations: DRG, dorsal root ganglia; VPL, ventral posterolateral nucleus.

► Dorsal Column–Medial Lemniscus

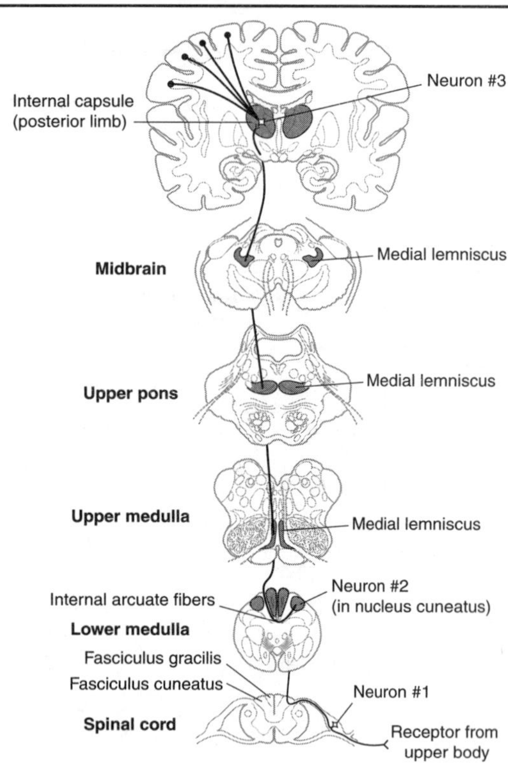

Pathway

1° neuron: cell body in **DRG**, synapses in **lower medulla**

- **Gracile fasciculus** from **lower** extremities; terminates in **gracile nucleus**
- **Cuneate fasciculus** from **upper** extremities; terminates in **cuneate nucleus**

2° neuron: decussates as **internal arcuate fibers**; ascends as **medial lemniscus**; synapses in **VPL** of the thalamus

3° neuron: VPL → somatosensory cortex

Clinical Correlation

If lesion is **above decussation** → **contralateral** loss of function

If lesion is in **spinal cord** → **ipsilateral** loss of function

Lesion can → **Romberg sign** (sways when standing, feet together, and eyes closed; swaying with eyes open indicates cerebellar dysfunction)

▶ Anterolateral (Spinothalamic)

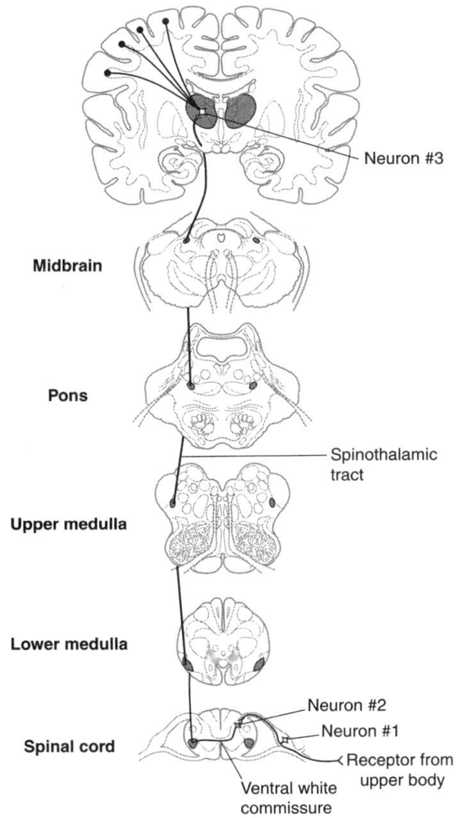

Pathway

1° neuron: cell body in **DRG**, enters cord via dorsolateral tract of Lissauer (ascends or descends one or two segments), **synapses in dorsal horn** of spinal cord. Fibers are **A-δ** (fast) or **C** (slow).

2° neuron: decussates as **ventral white commissure**; ascends in **lateral spinothalamic tract**; synapses in **VPL**

3° neuron: VPL → somatosensory cortex

Clinical Correlation

Lesion of lateral spinothalamic tract → loss of pain and temperature sensation on **contralateral** body, starting one or two segments below lesion

▶ Classic Spinal Cord Lesions

There are several classic and very testable spinal cord syndromes. An understanding of basic spinal cord anatomy makes the symptoms easy to predict.

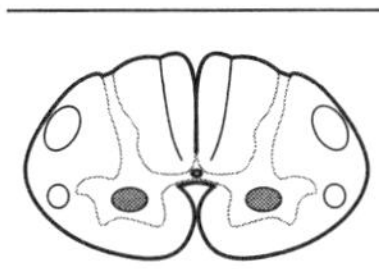

Polio
a. Flaccid paralysis
b. Muscle atrophy
c. Fasciculations
d. Areflexive

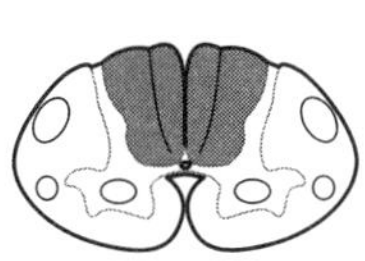

Tabes dorsalis
a. Bilateral dorsal column signs below lesions
b. Associated with late stage syphilis, plus Romberg sign: sways with eyes closed; Argyll Robertson pupils

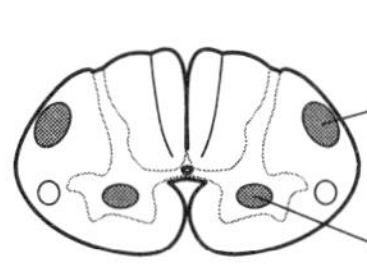

Amyotrophic lateral sclerosis (ALS)
a. Primary lateral sclerosis (corticospinal tract)
 • Spastic paralysis in lower limbs
 • Increased tone and reflexes
 • Flaccid paralysis in upper limbs
b. Progressive spinal muscular atrophy (ventral horn)

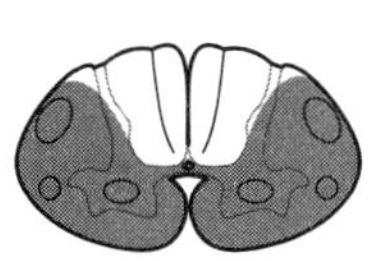

Anterior spinal artery (ASA) occlusion
a. DC spared
b. All else bilateral signs

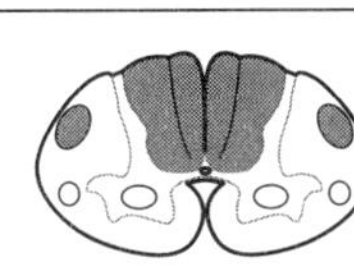

Subacute combined degeneration
a. Vitamin B_{12}, pernicious anemia; AIDS
b. Demyelination of the:
 • Dorsal columns
 • Corticospinal tracts (CST)

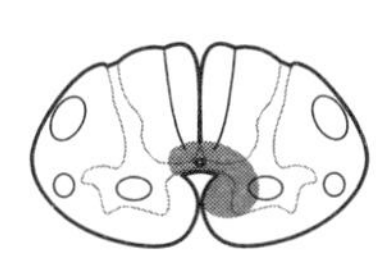

Syringomyelia
a. Cavitation of the cord (usually cervical)
b. Bilateral loss of pain and temperature at the level of the lesion
c. As the disease progresses, there is muscle weakness; eventually flaccid paralysis and atrophy of the upper limb muscles due to destruction of ventral horn cells

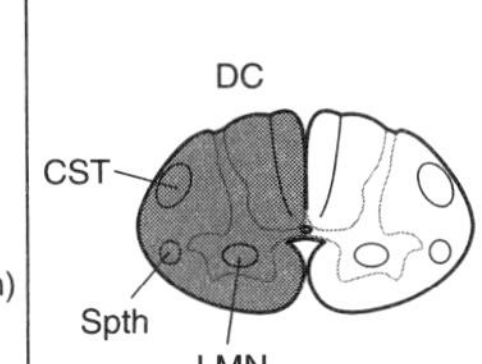

Hemisection: Brown-Séquard syndrome
a. DC: Ipsilateral loss of position and vibratory senses at and below level of the lesion
b. Spinothalamic tract: Contralateral loss of P&T below lesion and bilateral loss at the level of the lesion
c. CST: Ipsilateral paresis below the level of the lesion
d. LMN: Flaccid paralysis at the level of the lesion
e. Descending hypothalamics: Ipsilateral Horner syndrome (if cord lesion is above T_1)
 • Facial hemianhydrosis
 • Ptosis (slight)
 • Miosis

Definition of abbreviations: DC, dorsal column; LMN, lower motor neuron.

Cranial Nerves and Brain Stem

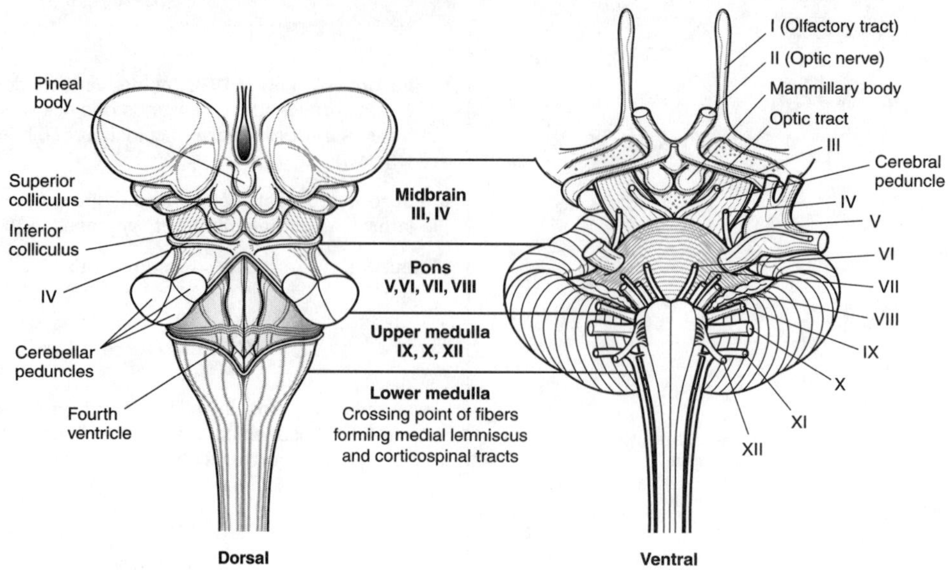

► Cranial Nerves: Functional Features

CN	Name	Type	Function	Results of Lesions
I	Olfactory	Sensory	Smells	Anosmia
II	Optic	Sensory	Sees	Visual field deficits (anopsia) Loss of light reflex with III Only nerve to be affected by MS
III	Oculomotor	Motor	Innervates SR, IR, MR, IO extraocular muscles: adduction (MR) most important action Raises eyelid (levator palpebrae superioris)	Diplopia, external strabismus Loss of parallel gaze Ptosis
			Constricts pupil (sphincter pupillae) Accommodates (ciliary muscle)	Dilated pupil, loss of light reflex with II Loss of near response
IV	Trochlear	Motor	Superior oblique—depresses and abducts eyeball (makes eyeball look down and out) Intorts	Weakness looking down with adducted eye Trouble going down stairs Head tilts away from lesioned side
V	Trigeminal	Mixed		
	Ophthalmic (V1)		General sensation (touch, pain, temperature) of forehead/scalp/cornea	V1—loss of general sensation in skin of forehead/scalp Loss of blink reflex with VII
	Maxillary (V2)		General sensation of palate, nasal cavity, maxillary face, maxillary teeth	V2—loss of general sensation in skin over maxilla, maxillary teeth
	Mandibular (V3)		General sensation of anterior two thirds of tongue, mandibular face, mandibular teeth	V3—loss of general sensation in skin over mandible, mandibular teeth, tongue, weakness in chewing
			Motor to muscles of mastication (temporalis, masseter, medial and lateral pterygoids) and anterior belly of digastric, mylohyoid, tensor tympani, tensor palati	Jaw deviation toward weak side Trigeminal neuralgia—intractable pain in V2 or V3 territory

Definition of abbreviations: IO, inferior oblique; MR, medial rectus; IR, inferior rectus; MS, multiple sclerosis; SR, superior rectus.

(*Continued*)

▶ Cranial Nerves: Functional Features (*Cont'd.*)

CN	Name	Type	Function	Results of Lesions
VI	Abducens	Motor	Lateral rectus—abducts eyeball	Diplopia, internal strabismus Loss of parallel gaze, "pseudoptosis"
VII	Facial	Mixed	To muscles of facial expression, posterior belly of digastric, stylohyoid, stapedius Salivation (submandibular, sublingual glands) Taste in anterior two thirds of tongue/palate Tears (lacrimal gland)	Corner of mouth droops, cannot close eye, cannot wrinkle forehead, loss of blink reflex, hyperacusis; Bell palsy—lesion of nerve in facial canal Alteration or loss of taste (ageusia) Eye dry and red
VIII	Vestibulocochlear	Sensory	Hearing Angular acceleration (head turning) Linear acceleration (gravity)	Sensorineural hearing loss Loss of balance, nystagmus
IX	Glossopharyngeal	Mixed	Sense of pharynx, carotid sinus/body Salivation (parotid gland) Taste and somatosensation of posterior one third of tongue Motor to one muscle—stylopharyngeus	Loss of gag reflex with X
X	Vagus	Mixed	To muscles of palate and pharynx for swallowing except tensor palati (V) and stylopharyngeus (IX) To all muscles of larynx (phonates) Sensory of larynx and laryngopharynx Sensory of GI tract To GI tract smooth muscle and glands in foregut and midgut	Nasal speech, nasal regurgitation Dysphagia, palate droop Uvula pointing away from affected side Hoarseness/fixed vocal cord Loss of gag reflex with IX Loss of cough reflex
XI	Accessory	Motor	Head rotation to opposite side (sternocleidomastoid) Elevates and rotates scapula (trapezius)	Weakness turning head to opposite side Shoulder droop
XII	Hypoglossal	Motor	Tongue movement (styloglossus, hyoglossus, genioglossus, and intrinsic tongue muscles—palatoglossus is by X)	Tongue pointing toward same (affected) side on protrusion

▶ Skull Base Anatomy

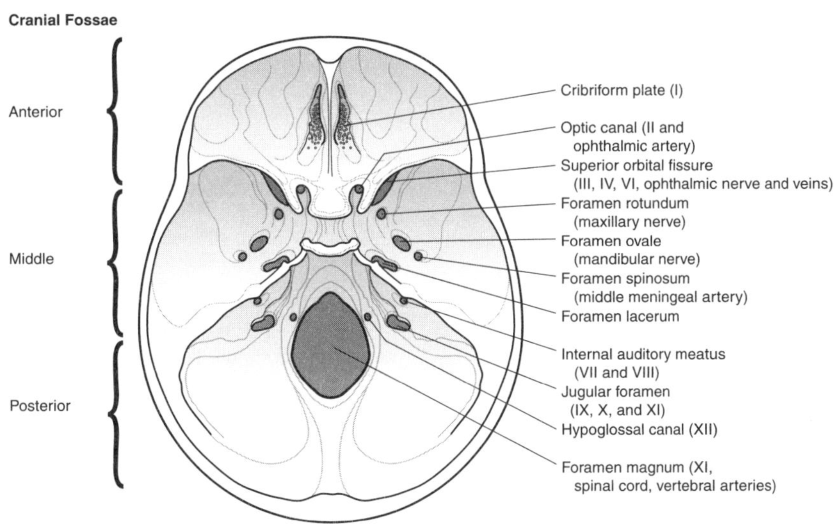

Visual System

▶ Visual Field Defects

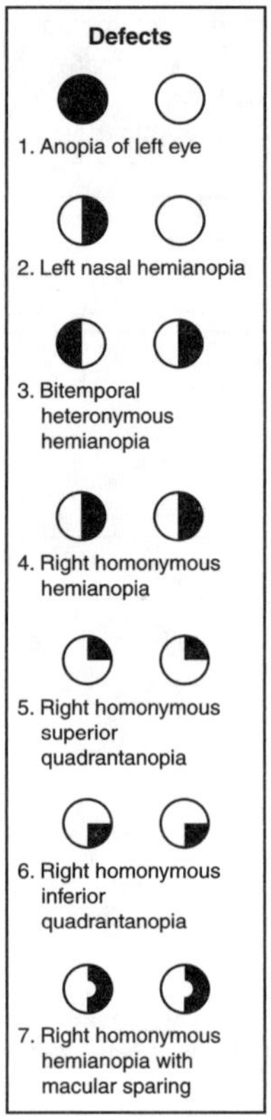

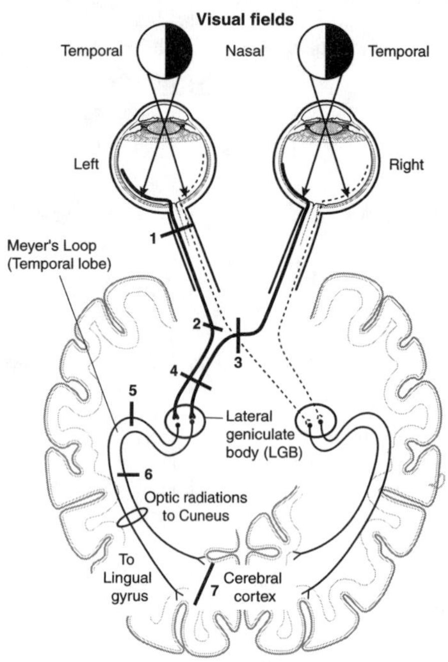

Notes

Like a camera, the lens inverts the image of the visual field, so the nasal retina receives information from the temporal visual field, and the temporal retina receives information from the nasal visual field.

At the **optic chiasm**, optic nerve fibers from the nasal half of each retina cross and project to the contralateral optic tract.

Most fibers from the **optic tract** project to the **lateral geniculate body (LGB)**; some also project to the pretectal area (light reflex), the superior colliculi (reflex gaze), and the suprachiasmatic nuclei (circadian rhythm). The LGB projects to the **primary visual cortex** (striate cortex, Brodmann area 17) of the occipital lobe via the optic radiations.

- Visual information from the lower retina (upper contralateral visual field) → temporal lobe (**Meyer loop**) → **lingual gyrus**
- Visual information from the upper retina (lower contralateral visual field) → parietal lobe → **cuneus gyrus**

Clinical Correlate (Some Causes of Lesions)

1. Optic neuritis, central retinal artery occlusion
2. Internal carotid artery aneurysm
3. Pituitary adenoma, craniopharyngioma
5. Middle cerebral artery (MCA) occlusion
6, 7. Posterior cerebral artery occlusion
Macula is spared in 7 due to collateral blood supply from MCA.

▶ Anatomy of the Eye and Glaucoma

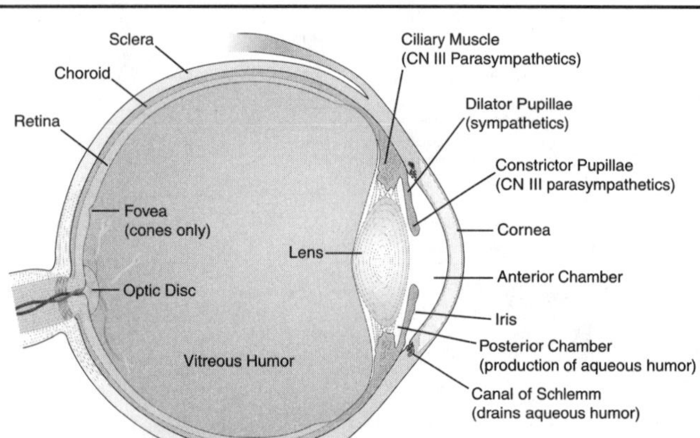

Open-Angle Glaucoma

A chronic condition (often with increased intraocular pressure [IOP]) due to decreased reabsorption of aqueous humor, leading to progressive (painless) visual loss and, if left untreated, blindness. IOP is a balance between fluid formation and its drainage from the globe.

Narrow-Angle Glaucoma

An acute (painful) or chronic (genetic) condition with increased IOP due to blockade of the canal of Schlemm. Emergency treatment prior to surgery often involves cholinomimetics, carbonic anhydrase inhibitors, and/or mannitol.

▶ Pharmacology of the Eye

The eye is predominantly innervated by the parasympathetic nervous system. Therefore, application of muscarinic antagonists or ganglionic blockers has a large effect by blocking the parasympathetic nervous system.

Structure	Predominant Receptor	Receptor Stimulation	Receptor Blockade
Pupillary sphincter ms. (iris)	M_3 receptor (PANS)	Contraction → miosis	Relaxation → mydriasis
Radial dilator ms. (iris)	α receptor (SANS)	Contraction → mydriasis	Relaxation → miosis
Ciliary ms.	M_3 receptor (PANS)	Contraction → accommodation for near vision	Relaxation → focus for far vision
Ciliary body epithelium	β receptor (SANS)	Secretion of aqueous humor	Decreased aqueous humor production

Definition of abbreviations: ms., muscle; PANS, parasympathetic nervous system; SANS, sympathetic nervous system.

▶ Drugs Used to Treat Glaucoma

Drug Class	Drug	Mechanism
Cholinomimetics (miotics)	Pilocarpine (M agonist) Carbachol (M agonist) Physostigmine (AChEI) Echothiophate (AChEI)	Contracts ciliary muscle and opens trabecular meshwork, increasing the outflow of aqueous humor through the canal of Schlemm
Beta blockers	Timolol (nonselective) Betaxolol (β_1)	Blocks actions of NE at ciliary epithelium to ↓ aqueous humor secretion
Prostaglandins	Latanoprost ($PGF_{2\alpha}$ analog)	↑ aqueous humor outflow; can darken the iris
Alpha agonists	Epinephrine Dipivefrin	↑ aqueous humor outflow
Alpha-2 agonists	Apraclonidine Brimonidine	↓ aqueous humor secretion
Diuretics	Acetazolamide (oral; CAI) Dorzolamide, brinzolamide (topical; CAI) Mannitol (for narrow-angle; osmotic)	CAI: ↓ HCO_3^- → ↓ aqueous humor secretion

Definition of abbreviations: AChEI, acetylcholinesterase inhibitor; CAI, carbonic anhydrase inhibitor; M, muscarinic cholinergic receptor.

▶ Pupillary Light Reflex Pathway

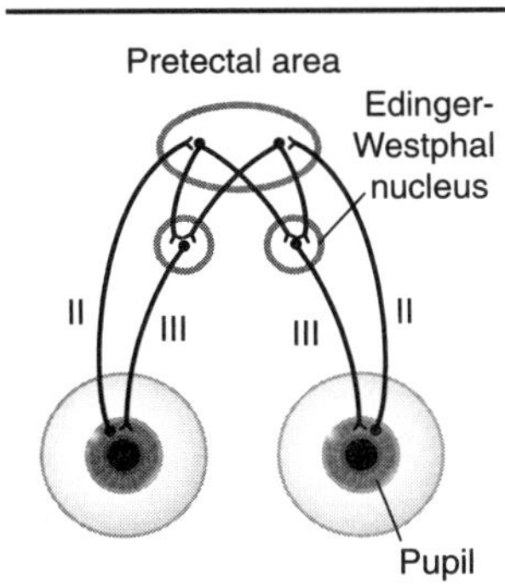

Afferent Limb: CN II

Light stimulates ganglion retinal cells → impulses travel up **CNII**, which projects **bilaterally** to the **pretectal nuclei** (midbrain)

The pretectal nucleus projects **bilaterally** → **Edinger-Westphal nuclei (CN III)**

Efferent Limb: CN III

Edinger-Westphal nucleus (preganglionic parasympathetic) → **ciliary ganglion** (postganglionic parasympathetic) → **pupillary sphincter muscle** → **miosis**

Note: This is a simplified diagram; the ciliary ganglion is not shown.

Because cells in the pretectal area supply the Edinger-Westphal nuclei bilaterally, shining light in one eye → constriction in the ipsilateral pupil (direct light reflex) and the contralateral pupil (consensual light reflex).

Because this reflex does not involve the visual cortex, a person who is cortically blind can still have this reflex.

▶ Accommodation–Convergence Reaction

When an individual focuses on a nearby object after looking at a distant object, three events occur:

1. **Accommodation**
2. **Convergence**
3. **Pupillary constriction (miosis)**

In general, stimuli from light → visual cortex → superior colliculus and pretectal nucleus → Edinger-Westphal nucleus (1, 3) and oculomotor nucleus (2).

Accommodation: Parasympathetic fibers contract the ciliary muscle, which relaxes suspensory ligaments, allowing the lens to increase its convexity (become more round). This increases the refractive index of the lens, thereby focusing a nearby object on the retina.

Convergence: Both medial rectus muscles contract, adducting both eyes.

Pupillary constriction: Parasympathetic fibers contract the pupillary sphincter muscle → miosis.

▶ Clinical Correlations

Pupillary Abnormalities	
Argyll Robertson pupil (pupillary light-near dissociation)	No direct or consensual light reflex; accommodation-convergence intact Seen in **neurosyphilis**, diabetes
Relative afferent (Marcus Gunn) pupil	Lesion of afferent limb of pupillary light reflex; diagnosis made with swinging flashlight Shine light in Marcus Gunn pupil → pupils do not constrict fully Shine light in normal eye → pupils constrict fully Shine light immediately again in affected eye → apparent dilation of both pupils because stimulus carried through that CN II is weaker; seen in multiple sclerosis
Horner syndrome	Caused by a lesion of the oculosympathetic pathway; syndrome consists of miosis, ptosis, apparent enophthalmos, and hemianhidrosis
Adie pupil	Dilated pupil that reacts sluggishly to light, but better to accommodation; often seen in women and often associated with loss of knee jerks
Transentorial (uncal) herniation	Increased intracranial pressure → leads to uncal herniation → CN III compression → fixed and dilated pupil, "down-and-out" eye, ptosis

► Eye Movement Control Systems

Extraocular Muscles: Function and Innervation

CN III	**Medial rectus:** adducts eye **Superior rectus:** elevates, intorts, adducts eye **Inferior rectus:** depresses, extorts, adducts eye **Inferior oblique:** elevates, extorts, abducts eye	**CN IV**	**Superior oblique:** depresses, intorts, abducts eye
		CN VI	**Lateral rectus:** Abducts eye

Two important eye movements are **abduction** (away from nose, **CN VI**) and **adduction** (toward nose, **CN III**).

For the eyes to move together **(conjugate gaze)**, the oculomotor nuclei and abducens nuclei are interconnected by the **medial longitudinal fasciculus (MLF)**.

Horizontal gaze is controlled by two gaze centers:

1. **Frontal eye field** (contralateral gaze)
2. **PPRF** (paramedial pontine reticular formation, ipsilateral gaze)

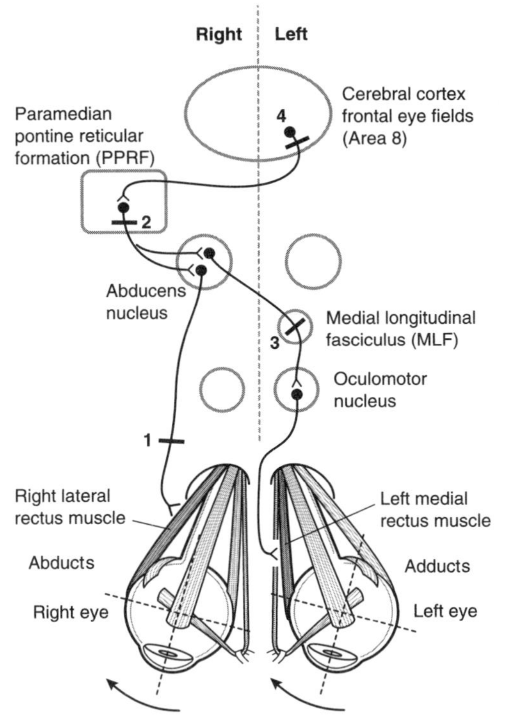

(Lesion sites are indicated by 1-4)

Clinical Correlation

Lesion Examples	Symptoms
1. Right CN VI	Right eye cannot look right
2. Right PPRF	Neither eye can look right
3. Left MLF	**Internuclear ophthalmoplegia (INO)** Left eye cannot look right; convergence is intact (this is how to distinguish an INO from an oculomotor lesion); right eye has nystagmus; seen in multiple sclerosis
4. Left frontal eye field	Neither eye can look right; but slow drift to left

▶ Trigeminal Nerve (V)

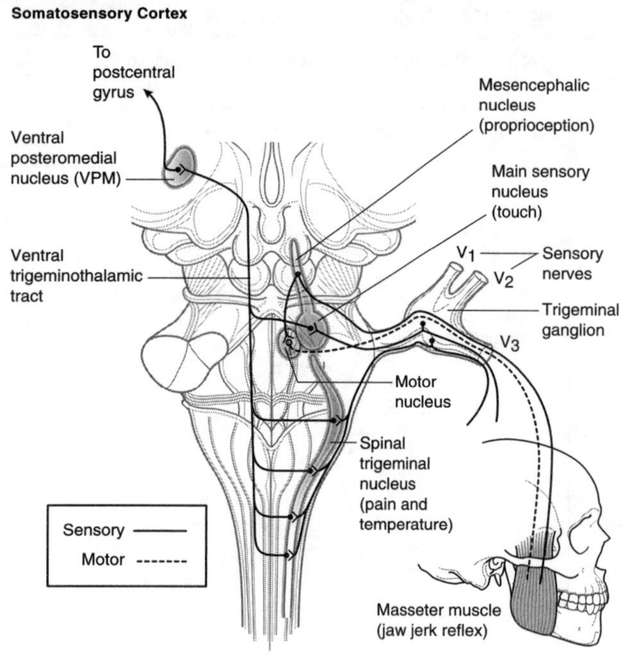

▶ Facial Nerve (VII)

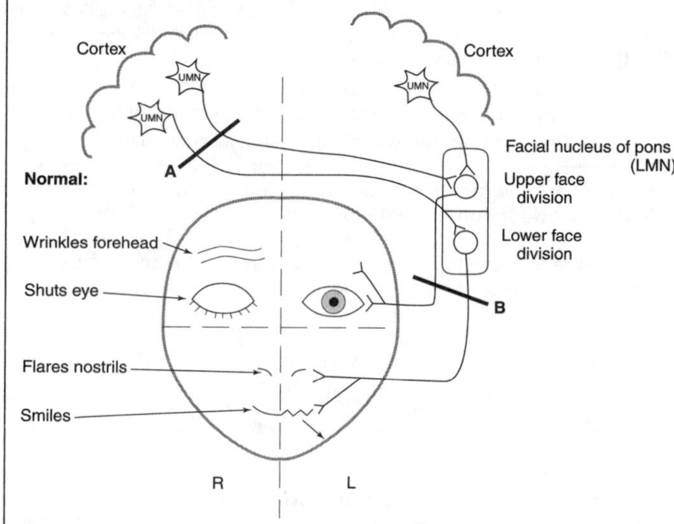

A. **Upper motor neuron lesion** → weakness of **contralateral lower face**
B. **Lower motor neuron lesion** → paralysis of **ipsilateral upper and lower face (Bell palsy)**

▶ Vestibular System (VIII)

Three semicircular ducts respond to **angular acceleration and deceleration** of the head. The **utricle** and **saccule** respond to **linear acceleration** and the pull of **gravity**. There are four **vestibular nuclei** in the medulla and pons, which receive information from CN VIII. Fibers from the vestibular nuclei join the MLF and supply the motor nuclei of CNs III, IV, and VI, thereby regulating conjugate eye movements. Vestibular nuclei also receive and send information to the **flocculonodular lobe** of the cerebellum.

Vestibulo-Ocular Reflex

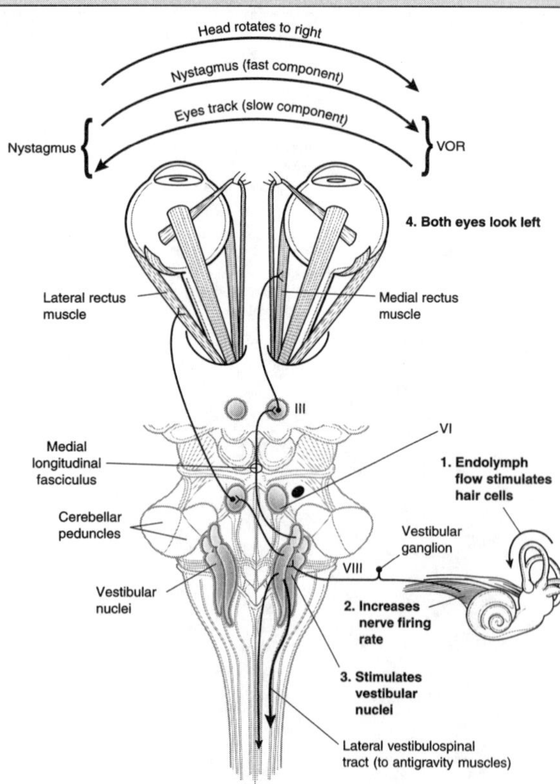

Caloric Test

This stimulates the horizontal semicircular ducts; can be used as a test of brain stem function in unconscious patients.

Normal results:

- **Cold water** irrigation of ear → nystagmus to opposite side
- **Warm water** irrigation of ear → nystagmus to same side
- **COWS:** cold opposite, warm same

Clinical Correlation

Vertigo: the perception of rotation. Usually severe in peripheral disease and mild in brain stem disease. Chronic vertigo suggests a central lesion.

Ménière disease: characterized by abrupt, recurrent attacks of vertigo lasting minutes to hours; accompanied by deafness or tinnitus and is usually in one ear. Nausea and vomiting may occur. Due to distention of fluid spaces in the cochlear and vestibular parts of the labyrinth.

▶ Auditory System (VIII)

Inner Ear

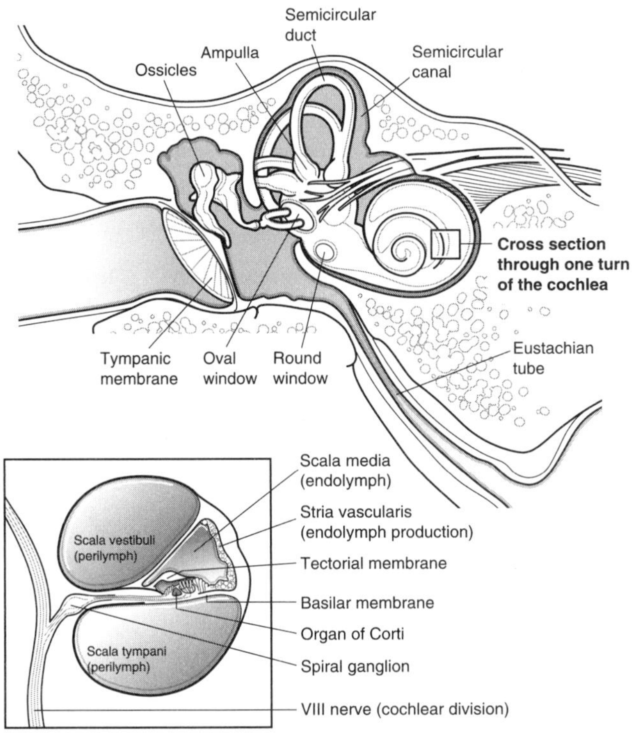

Auditory Pathways

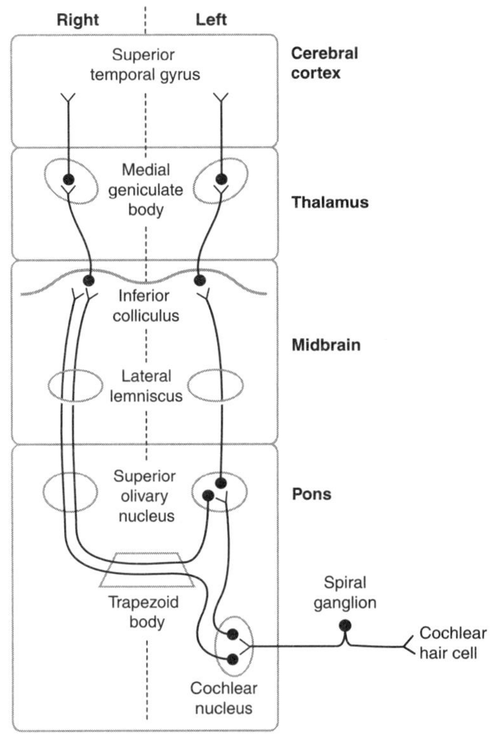

Deafness

Conduction deafness: passage of sound waves through external or middle ear is interrupted

Causes: obstruction, otosclerosis, otitis media

Sensorineural deafness: damage to cochlea, CN VIII, or central auditory connections

- Lesions to CN VIII or cochlear nuclei → **ipsilateral** sensorineural hearing loss
- Lesions to all other auditory structures in brainstem, thalamus, or cortex → **bilateral** ↓ in hearing and ↓ ability to localize sound

Auditory Tests

Weber test: place tuning fork on vertex of skull. If **unilateral conduction deafness** → vibration is louder in affected ear; if **unilateral sensorineural deafness** → vibration is louder in normal ear

Rinne test: place tuning fork on mastoid process (bone conduction) until vibration is not heard, then place fork in front of ear (air conduction). If **unilateral conduction deafness** → no air conduction after bone conduction is gone; if **unilateral sensorineural deafness** → air conduction present after bone conduction is gone

Brain Stem Lesions

▶ Medulla

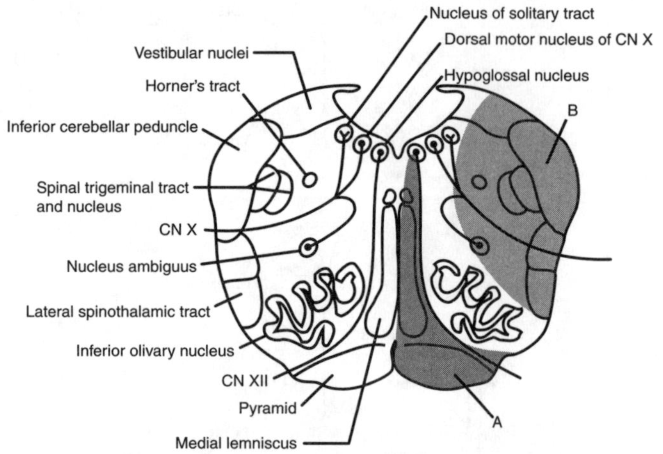

Medial Medullary Syndrome (A)
Anterior Spinal Artery

Pyramid: contralateral spastic paresis (body)

Medial lemniscus: contralateral loss of tactile, vibration, conscious proprioception (body)

XII nucleus/fibers: ipsilateral flaccid paralysis of tongue

Lateral Medullary Syndrome (B)
PICA, Wallenberg Syndrome

Inferior cerebellar peduncle: ipsilateral limb ataxia
Vestibular nuclei: vertigo, nausea/vomiting, nystagmus (away from lesion)
Nucleus ambiguus (CN IX, X, XI): ipsilateral paralysis of larynx, pharynx, palate → dysarthria, dysphagia, loss of gag reflex
Spinal V: ipsilateral pain/temperature loss (face)
Spinothalamic tract: Contralateral pain/temperature loss (body)
Descending hypothalamics: ipsilateral Horner syndrome

▶ Pons

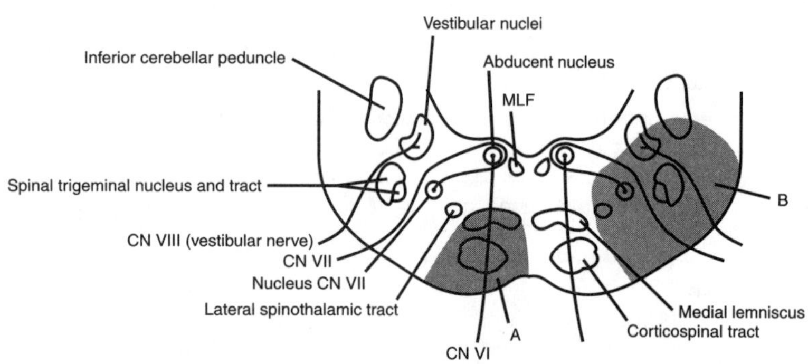

Medial Pontine Syndrome (A)
Paramedian Branches of Basilar Artery

Corticospinal tract: contralateral spastic hemiparesis

Medial lemniscus: contralateral loss of tactile/position/vibration sensation on body

Fibers of VI: medial strabismus

Lateral Pontine Syndrome (B)
AICA

Middle cerebellar peduncle: ipsilateral ataxia
Vestibular nuclei: vertigo, nausea and vomiting, nystagmus
Facial nucleus and fibers: ipsilateral facial paralysis; ipsilateral loss of taste (anterior 2/3 tongue), lacrimation, salivation, and corneal reflex; hyperacusis
Spinal trigeminal nucleus/tract: ipsilateral pain/temperature loss (face)
Spinothalamic tract: contralateral pain/temperature loss (body)
Cochlear nucleus/VIII fibers: ipsilateral hearing loss
Descending sympathetics: ipsilateral Horner syndrome

▶ Midbrain

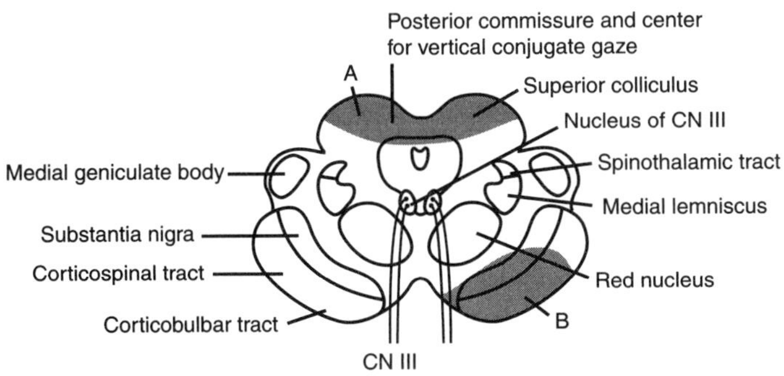

Dorsal Midbrain (Parinaud) Syndrome (A) Tumor in Pineal Region
Superior colliculus/pretectal area: paralysis of upward gaze, various pupillary abnormalities **Cerebral aqueduct:** noncommunicating hydrocephalus

Medial Midbrain (Weber) Syndrome (B) Branches of PCA
Fibers of III: ipsilateral oculomotor palsy (lateral strabismus, dilated pupil, ptosis) **Corticospinal tract:** contralateral spastic hemiparesis **Corticobulbar tract:** contralateral spastic hemiparesis of lower face

Cerebellum

The cerebellum controls posture, muscle tone, learning of repeated motor functions, and coordinates voluntary motor activity. Diseases of the cerebellum result in disturbances of gait, balance, and coordinated motor actions, but there is no paralysis or inability to start or stop movement.

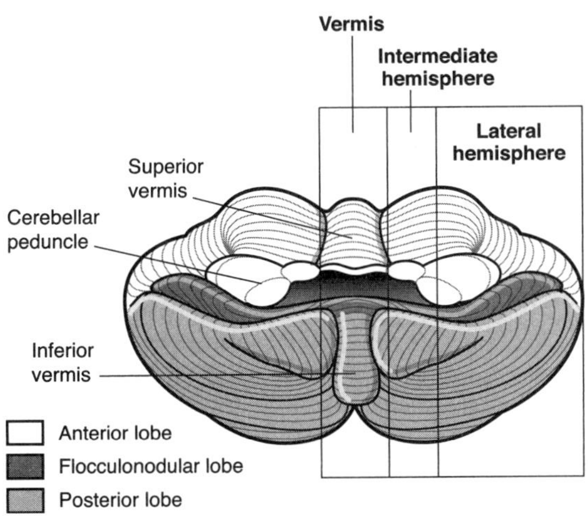

Input
Climbing fibers (from inferior olivary nucleus of medulla), **mossy fibers** (from vestibular nucleus, spinal cord, pons); most input via **ICP** and **MCP**

Output
From deep cerebellar nucleus (fastigial, interpositus, dentate); most output via **SCP**

Three Layers
Molecular, Purkinje, granule cell

Major Pathway	Dysfunction
Purkinje cells → deep cerebellar nucleus; dentate nucleus → contralateral VL → 1° motor cortex → pontine nuclei → contralateral cerebellar cortex	• **Hemisphere lesions** → ipsilateral symptoms; **intention** tremor, dysmetria, dysdiadochokinesia, scanning dysarthria, nystagmus, hypotonia • **Vermal lesions** → truncal ataxia

Definition of abbreviations: ICP, inferior cerebellar peduncle; MCP, middle cerebellar peduncle; SCP, superior cerebellar peduncle; VL, ventral lateral nucleus.

Diencephalon

Thalamus, Hypothalamus, Epithalamus, Subthalamus

Thalamus—serves as a major sensory relay for information that ultimately reaches the neocortex. Motor control areas (basal ganglia, cerebellum) also synapse in the thalamus before reaching the cortex. Other nuclei regulate states of consciousness.

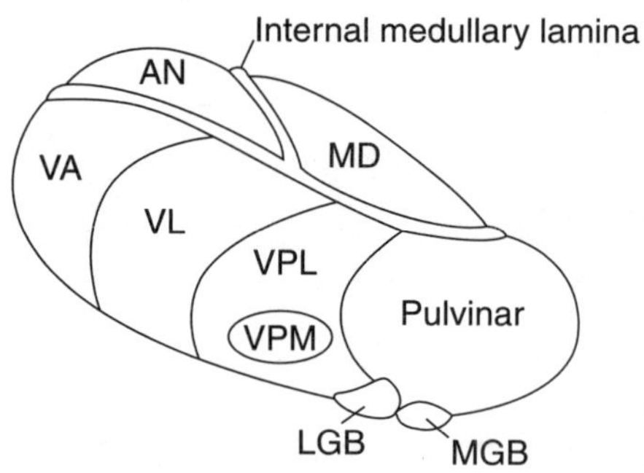

THALAMIC NUCLEI	INPUT	OUTPUT
VPL	Sensory from **body and limbs**	Somatosensory cortex
VPM	Sensory from **face**	Somatosensory cortex
VA/VL	**Motor** info from BG, cerebellum	Motor cortices
LGB	**Visual** from optic tract	1° visual cortex
MGB	**Auditory** from inferior colliculus	1° auditory cortex
AN	Mammillary nucleus (via mamillothalamic tract)	Cingulate gyrus (part of **Papez** circuit)
MD	(Dorsomedial nucleus). Involved in **memory** Damaged in **Wernicke-Korsakoff** syndrome	
Pulvinar	Helps integrate somesthetic, visual, and auditory input	
Midline/intralaminar	Involved in **arousal**	

Hypothalamus—helps maintain homeostasis; has roles in the autonomic, endocrine, and limbic systems

HYPOTHALAMIC NUCLEI	FUNCTIONS AND LESIONS
Lateral hypothalamic	**Feeding center;** lesion → starvation
Ventromedial	**Satiety center;** lesion → hyperphagia, obesity, savage behavior
Suprachiasmatic	Regulates circadian rhythms
Supraoptic and paraventricular	Synthesizes **ADH** and **oxytocin; regulates water balance** Lesion → **diabetes insipidus**, characterized by polydipsia and polyuria
Mammillary body	Input from hippocampus; damaged in Wernicke encephalopathy
Arcuate	Produces hypothalamic releasing and inhibiting factors and gives rise to tuberohypophysial tract Has neurons that produce dopamine (prolactin-inhibiting factor)
Anterior	**Temperature regulation;** lesion → hyperthermia Stimulates the parasympathetic nervous system
Posterior	**Temperature regulation;** lesion → poikilothermia (inability to thermoregulate) Stimulates sympathetic nervous system
Preoptic area	Regulates release of gonotrophic hormones; contains sexually dimorphic nucleus Lesion before puberty → arrested sexual development; lesion after puberty → amenorrhea or impotence
Dorsomedial	Stimulation → savage behavior

Epithalamus—Consists of pineal body and habenular nuclei. The **pineal body** aids in the regulation of **circadian rhythms**.

Subthalamus—The **subthalamic nucleus** is involved in **basal ganglia** circuitry. Lesion → **hemiballismus** (contralateral flinging movements of one or both extremities)

Definition of abbreviations: ADH, antidiuretic hormone; AN, anterior nuclear group; BG, basal ganglia; LBG, lateral geniculate body; MD, mediodorsal nucleus; MGB, medial geniculate body; VA, ventral anterior nucleus; VL, ventral lateral nucleus; VLP, ventroposterolateral nucleus; VPM, ventroposteromedial nucleus.

Basal Ganglia

The basal ganglia initiate and provide gross control over skeletal muscle movements. The basal ganglia are sometimes called the **extrapyramidal** nervous system because they modulate the pyramidal (corticospinal) nervous system.

► Basal Ganglia Components

Striatum (caudate and putamen)	**Subthalamic nucleus** (diencephalon)
Globus pallidus (external and internal segments)	**Lentiform nucleus** (globus pallidus and putamen)
Substantia nigra (midbrain)	**Corpus striatum** (lentiform nucleus and caudate)

Together with the cerebral cortex and **VA/VL** thalamic nuclei, these structures form two parallel but antagonistic circuits known as the **direct** and **indirect pathways**. The direct pathway increases cortical excitation and promotes movement, and the indirect pathway decreases cortical excitation and inhibits movement. Hypokinetic movement disorders (e.g., Parkinson disease) result in a lesion of the direct pathway, and hyperkinetic movement disorders (e.g., Huntington disease, hemiballismus) result from indirect pathway lesions.

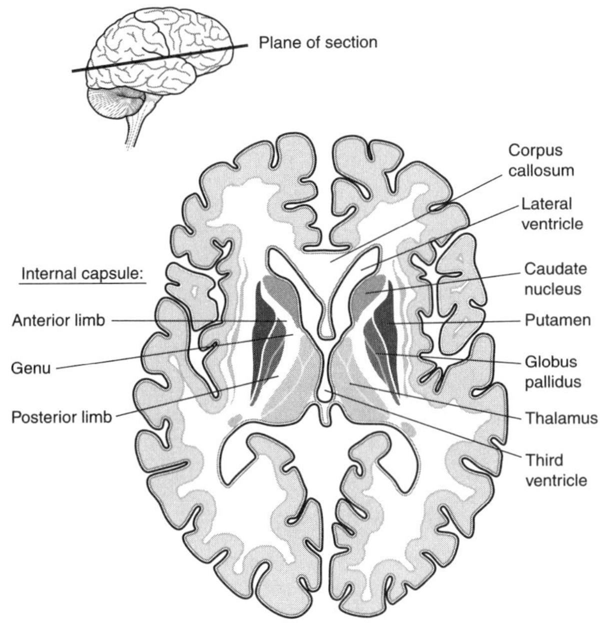

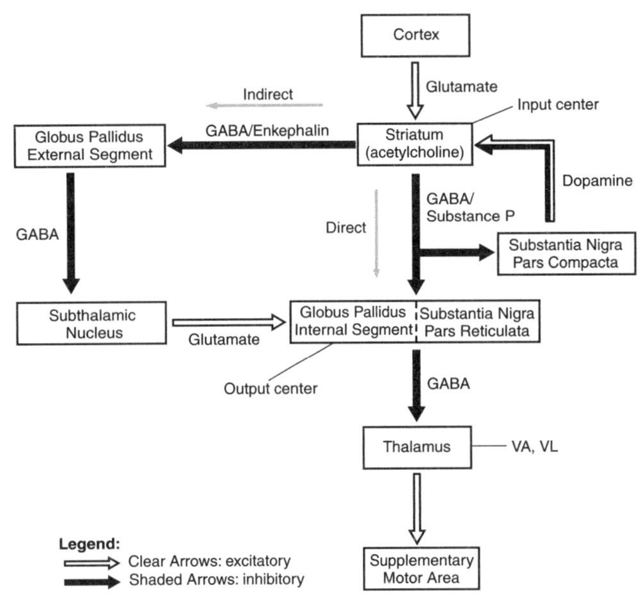

Definition of abbreviation: VA/VL, ventral anterior/ventral lateral thalamic nuclei.

► Diseases of the Basal Ganglia

Disease	Clinical Manifestations	Notes
Parkinson disease	Bradykinesia, cogwheel rigidity, pill rolling (resting) tremor, shuffling gate, stooped posture, masked facies, depression, dementia	**Loss of pigmented dopaminergic neurons from substantia nigra** **Lewy bodies:** intracytoplasmic eosinophilic inclusions, contain α-synuclein Known causes of parkinsonism: infections, vascular, and toxic insults (e.g., **MPTP**)
Huntington disease	Chorea (multiple, rapid, random movements), athetosis (slow writhing, movements), personality changes, dementia Onset: 20–40 years	**Degeneration** of GABAergic neurons in **neostriatum**, causing atrophy of neostriatum (and ventricular dilatation) **Autosomal dominant** **Unstable nucleotide repeat** on gene in chromosome 4, which codes for huntingtin protein Disease shows **anticipation** and **genomic imprinting** **Treatment:** antipsychotic agents, benzodiazepines, anticonvulsants
Wilson disease (hepatolenticular degeneration)	Tremor, asterixis, parkinsonian symptoms, chorea, neuropsychiatric symptoms; fatty change, hepatitis, or cirrhosis of liver	**Autosomal recessive defect in copper transport** Accumulation of copper in liver, brain, and eye (Descemet membrane, producing **Kayser-Fleischer ring**) Lesions in basal ganglia (especially putamen) **Treatment: penicillamine** (a chelator), zinc acetate (blocks absorption)
Hemiballism	Wild flinging movements of half the body	Hemorrhagic destruction of **contralateral subthalamic nucleus** Hypertensive patients
Tourette syndrome	Motor tics and vocal tics (e.g., snorting, sniffing, uncontrolled and often obscene vocalizations), commonly associated with OCD and ADHD	**Treatment:** Antipsychotic agents

Definition of abbreviations: ADHD, attention deficit hyperactivity disorder; MPTP, 1-methyl-4-phenyl-1,2,3,6-tetrahydropyridine; OCD, obsessive-compulsive disorder.

► Treatment for Parkinson Disease

The pharmacologic goal in the treatment of Parkinson disease is to **increase DA and/or decrease ACh** activity in the striatum, thereby correcting the DA/ACh imbalance. Additional treatment strategies include surgical intervention, such as pallidotomy, thalamotomy, deep brain stimulation, and transplantation.

Agents	Mechanism	Notes
Dopamine precursor: L-dopa	Dopamine precursor that crosses the blood–brain barrier (BBB) Converted to DA by DOPA decarboxylase (L-aromatic amino acid decarboxylase)	Side effects include on/off phenomena, dyskinesias, psychosis, postural hypotension, nausea/vomiting
DOPA decarboxylase inhibitor: carbidopa	Inhibits DOPA decarboxylase in the periphery, preventing L-dopa from being converted to dopamine in the periphery; instead, L-dopa crosses the BBB and is converted to dopamine in the brain	Often given in combination with L-dopa (Sinemet®)
DA agonists: bromocriptine pramipexole ropinirole	Stimulates D_2 receptors in the striatum; pramipexole and ropinirole are also D_3 agonists	Pramipexole and ropinirole now considered first-line drugs in the initial management of PD; pramipexole and ropinirole are also used in **restless legs syndrome**
MAO B inhibitor: selegiline rasagiline	Inhibits MAO type B, which preferentially metabolizes dopamine	Not to be taken with SSRIs (serotonin syndrome) or meperidine
Antimuscarinics: benztropine trihexyphenidyl biperiden	Blocks muscarinic receptors in the striatum	↓ tremor and rigidity, have little effect on bradykinesia Antimuscarinic side effects
COMT inhibitors: entacapone tolcapone	COMT inhibitors increase the efficacy of L-dopa. COMT metabolizes L-dopa to 3-*O*-methyldopa (3OMD), which competes with L-dopa for active transport into the CNS	Used as an adjunct to L-dopa/carbidopa, increases the “on” time
Amantadine	Increases dopaminergic neurotransmission, antimuscarinic; also an antiviral	Antimuscarinic effects, livedo reticularis

Limbic System

The limbic system is involved in emotion, memory, attention, feeding, and mating behaviors. It consists of a core of cortical and diencephalic structures found on the medial aspect of the hemisphere. The limbic system modulates feelings, such as fear, anxiety, sadness, happiness, sexual pleasure, and familiarity.

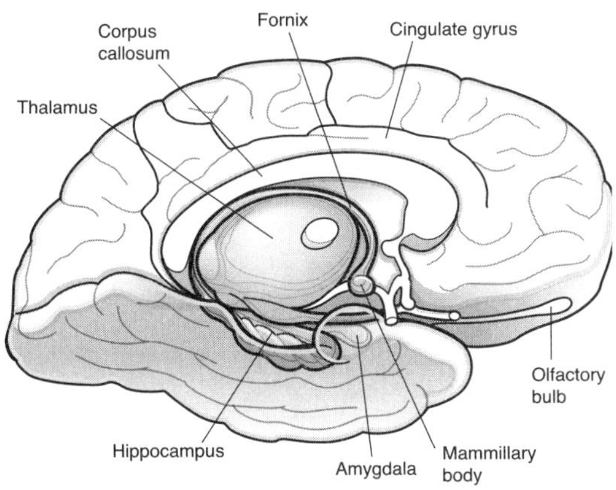

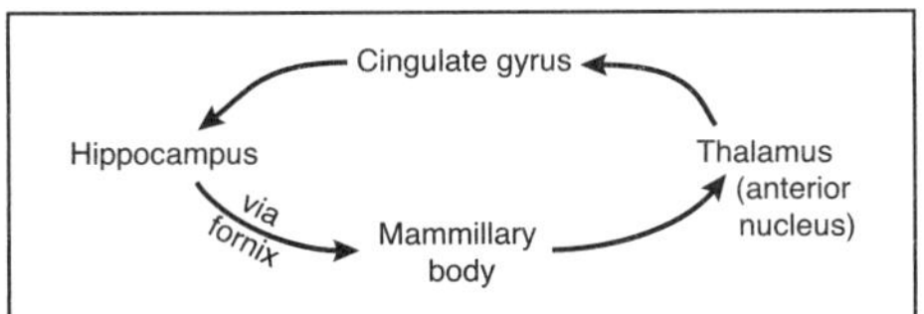

Papez Circuit

Limbic Structures and Function

- Hippocampal formation (hippocampus, dentate gyrus, the subiculum, and entorhinal cortex)
- Amygdala
- Septal nuclei
- The hippocampus is important in learning and memory. The amygdala attaches an emotional significance to a stimulus and helps imprint the emotional response in memory.

Limbic Connections

- The limbic system is interconnected with anterior and dorsomedial nuclei of the thalamus and the mammillary bodies.
- The cingulate gyrus is the main limbic cortical area.
- Limbic-related structures also project to wide areas of the prefrontal cortex.
- Central projections of olfactory structures reach parts of the temporal lobe and the amygdala.

Papez Circuit

Axons of hippocampal pyramidal cells converge to form the fimbria and, finally, the fornix. The fornix projects mainly to the mammillary bodies in the hypothalamus. The mammillary bodies project to the anterior nucleus of the thalamus (mammillothalamic tract). The anterior nuclei project to the cingulate gyrus, and the cingulate gyrus projects to the entorhinal cortex (via the cingulum). The entorhinal cortex projects to the hippocampus (via the perforant pathway).

► Clinical Correlations

Anterograde Amnesia

Bilateral damage to the medial temporal lobes, including the **hippocampus**, results in a profound loss of the ability to acquire new information.

Wernicke Encephalopathy and Korsakoff Syndrome

Wernicke encephalopathy typically occurs in alcoholics who have a **thiamine deficiency**. Patients present with ocular palsies, confusion, and gait ataxia. If the thiamine deficiency is not corrected in time, patients can develop **Korsakoff syndrome**, characterized by **anterograde amnesia**, retrograde amnesia, and confabulation. Lesions are found in the **mammillary bodies** and the **dorsomedial nuclei of the thalamus**. Wernicke encephalopathy is reversible; Korsakoff syndrome is not.

Klüver-Bucy Syndrome

Klüver-Bucy syndrome results from bilateral lesions of the anterior temporal lobes, including the **amygdala**. Symptoms include placidity (decrease in aggressive behavior), psychic blindness (visual agnosia), increased oral exploratory behavior, hypersexuality and loss of sexual preference, hypermetamorphosis (visual stimuli are repeatedly approached as if they were new), and anterograde amnesia.

Cerebral Cortex

The cerebral cortex is highly convoluted with bulges (**gyri**) separated by spaces (**sulci**). Several prominent sulci separate the cortex into four lobes: **frontal**, **parietal**, **temporal**, and **occipital**. The figures below show the lateral and medial views of the right cerebral hemispheres.

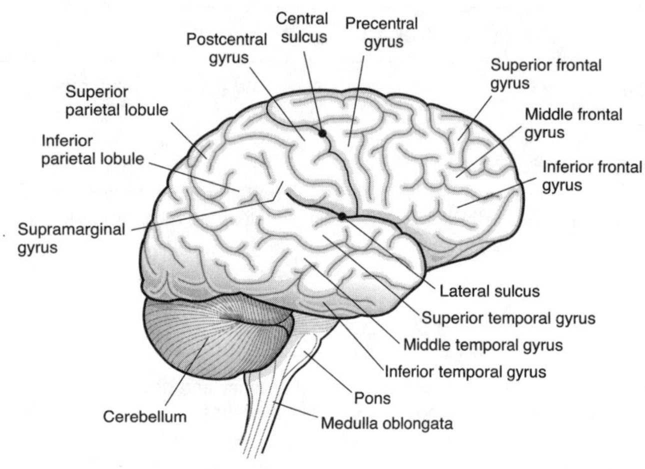

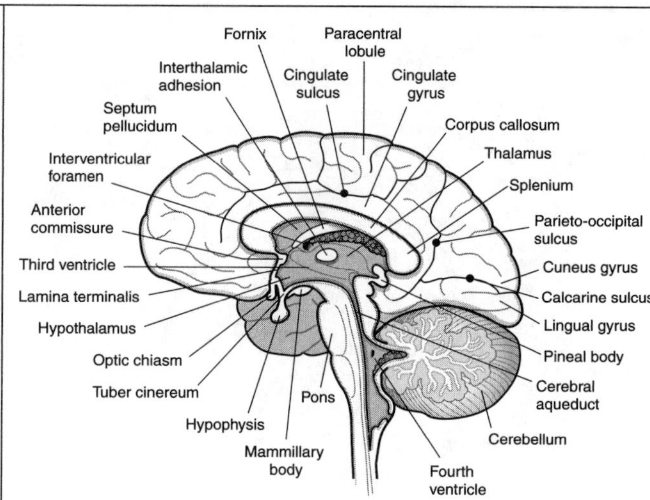

Most of the cortex has **six layers** (**neocortex**). The olfactory cortex and hippocampus have **three layers** (**allocortex**). The figure below shows the six-layered cortex:

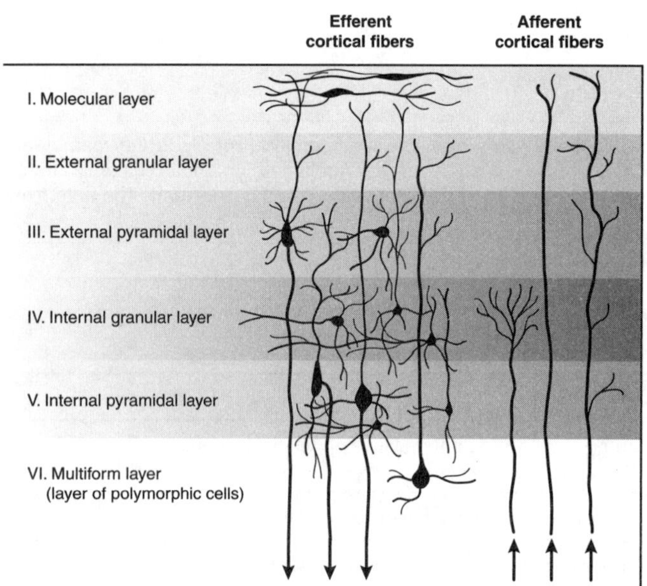

Key Afferents/Efferents

Layer IV receives thalamocortical inputs.

Layer V gives rise to corticospinal and corticobulbar tracts.

► Key Features of Lobes

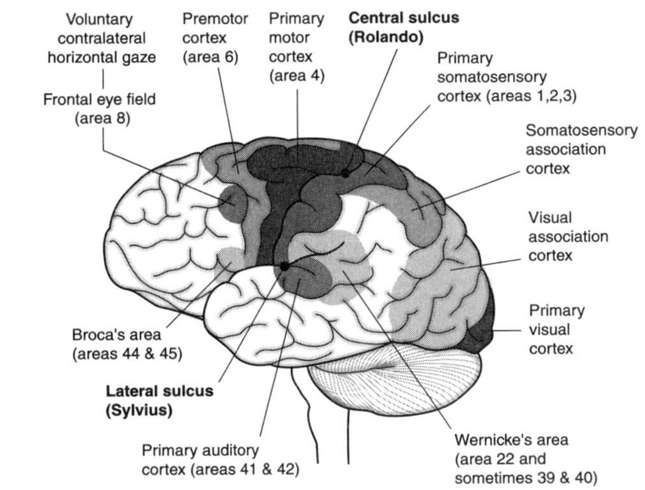

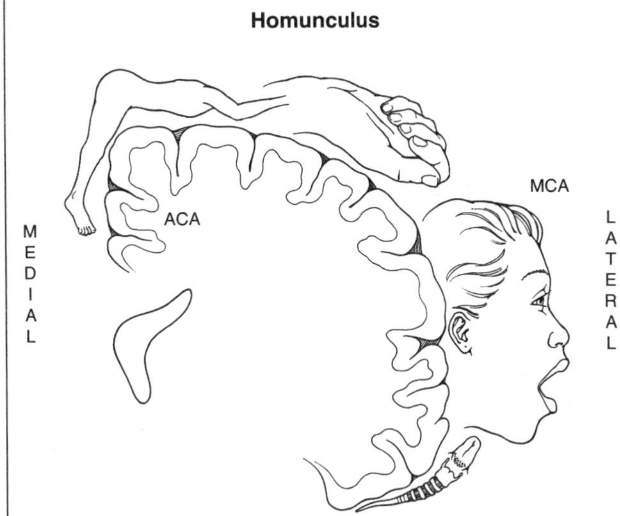

Lobes	Important Regions	Deficit After Lesion
Frontal	Primary motor and premotor cortex	Contralateral spastic paresis (region depends on area of homunculus affected; see figure above)
	Frontal eye fields	Eyes deviate to ipsilateral side
	Broca speech area*	**Broca aphasia (expressive, nonfluent aphasia):** patient can understand written and spoken language, but speech and writing are slow and effortful; patients are aware of their problem; often associated with contralateral facial and arm weakness
	Prefrontal cortex	**Frontal lobe syndrome:** symptoms can include poor judgment, difficulty concentrating and problem solving, apathy, inappropriate social behavior
Parietal	Primary somatosensory cortex	Contralateral hemihypesthesia (region depends on area of homunculus affected)
	Superior parietal lobule	Contralateral astereognosis and sensory neglect, apraxia
	Inferior parietal lobule	**Gerstmann syndrome** (if dominant hemisphere): right/left confusion, dyscalculia and dysgraphia, finger agnosia, contralateral hemianopia or lower quadrantanopia
Temporal	Primary auditory cortex	Bilateral damage → deafness Unilateral leads to slight hearing loss
	Wernicke area*	**Wernicke aphasia (receptive, fluent aphasia):** patient cannot understand any form of language; speech is fast and fluent, but not comprehensible
	Hippocampus	Bilateral lesions lead to inability to consolidate short-term to long-term memory
	Amygdala	**Klüver-Bucy syndrome:** hyperphagia, hypersexuality, visual agnosia
	Olfactory bulb, tract, primary cortex	Ipsilateral anosmia
	Meyer loop (visual radiations)	Contralateral upper quadrantanopia ("pie in the sky")
Occipital	Primary visual cortex	Blindness

*In the dominant hemisphere. Eighty percent of people are left-hemisphere dominant.

► Alzheimer Disease

- Alzheimer disease accounts for 60% of all cases of dementia. The incidence increases with age.
- **Clinical:** insidious onset, progressive memory impairment, mood alterations, disorientation, aphasia, apraxia, and progression to a bedridden state with eventual death
- Five to 10% of AD cases are hereditary, early onset, and transmitted as an autosomal dominant trait.

Genetics of Alzheimer Disease

Gene	Location	Notes
Amyloid precursor protein (*APP*) gene	Chromosome 21	Virtually all Down syndrome patients are destined to develop AD in their forties. Down patients have triple copies of the *APP* gene.
Presenilin-1 gene	Chromosome 14	Majority of hereditary AD cases—early onset
Presenilin-2 gene	Chromosome 1	Early onset
Apolipoprotein E gene	Chromosome 19	Three allelic forms of this gene: epsilon 2, epsilon 3, and epsilon 4 The allele epsilon 4 of apolipoprotein E (*ApoE*) increases the risk for AD, epsilon 2 confers relative protection

Pathology of Alzheimer Disease

Lesions involve the neocortex, hippocampus, and subcortical nuclei, including forebrain cholinergic nuclei (i.e., basal nucleus of Meynert). These areas show atrophy, as well as characteristic microscopic changes. The earliest and most severely affected areas are the hippocampus and temporal lobe, which are involved in learning and memory.

Intra- and extracellular accumulation of abnormal proteins	**Aβ amyloid:** 42-residue peptide from a normal transmembrane protein, the amyloid precursor protein (APP) **Abnormal *tau*** (a microtubule-associated protein)
Senile plaques	Core of Aβ amyloid surrounded by dystrophic neuritic processes associated with microglia and astrocytes
Neurofibrillary tangles (NFT)	Intraneuronal aggregates of insoluble cytoskeletal elements, mainly composed of abnormally phosphorylated tau forming **paired helical filaments** (PHF)
Cerebral amyloid angiopathy (CAA)	Accumulation of Aβ amyloid within the media of small and medium-sized intracortical and leptomeningeal arteries; associated with intracerebral hemorrhage
Granulovacuolar degeneration (GVD) and Hirano bodies (HBs)	GVD and HBs develop in the hippocampus and are less significant diagnostically

Treatment of Alzheimer Disease

AChE Inhibitors
(rivastigmine, donepezil, galantamine, tacrine)

These agents prevent the metabolism of ACh to counteract the depletion in ACh in the cerebral cortex and hippocampus. Rivastigmine and tacrine also inhibit BuChE. Indicated for mild to moderate AD.

NMDA Antagonist
(memantine)

This is the newest class of agents used for the treatment of AD. It is hypothesized that overstimulation of NMDA receptors contributes to the symptomatology of AD. Indicated for moderate to severe AD. Often used in combination with the AChEIs.

Definition of abbreviations: AChE, acetylcholinesterase; BuChE, butyrylcholinesterase; NMDA, *N*-methyl-D-aspartate.

▶ Creutzfeldt-Jakob Disease (CJD)

Mechanism of Disease

Caused by a **prion protein** (PrP = 30-kD protein normally present in neurons encoded by gene on chromosome 20);
PrP^{c} = normal conformation = alpha-helix; PrP^{sc} = abnormal conformation = beta-pleated sheet. PrP^{sc} facilitates conformational change of other PrP^{c} molecules into PrP^{sc}.

Spontaneous change from one form to another → sporadic cases (85% of total) of CJD

Mutations of PrP → hereditary cases (15% of total) of CJD

Pathology

Spongiform change: vacuolization of the neuropil in gray matter (especially cortex) due to large membrane-bound vacuoles within neuronal processes

- Associated with neuronal loss and astrogliosis
- **Kuru plaques** are deposits of amyloid of altered PrP protein

Clinical Manifestations

Rapidly progressive dementia, memory loss, startle myoclonus or other involuntary movements. EEG changes. Death within 6–12 months.

Variant CJD (vCJD)

Affects young adults. May be related to bovine spongiform encephalopathy (BSE; mad cow disease). Pathologically similar to CJD.

▶ Pick Disease (Lobar Atrophy)

- Rare cause of dementia
- Striking **atrophy of frontal and temporal lobes** with sparing of posterior structures
- Microscopic: swollen neurons (Pick cells) or neurons containing **Pick bodies** (round to oval inclusions that stain with silver stains)

▶ CNS Trauma

Concussion	Occurs with a change in momentum of the head (impact against a rigid surface) Loss of consciousness and reflexes, temporary respiratory arrest, and amnesia for the event
Contusion	Bruising to the brain resulting from impact of the brain against inner calvarial surfaces, especially along crests of orbital gyri (frontal lobe) and temporal poles Coup (site of injury) and contrecoup (site diametrically opposite) develop when the head is **mobile** at the time of impact.
Diffuse axonal injury	Injury to white matter due to acceleration/deceleration produces damage to axons at nodes of Ranvier with impairment of axoplasmic flow Poor prognosis, related to duration of coma

▶ Cerebral Herniations

Subfalcine (cingulate)	Cingulate gyrus displaced underneath the falx to the opposite side with compression of anterior cerebral artery
Transtentorial (uncal)	The uncus of the temporal lobe displaced over the free edge of the tentorium Compression of the third nerve, with pupillary dilatation on the same side Infarct in dependent territory Advanced stages: **Duret hemorrhage** within the central pons and midbrain
Cerebellar tonsillar	Displacement of cerebellar tonsils through the foramen magnum Compression of medulla leads to cardiorespiratory arrest

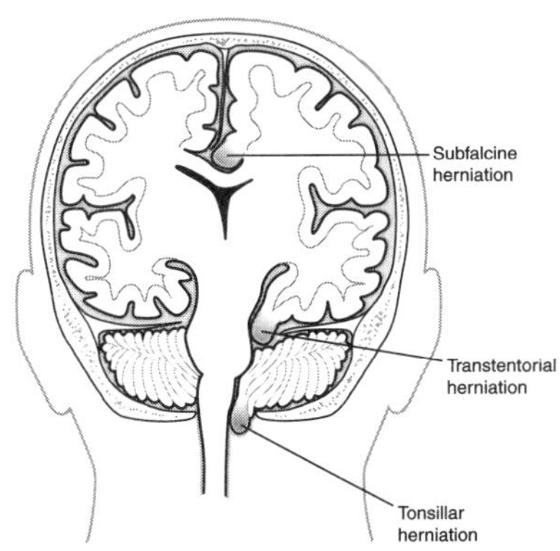

Blood Supply

The cortex is supplied by branches of the **two internal carotid arteries** and **two vertebral arteries**.

- On the ventral surface of the brain, the anterior cerebral and middle cerebral branches of the internal carotid arteries connect with the posterior cerebral artery (derived from the basilar artery) and form the **circle of Willis**. This circle of vessels is completed by the anterior and posterior communicating arteries.
- The **middle cerebral artery** mainly supplies the lateral surface of the frontal, parietal, and upper aspect of the temporal lobe. Deep branches also supply part of the basal ganglia and internal capsule.
- The **anterior cerebral artery** supplies the medial aspect of the frontal and parietal lobes.
- The entire occipital lobe, lower aspect of temporal lobe, and the midbrain are supplied by the **posterior cerebral artery**.

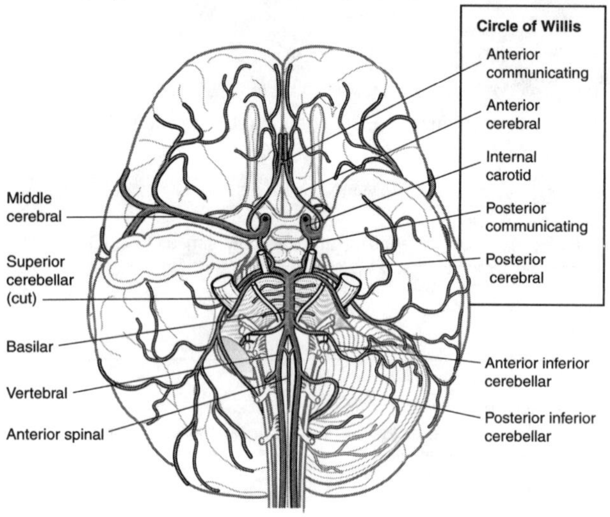

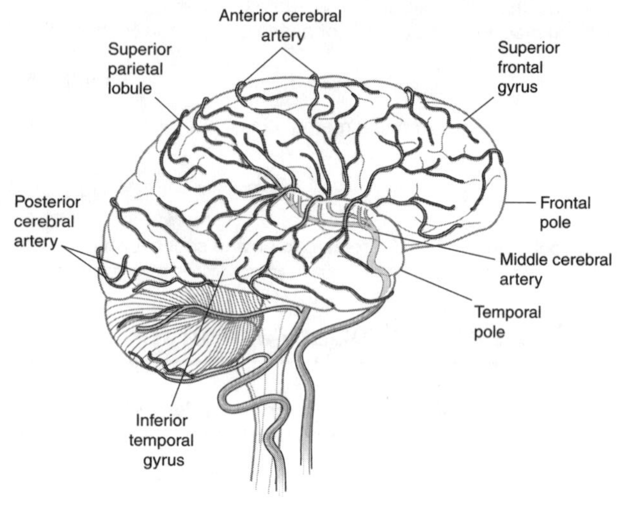

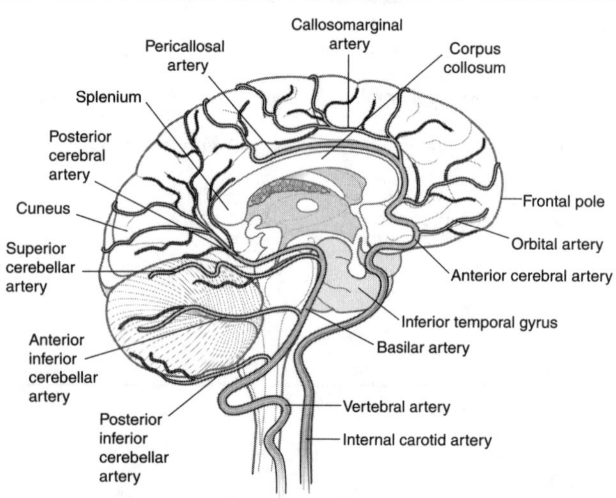

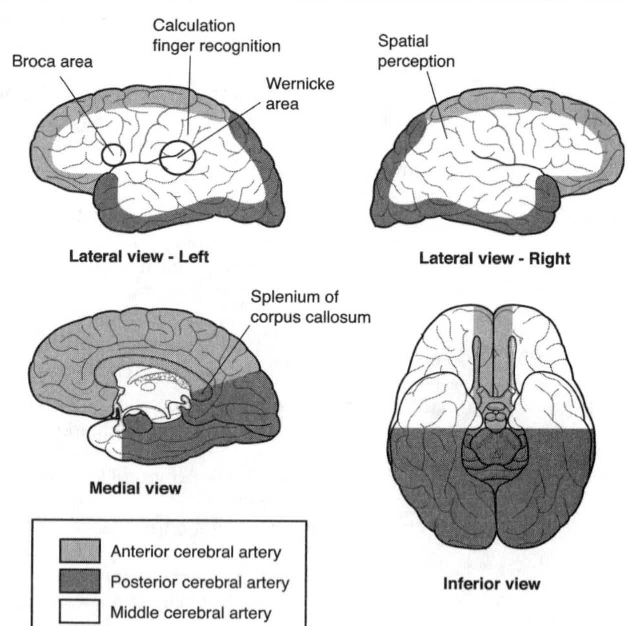

(*Continued*)

► Blood Supply (*Cont'd.*)

System	Primary Arteries	Branches	Supplies	Deficits after Stroke
Vertebrobasilar (posterior circulation)	**Vertebral arteries**	**Anterior spinal artery**	Anterior 2/3 of spinal cord	Dorsal columns spared; all else bilateral
		Posterior cerebellar (PICA)	Dorsolateral medulla	See brain stem lesions on pages 212–213.
	Basilar artery	Pontine arteries	Base of pons	
		Anterior inferior cerebellar (AICA)	Inferior cerebellum, cerebellar nuclei	
		Superior cerebellar artery	Dorsal cerebellar hemispheres; superior cerebellar peduncle	
		Labyrinthine artery (sometimes arises from AICA)	Inner ear	
	Posterior cerebral arteries	—	Midbrain, thalamus, occipital lobe	**Contralateral hemianopia with macular sparing** Alexia without agraphia*
Internal carotid (anterior circulation)	Ophthalmic artery	Central artery of retina	Retina	Blindness
	Posterior communicating artery	—	—	Second most common **aneurysm** site (often with CN III palsy)
	Anterior cerebral artery	—	Primary motor and sensory cortex (leg/foot)	Contralateral spastic paralysis and anesthesia of **lower limb** Frontal lobe abnormalities
	Anterior communicating artery	—	—	Most common site of **aneurysm**
	Middle cerebral artery	Outer cortical	Lateral convexity of hemispheres	Contralateral spastic paralysis and anesthesia of **upper limb/face** **Gaze palsy** **Aphasia*** Gerstmann syndrome* Hemi inattention and neglect of contralateral body†
		Lenticulostriate	Internal capsule, caudate, putamen, globus pallidus	

*If dominant hemisphere is affected (usually the left).

†Right parietal lobe lesion

► Cerebrovascular Disorders

Disorder	Types	Key Concepts
Cerebral infarcts	Thrombotic	**Anemic/pale** infarct; usually atherosclerotic complication
	Embolic	**Hemorrhagic/red** infarct; from heart or atherosclerotic plaques; **middle cerebral artery** most vulnerable to emboli
	Hypotension	**"Watershed"** areas and **deep cortical layers** most affected
	Hypertension	**Lacunar** infarcts; **basal ganglia** most affected
Hemorrhages	Epidural hematoma	Almost always traumatic Rupture of **middle meningeal artery** after skull fracture Lucid interval before loss of consciousness ("talk and die" syndrome)
	Subdural hematoma	Usually caused by trauma Rupture of **bridging veins** (connect brain and sagittal sinus)
	Subarachnoid hemorrhage	**Ruptured berry aneurysm** is most frequent cause Predisposing factors: Marfan syndrome, Ehlers-Danlos type 4, adult polycystic kidney disease, hypertension, smoking
	Intracerebral hemorrhage	Common causes: hypertension, trauma, infarction

Seizures and Anticonvulsants

► Seizures

Partial	Occur in localized region of brain; can become secondarily generalized **Drugs of choice:** carbamazepine, phenytoin, valproic acid **Backup and adjuvants:** most newer drugs are also effective
Simple	• **Consciousness unaffected** • Can be motor, somatosensory or special sensory, autonomic, psychic
Complex	• Consciousness is impaired • The four "A"s: aura, alteration of consciousness, automatisms, amnesia • Often called "psychomotor" or "temporal lobe seizures"
Generalized	Affects **entire brain**
Absence	• Impaired consciousness (usually abrupt onset and brief); automatisms sometimes occur • Begin in childhood, often end by age 20 • Also called **petit mal** • **Drugs of choice:** ethosuximide (1st line if only absence is present), valproic acid • **Backup and adjuvants:** clonazepam, lamotrigine, topiramate
Tonic-clonic	• Alternating tonic (stiffening) and clonic (movements); loss of consciousness • Also called grand mal • **Drugs of choice:** valproic acid, carbamazepine, phenytoin, phenobarbital • **Backup and adjuvants:** lamotrigine, topiramate, levetiracetam, phenobarbital, others
Myoclonic	Single or multiple myoclonic jerks • **Drug of choice:** valproic acid • **Backup and adjuvants:** clonazepam, topiramate, lamotrigine, levetiracetam
Status epilepticus	• Seizure activity (often tonic-clonic), continuous or intermittent (without recovery of consciousness) for at least 30 minutes; life-threatening • **Drugs of choice:** diazepam, lorazepam, phenytoin, fosphenytoin • **Backup and adjuvants:** phenobarbital, general anesthesia

► Anticonvulsants

Drug	Mechanism	Notes
Benzodiazepines	↑ frequency of $GABA_A$ (Cl^-) receptor opening	Sedation, dependence, tolerance
Carbamazepine	Blocks Na^+ channels	Diplopia, ataxia, blood dyscrasias (agranulocytosis, aplastic anemia), P450 induction, teratogenic
Ethosuximide	Blocks T-type Ca^{2+} channels (thalamus)	GI distress, headache, lethargy, hematotoxicity, Stevens-Johnson syndrome
Phenobarbital	↑ duration of $GABA_A$ (Cl^-) receptor opening	Induction of cytochrome P450, sedation, dependence, tolerance
Phenytoin	Blocks Na^+ channels	Gingival hyperplasia, hirsutism, sedation, anemia, nystagmus, diplopia, ataxia, teratogenic (fetal hydantoin syndrome), P450 induction, zero-order kinetics
Valproic acid	Blocks Na^+ channels, inhibits GABA transaminase	GI distress, hepatotoxic (rare but can be fatal), inhibits drug metabolism, neural tube defects

► Newer Agents

Drug	Side Effects
Felbamate	Aplastic anemia, hepatoxicity
Gabapentin	Sedation, dizziness
Lamotrigine	Life-threatening rash, Stevens-Johnson syndrome
Levetiracetam	Neuropsychiatric effects, sedation
Tiagabine	Sedation, dizziness
Topiramate	Sedation, dizziness, ataxia, anomia, renal stones, weight loss
Vigabatrin	Sedation, dizziness, visual field defects, psychosis

Opioid Analgesics and Related Drugs

Opioid analgesics act by stimulating receptors for endogenous opioid peptides (e.g., enkephalins, β-endorphin, dynorphins). Opioid receptors are G-protein coupled, and the three major classes are μ **(mu)**, κ **(kappa)**, and δ **(delta)**. β-Endorphin has the greatest affinity for the μ receptor, dynorphins for the κ receptor, and enkephalins for the δ receptor. The effects of specific drugs depend on the receptor subtype with which they interact, and whether they act as full agonists, partial agonists, or antagonists. The μ receptor is primarily responsible for analgesia, respiratory depression, euphoria, and physical dependence.

► Individual Agents

	Strong Agonists	
Morphine	Full μ agonist	Prototype of this class; poor oral bioavailability; histamine release
Methadone		Orally active; long duration; useful in maintenance
Meperidine		Muscarinic antagonist (no miosis or smooth muscle contraction); forms normeperidine → possible seizures; do not combine with MAO inhibitors or SSRIs
	Additional strong agonists: fentanyl, heroin (schedule I), levorphanol	
	Moderate Agonist	
Codeine	Partial μ agonist	Antitussive, often given in combination with NSAIDs
	Additional moderate agonists: oxycodone, hydrocodone	
	Partial Agonist	
Buprenorphine	Partial μ agonist	Binds tightly to receptor, so is more resistant to naloxone reversal
	Mixed Agonist–Antagonists	
Pentazocine **Nalbuphine** **Butorphanol**	κ agonist/ μ antagonist	In general, less analgesia than morphine Can cause hallucinations and nightmares Has less respiratory depression and abuse liability than the pure agonists
	Antitussives	
Codeine **Dextromethorphan**	Codeine is by prescription; dextromethorphan is available OTC	
	Antidiarrheals	
Diphenoxylate **Loperamide**	Diphenoxylate used in combination with atropine to prevent abuse Loperamide available OTC	
	Antagonists	
Naloxone (IV) **Naltrexone (PO)** **Nalmefene (IV)**	All are used in the management of acute opioid overdose. Naloxone has a short half-life and may require multiple doses. Naltrexone ↓ craving for ethanol and is used in alcohol dependency programs.	

► Characteristics of Opioid Analgesics

Effects and Side Effects

- Analgesia
- Sedation
- Respiratory depression
- Constipation
- Smooth muscle: (except meperidine)
  ↑ tone: biliary tract (biliary colic), bladder, ureter
  ↓ tone: uterus (prolongs labor), vascular
- Euphoria
- Cough suppression
- Nausea and vomiting
- Pupillary miosis (except meperidine)
- Cardiovascular:
  Cerebrovascular dilation (esp. with ↑ P_{CO_2}) leads to ↑ intracranial pressure
  ↓ BP may occur; bradycardia

Clinical Uses

Analgesia, cough suppression, treatment of diarrhea, preoperative medications and adjunct to anesthesia, management of pulmonary edema

Overdose

- **Classic triad:** Respiratory depression, miosis (pinpoint pupils), coma
- Diagnosis confirmed with naloxone (short duration, may need repeat dosing); give supportive care

Chronic Effects

- Pharmacodynamic tolerance (tolerance does not develop to constipation or miosis)
- **Dependence:** Psychological and physical
- **Abstinence syndrome (withdrawal):** anxiety, hostility, GI distress (cramps and diarrhea) gooseflesh ("cold turkey"), muscle cramps and spasms ("kicking the habit"), rhinorrhea, lacrimation, sweating, yawning
- Abstinence syndrome can be precipitated in tolerant individuals by administering an opioid antagonist

Contraindications and Cautions

- Use of full agonists with weak partial agonists. Weak agonists can precipitate withdrawal from the full agonist.
- Use in patients with pulmonary dysfunction (acute respiratory failure). Exception: pulmonary edema
- Use in patients with head injuries (possible increased intracranial pressure)
- Use in patients with hepatic/renal dysfunction (drug accumulation)
- Use in patients with adrenal or thyroid deficiencies (prolonged and exaggerated responses)
- Use in pregnant patients (possible neonatal depression or dependence)

Local Anesthetics

Local anesthetics **block voltage-gated sodium channels**, preventing sensory information from being transmitted from a local area to the brain. These agents are initially uncharged and diffuse across the axonal membrane to enter the cytoplasm. Once inside, they become ionized and block the Na^+ channels from the **inside**. These agents bind best to channels that are open or recently inactivated, rather than resting, and therefore work better in rapidly firing fibers (**use-dependence**). Infection leads to a more acidic environment, making the basic local anesthetic more likely to be ionized, therefore higher doses may be required. **Order of blockade:** small fibers > larger fibers; myelinated fibers > unmyelinated fibers. **Modality blocked:** autonomic and pain > touch/pressure > motor. There are two main classes: **amides** and **esters**.

Amides (metabolized in **liver**)	**Esters** (metabolized by **plasma cholinesterases**)	**Side Effects**
Bupivacaine (L) Etidocaine (L) Ropivacaine (L) Lidocaine (M)* Mepivacaine (M) Prilocaine (M)	Tetracaine (L) Cocaine (M)† Procaine (S) Benzocaine‡	1. **Neurotoxicity:** lightheadedness, nystagmus, restlessness, convulsions 2. **Cardiovascular toxicity**: ↓ CV parameters (except cocaine which ↑ HR and BP); bupivacaine especially notable for CV toxicity 3. **Allergic reaction:** esters via PABA formation; switch to amides if allergic to esters

Notes

Duration of action can be increased by coadministration of a vasoconstrictor (e.g., epinephrine) to limit blood flow

Hint: Amide drugs have two "i"s, and ester drugs have one "i" in their names.

Definition of abbreviations: L, long acting; M, medium acting; S, short acting.
*Also a IB antiarrhythmic
†Primarily used topically; sympathomimetic; drug of abuse (schedule II)
‡Topical only

The Cardiovascular System

Chapter 2

Cardiovascular Embryology

► Development of the Heart Tube

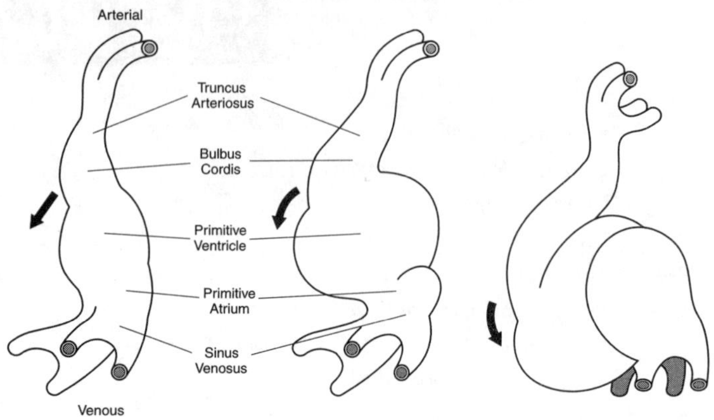

The primitive heart tube is formed from lateral plate mesoderm. The primitive heart tube undergoes dextral looping (bends to the right) and forms five dilatations. Four of the five dilatations become subdivided by a septum. Most of the common congenital cardiac anomalies result from defects in the formation of these septa.

► Adult Structures Derived from the Dilatations of the Primitive Heart

Embryonic Dilatation	Adult Structure
Truncus arteriosus (neural crest)	Aorta Pulmonary trunk
Bulbus cordis	Smooth part of right ventricle (**conus arteriosus**) Smooth part of left ventricle (**aortic vestibule**)
Primitive ventricle	Trabeculated part of right ventricle Trabeculated part of left ventricle
Primitive atrium	Trabeculated part of right atrium Trabeculated part of left atrium
Sinus venosus (the only dilatation that does not become subdivided by a septum)	Right—smooth part of right atrium (**sinus venarum**) Left—coronary sinus Oblique vein of left atrium

► Atrial Septum

Formation of the Atrial Septum

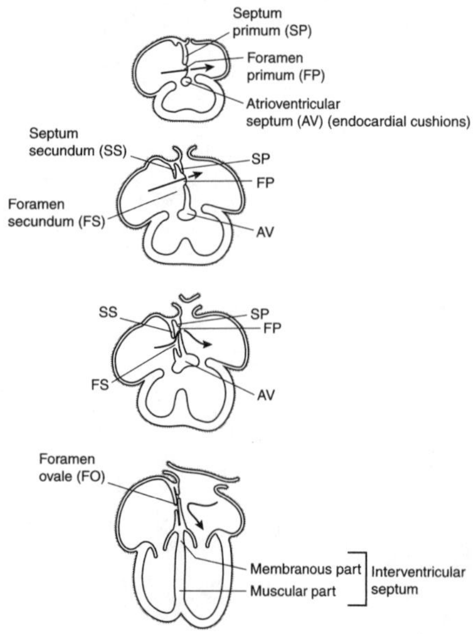

Atrial septal defects are called **ASDs**.

Secundum-type ASDs are caused by excessive resorption of the SP or reduced size of the SS or both. This results in an opening between the right and left atria. If the ASD is small, clinical symptoms may be delayed as late as age 30. This is the most clinically significant ASD.

The **foramen ovale** (FO) is the fetal communication between the right and left atria. It remains patent in up to 25% of normal individuals throughout life, although paradoxical emboli may pass through a large patent FO. **Premature closure of the FO** is the closure of the FO during prenatal life. This results in hypertrophy of the right side of the heart and underdevelopment of the left side.

► Ventricular Septum

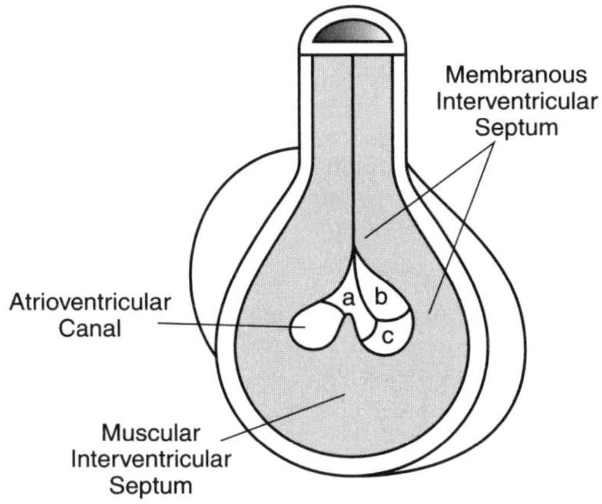

A **membranous ventricular septal defect (VSD)** is caused by the failure of the membranous interventricular septum to develop, and it results in **left-to-right shunting** of blood through the interventricular foramen. Patients with left-to-right shunting complain of **excessive fatigue upon exertion**.

Left-to-right shunting of blood is not cyanotic but causes increased blood flow and pressure to the lungs (pulmonary hypertension). Pulmonary hypertension causes marked proliferation of the tunica intima and media of pulmonary muscular arteries and arterioles. Ultimately, the pulmonary resistance becomes higher than systemic resistance and causes **right-to-left shunting** of blood and "late" **cyanosis**. At this stage, the condition is called **Eisenmenger complex**. VSD is the most common congenital cardiac anomaly.

Figure legend: a, right bulbar ridge; b, left bulbar ridge; c, AV cushions.

► Aorticopulmonary Septum

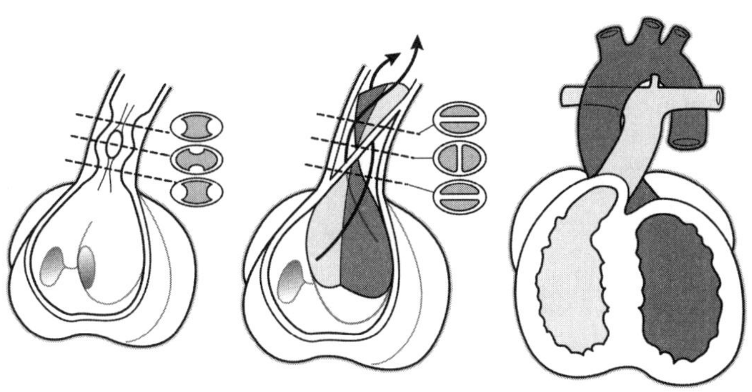

Neural crest cells migrate into the truncal and bulbar ridges of the truncus arteriosus, which grow in a spiral fashion and fuse to form the aorticopulmonary (AP) septum. The AP septum divides the truncus arteriosus into the **aorta** (dark gray) and **pulmonary trunk** (light gray).

Transposition of the Great Vessels
Occurs when the AP septum fails to develop in a spiral fashion and results in the aorta opening into the right ventricle and the pulmonary trunk opening into the left ventricle. This causes **right-to-left** shunting of blood with resultant **cyanosis**. Infants born alive with this defect must have other defects (like a PDA or VSD) that allow mixing of oxygenated and deoxygenated blood.
Tetralogy of Fallot
Occurs when the AP septum fails to align properly and results in (1) pulmonary stenosis, (2) overriding aorta, (3) interventricular septal defect, and (4) right ventricular hypertrophy. This causes **right-to-left** shunting of blood with resultant "early" **cyanosis**, which is usually present at birth. Tetralogy of Fallot is the most common congenital cyanotic cardiac anomaly.
Persistent Truncus Arteriosus
Occurs when there is only partial development of the AP septum. This results in a condition in which only one large vessel leaves the heart and receives blood from both the right and left ventricles. This causes **right-to-left** shunting of blood with resultant **cyanosis**. This defect is always accompanied by membranous ventricular septal defect.

Definition of abbreviation: PDA, patent ductus arteriosus.

▶ Fetal Circulation

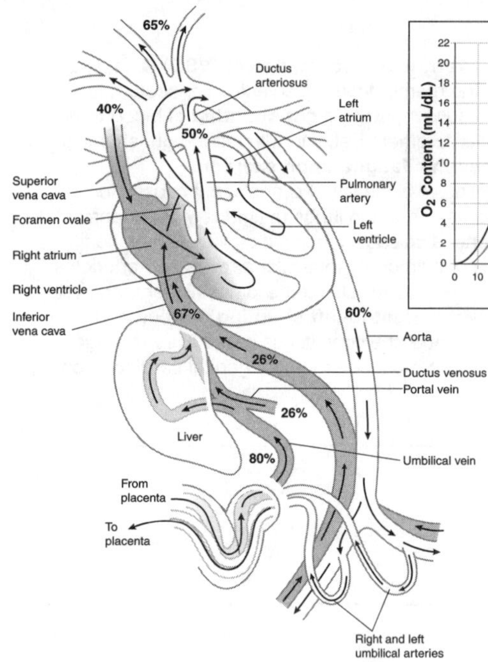

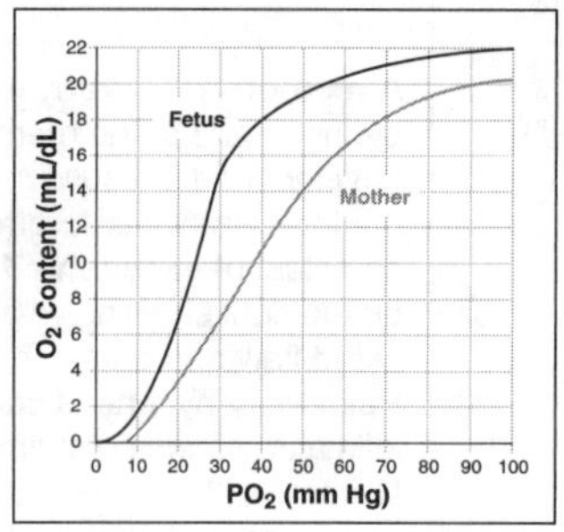

In the fetal circulation, the ductus venosus allows fetal blood to bypass the liver, and the foramen ovale and the ductus arteriosus allow fetal blood to bypass the lungs. Note the sites where the oxygen saturation level of fetal blood is the highest (umbilical vein) and the lowest (ductus arteriosus).

Clinical Correlation

Normally, the ductus arteriosus closes within a few hours after birth, via smooth muscle contraction, to form the ligamentum arteriosum. **Patent ductus arteriosus (PDA)** occurs when the ductus arteriosus (connection between the pulmonary trunk and aorta) fails to close after birth.

Prostaglandin E and intrauterine or neonatal asphyxia **sustain the patency** of the ductus arteriosus.

Prostaglandin inhibitors (e.g., indomethacin), acetylcholine, histamine, and catecholamines **promote closure** of the ductus arteriosus.

PDA is common in premature infants and cases of maternal rubella infection. It causes a left-to-right shunting of blood. (Note: During fetal development, the ductus arteriosus is a right-to-left shunt).

Cardiovascular Anatomy

▶ Structures of the Mediastinum

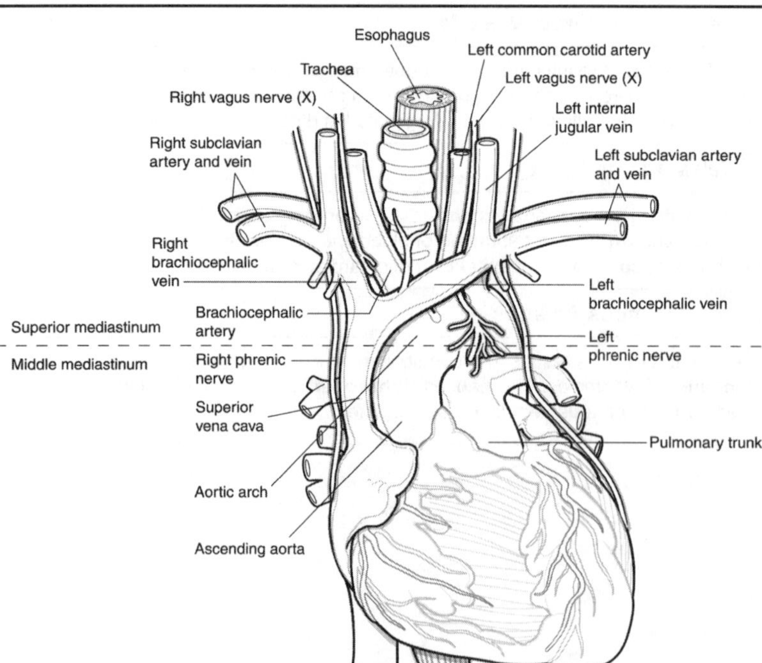

The thoracic cavity is divided into the **superior mediastinum** above the plane of the sternal angle and the **inferior mediastinum** (anterior, middle, and posterior mediastina) below that sternal plane. The superior mediastinum contains the thymic remnants, superior vena cava and its brachiocephalic tributaries, aortic arch and its branches, trachea, esophagus, thoracic duct, and the vagus and phrenic nerves.

The **anterior mediastinum** is anterior to the heart and contains remnants of the thymus. The **middle mediastinum** contains the heart and great vessels, and the **posterior mediastinum** contains the thoracic aorta, esophagus, thoracic duct, azygos veins, and the vagus nerves. The inferior vena cava passes through the diaphragm at the caval hiatus at the level of the eighth thoracic vertebra; the esophagus through the esophageal hiatus at the tenth thoracic vertebra; and the aorta courses through the aortic hiatus at the level of the twelfth thoracic vertebra.

▶ Arterial Supply to the Heart

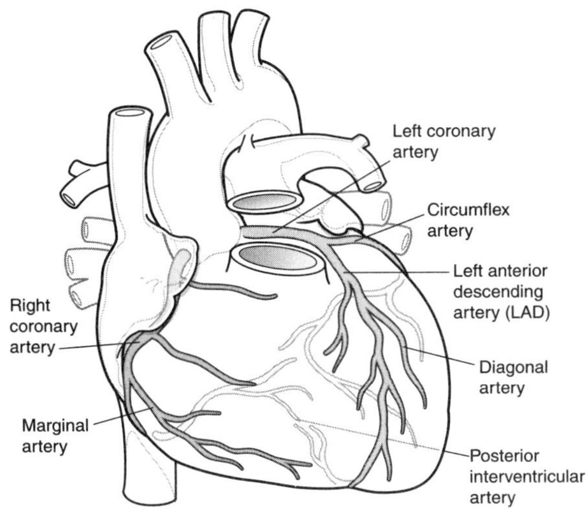

Arterial supply to the heart muscle is provided by the **right and left coronary arteries**, which are branches of the ascending aorta. The **right coronary artery** supplies the right atrium, the right ventricle, the sinoatrial and atrioventricular nodes, and parts of the left atrium and left ventricle. The distal branch of the right coronary artery (in 70% of subjects, "right dominant") is the **posterior interventricular artery** that supplies, in part, the posterior aspect of the interventricular septum. The **left coronary artery** supplies most of the left ventricle, the left atrium, and the anterior part of the interventricular septum. The two main branches of the left coronary artery are the anterior interventricular artery (LAD) and the circumflex artery.

In a myocardial infarction, the LAD is obstructed in 50% of cases, the right coronary in 30%, and the circumflex artery in 20% of cases.

▶ Chambers and Valves of the Heart

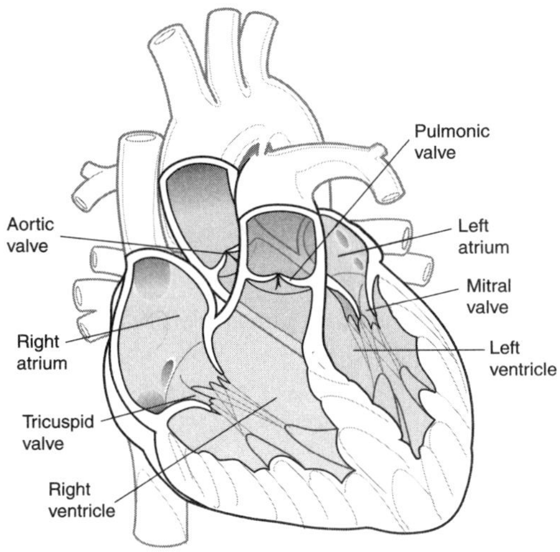

Right Atrium

The right atrium receives venous blood from the entire body (except for blood from the pulmonary veins).

The **auricle** is derived from the fetal atrium; it has rough myocardium known as pectinate muscles.

The **sinus venarum** is the smooth-walled portion of the atrium, which receives blood from the superior and inferior venae cavae.

The **crista terminalis** is the vertical ridge that separates the smooth from the rough portion of the right atrium; it extends longitudinally from the superior vena cava to the inferior vena cava. The SA node is in the upper part of the crista terminalis.

The right AV **(tricuspid valve)** communicates with the right ventricle.

Right Ventricle

The right ventricle receives blood from the right atrium via the tricuspid valve; outflow is to the pulmonary trunk via the pulmonary semilunar valve.

The **trabeculae carneae** are the ridges of myocardium in the ventricular wall.

The **papillary muscles** project into the cavity of the ventricle and attach to cusps of the AV valve by the strands of the chordae tendineae. Papillary muscles contract during ventricular contraction to keep the cusps of the AV valves closed.

The **chordae tendineae** control closure of the valve during contraction of the ventricle.

The **infundibulum** is the smooth area of the right ventricle leading to the pulmonary valve.

Left Atrium

The left atrium receives oxygenated blood from the lungs via the pulmonary veins. There are four openings: the upper right and left and the lower right and left pulmonary veins.

The left AV orifice is guarded by the **mitral (bicuspid) valve**; it allows oxygenated blood to pass from the left atrium into the left ventricle.

(Continued)

► Chambers and Valves of the Heart (*Cont'd.*)

Left Ventricle
Blood enters from the left atrium through the mitral valve and is pumped out to the aorta through the aortic valve. **Trabeculae carneae**, the ridges of myocardium in the ventricular wall, are normally three times thicker than those of the right ventricle. **Papillary muscles** (usually two large ones) are attached by the chordae tendineae to the cusps of the bicuspid valve. The **aortic vestibule** leads to the aortic semilunar valve and ascending aorta; the right and left coronary arteries originate from the right and left aortic sinuses at the root of the ascending aorta.

Clinical Correlation
Murmurs
Murmurs in valvular heart disease result when there is valvular insufficiency or a stenotic valve. For most of **ventricular systole**, the mitral valve should be closed and the aortic valve should be open, so that "common systolic valvular defects" include mitral insufficiency and aortic stenosis. For most of **ventricular diastole**, the mitral valve should be open and the aortic valve should be closed, so that "common diastolic valvular defects" include mitral stenosis and aortic insufficiency.

► Borders of the Heart

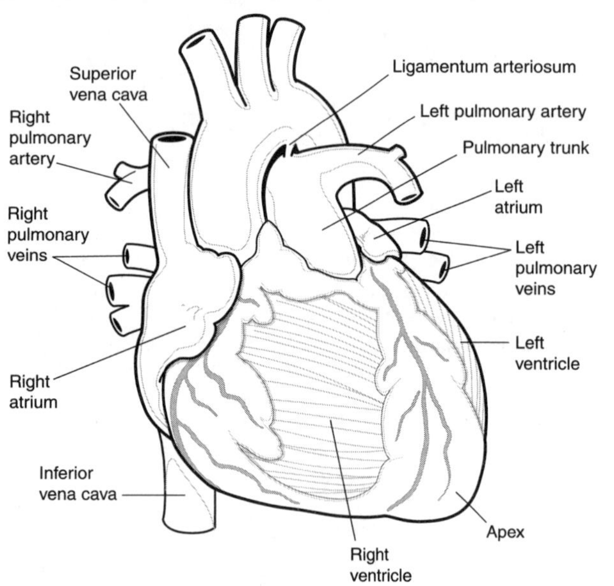

The **external** surface of the heart consists of several borders:

- the right border is formed by the right atrium
- the left border is formed by the left ventricle
- the base formed by the two atria
- the apex at the tip of the left ventricle

The **anterior** surface is formed by the right ventricle.

The **posterior** surface is formed mainly by the left atrium.

A **diaphragmatic** surface is formed primarily by the left ventricle.

▶ Cross-Sectional Anatomy of the Thorax

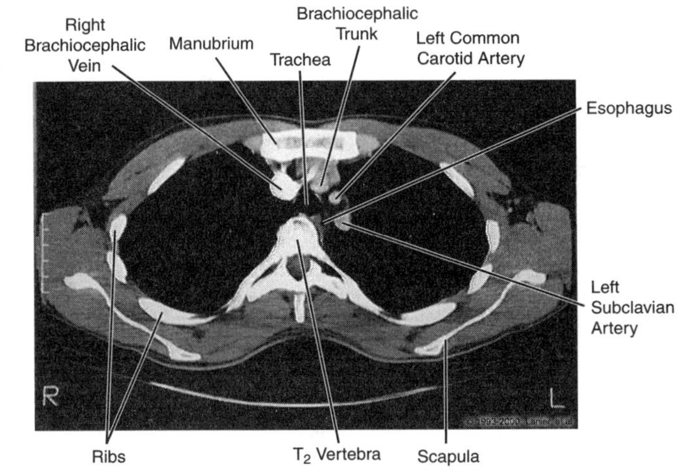

Chest: CT, T2

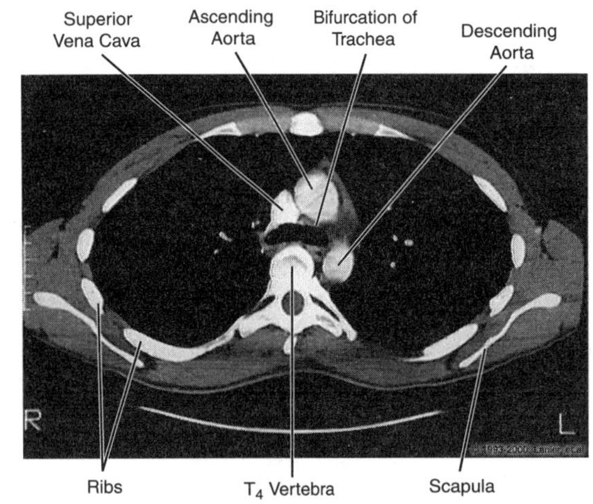

Chest: CT, T4

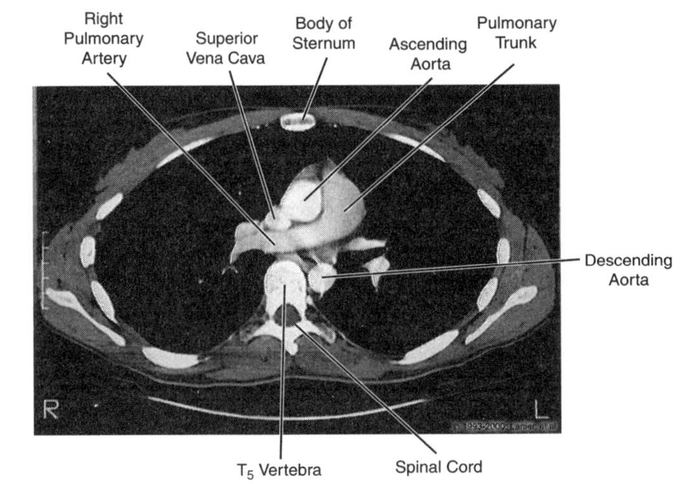

Chest: CT, T5

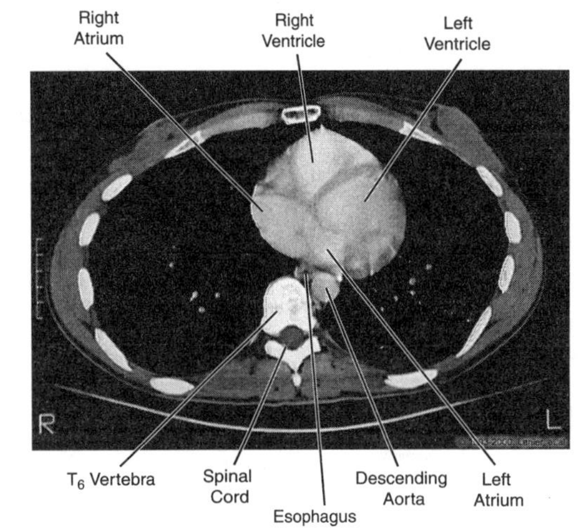

Chest: CT, T6

► Conducting System of the Heart

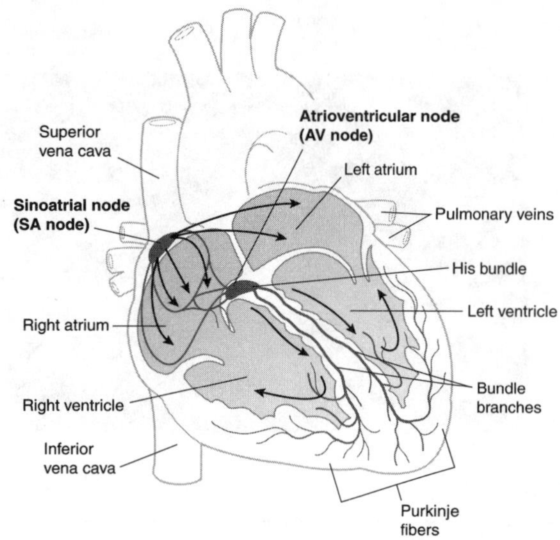

The **sinoatrial node** initiates the impulse for cardiac contraction. The **atrioventricular node** receives the impulse from the sinoatrial node and transmits that impulse to the ventricles through the **bundle of His**. The bundle divides into the **right and left bundle branches** and **Purkinje fibers** to the two ventricles.

Sympathetic innervation from the T1 to T5 spinal cord segments increases the heart rate, while the **parasympathetics** by way of the vagus nerves slow the heart rate..

► Associations of Common Traumatic Injuries with Vessel and Nerve Damage

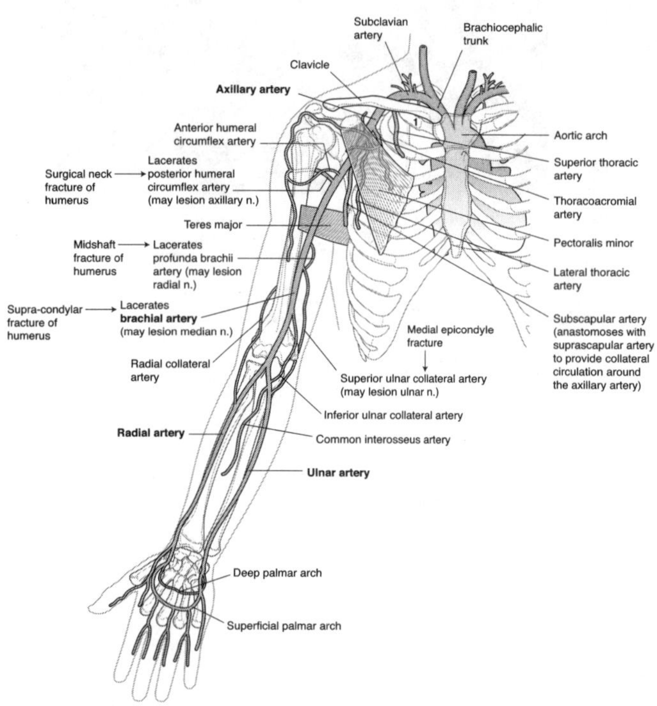

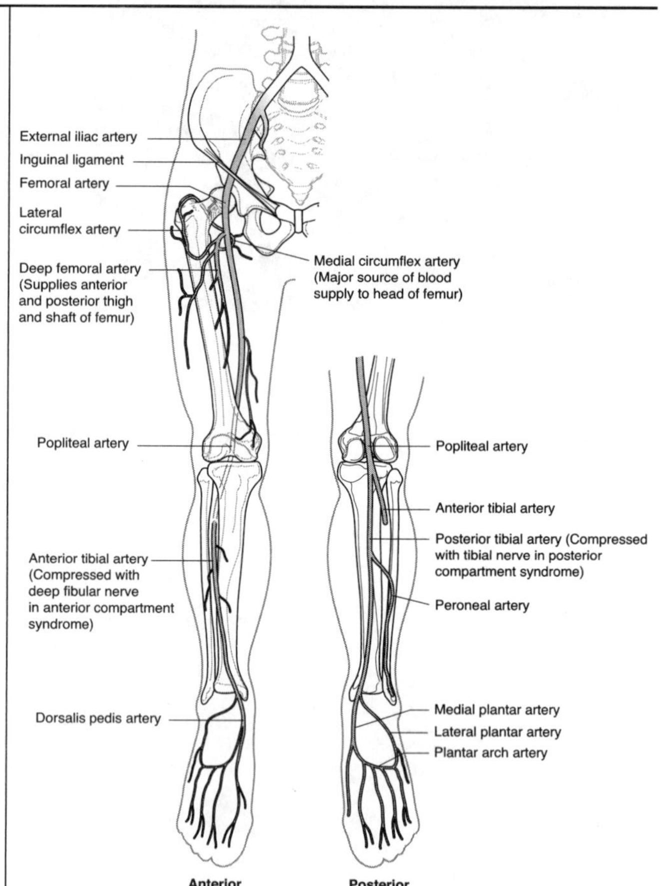

Cardiovascular Physiology

► Comparison of Cardiac Action Potentials

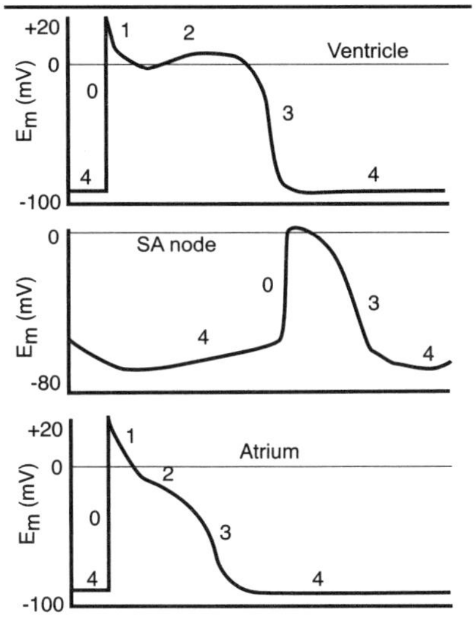

► Important Implications of Ion Currents

Force development
Ca^{2+} current of plateau (phase 2) has major influence

Timing/heart rate
i_f is increased by sympathetics → increased heart rate; parasympathetics increase gK^+ → decreased heart rate

Premature beats
Action potential amplitude and shape not all-or-none; early beats abnormal with low force

Susceptible period
Arrhythmia risk high during relative refractory period

► Cardiac Action Potentials—Ionic Mechanisms

Unique Cardiac Ion Channels

iK	Delayed rectifier; slow to open/close; depolarization opens
iK_1	Inward rectifier; open at rest; depolarization closes it
L-type	Ca^{2+}, slow channel, long acting; depolarization opens
i_f	Na^+; "funny channel"; repolarization opens it; causes the pacemaker spontaneous depolarization

Ionic Basis of Ventricular AP

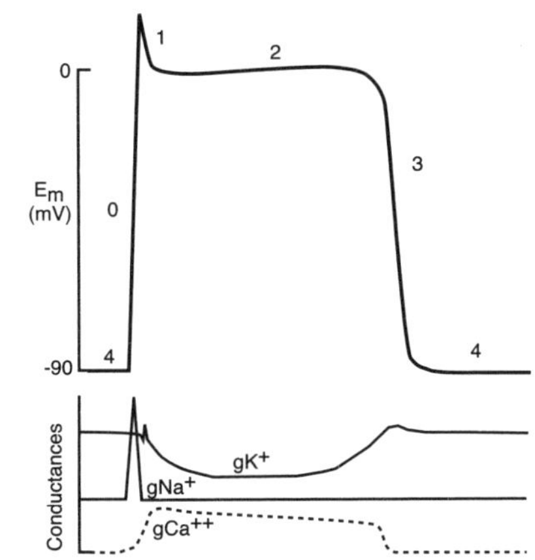

Conductances show changes only and do not reflect absolute values of different ions.

Ionic Basis of SA Node AP

Slow Response (SA node) Cell Action Potential and its Ionic Basis

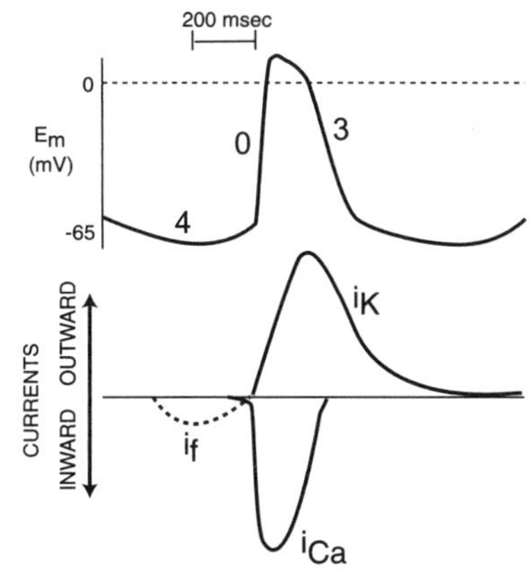

Ventricles and Atria

Phase 4—resting potential
↑ gK^+ occurs via iK_1 channels
iK channels are closing or closed

Phase 0—upstroke
↑ gNa^+ via typical fast Na^+ channels
↓ gK^+ as iK_1 channels close

Phase 1—rapid partial repolarization
↓ gNa^+ as fast channels close
↑ gK^+ transiently via iK_{to}

Phase 2—plateau
↑ gCa^{2+}: slow (L-type) channels
at end of phase 2, ↑ gK^+ via iK channels

Phase 3—repolarization
↓ gCa^{2+} as L-type channels close
↑ gK^+ via iK; then iK_1 opens

SA Node and AV Node

Phase 4—pacemaker
↑ gNa^+ via i_f "funny channel"
High gK^+ but ↓ as iK channels close

Phase 0—upstroke
↑ gCa^{2+} via T-type (fast, transient) channels, then L-type (slow) open

No **phase 1** because no fast sodium channels

Phase 2 usually absent

Phase 3—repolarization
↓ gCa^{2+} as slow channels close
↑ gK^+ via iK channels

► Refractory Periods

Summation is difficult to achieve in cardiac muscle and tetany does not occur. In fact, the abnormal shape of action potentials initiated during the relative refractory period reduces calcium influx and thus contractile force, as shown.

Muscle Twitch Versus Refractory Periods

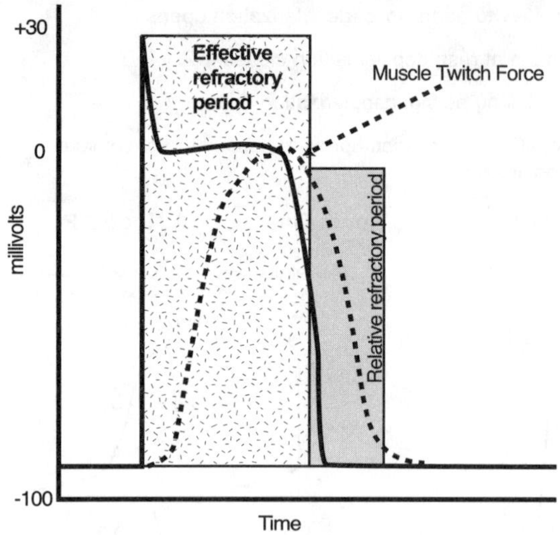

Effect of AP Initiation During the Relative Refractory Period

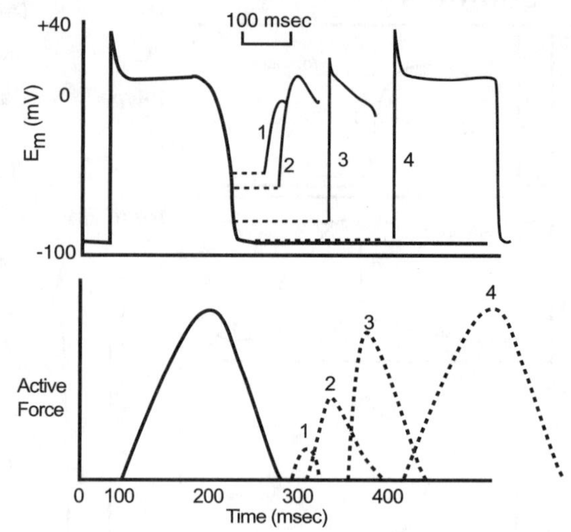

► Basic Principles of the Electrocardiogram

A moving wave of depolarization in the heart produces a positive deflection as it moves toward the positive terminals of the ECG electrodes. A depolarizing wave moving away from the positive (toward the negative) terminals produces a negative deflection. A wave of depolarization moving at right angles to the axis of the electrode terminals produces no deflection. Upon repolarization, the reverse occurs.

► Sequence of Myocardial Excitation and Conduction

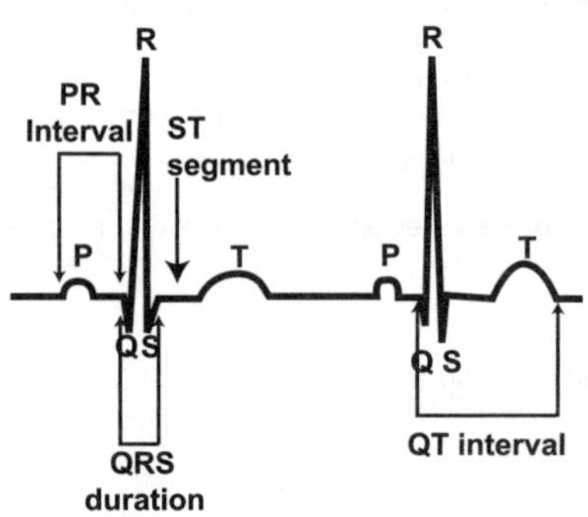

Event/Tissue	Electrocardiogram
Sinoatrial node (SA) depolarizes (primary pacemaker)	Beginning of P wave
Conduction of depolarization through atrial muscle	P wave
Conduction through atrioventricular node (AV)	Between P wave and QRS complex (PR interval)
Conduction through His-Purkinje system and ventricular septum	QRS complex begins
Ventricular depolarization apex to base; septum to lateral wall; endocardial to epicardial	QRS complex
Ventricles are in the plateau phase of depolarization	ST segment
Repolarization of ventricles in reverse sequence	T wave

Important ECG Values		
PR interval	0.12–0.20 sec	Length measures AV conduction time
QRS duration	<0.12 sec	Measures ventricular conduction time
QT interval	0.35–0.45 sec	Total time of ventricular depolarization and repolarization Varies with heart rate, age
Heart rate, normal resting	60–100 beats/min	<60/min = bradycardia; >100/min = tachycardia

▶ Principles of the Electrocardiogram (EKG or ECG)

Moving Electrical Charge		Creates Electrical Field Movement That Causes Ion Currents in Skin
Standard limb leads (frontal plane)	I	⊖ right arm; ⊕ left arm; positive lead at 0°
	II	⊖ right arm; ⊕ left leg; positive lead at +60°
	III	⊖ left arm; ⊕ left leg; positive lead at +120°
Augmented limb leads (frontal plane)	aVR; aVL, aVF	aVR positive lead at –150°; aVL positive lead at –30°; aVF positive lead at +90°
Precordial	V_1–V_6 (chest)	Horizontal plane; positive leads front; negative leads back of chest
Chart speed	25 mm/sec	Each horizontal mm = 0.04 sec (40 msec)
Voltage	1 mV/10 mm	Measure ± voltages of QRS, add to get net voltage of each lead
Mean electrical axis	Vector sum of two leads	Measure of overall wave of ventricular depolarization: normal axis, left or right axis deviation

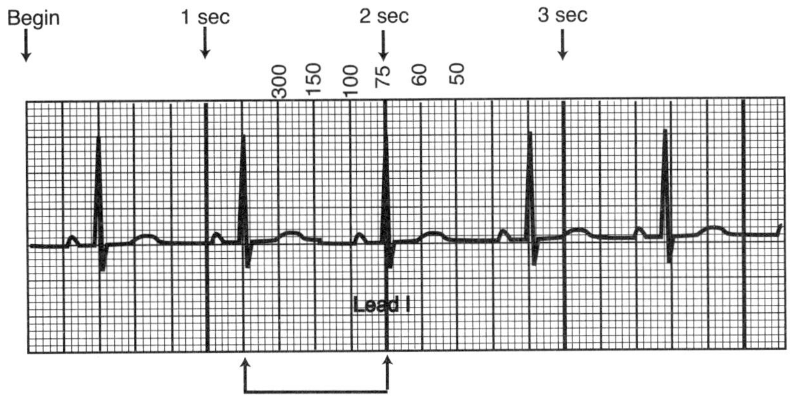

Four intervals = 75 beats/min
OR
Four beats in 3 sec = 4 X 20 = 80 beats/min

Estimation of Heart Rate	
Triplet Method	**Interval**
How many dark lines are between R waves (5 mm apart)? 1 = 300/min; 2 = 150; 3 = 100; 4 = 75; 5 = 60; 6 = 50	Measure time interval (longer interval is better) Count R waves Multiply count to convert to 1 minute e.g., four R waves in 3 sec = 4 × 20 = 80 beats/min

► Important Rhythms to Recognize

Rhythm	Characteristics
Sinus rhythm Normal rate = 60–100 Bradycardia rate <60 Tachycardia rate >100	Each beat originates in the SA node; therefore, the P wave precedes each QRS complex; PR interval is normal
AV conduction block	Abnormal conduction through AV node
First degree	PR interval (> 0.20 sec); 1:1 correspondence; P wave:R wave
Second degree Mobitz I (Wenckebach)	Progressively increased PR interval; then dropped (missing) QRS and then repeat of sequence
Second degree Mobitz II	Regular but prolonged PR interval; unexpected dropped QRS; may be a regular pattern, such as 2:1 = 2 P waves:1 QRS complex or 3:1, etc.
Third degree (complete)	No correlation of P waves and QRS complexes; usually high atrial rate and lower ventricular rate
Premature ventricular contraction (PVC)	Large, wide QRS complex originates in ectopic focus of irritability in ventricle; may indicate hypoxia
Ventricular tachycardia	Repeated large, wide QRS complexes like PVCs; Rate 150–250/min; acts like prolonged sequence of PVCs
Ventricular fibrillation	Total loss of rhythmic contraction; totally erratic shape

► Evolution of an Infarction: Signs on the EKG

Features to observe	QRS complex	Presence of prominent Q waves in leads where normally absent: infarct damage
	ST segment	Elevation or depression: acute injury
	T wave	Inversion; e.g., downward in lead where usually positive: acute ischemia
Acute myocardial infarction (MI)	Minutes to a few days	ST segment elevation or depression Inverted T waves Prominent Q waves
Resolving infarction (healing)	Weeks to months	Inverted T waves Prominent Q waves
Stable (old) MI	Months to years	Prominent Q waves as result of MI persist for the rest of life

Caution: Not all infarctions produce Q waves. Inverted T waves and/or ST abnormalities should always be investigated, even in absence of significant Q waves.

► Identifying Location of an Infarction

Location	Principal Feature of ECG	Vessel Involvement
Posterior	Large R with ST depression in V1 and V2: Mirror test or reversed transillumination	Right coronary artery
Lateral	Q waves in lateral leads I and AVL	Circumflex coronary artery
Inferior	Q waves in inferior leads II, III & AVF	Right or left coronary artery
Anterior	Q waves in V1, V2, V3 & V4	Anterior descending coronary artery

▶ Mean Electrical Axis (MEA)

Definition	• Overall direction and force (vector) of the events of ventricular depolarization: obtained by vector sum of net voltage of two leads or by quadrant method using leads I and aVF • MEA tends to shift toward large mass and away from an MI
Normal axis	• Expected in the absence of cardiac disease • R wave: lead I, +; lead II, +; lead III, +
Left axis deviation	• May indicate left heart enlargement, as in hypertrophy or left dilated failure • Abnormally prolonged (slow) left ventricular conduction • Right heart MI, expiration, obesity, lying down • R wave: lead I, +; lead II, +; lead III, –
Right axis deviation	• Right ventricular hypertrophy or dilation • Prolonged right conduction • Left heart MI, inspiration, tall lanky people, standing up • R wave: lead I, –; lead II, +; lead III, +
Extreme right axis deviation	Difficult interpretation; one example: depolarization proceeding from abnormal focus in LV apex

Einthoven's Triangle: Leads I, II, and III*

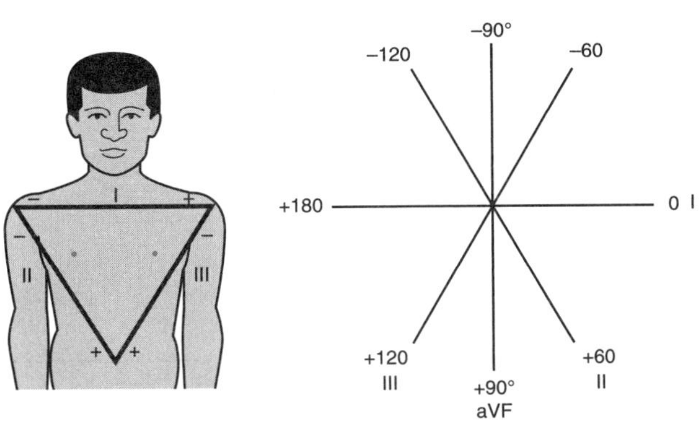

Vector Cardiogram

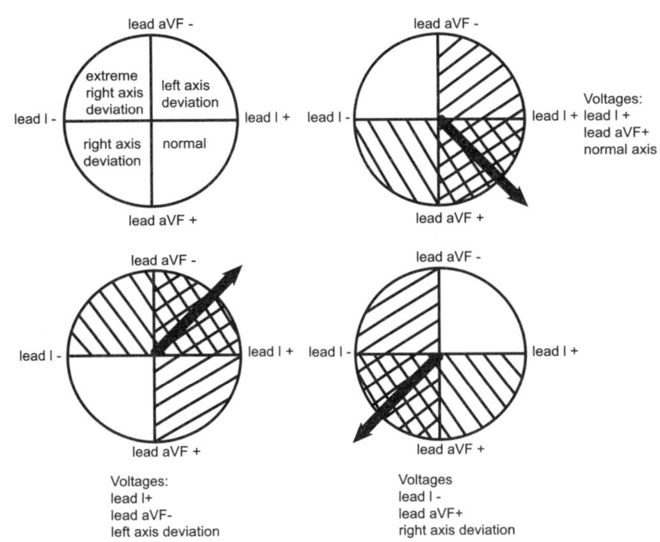

Essentials of the EKG

Heart rate

Rhythm

Axis deviation

Hypertrophy

Infarction

*The figure adds aVF because the quadrant method of determining axis uses leads I and aVF.

► Cardiac Mechanical Performance

Factor	Definition	Effects
Preload	Cardiac muscle cell length (sarcomere length) **before contraction begins**	↑ preload causes ↑ active force development up to a limit
Afterload	Load on the heart during ejection of blood from the ventricle	↑ afterload ↓ the volume of blood ejected during a beat
Contractility	Capacity of the heart to produce active force at a specified preload	High contractility ↑ ability to work Low contractility ↓ ability to work
Rate	Heart rate (HR): number of cardiac cycles per minute	↑ output of blood per minute, but ↓ output per beat; very high rate (>≈150/min) ↓ output

► Cardiac Performance: Definitions

Stroke volume (SV)	Blood ejected from ventricle per beat = EDV – ESV
End diastolic volume (EDV)	Volume of blood in ventricle at end of diastole; the preload
End systolic volume (ESV)	Volume of blood remaining in ventricle at end of systole
Cardiac output (CO)	Volume of blood per minute pumped by the heart; CO = SV × HR
Ejection fraction (EF)	Measure of contractility: EF = SV/EDV
Left ventricular dP/dT (mm Hg/sec)	Measure of contractility: maximum rate of change of pressure during isovolumic contraction

► Cardiac and Vascular Function Curves

Cardiac function curve (CFC)	• CFC generated by controlling preload and measuring cardiac output, stroke volume or other measure of systolic performance • ↑ preload improves actin-myosin interdigitation and thus ↑ SV, CO, etc. • CFC shifts **up** with ↑ **contractility; down** with ↓ **contractility**; so a new curve is produced when contractility changes • Moving to a **different point on the same CFC** is a change only of **preload:** moving to a **different CFC** is change of **contractility**
Vascular function curve (VFC)	• VFC relates venous return to right atrial pressure • ↑ **blood volume shifts VFC up,** ↓ **volume shifts VFC down**
Equilibrium point	Cardiac output is determined by both CFC and VFC. Intersection of the CFC and VFC is the stable operating point; if contractility or blood volume changes, the system will operate at the intersection of the two new curves.

► Cardiovascular Responses in Exercise

	Heart Rate	TPR	MAP	Cardiac Output
Aerobic, Dynamic	Increased	Decreased	Minimal change	Increased
Anaerobic, Static	Increased	Increased	Increased	Increased, unchanged, or decreased*

*Cardiac output during static or anaerobic exercise is highly dependent on the type and intensity of exercise.

Definition of abbreviations: MAP, mean arterial pressure; TPR, total peripheral resistance.

▶ Cardiac and Vascular Function Curves: Examples

Stability of Typical CFC and VFC

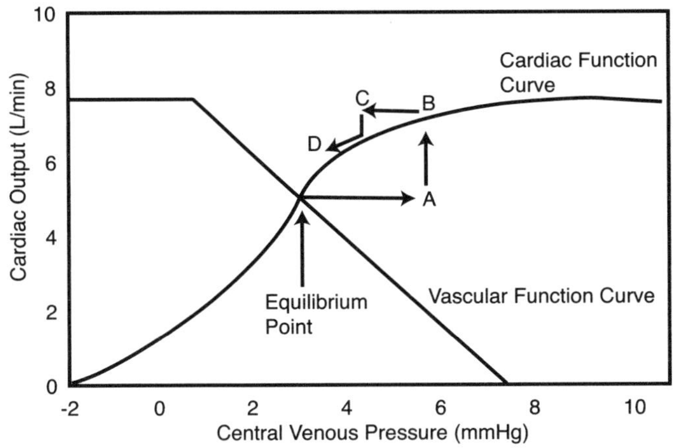

Diagram shows that cardiac output (CO, 5 L/min) changes only transiently when CFC and VFC are not changed. **Point A:** venous pressure is increased from 3 to 6 mm Hg because of sudden removal of blood from arterial system and injection into venous system. This causes **CO** to increase to **point B**. CO then returns to **equilibrium point** in steps (B → C, C → D) as blood is pumped from venous system back to arterial system.

Changes in Blood Volume

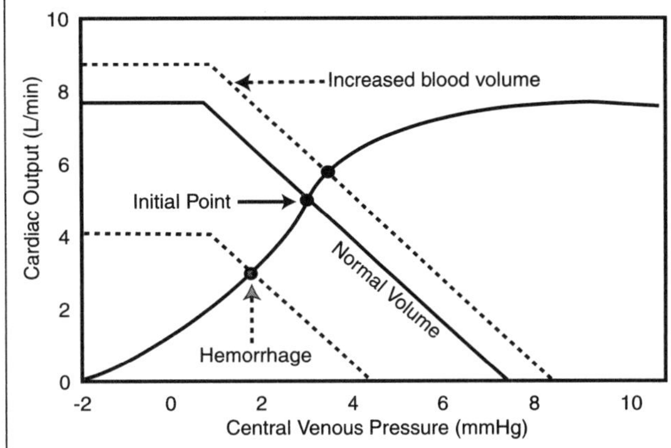

Increased blood volume (e.g., transfusion) shifts the VFC upward, which increases preload. Increased CO follows. Decreased blood volume (e.g., hemorrhage) shifts the VFC downward, which decreases preload. Decreased CO follows. Increases and decreases in preload produce increases and decreases in CO by the **Frank-Starling** mechanism.

Sympathetic Stimulation of Heart

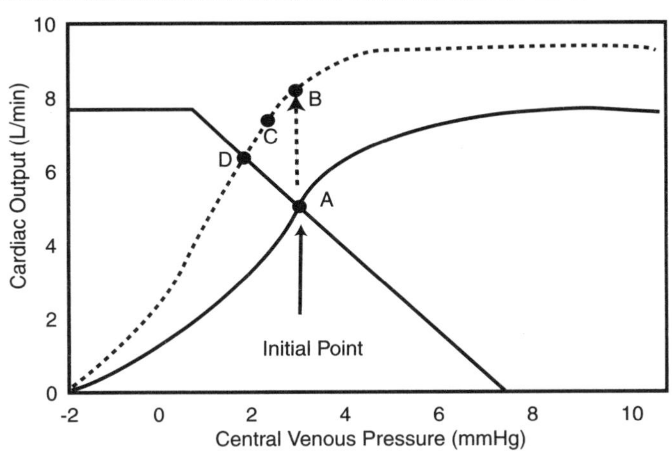

Increased contractility by cardiac sympathetic nerve stimulation shifts the CFC upward *(dashed line)*; however, this does not change the VFC. The initial large increase in CO *(point B)* returns to **point D** on the VFC as blood is transferred from the venous system to the arterial system.

Changes in CO After Heart Failure

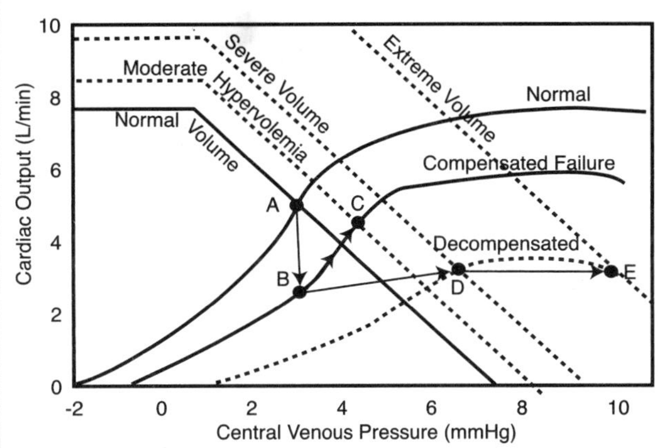

Reduced contractility shifts CO down **(point B)**, but preload immediately increases to intersect with the normal volume curve as shown. Within hours to days, blood volume increases, shifting VFC upward, and **point C** becomes the equilibrium point. With progressive failure, blood volume cannot increase enough to maintain CO at a normal level. **(point D)**. Blood volume continues to increase, which overstretches the heart **(point E)**.

► The Cardiac Cycle: The Wigger's Diagram

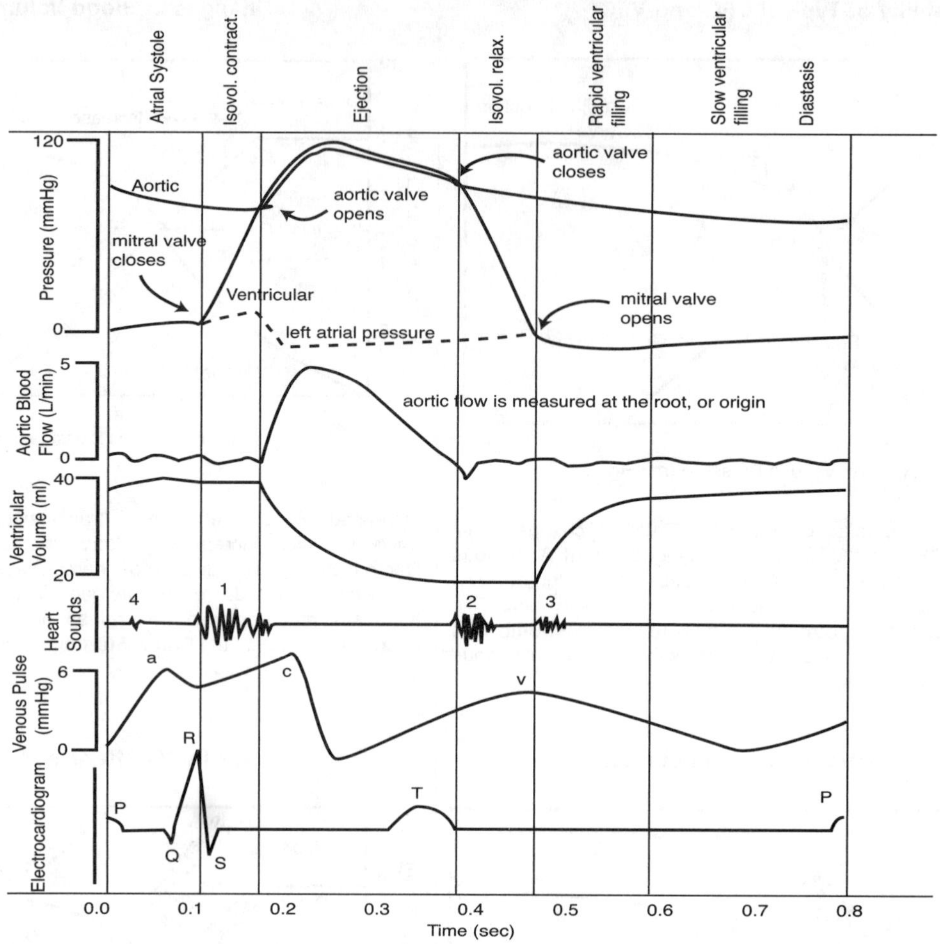

Left ventricular pressure	**Systole:** begins at isovolumic contraction, ends at beginning of isovolumic relaxation: two phases are isovolumic contraction and ventricular ejection	**Diastole:** begins at beginning of isovolumic relaxation and ends at onset of isovolumic contraction: two phases are isovolumic relaxation and ventricular filling
Aortic pressure	Maximum is systolic pressure. During ejection, aortic pressure is slightly below ventricular pressure.	Minimum is diastolic pressure. Pressure falls during diastole as blood flows from aorta into capillaries and then veins.
Left atrial pressure	Systole; isolated from ventricular pressure because mitral valve is closed	Diastole, blood flows from atrium into ventricle because mitral valve is open. Note mitral closed during isovolumic relaxation.
Aortic flow (measured at root)	Systolic ejection begins when ventricular pressure exceeds aortic diastolic and aortic valve opens.	Ejection ends when rapidly falling ventricular pressure causes aortic valve to close.
Ventricular volume	Maximum at end of diastole; does not change during isovolumic contraction because mitral and aortic valves are closed.	Minimum at end of ejection phase; does not change during isovolumic relaxation (both valves closed).
Heart sounds	Systole: S_1 caused by sound of mitral closure	S_2 caused by sound of aortic valve closure
Venous pulse	Rises with atrial systole	Drops as atrium fills
EKG	QRS begins before isovolumic contraction	T wave begins during late ejection phase

▶ Cardiac Pressure–Volume Loops (PV Loops)

Phase	Pressure	Volume
Filling	Slightly ↑	Large ↑; point C = EDV
Isovolumic contraction	Rapid ↑; maximum dp/dt	No change, valves closed
Ejection	Continues to rise	↓ as ejection proceeds
Isovolumic relaxation	Rapid ↓	No change, valves closed

Applications	
Area within loop = stroke work output	Increase work by ↑ stroke volume (volume work) or by ↑ LVP (pressure work)
Decreased blood volume (hemorrhage, dehydration, urination)	Line C–D shift left (↓ preload); ↓ stroke volume ↓ stroke work
Increase in contractility (sympathetics, or β-adrenergic drugs, digitalis)	Line F–A shifts left (↓ ESV) a major effect; slight ↓ EDV; overall ↑ stroke volume, ↑ stroke work
Decreased contractility, as in heart failure	Loop shifts to right and systolic pressure is lower: ↑↑ ESV, ↑ EDP, ↓ SV, ↓ stroke work
Volume expansion (normal heart)	Line C–D shifts right (↑ EDV); ↑ SV; ↑ stroke work

Normal PV Curve	Blood Volume Changes

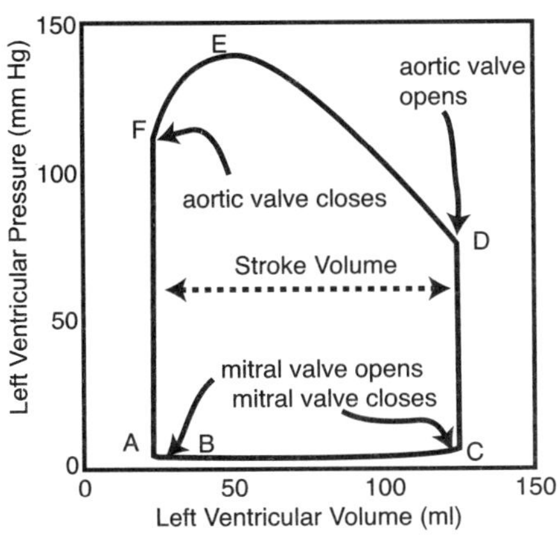

A–B: rapid filling
B–C: reduced or slower filling
C: end diastolic volume (EDV)
C–D: isovolumic contraction
D–F: ejection phase
F: end systolic volume (ESV)
F–A: isovolumic relaxation

- Area within loop = **stroke work**
- Increase work by ↑ stroke volume (volume work) or by ↑ LVP (pressure work)

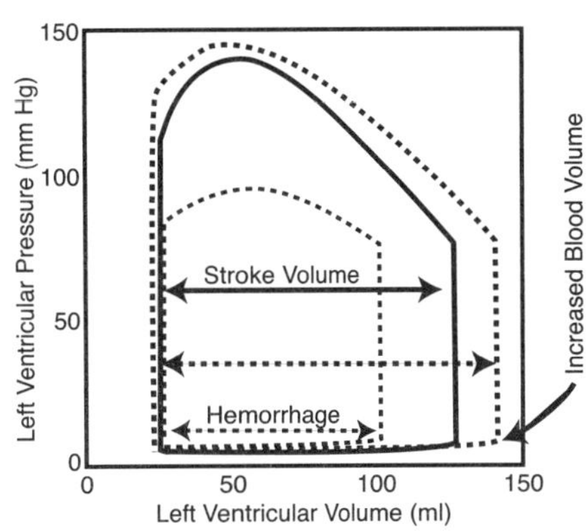

- **Decreased blood volume** (hemorrhage, dehydration): Line C–D shifts **left** (↓ preload); ↓ stroke volume, ↓ stroke work
- **Volume expansion** (normal heart): Line C–D shifts **right** (↑ EDV), ↑ SV, ↑ stroke work
- Diastolic dysfunction tends to ↓ EDV despite ↑ EDP
- Systolic dysfunction tends to ↑ ESV and ↓ systolic LVP

(Continued)

► Cardiac Pressure–Volume Loops (PV Loops; *Cont'd.*)

Increased Afterload

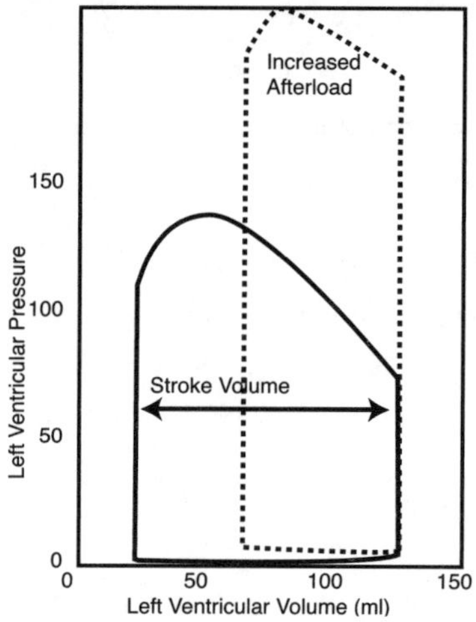

With increased afterload (e.g., ↑ aortic pressure), the velocity of shortening and the distance shortened are both decreased. Thus, ESV increases, causing SV to decrease.

Decreased Afterload

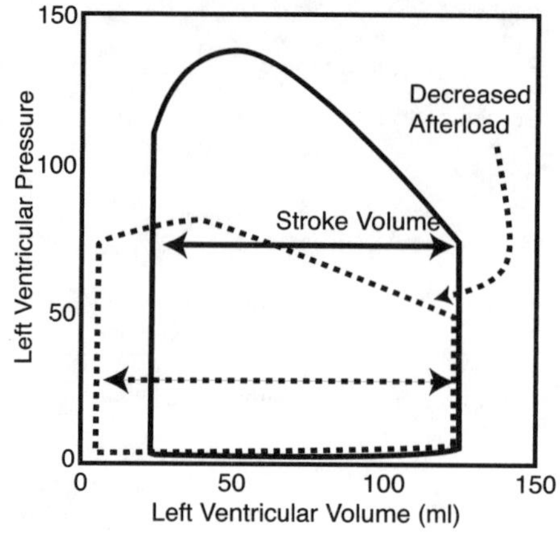

Decreased afterload produces the opposite changes as increased afterload. Thus, ESV decreases and SV increases.

Progressive Heart Failure

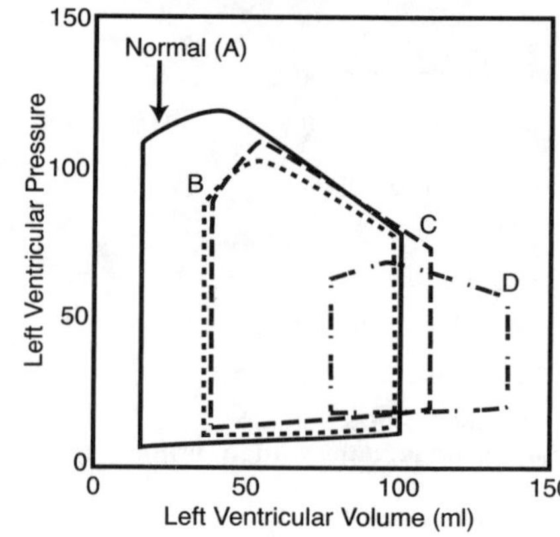

A: Normal
B: Acute loss of contractility without compensation
C: Compensated LV failure (SV partially restored because of moderate increase in preload)
D: Decompensated failure (SV remains low despite ↑↑↑ in preload)
Overall: Curves shift to the right and systolic pressures ↓.
Heart failure: ↑↑↑ ESV, ↑ EDV, ↓ SV, ↓ stroke work

► The Cardiac Valves

Mitral	Between LA and LV	Open during filling	Closed during ventricular systole and isovolumic relaxation
Aortic	Between LV and aorta	Open during ejection	Closed during diastole and isovolumic contraction
Tricuspid	Between RA and RV	Open during filling	Closed during ventricular systole and isovolumic relaxation
Pulmonic	Between RV and pulmonary artery	Open during ejection	Closed during diastole and isovolumic contraction

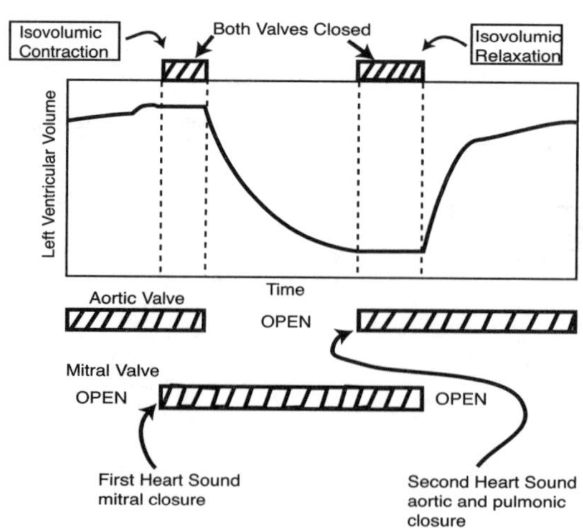

▶ Valvular Disorders

Aortic Stenosis

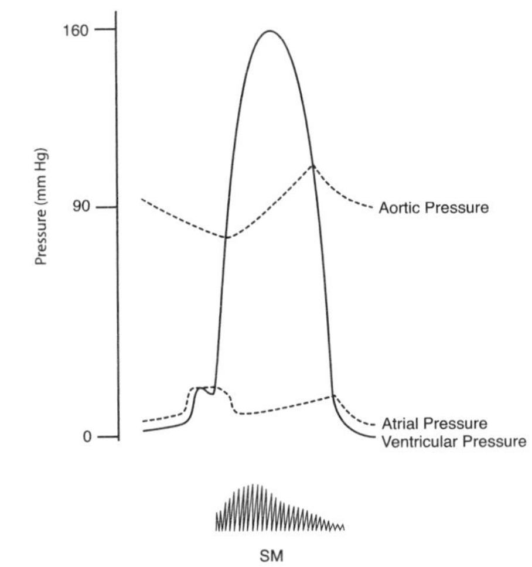

- Discrepancy of systolic LV and systolic aortic pressures
- Causes crescendo-decrescendo systolic murmur

Aortic Regurgitation

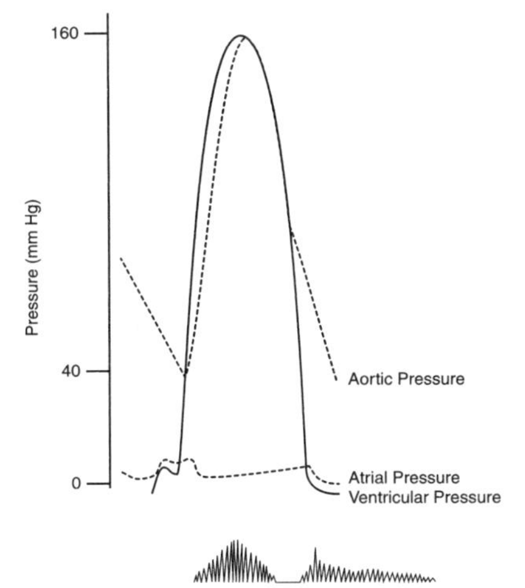

- Diastolic aortic P decreases rapidly as blood flows back into ventricle; ventricular diastolic P is elevated.
- Causes diastolic murmur

Mitral Valve Stenosis

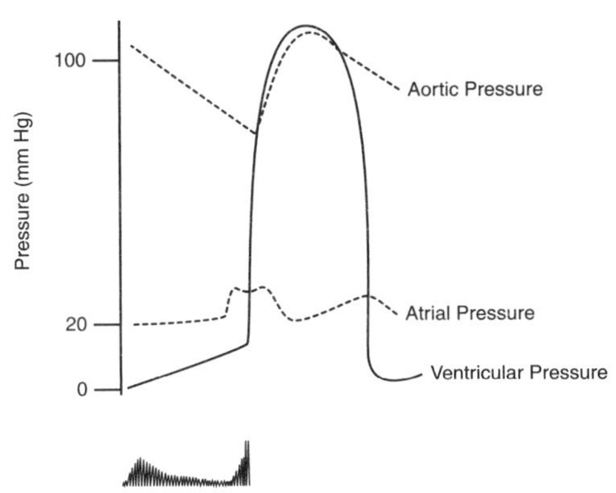

- Discrepancy of diastolic LVP and left atrial P during filling
- Causes diastolic murmur

Mitral Regurgitation

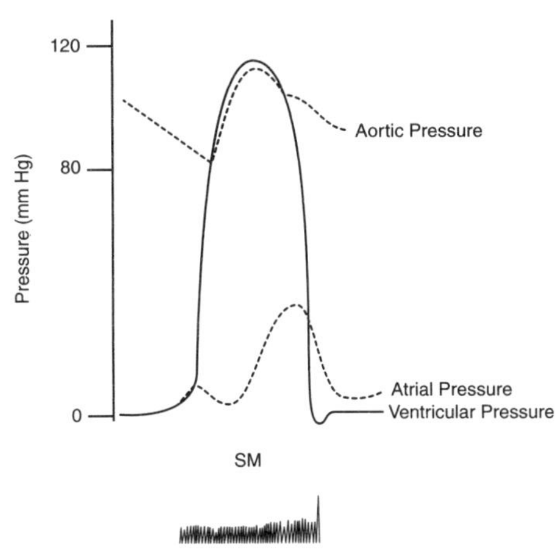

- Incompetent valve allows backflow into left atrium during ventricular systole
- Causes systolic murmur

Definition of abbreviation: SM, systolic murmur.

▶ Hemodynamics

Poiseuille's equation:

$Q = (P_1 - P_2)/R$

- Flow (Q); P_1 (input pressure); P_2 (output pressure); R (resistance); $(P_1 - P_2)$ = pressure gradient
- ↑ pressure gradient → ↑ flow
- ↑ resistance → ↓ flow

Series circuits:

$R_T = R_1 + R_2 + R_3 .....R_n$

- R_T = total resistance
- Flow is equal at all points in series circuit; pressure drops across each resistor
- **Adding more resistors in series increases R_T.** Pressure drop increases along circuit with constant flow, and flow decreases with constant input pressure (P_1).
- Various types of blood vessels lie in series.

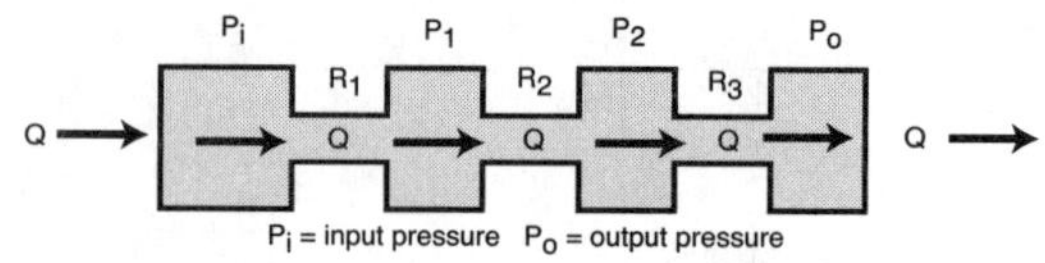

Parallel circuits:

$1/R_T = 1/R_1 + 1/R_2 + 1/R_3 ... ..1/R_n$

- Flow divided between parallel resistors
- R_T is always lower than the lowest resistor
- **Adding more resistors in parallel decreases R_T.**
- Produces low resistance circuit
- Organs lie in parallel

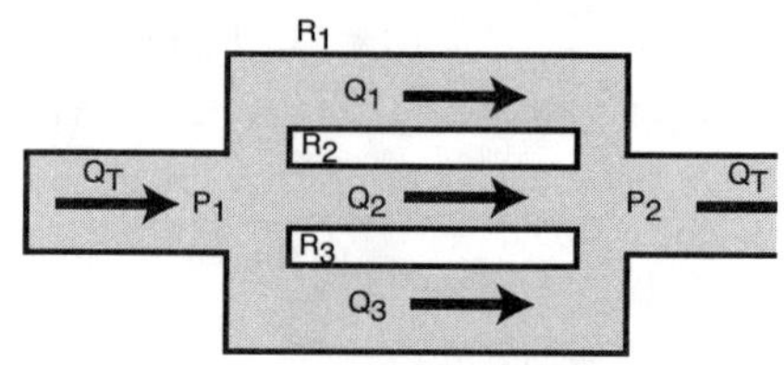

$$Q_T = Q_1 + Q_2 + Q_3$$

$$\frac{1}{R_T} = \frac{1}{R_1} + \frac{1}{R_2} + \frac{1}{R_3}$$

Hydraulic Resistance Equation:

$R = (P_1 - P_2)/Q = 8\eta l/\pi r^4$

- η = viscosity; l = length; r = radius
- **Viscosity ↑ by ↑ hematocrit**
- **Viscosity ↓ in anemia**
- l is usually constant; r changes greatly for normal regulation and in disease.
- 2× radius = 1/16 R → 16 × flow
- ½ radius = 16 × R → 1/16 × flow
- **Control of radius is the dominant mechanism to control resistance.**

Total peripheral resistance (TPR)

- Resistance of peripheral circuit: aorta → right atrium
- **TPR ↑ by sympathetics, angiotensin II, and other vasoconstrictors**
- Highest TPRs in **arterioles**; also main site of blood flow regulation

Total peripheral resistance equation

TPR = (MAP – RAP)/CO

- Mean arterial pressure (MAP); right atrial pressure (RAP)
- Pressure gradient is between aorta and right atrium.
- TPR is calculated from MAP and cardiac output (CO). RAP is assumed to be 0 mm Hg, unless specified.
- TPR is also known as SVR (systemic vascular resistance)

Compliance (C):

C = ΔV / ΔP

- ΔV = volume change; ΔP = pressure change
- High **compliance** means vessels easily distended by blood.
- **Elasticity** is inverse of compliance; vessels are stiff when elasticity is high

Pulse pressure (PP):

PP = SP – DP

- SP = systolic pressure; DP = diastolic pressure

↓ compliance (e.g., arteriosclerosis) → ↑ SP and ↓ DP, so PP ↑

- **Compliance:** systemic veins > pulmonary circuit > systemic arteries (volume of blood is in same order)

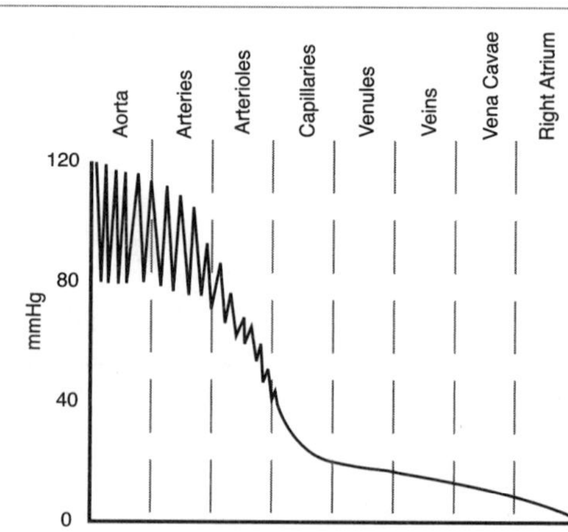

- **MAP = diastolic + 1/3 (pulse pressure)**
- MAP = 80 + 1/3(120 – 80) = 80 = 13 = 93 mm Hg

(Continued)

▶ Hemodynamics (CONT'D.)

Cardiac output (Fick method)	• $CO = \dot{V}O_2/(Ca - Cv)$ • $\dot{V}O_2$ = oxygen consumption, Ca = arterial oxygen content, Cv = venous oxygen content	• Used to measure cardiac output; most accurate if Ca is pulmonary venous and Cv is pulmonary arterial

▶ Area-Velocity Relationship

- **V∝ 1/cross sectional area**
- **$V \propto 1/r^2$,**
- V = velocity; r = radius
- **Assuming total flow is equal in all vessel types, velocity increases as radius decreases.**
- **The aorta is a single large vessel, but its total area is small compared with numerous capillaries in parallel.**
- If low capillary velocity allows adequate time for diffusion, exchange is **perfusion limited**.
- If velocity is high, metabolic exchange may become **diffusion limited**.

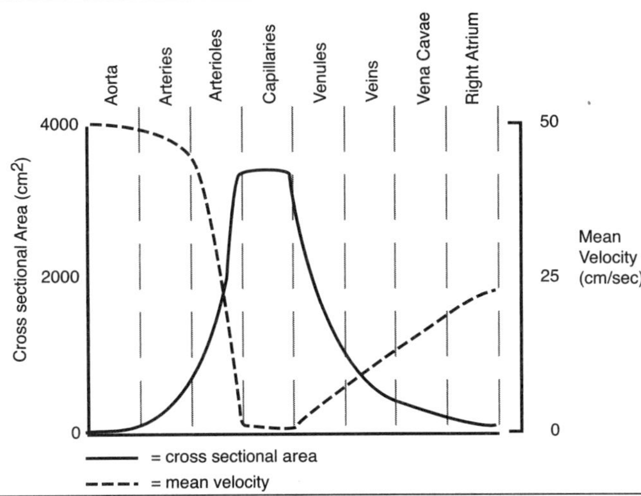

▶ Pressures of the Cardiovascular System

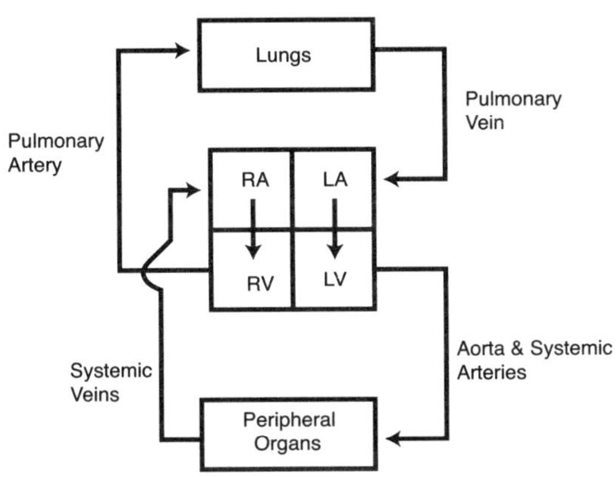

- The cardiac output and stroke volume of the left and right heart are nearly equal.
- The mean pressures are different because the systemic resistance is about 6× higher.
- The pulse pressure in the pulmonary circulation is lower because its compliance is higher.

Pressures in the Pulmonary Circulation (mm Hg)	
Right ventricle	25/0
Pulmonary artery	25/8
Mean pulmonary artery	14
Capillary	7–9
Pulmonary vein	5
Left atrium	<5
Pressure gradient	15 – 5 = 10

Pressures in the Systemic Circulation (mm Hg)	
Left ventricle	120/0
Aorta	120/80
MAP	93
Capillary: skeletal Renal glomerular	<30 45–50
Peripheral veins	<15
Right atrium	0
Pressure gradient	93 – 0 = 93

► Factors That Control Filtration and Reabsorption in Capillaries

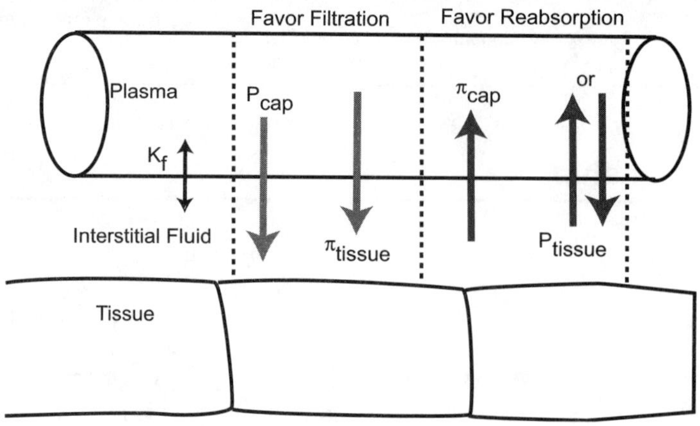

Filtration = K_f (forces favor – forces opposed)
Filtration = K_f [($P_{capillary} + \pi_{tissue}$) – ($P_{tissue} + \pi_{capillary}$)]

Ultrafiltration coefficient (K_f)	• Related to surface area, capillary porosity; different in each tissue/organ • Determines amount of ultrafiltration to given filtration pressure
Capillary hydrostatic pressure (P_{cap})	• **Favors filtration;** ↑ P_{cap} → ↑ filtration • Controlled by input pressure, arteriolar diameter, venous pressure
Tissue (interstitial) oncotic pressure (π_{tissue})	• **Favors filtration;** ↑ π_{tissue} →↑ filtration • Directly related to [protein] in interstitial fluid • **Example:** ↑ permeability (e.g., sepsis) →↑ π_{tissue} →↑ filtration
Capillary (plasma) oncotic pressure (π_{cap})	• **Opposes filtration;** ↑π_{cap} →↓ filtration • Directly related to [protein] in plasma • **Examples:** – Liver failure ↓π_{cap} → edema – Dehydration ↑π_{cap} → reabsorption
Tissue (interstitial) hydrostatic pressure (P_{tissue})	• Increases filtration when negative (is normally negative in many but not all tissues) • Opposes filtration when positive; edema causes positive pressure in interstitium, even when pressure is normally negative.

▶ Factors That Alter Capillary Flow and Pressure

	Resistance	Capillary Flow	Capillary Pressure	Example
Arteriole dilation	↓	↑	↑	β-adrenergic agonist, α-adrenergic blocker, decreased sympathetic nervous system activity, metabolic dilation, ACE inhibitors
Arteriole constriction	↑	↓	↓	α-adrenergic agonist, β-adrenergic blocker, increased sympathetic nervous system activity, angiotensin II
Venous dilation	↓	↑	↓	Increased metabolism of tissue
Venous constriction	↑	↓	↑	Physical compression, increased sympathetic activity
Increased arterial pressure	N	↑	↑	Increased cardiac output, volume expansion
Decreased arterial pressure	N	↓	↓	Decreased cardiac output, hemorrhage, dehydration
Increased venous pressure	N	↓	↑	Congestive heart failure, physical compression
Decreased venous pressure	N	↑	↓	Hemorrhage, dehydration

▶ Wall Tension: Law of Laplace

T = P × r

- Tension (T) in wall
- **↑ pressure and ↑ radius → ↑ tension**

Applications

Arterial aneurysm:

- Weak wall balloons
- Vessel radius ↑, causing ↑ wall tension.
- ↑ tension causes ↑ radius (vicious cycle), increasing risk of rupture

Dilated heart failure:

- ↑ ventricular volume → ↑ ventricular radius, which in turn causes ↑ wall tension.
- Thus, dilated ventricle must work harder than normal heart

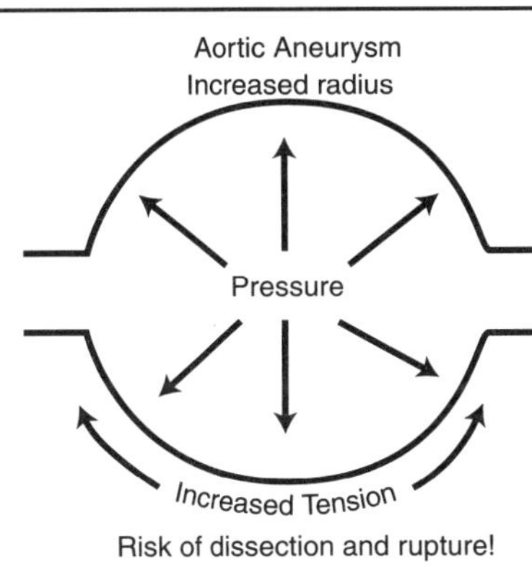

► Autonomic Control of Heart and Circulation

	Sympathetic	Parasympathetic
Heart		
Transmitter-receptor	Norepinephrine: β_1-adrenergic	Acetylcholine: muscarinic
Heart rate	↑ rate (i_f and Ca^{2+} currents): ⊕ chronotropic	↓ rate (↑ gK, ↓ i_f): ⊖ chronotropic
Contractility	↑ force (dp/dt, EF): ⊕ inotropic ↑ gCa^{2+}, ↑ cAMP, ↑ Ca^{2+} release from SR, ↓ duration: fast, strong, short duration	Modest effects: ⊖ inotropic ↓cAMP; ↓gCa^{2+} mainly at very high levels of activity only
Conduction	↑ atrial and ventricular conduction ↑ conduction AV node ↓ PR interval of EKG	↓ atrial and ventricular conduction ↓ conduction AV node ↑ PR interval of EKG
Arteries/arterioles	Norepinephrine: α_1 (mainly) constriction Epinephrine (adrenal): β_2 dilation High levels: α_1 constriction	No direct innervation of vascular smooth muscle
Veins	Norepinephrine: α_1 (mainly) constriction but not usually much ↑ resistance, rather, ↓ capacitance shifts blood toward heart	No direct innervation

► Control of Organ Blood Flow

Organ/Tissue	Neural	Metabolic/Other
Skeletal muscle	**Resting:** α-adrenergic constriction **Exercising:** β-adrenergic dilation (epinephrine, adrenal medulla)	• **Metabolic vasodilation dominates in exercise** • Compression during static exercise blocks flow
Skin	• Thermoregulatory center • α-adrenergic constriction only	• Heat dilates, cold constricts, a direct effect
Heart	• α-adrenergic constriction • β-adrenergic dilation • Overridden by metabolism	• **Metabolic dilation is dominant** • ↑ Cardiac work → ↑ O_2 consumption →↑ coronary flow • Compression during systole, so most coronary flow is during diastole
Brain	Not generally under neural control: autoregulation	• **Metabolism dominates:** ↑ CO_2 → dilation

► Autoregulation

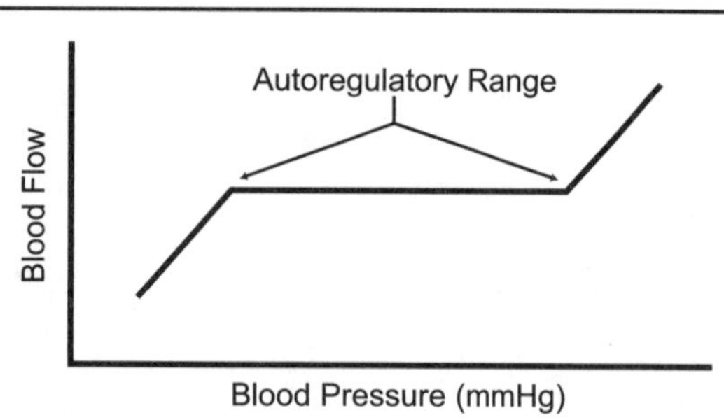

Regulation of blood flow within the organ itself

Autoregulating Organs

- Cerebrum
- Heart
- Exercising muscle
- Gastrointestinal tract
- Kidney (not metabolic autoregulation)

▶ Basics of Integrated Control of Arterial Pressure and Cardiac Output

	Control	Major Actions
Baroreceptors: Carotid sinus (primary) Aortic arch (secondary)	↑ pressure →↑ activity ↓ pressure →↓ activity	↑ activity → ↑ PNS and ↓ SNS ↓ activity → ↓ PNS and ↑ SNS
Sympathetic (SNS)	↑ pressure → ↓ SNS ↓ pressure → ↑ SNS	• Vasoconstriction (↑ α-adrenergic) → ↑ TPR • ↑ Contractility heart (↑ β-adrenergic) → ↓ ESV → ↑ SV • ↑ Heart rate (β-adrenergic) • ↑ Cardiac output (CO)
Parasympathetic (PNS)	↑ pressure → ↑ PNS ↓ pressure → ↓ PNS	• ↓ heart rate (major); ↓ contractility (minor) • At rest, PNS dominant control of heart rate • ↓ cardiac output
Renal	↑ MAP → ↓ renin, angiotensin II (AII) ↑ MAP →↑ urination →↓ volume →↓ preload	• All vasoconstricts • **Renal control of blood volume and TPR dominant long-term control of blood pressure and CO**

▶ Selected Applications of the Diagram

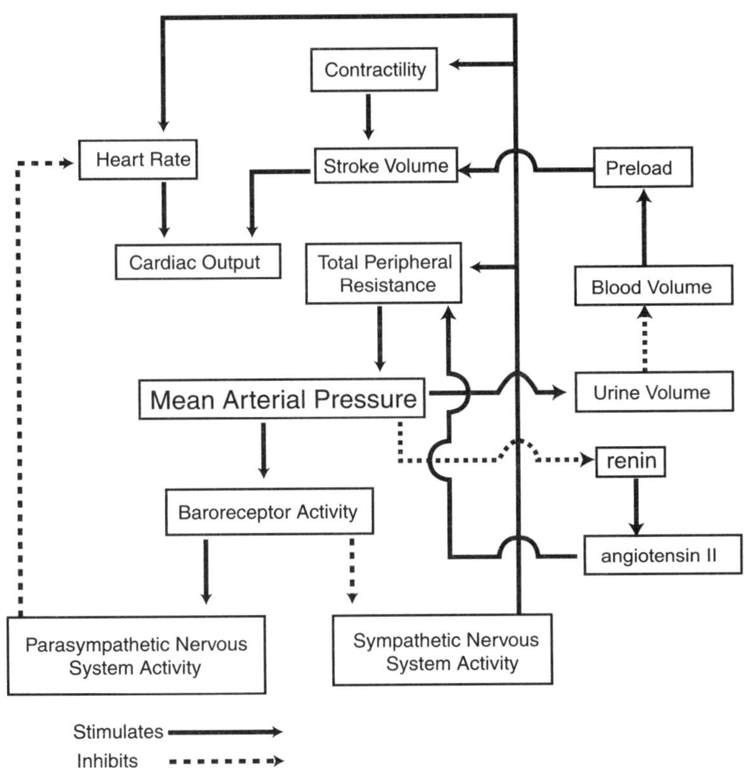

Hemorrhage—enter at blood volume (↓)

Heart failure—enter at contractility (↓)

Vasodilator drug—enter at TPR (↓)

Vasoconstrictor drug—enter at TPR (↑)

Diuretics—enter at urine volume (↑)

Carotid massage—enter at baroreceptor (↑)

ACE inhibitor—enter at angiotensin II* (↓)

**Note:* also would increase urine flow through reduction of aldosterone (not shown in figure)

Cardiovascular Pathology

► Congenital Abnormalities of the Heart

- Congenital abnormalities occur before the end of week 16 (completion of heart development).
- Clinical significance depends on degree of shunt.
- Up to 90% of congenital heart disease is of unknown etiology.
- **Maternal rubella:** exposure at fifth to tenth week can lead to PDA, ASDs, and VSDs.
- **Fetal alcohol syndrome:** cardiovascular defects, including VSD

Acyanotic (Late Cyanosis) Congenital Heart Disease (Left-to-Right Shunts)	
Initially a left-to-right shunt; causes chronic right heart failure and secondary pulmonary hypertension. Increased pressure causes **reversal of shunt flow** with late onset cyanosis: **Eisenmenger syndrome**	
Ventricular septal defect (VSD)	• Usually of membranous interventricular septum • Often associated with other defects, including **trisomy 21**
Atrial septal defect (ASD)	**Ostium primum defect (5% of ASDs):** • Defect in lower atrial septum above the atrioventricular valves • Associated with anomaly of AV valves • Requires antibiotic prophylaxis for invasive procedures **Ostium secundum defects (90% of ASDs):** • Defect is in center of the atrial septum at the foramen ovale • Results from abnormalities of septum primum and/or septum secundum • AV valves normal • Antibiotic prophylaxis not needed
Complete endocardial cushion defect	Combination of ASD, VSD, and a common atrioventricular valve
Sinus venosus	• Defect in the upper part of the atrial septum • May cause anomalous pulmonary venous return into superior vena cava or right atrium
Patent foramen ovale	• Remnant of the foramen ovale, usually not of clinical significance • Risk of paradoxical emboli
Patent ductus arteriosus (PDA)	In the fetal circulation, the PDA shunts blood from the pulmonary artery into aorta. At birth, the pressure differential changes, and the flow is reversed (from aorta to pulmonary artery). This leads to pulmonary hypertension due to excess blood flowing through pulmonary artery. **Pharmacology:** • Indomethacin: closes PDA • Prostaglandin E: keeps PDA open
Cyanotic Congenital Heart Disease (Right-to-Left Shunts)	
• Right-to-left shunt bypasses the lungs and hence produces cyanosis as early as birth. • Paradoxical embolism (DVT causes systemic infarct) may occur.	
Tetralogy of Fallot	• **Most common cyanotic congenital heart disease in older children and adults** • Associated with trisomy 21 • Four lesions: *1)* VSD *2)* An overriding aorta that receives blood from both ventricles *3)* Right ventricular hypertrophy *4)* Pulmonic stenosis (right ventricular outflow obstruction)

(Continued)

Cyanotic Congenital Heart Disease (Right-To-Left Shunts; *Cont'd.*)	
Transposition of the great vessels	• Failure of the **truncoconal septum** to spiral • The aorta arises from the right ventricle, and the pulmonary artery arises from the left ventricle, producing two closed loops. This is fatal if a shunt (e.g., PDA, VSD, ASD, patent foramen ovale) is not present to mix the venous and systemic blood.
Persistent truncus arteriosus	• Failure of the truncus arteriosus to separate into the aorta and pulmonary arteries • Usually a membranous VSD • Truncus arteriosus receives blood from both ventricles, so cyanosis results.

Definition of abbreviation: DVT, deep venous thrombosis.

▶ Obstructive Congenital Heart Disease

Does not usually cause cyanosis	
Coarctation of the aorta	**Preductal (infantile) type:** • Narrowing of the aorta proximal to the opening of the ductus arteriosus • May be associated with cyanosis of the lower half of the body • Often requires surgery **Postductal (adult) type:** • Narrowing of the aorta distal to the opening of the ductus arteriosus • **Most common type**; allows survival into adulthood • **Disparity in pressure between the upper and lower extremities** • Collateral circulation leads to rib notching
Pulmonic valve stenosis or atresia	• Unequal division of the truncus arteriosus so that the pulmonary trunk has no lumen or opening at the level of the pulmonary valve • May cause cyanosis if severe
Aortic valve stenosis or atresia	**Complete atresia:** incompatible with life **Bicuspid aortic valves:** asymptomatic, can lead to infective endocarditis, left ventricular overload, and sudden death • Calcify fifth to sixth decade (tricuspid aortic valves usually calcify 10 years later) • Most common cause of aortic stenosis (more than rheumatic fever)

Diseases Associated with Congenital Heart Defects
Marfan syndrome: 1/3 patients have aortic dilatation and incompetence, aortic dissection, and ASD
Down syndrome: 20% of patients may have congenital cardiovascular disease
Turner syndrome: Coarctation of the aorta
22q11 syndromes (DiGeorge syndrome and velocardial facial syndrome): Truncus arteriosus and tetralogy of Fallot
Congenital rubella: Septal defects, patent ductus arteriosus, pulmonary artery stenosis
Maternal diabetes: Transposition of great vessels

▶ Ischemic Heart Disease

- **Leading cause of death**
- Most angina pectoris caused by severe atherosclerotic narrowing of coronary arteries
- Result of decreased supply (anemia, carbon monoxide, pulmonary disease) and/or increased demand (exertion, hypertrophy)
- Sudden cardiac death the presenting symptom in 25% of patients with IHD

Angina pectoris	• Paroxysmal substernal or precordial chest pain • Transient **myocardial ischemia** without myocardial infarction
Stable angina pectoris	• Paroxysms are associated with a **fixed** amount of exertion, e.g., after walking three blocks • Typical attacks last less than 10 minutes and are **relieved with rest** or sublingual nitroglycerin • ECG may show **ST segment depression** (ischemia limited to subendocardium)
Prinzmetal angina	• Vasospasm causes decreased blood flow through atherosclerotic vessels • This form of attack frequently occurs at rest with **ST-segment elevation** on ECG • Treat with calcium channel blockers
Unstable angina	• Chest pain with progressively less exertion, then occurring at rest, **often precedes myocardial infarction** • May be unresponsive to nitroglycerin

▶ Myocardial Infarction

- Ischemic necrosis of myocardium, most commonly transmural, but can be subendocardial
- Highest incidence of fatal MI: 55 to 64 years old
- Risk factors: male sex, hypertension, hypercholesterolemia, cigarette smoking, family history, diabetes mellitus, oral contraceptive use, sedentary lifestyle, type A personality, family history of MI in men under 45, women under 55 years of age

Clinical features	• Acute, severe, crushing chest pain, often radiating to the jaw or left arm; diaphoresis; little or no chest pain may be present in diabetic and elderly patients • ECG: **ST elevation and T-wave inversion** with or without Q-waves • **Elevated cardiac enzymes**
Prognosis	• Sudden cardiac death: secondary to a fatal arrhythmia, occurs in 25% • Mortality after myocardial infarction: 35% in the first year, 45% in second year, and 55% in third year • Complications: arrhythmias, CHF, cardiogenic shock, systemic emboli from mural thrombi, aneurysm • Wall/papillary muscle rupture (3–7 days after infarct), postinfarction pericarditis (Dressler syndrome; 2–10 weeks postinfarction)
Treatment and management	• **Coronary artery bypass:** saphenous vein or internal mammary artery grafts restore circulation; grafts last approximately 10 years before restenosis typically occurs • **Angioplasty** (balloon dilatation) also restores circulation, half re-stenose in 1 year • **Fibrinolytic therapy** (e.g., tissue plasminogen activators): highly effective in reducing mortality if administered early in the course of the MI.

▶ Appearance of Infarcted Myocardium

Time	Gross	Histologic
1 hour	No gross changes evident	Intracellular edema
6–12 hours		Wavy myocardial fibers, vacuolar degeneration, contraction band necrosis, beginning neutrophilic infiltrate
12–24 hours	Pale, cyanotic, edematous	
24–48 hours	Well-demarcated, soft, pale	Neutrophilic infiltrate, increased cytoplasmic eosinophilia, and coagulation necrosis become evident
3–10 days	Infarct becomes soft, yellow, surrounded by hyperemic rim	Monocytic infiltrate predominates at 72 hours
2 weeks	Infarct area is surrounded by granulation tissue that is gradually replaced by scar tissue.	

Cardiac Enzymes

Troponin I peaks first (4 h): remains elevated 7–10 days

CK-MB peaks within 24 h: remains elevated 2–3 days

LDH peaks later (about 2 days): remains elevated 8–14 days

AST also rises and falls predictably in myocardial infarction, but may indicate liver damage instead

Definition of abbreviations: AST, aspartate aminotransferase; CK-MB, creatine kinase MB fraction; LDH, lactate dehydrogenase.

▶ Rheumatic Fever and Rheumatic Heart Disease

Acute rheumatic fever	• Onset is typically 1–3 weeks after group A β-hemolytic streptococcal pharyngitis, otitis media • Children: 5–15 years old • Declining incidence secondary to penicillin use • Antistreptococcal antibodies cross-react with host connective tissue • Diagnosed using Jones criteria (two major or one major and two minor)	
Jones Criteria	**Major**	**Minor**
Mnemonic: **J**ones ♥ carditis **N**odules **E**rythema marginatum **S**ydenham chorea	• **Migratory polyarthritis**—large joints that become red, swollen, and painful • **Erythema marginatum**—macular skin rash, often in "bathing suit" distribution • **Sydenham chorea**—involuntary, choreiform movements of the extremities • **Subcutaneous nodules** • **Carditis**—may affect the endocardium, myocardium, or pericardium; myocarditis causes most deaths during the acute stage	• Previous rheumatic fever • Fever • Arthralgias • Prolonged PR interval • Elevated ESR • Leukocytosis • Elevated C-reactive protein
Rheumatic heart disease	• Repeated bouts of endocarditis and inflammatory insult lead to scarring and thickening of the valve leaflets with nodules along lines of closure • **Mitral valve** most commonly (75–80%) affected; fibrosis and deformity lead to "fish mouth" or "buttonhole" stenosis. Next in frequency are the aortic and mitral valves together. Tricuspid and pulmonic valves are rarely affected. • **Aschoff bodies** are pathognomonic lesions; focal collections of perivascular fibrinoid necrosis surrounded by inflammatory cells including large histiocytes (**Anitschkow cells**) • Left atrial dilatation, mural thrombi, and right ventricular hypertrophy • Predisposes to infective endocarditis	

► Congestive Heart Failure (CHF)

Types	Etiology	Comments
Left-sided heart failure	• Ischemic heart disease • Aortic stenosis • Aortic insufficiency • Hypertension • Cardiomyopathies	• Increased back pressure produces pulmonary congestion and edema • Dyspnea, orthopnea, paroxysmal nocturnal dyspnea, and cough • Renal hypoperfusion stimulates renin-angiotensin-aldosterone axis • Retention of salt and water compounds the pulmonary edema
Right-sided heart failure	• Left-sided heart failure • Cor pulmonale • Pulmonary stenosis • Pulmonary insufficiency	• Chronic passive congestion of the liver (**nutmeg liver**), peripheral edema, ascites, jugular venous distension • Renal hypoperfusion with salt and water retention
Cor pulmonale	• Parenchymal disease (e.g., COPD, causing increased pulmonary vascular resistance) • Vascular disease (e.g., vasculitis, shunts, multiple emboli)	• Cor pulmonale is right ventricular failure, resulting specifically from pulmonary hypertension • May be acute (massive pulmonary embolus) or chronic.

► Shock

Decreased Effective Circulatory Volume

Causes	• Decreased cardiac output (myocardial infarction, arrhythmia, tamponade) • Reduction of blood volume (hemorrhage, adrenal insufficiency, fluid loss) • Pooling in periphery: massive vasodilation caused by bacterial toxins and vasoactive substances
Complications	• Cellular hypoxia, lactic acidosis • Encephalopathy • Myocardial necrosis and infarcts • Pulmonary edema, adult respiratory distress syndrome • Acute tubular necrosis
Stages	**Compensated:** reflex tachycardia, peripheral vasoconstriction **Decompensated:** ↓ blood pressure, ↑ tachycardia, metabolic acidosis, respiratory distress, and ↓ renal output **Irreversible:** irreversible cellular damage, coma, and death

▶ Endocarditis

Classic Signs	
Janeway lesions—erythematous, nontender lesions on palms and soles **Roth spots**—retinal hemorrhages **Osler nodes**—erythematous, tender lesions on fingers and toes (Also see anemia, **splinter hemorrhages)**	
Acute	• Organism—high virulence; *Staphylococcus aureus* (50%) and streptococci (35%) • Affects **previously normal valves** • Often involves the **tricuspid valve in intravenous drug users** • Vegetations may form myocardial abscesses, septic emboli, or destroy the HACEK valve, causing insufficiency. • High fever with chills
Subacute bacterial endocarditis	• Organism—low virulence. ***Streptococcus viridans***, gram-negative bacilli, *Staphylococcus epidermidis*, gram-negative bacilli (both are normal oral flora), *Staphylococcus epidermidis* (IV drug use) • *Candida* is a rare cause (associated with indwelling vascular catheters) • Affects **previously abnormal valves** • More insidious onset, with positive blood cultures, fatigue, low-grade fever without chills, splinter hemorrhages
Nonbacterial thrombotic (marantic) endocarditis	• Associated with chronic illness • Mitral valve most commonly affected • Sterile, small vegetations, loosely adhering along lines of closure • May embolize and provide a nidus for infective endocarditis
Nonbacterial verrucous (Libman-Sacks) endocarditis	• Mitral and tricuspid valvulitis in patients with systemic lupus erythematosus (SLE) • Small, warty vegetations on **both sides** of their valve leaflets • Does not embolize and rarely provides a nidus for infection

▶ Myocarditis

- May have dilatation and hypertrophy of all four chambers, diffuse or patchy pallor with foci of hemorrhage, peripheral edema
- Inflammatory lesions with characteristic cellular infiltrate:
    - Neutrophilic—bacterial myocarditis
    - Mononuclear—viral myocarditis
    - Eosinophilic—Fiedler myocarditis

Noninfectious myocarditis	Collagen vascular diseases, rheumatic fever, SLE, and drug allergies
Viral myocarditis	• **Most common form of myocarditis** • **Coxsackie B** (positive-sense RNA viruses, picornavirus family); also, polio, rubella, and influenza • Self-limited, but may be recurrent and lead to cardiomyopathy and death. • 1/3 of AIDS patients show focal myocarditis on autopsy
Bacterial myocarditis	Diphtheria (toxin-mediated), meningococci
Protozoal	• ***Trypanosoma cruzi***: Chagas disease; myocardial pseudocysts can lead to CHF • Toxoplasmosis also causes pseudocysts • Myocardial involvement appears days to weeks after the primary infection • May be asymptomatic versus acute onset of dyspnea, tachycardia, weakness, or severe CHF • Most recover fully

▶ Valvular Heart Disease

Mitral valve prolapse	• Mitral leaflets (usually posterior) project into left atrium during systole, leading to insufficiency • 7% of the United States population, most commonly in **young women** • Seen in most patients with **Marfan syndrome** • Characteristic **midsystolic click** and high-pitched murmur • Usually asymptomatic, but may have associated dyspnea, tachycardia, chest pain • *Complications:* atrial thrombosis, calcification, infective endocarditis, systemic embolization
Mitral stenosis	• Stenosis may be combined with mitral valve prolapse • Increased left atrial pressure and enlarged left atrium • Early diastolic **opening snap** • *Complications:* pulmonary edema, left atrial enlargement, chronic atrial fibrillation, atrial thrombosis and systemic emboli
Aortic valve insufficiency	• **Acute** (infective endocarditis) • Sudden left ventricular failure, increased left ventricular filling pressure, inadequate stroke volume • **Chronic** (aortic root dilation): – Volume overload, eccentric hypertrophy – Wide pulse pressure (**bounding pulse**) – Etiologies include congenitally bicuspid aortic valve, rheumatic heart disease, or syphilis
Aortic valve stenosis	• Rheumatic heart disease, bicuspid aortic valve • Thickening and fibrosis of valve cusps without fusion of valve commissures (fusion present in rheumatic heart disease) • Asymptomatic until late, presents with angina, syncope, and CHF • Systolic ejection click • *Complications:* sudden death, secondary to an arrhythmia or CHF

▶ Cardiomyopathies

Diseases Not Related to Ischemic Injury

Dilated (congestive) cardiomyopathy	• Gradual dilatation of all four chambers, producing cardiomegaly, ↓ contractility, stasis, formation of mural thrombi. • Death from progressive CHF, thromboembolism, or arrhythmia • *Etiologies:* idiopathic, alcohol (reversible), doxorubicin (irreversible), thiamine deficiency, pregnancy, postviral
Hypertrophic cardiomyopathy (idiopathic hypertrophic subaortic stenosis)	• Marked **asymmetric hypertrophy** of the ventricular septum, **left ventricular outflow obstruction** • Decreased cardiac output may cause dyspnea, angina, atrial fibrillation, syncope, sudden death • Classic case: **young adult athletes** who die during strenuous activity • *Etiologies:* genetic (50%, autosomal dominant pattern)
Restrictive (infiltrative) cardiomyopathy	• Diastolic dysfunction (impaired filling) • Infiltration of extracellular material within myocardium • *Etiologies:* elderly—cardiac amyloidosis (may induce arrhythmias); young (<25 years old)—sarcoidosis associated with systemic sarcoidosis • Secondary cardiomyopathy: metabolic disorders, nutritional deficiencies

▶ Pericardial Disease

- Usually secondary; local spread from adjacent mediastinal structures
- Primary pericarditis is usually due to systemic viral infection, uremia, and autoimmune diseases

Fibrinous pericarditis	• Exudate of fibrin • *Etiologies:* post myocardial infarction, trauma, rheumatic fever, radiation, SLE • Loud pericardial friction rub with chest pain, fever
Serous pericarditis	• Small exudative effusion with few inflammatory cells • *Etiologies:* nonbacterial, immunologic reaction (rheumatic fever, SLE), uremia, or viral • Usually asymptomatic
Suppurative pericarditis	• Purulent exudate; leads to constrictive pericarditis and cardiac insufficiency • *Etiologies:* bacterial, fungal, or parasitic infection • May have systemic signs of infection and a soft friction rub
Hemorrhagic pericarditis	• Exudate of blood with suppurative or fibrinous component • *Etiologies:* tuberculosis or a malignant neoplasm; organization • May lead to constrictive pericarditis
Caseous pericarditis	• Caseous exudate with fibrocalcific constrictive pericarditis • *Etiologies:* tuberculosis

▶ Pericardial Effusion

Pericardial effusion is leakage of fluid (transudate or exudate) into the limited pericardial space. It may result in cardiac tamponade. Generally, the rate of filling rather than the absolute volume determines the degree of tamponade.

Serous effusion	• *Etiology:* hypoproteinemia or CHF • Develops slowly, rarely causing cardiac compromise
Serosanguineous effusion	• *Etiology:* history of trauma (e.g., cardiopulmonary resuscitation), tumor, or TB • Develops slowly, rarely causing cardiac compromise
Hemopericardium	• *Etiology:* penetrating trauma, ventricular rupture (after myocardial infarction), or aortic rupture • Develops quickly; **can cause cardiac tamponade** and death

▶ Cardiac Neoplasms

Primary tumors (rare, majority benign)	**Myxoma: most common primary cardiac tumor in adults** • Most occur in the left atrium • May be any size; sessile or pedunculated • Complications include ball-valve obstructions of the mitral valve, embolization of tumor fragments **Rhabdomyoma: most common primary cardiac tumor in children** (especially those with **tuberous sclerosis**)
Metastases	Lung and lymphoma, predominantly involving the pericardium

▶ Vasculitides

Disease	Involvement	Clinical	Comments	Treatment
Buerger disease (thromboangiitis obliterans)	• Involves **small and medium-sized arteries** and veins in the **extremities** • **Microabscesses** and segmental **thrombosis** lead to vascular insufficiency, ulceration, **gangrene**	Causes severe pain (claudication) and Raynaud phenomenon in affected extremity	• Neutrophilic vasculitis that tends to involve the extremities of young men (usually under 40) who smoke heavily • Common in Israel, India, Japan, and South America	Smoking cessation
Churg-Strauss syndrome (allergic granulomatosis and angiitis)	Lung, spleen, kidney	Associated with bronchial **asthma**, **granulomas**, and **eosinophilia**	• Variant of polyarteritis nodosa • **P-ANCA** ⊕	Corticosteroids, occasionally immunosuppressants
Henoch-Schönlein purpura	• Affects small vessels, most commonly in the skin, joints, and gastrointestinal system	• Typically develops after a URI • "Palpable purpura" skin rash on buttocks and legs • Arthralgias • GI symptoms: abdominal pain, intestinal hemorrhage, melena • Nephritis in cases with IgA nephropathy	• Most common form of childhood systemic vasculitis (peak at age 5) • IgA-mediated leukocytoclastic vasculitis with circulating IgA immune complexes • Linked to HLA-B35 and human parvovirus	• Most patients treated with supportive therapy • Usually self-limited • Cyclophosphamide sometimes used in cases with severe IgA nephropathy
Kawasaki disease (mucocutaneous lymph node syndrome)	• Segmental necrotizing vasculitis involves large, medium-sized, and small arteries • **Coronary arteries** commonly affected (70%)	• Fever • Conjunctivitis • Erythema and erosions of the oral mucosa • Generalized maculopapular skin rash • Lymphadenopathy • Mortality rate is 1–2% due to rupture of a **coronary aneurysm** or coronary thrombosis	Commonly affects infants and **young children** (age <4) in **Japan**, Hawaii, and U.S. mainland	IV immunoglobulin (IVIG), aspirin, sometimes anticoagulants
Microscopic polyangiitis	• Involves small vessels in a pattern resembling Wegener granulomatosis, but without granulomas • Resembles polyarteritis nodosa in some vessels • Segmental fibrinoid necrosis of the media may be present • Some vessels show infiltration with fragmented neutrophils = **leukocytoclastic angiitis**	• Fever, malaise, myalgia, weight loss • Skin rash in 50%, including ulcerations and gangrene • Can affect vessels in many organ systems • Roughly ¾ of patients survive 5 years	• 80% are ANCA positive, with 60% P-ANCA positive and 40% C-ANCA positive • Immune complexes are rare • Etiology unclear	Prednisone and cyclophosphamide to induce remission or treat relapse; methotrexate or azathioprine to maintain remission

(Continued)

▶ Vasculitides (*Cont'd.*)

Disease	Involvement	Clinical	Comments	Treatment
Polyarteritis nodosa	• Small and medium-sized arteries in skin, joints, peripheral nerves, kidney, heart, and GI tract • Lesions will be at different stages (acute, healing, healed)	• Affects young adults (male > female) • Low-grade fever, weight loss, malaise • Hematuria, renal failure, hypertension • Abdominal pain, diarrhea, GI bleeding • Myalgia and arthralgia	• Hepatitis B antigen (HBsAg) ⊕ in 30% of cases	Corticosteroids and cyclophosphamide (often fatal without treatment)
Sturge Weber syndrome	• Congenital vascular disorder affecting capillary-type vessels • Angiomas of the leptomeninges and skin • Cutaneous angiomas (**port-wine stains**) involving the skin of the face in the distribution of ophthalmic and maxillary divisions of trigeminal nerve • Leptomeningeal angiomatosis	• Seizures and other neurologic manifestations due to altered blood flow ("vascular steal") in brain adjacent to leptomeningeal angiomas • Glaucoma, blindness • Mental deficiency may be present • May have hemiparesis contralateral to leptomeningeal angiomatosis	• Thought to be due to a failure of regression of embryonal vessels that normally occurs around the ninth week of gestation • Microscopically, the port-wine stain, which is a type of nevus flammeus, shows dilated and ectatic capillaries	• Laser therapy can ameliorate the port-wine stain • Medical treatment of secondary conditions such as seizures, glaucoma, and headaches • Some patients require surgery for intractable seizures or other major neurologic problems
Takayasu arteritis (pulseless disease)	• Granulomatous vasculitis with massive intimal fibrosis that tends to involve **medium-sized to large arteries**, including the aortic arch and major branches • Produces characteristic narrowing of arterial orifices	• Fever, night sweats, muscle and joint aches, loss of pulse in upper extremities • May lead to visual loss and other neurologic abnormalities	Most common in **Asia, especially in young and middle-aged women** (ages 15–45)	Corticosteroids
Temporal arteritis (giant cell arteritis)	• Usually segmental granulomatous involvement of small and medium-sized arteries, esp. the **cranial arteries** (temporal, facial, and ophthalmic arteries) • Multinucleated giant cells and **fragmentation of the internal elastic lamina** seen in affected segments.	• Headache, facial pain, tenderness over arteries, and visual disturbances (**can progress to blindness**) • Fever, malaise, weight loss, muscle aches, anemia • Patient usually middle-aged to elderly female • Elevated ESR	• Most common form of vasculitis • Associated with HLA-DR4 • **Polymyalgia rheumatica:** systemic flu-like symptoms; joint involvement also present	Corticosteroids (important to avoid blindness)
Wegener granulomatosis	• Necrotizing granulomatous vasculitis that affects small arteries and veins • Classically involves **nose**, **sinuses**, **lungs**, and **kidneys**	• Middle-aged adults, males > females • Bilateral pneumonitis with nodular and cavitary pulmonary infiltrates • Chronic sinusitis • Nasopharyngeal ulcerations • Renal disease (focal necrotizing glomerulonephritis)	Associated with **C-ANCA** (autoantibody against **proteinase 3**)	Corticosteroids, immunosuppressants

▶ Additional Vascular Diseases

Arteriolosclerosis

- Refers to small artery and arteriolar changes, leading to luminal narrowing that are most often seen in patients with diabetes, hypertension, and aging
- Hyaline and hyperplastic (onion-skinning) types

Atherosclerosis

Characterized by lipid deposition and intimal thickening of large and medium-sized arteries. Abdominal aorta more likely involved than the thoracic aorta. Within the abdominal aorta, lesions tend to be more prominent around the ostia. After the abdominal aorta, others commonly affected are the coronary, popliteal, and internal carotid arteries.

Key process: intimal thickening and lipid accumulation produces atheromatous plaques

The earliest lesion is the **fatty streak**, which is seen almost universally in children and may represent reversible precursor. The progression of the disease is thought in part due to a response to injury from such agents as hypertension, hyperlipidemia, and tobacco smoke. This leads to inflammatory cell adherence, migration, and proliferation of smooth muscle cells from the media into the intima.

The **mature plaque** has a **fibrous cap**, a cellular zone composed of **smooth muscle cells**, **macrophages**, and lymphocytes and a **central core** composed of necrotic cells, **cholesterol clefts, and lipid-filled foam cells** (macrophages). **Complicated plaques** are seen in advanced disease. These plaques may rupture, form fissures or ulcerate, leading to myocardial infarcts, strokes, and mesenteric artery occlusion. Damage to the cell wall predisposes to aneurysm formation.

Major Risk Factors	Minor Risk Factors
Hyperlipidemia, hypertension, smoking, diabetes	Male sex, obesity, sedentary lifestyle, stress, elevated homocysteine, oral contraceptive use, increasing age, familial/genetic factors

Mönckeberg Medial Calcific Sclerosis

Asymptomatic medial calcification of medium-sized arteries

Raynaud Disease

An idiopathic small artery vasospasm that causes **blanching and cyanosis of the fingers and toes**; the term Raynaud phenomenon is used when similar changes are observed secondary to a systemic disease, such as scleroderma or systemic lupus erythematosus.

▶ Hypertension

Most cases (90%) are idiopathic and termed essential hypertension. The majority of the remainder is secondary to intrinsic renal disease; less commonly, narrowing of the renal artery. Infrequent secondary causes include primary aldosteronism, Cushing disease, and pheochromocytoma.

Renal causes of hypertension can usually be attributed to increased renin release. This converts angiotensinogen to angiotensin I, which is converted to angiotensin II in the lung. Angiotensin II causes arteriolar constriction and stimulates aldosterone secretion and therefore sodium retention, which leads to an increased intravascular volume.

Classification of Blood Pressure for Adults*

BP Classification	Systolic BP (mm Hg)	Diastolic BP (mmHg)
Normal	< 120	and < 80
Prehypertension	120-139	or 80-89
Stage 1 Hypertension	140-159	or 90-99
Stage 2 Hypertension	≥ 160	or ≥ 100

*Guidelines from 7th Report of the Joint National Committee on Prevention, Detection, Evaluation, and Treatment of High Blood Pressure (JNC 7)

▶ Aneurysm

- A congenital or acquired weakness of the vessel wall media, resulting in a localized dilation or outpouching
- *Complications:* thrombus formation, compression of adjacent structures, and rupture with risk of sudden death

Type of Aneurysm	Associations	Anatomic Location	Comments
Atherosclerotic	Atherosclerosis, hypertension	Usually involve **abdominal aorta**, often below renal arteries	Half of aortic aneurysms >6 cm in diameter will rupture within 10 years
Syphilitic	Syphilitic obliterative endarteritis of vasa vasorum	**Ascending aorta** (aortic root)	May dilate the aortic valve ring, causing aortic insufficiency
Marfan syndrome	Lack of **fibrillin** leads to poor elastin function	Ascending aorta (aortic root)	May dilate the aortic valve ring, causing aortic insufficiency
Dissecting aneurysm (aortic dissection)	**Hypertension, cystic medial necrosis** (e.g., Marfan syndrome)	Blood enters intimal tear in aortic wall and spreads through media	Presents with severe tearing pain
Berry aneurysm	Congenital; some associated with **adult polycystic kidney disease**	Classic location: **Circle of Willis**	Rupture leads to **subarachnoid hemorrhage**

▶ Venous Disease

Deep vein thrombosis	Involves deep leg veins	Major complication: **pulmonary embolus**
Varicose veins	Dilated, tortuous veins caused by increased intraluminal pressure	• Superficial veins of legs • Hemorrhoids • **Esophageal varices**

► Vascular Tumors

Angiosarcoma	• Malignant vascular tumor with a high mortality • Occurs most commonly in skin, breast, liver, soft tissues
Glomus tumor	• Small, painful tumors most often found under fingernails
Hemangioma	• Common, benign tumors that may involve skin, mucous membranes, or internal organs
Hemangioblastoma	• Associated with **von Hippel-Lindau disease** • Tends to involve the central nervous system and retina
Kaposi sarcoma	• Low-grade malignancy of endothelial cells • Viral etiology: **human herpesvirus 8** (HHV8) • Most often seen in AIDS patients in the U.S.

► Edema and Shock

Edema	• Fluid is maintained with vessels via balance between hydrostatic pressure ("pushing fluid out") and oncotic pressure ("pulling fluid in"). • Most causes of edema can be related to either increased hydrostatic pressure or reduced plasma osmotic pressure. Other causes included lymphatic obstruction, sodium retention. • Clinically, may see pitting edema in extremities (dependent) or massive generalized edema (**anasarca**).

Increased Hydrostatic Pressure	Reduced Plasma Osmotic Pressure
Local: deep vein thrombosis *Generalized:* congestive heart failure	Cirrhosis, nephrotic syndrome, protein losing enteropathy

Shock	Three major variants: cardiogenic, septic, and hypovolemic

Type	Comments	Heart Rate	Systemic Vascular Resistance	Cardiac Output
Cardiogenic	Intrinsic pump failure. As the heart fails, stroke volume decreases, with compensatory increases in heart rate and systemic vascular resistance.	↑	↑	↓
Septic	Endotoxin mediated. Massive peripheral vasodilation with a decrease in systemic vascular resistance. There is peripheral pooling of blood (decreased effective circulatory volume). The heart compensates with an increase in heart rate.	↑	↓	↑
Hypovolemic	Blood loss. The effective circulatory volume decreases through actual loss. The heart is able to attempt to compensate with an increase in heart rate.	↑	↑	Unchanged

The Respiratory System

Chapter 3

Respiratory Embryology and Histology

▶ Development of the Respiratory System

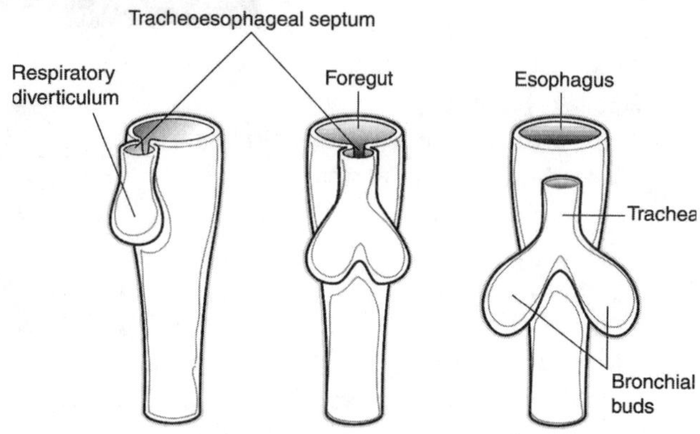

The **respiratory (laryngotracheal) diverticulum** forms in the ventral wall of the foregut. The lung bud forms at the distal end of the diverticulum and divides into two **bronchial buds**. These branch into the **main bronchi**, **lobar bronchi**, and **segmental bronchi**. The right bud divides into three main bronchi, and the left divides into two.

The **tracheoesophageal septum** divides the foregut into the esophagus and trachea.

Clinical Correlate

A **tracheoesophageal fistula** is an abnormal communication between the trachea and esophagus caused by a malformation of the tracheoesophageal septum. 90% occur between the esophagus and **distal third of the trachea**. It is generally associated with **esophageal atresia** and **polyhydramnios**. Symptoms include gagging and cyanosis after feeding and the reflux of gastric contents into the lungs, causing pneumonitis.

▶ The Alveoli and Blood-Gas Barrier

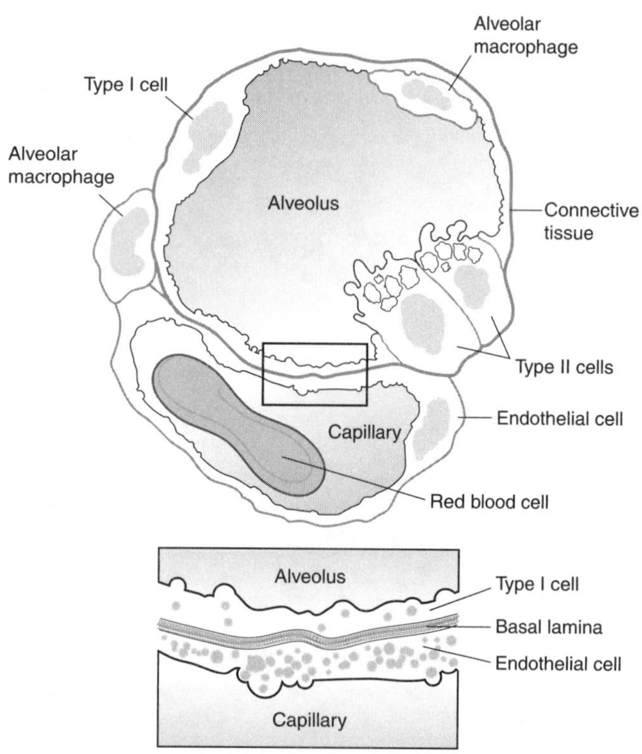

The **conducting zone** of the lungs does not participate in gas exchange and is **anatomic dead space**. It is composed of the trachea, bronchi, bronchioles, and terminal bronchioles. The trachea and bronchi contain pseudostratified ciliated columnar cells and goblet cells (secrete mucous). Bronchioles and terminal bronchioles contain ciliated epithelial cells and Clara cells (which secrete a surfactant-like substance, aid in detoxification, and are stem cells for the ciliated cells).

The **respiratory zone** carries out gas exchange and consists of respiratory bronchioles, alveolar ducts, and alveoli.

Terminal bronchioles divide into **respiratory bronchioles**, which contain alveoli and branch to form alveolar ducts. The ducts terminate in alveolar sacs and are lined by squamous alveolar epithelium.

Alveoli are thin-walled sacs responsible for gas exchange. They contain:

- **Type I epithelial cells**, which provide a thin surface for gas exchange.
- **Type II epithelial cells**, which produce **surfactant**.
- **Alveolar macrophages**, which are derived from monocytes and remove particles and other irritants via phagocytosis.

There are approximately 300 million alveoli in **each** lung.

Gross Anatomy

▶ Pharynx and Related Areas

The **pharynx** is a passageway shared by the digestive and respiratory systems. It has lateral, posterior, and medial walls throughout but is open anteriorly in its upper regions (**nasopharynx**, **oropharynx**), communicating with the nasal cavity and the oral cavity.

The **nasopharynx** is the region of the pharynx located directly posterior to the nasal cavity. It communicates with the nasal cavity through the **choanae** (i.e., posterior nasal apertures).

The **oropharynx** is the region of the pharynx located directly posterior to the oral cavity. It communicates with the oral cavity through a space called the **fauces**. The fauces are bounded by two folds, consisting of mucosa and muscle, known as the **anterior and posterior pillars**.

- The **anterior pillar of the fauces**, also known as the **palatoglossal fold**, contains the **palatoglossus muscle**.
- The **posterior pillar of the fauces**, also known as the **palatopharyngeal fold**, contains the **palatopharyngeus muscle**.
- The **tonsillar bed** is the space between the pillars that houses the **palatine tonsil**.

The **laryngopharynx** is the region of the pharynx that surrounds the larynx. It extends from the tip of the epiglottis to the cricoid cartilage. Its lateral extensions are known as the **piriform recesses**.

▶ The Larynx

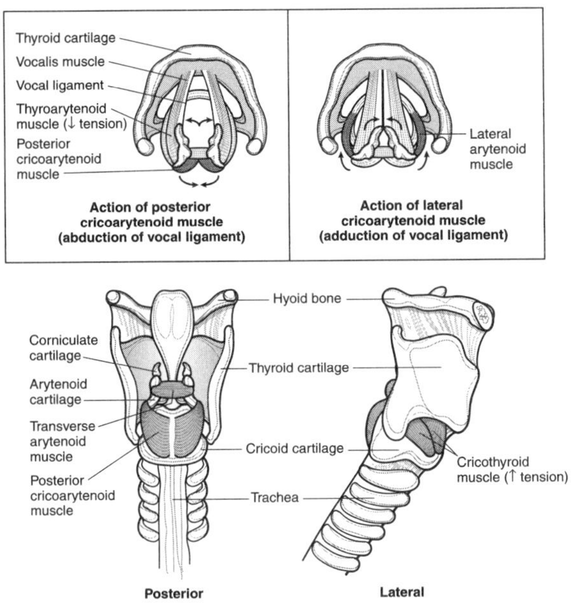

The larynx is the **voice box**. It also maintains a patent airway and acts as a sphincter during lifting and pushing.

Skeleton of the larynx:

- Three unpaired laryngeal cartilages (i.e., thyroid, cricoid, epiglottis) and three paired cartilages (i.e., arytenoid, cuneiform, corniculate)
- The fibroelastic membranes include the thyrohyoid membrane and the cricothyroid membrane (conus elasticus).The free, upper border of the latter is specialized to form the vocal ligament on either side.

▶ Intrinsic Muscles of the Larynx*

Muscle	Function
Posterior cricoarytenoid	Abducts vocal fold
Lateral cricoarytenoid	Adducts vocal fold
Cricothyroid	Tenses vocal fold
Thyroarytenoid (including vocalis)	Relaxes vocal fold
Thyroepiglotticus	Opens laryngeal inlet
Aryepiglotticus	Closes laryngeal inlet
Oblique and transverse arytenoids	Close laryngeal inlet

*Note that the cricothyroid is innervated by the external laryngeal nerve, a branch of the superior laryngeal branch of the vagus nerve. All other intrinsic laryngeal muscles are supplied by the recurrent laryngeal branch of the vagus nerve.

► Pleura and Pleural Cavities

Parietal pleura lines the inner surface of the thoracic cavity; **visceral pleura** follows the contours of the lung itself. Inflammation of the central part of the diaphragmatic pleura may produce pain referred to the shoulder (phrenic nerve; C3, C4, and C5).

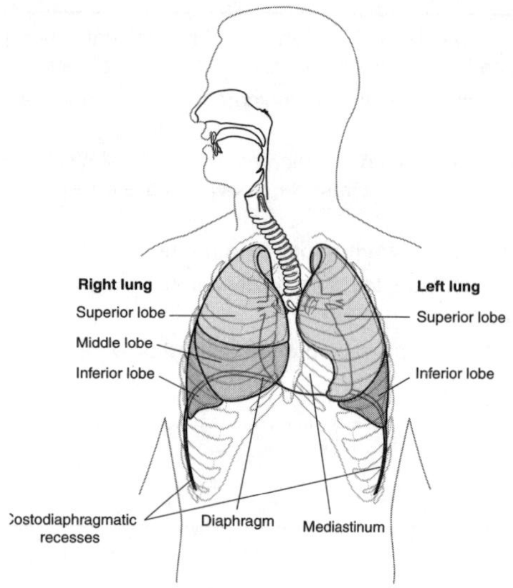

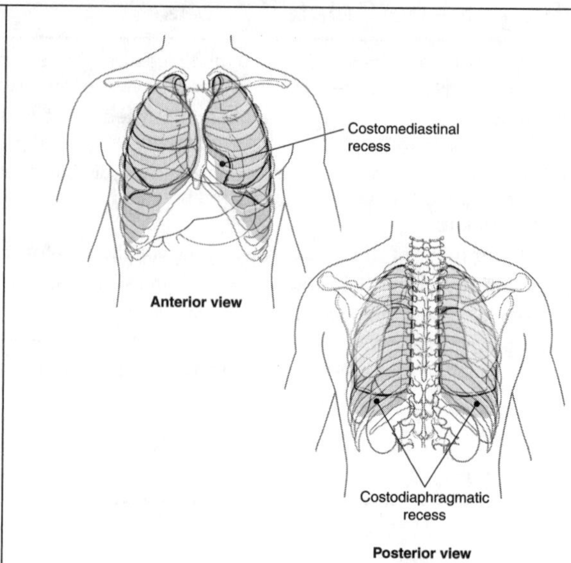

- The **costal line of reflection** is where the costal pleura becomes continuous with the diaphragmatic pleura from Rib 8 in the midclavicular line, to Rib 10 in the midaxillary line, and to Rib 12 lateral to the vertebral column.
- **Costodiaphragmatic recesses** are spaces below the inferior borders of the lungs where costal and diaphragmatic pleurae are in contact.
- The **costomediastinal recess** is a space where the left costal and mediastinal parietal pleurae meet, leaving a space due to the cardiac notch of the left lung. This space is occupied by the lingula of the left lung during inspiration.

Structure of the Lungs

- The **right lung** is divided by the oblique and horizontal fissures into three lobes: superior, middle, and inferior.
- The **left lung** has only one fissure, the oblique, which divides the lung into upper and lower lobes. The **lingula** of the upper lobe corresponds to the middle lobe of the right lung.
- **Bronchopulmonary segments** of the lung are supplied by the segmental (tertiary) bronchus, artery, and vein. There are 10 on the right and eight on the left.

Arterial Supply

- **Right and left pulmonary arteries** arise from the pulmonary trunk. The pulmonary arteries deliver deoxygenated blood to the lungs from the right side of the heart.
- **Bronchial arteries** supply the bronchi and nonrespiratory portions of the lung. They are usually branches of the thoracic aorta.

Venous Drainage

- There are **four pulmonary veins**: superior right and left and inferior right and left.
- Pulmonary veins carry oxygenated blood to the left atrium of the heart.
- The **bronchial veins** drain to the azygos system. They share drainage from the bronchi with the pulmonary veins.

Lymphatic Drainage

- Superficial drainage is to the bronchopulmonary nodes; from there, drainage is to the tracheobronchial nodes.
- Deep drainage is to the pulmonary nodes; from there, drainage is to the bronchopulmonary nodes.
- Bronchomediastinal lymph trunks drain to the right lymphatic and the thoracic ducts.

Innervation of Lungs

- Anterior and posterior pulmonary plexuses are formed by vagal (parasympathetic) and sympathetic fibers.
- Parasympathetic stimulation has a bronchoconstrictive effect.
- Sympathetic stimulation has a bronchodilator effect.

Respiratory Physiology

▶ Lung Volumes and Capacities

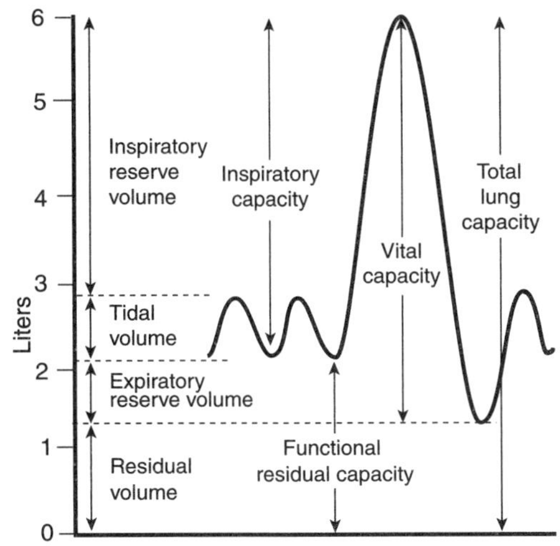

V_T	Tidal volume	Air inspired and expired in normal breathing
TLC	Total lung capacity	Volume in lungs with maximal inspiration
FRC	Functional residual capacity	Volume in lungs at end of quiet, passive expiration; the equilibrium point of the system
RV	Residual volume	Volume at end of maximal forced expiration
VC	Vital capacity	Volume expired from maximal inspiration to maximal expiration
IRV	Inspiratory reserve volume	The volume inspired with a maximal inspiratory effort in excess of the tidal volume
ERV	Expiratory reserve volume	The volume expelled with an active expiratory effort after passive expiration
IC	Inspiratory capacity	The volume of air inspired with a maximal inspiratory effort after passive expiration

Note: **FRC** and **RV** cannot be measured with a spirometer. Spirometry can only measure changes in volume.

▶ Dead Space and Ventilation

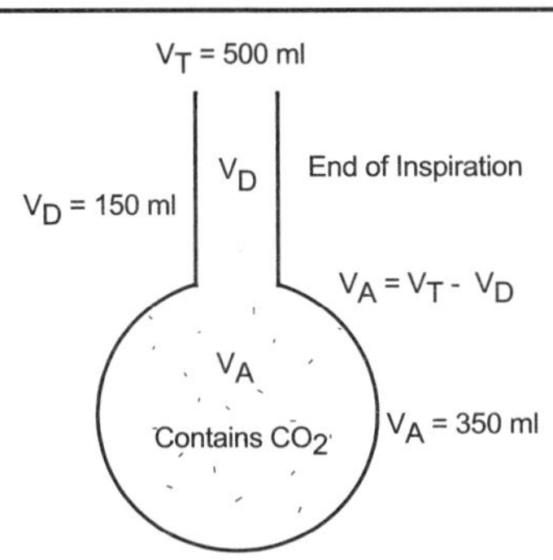

V_D = dead space (no gas exchange)

Anatomic V_D = conducting airways

Alveolar V_D = alveoli with poor blood flow (ventilated but not perfused)

Physiologic V_D = anatomic + alveolar dead space

Standard Symbols

- A = alveolar
- a = arterial
- V = volume
- $\dot{V}$ = minute ventilation
- P = pressure
- P_{ACO_2} = alveolar pressure of CO_2
- P_{aCO_2} = arterial pressure of CO_2
- P_{ECO_2} = P_{CO_2} in expired air

Abbreviation	Name	Definition	Normal Values
V_D	Dead space	Volume that does not exchange gas with blood	150 mL
V_A	Alveolar volume	Portion of tidal volume that reaches alveoli during inspiration	350 mL
V_T	Tidal volume: $V_T = V_A + V_D$	Amount of gas inhaled and exhaled during normal breathing – the sum of dead space volume and alveolar volume	500 mL
n	Respiratory frequency	Breaths/minute	15/min
$\dot{V}_E$	Total ventilation: $V_Tn = V_An + V_Dn$ $\dot{V}_E = \dot{V}_A + \dot{V}_D$	Total ventilation per minute V_Tn = (350 mL × 15/min) + (150 mL × 15/min) = 7,500 mL/min $\dot{V}_E$ = 5,250 mL/min + 2,250 mL/min = 7,500 mL/min	7,500 mL/min

(Continued)

▶ Dead Space and Ventilation *(Cont'd.)*

$\dot{V}_A$	Alveolar ventilation $\dot{V}_A = (V_T - V_D) \times n$	Amount of inspired air that reaches the alveoli each minute. It is the effective part of ventilation.	5,250 mL/min
	$\dot{V}_A = \frac{\dot{V}_{CO_2}}{P_{CO_2}} \times K$	The adequacy of alveolar ventilation can be determined from the concentration of expired carbon dioxide. • $\dot{V}_{CO_2}$ = CO_2 production (generally assume is normal and constant) • **↑ alveolar ventilation → ↓ Pa_{CO_2}** • **↓ alveolar ventilation → ↑ Pa_{CO_2}**	
Physiologic Dead Space			
$\frac{V_D}{V_T} = \frac{Pa_{CO_2} - PE_{CO_2}}{Pa_{CO_2}}$	All expired CO_2 comes from alveolar gas, not from dead space gas. Therefore, the fraction shows the dilution of CO_2 by the dead space. In the normal individual, anatomic dead space = physiologic dead space, and V_D/V_T = 0.2–0.35. In lung disease, this number can increase.		

Mechanics of Breathing

▶ Muscles of Breathing

Muscles of inspiration	• **Diaphragm—most important** • Other muscles of inspiration are used primarily during exercise or in diseases that increase airway resistance (e.g., asthma): – **External intercostal muscles** (move ribs upward and outward) – **Accessory muscles** (elevate first two ribs and sternum)
Muscles of expiration	• Expiration is **passive** during quiet breathing. • Muscles of expiration are used during exercise or increased airway resistance (e.g., asthma): – **Abdominal muscles** (help push diaphragm up during exercise or increased airway resistance) – **Internal intercostal muscles** (pull ribs downward and inward)

▶ Elastic Properties of the Lung

Pressure-Volume Curve

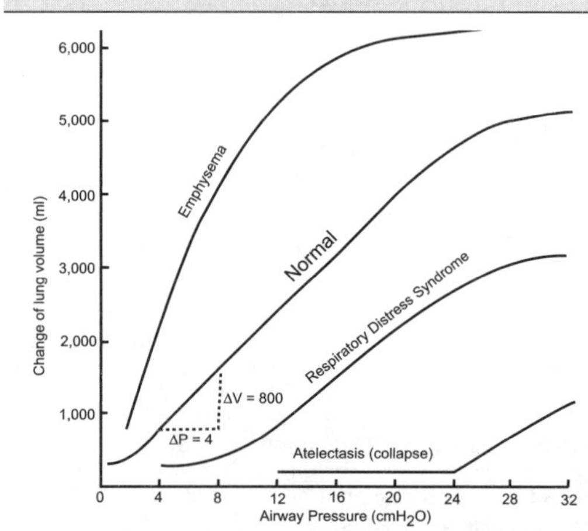

- **Compliance (ΔV/ΔP)** is used to estimate the distensibility of the lungs. It is inversely related to **elasticity** (tendency of a material to recoil when stretched).
- The steeper the slope, the higher the compliance. The flatter the slope, the lower the compliance (stiffer).
- Normal curve: Compliance = ΔV/ΔP = 800 mL/4 cm H_2O = 200 mL/cm H_2O
- Atelectasis requires an extreme effort to open collapsed alveoli.
- Compliance of lungs also ↑ with age.

Clinical Correlation: Changes in Lung Compliance		
↑ Compliance	Emphysema	• Less elastic recoil of lungs, so FRC ↑ • Chest wall expands and becomes **barrel-shaped** • Also, ↑ RV, ↑ TLC, ↓ FVC, ↑ R_{aw}
↓ Compliance*	Fibrosis, respiratory distress syndrome	• Tendency of lungs to collapse ↑, so FRC ↓ • Also, ↓↓ TLC, ↓ RV, ↓↓ FVC

Definition of abbreviation: R_{aw}, airway resistance.
***Restrictive lung disease:** a condition that reduces the ability to inflate the lungs (e.g., ↓ compliance).

► Elastic Properties of the Lung and Chest Wall

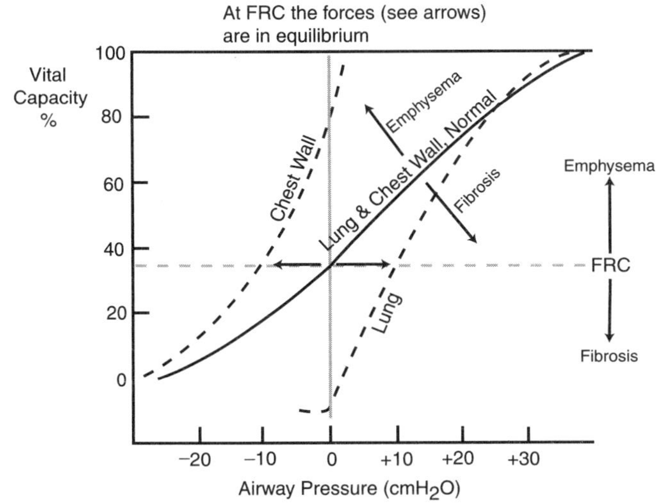

The figure to the left shows the pressure–volume relationships of the lung, the chest wall, and the lung and chest wall together.

- At FRC, the system is at equilibrium and the airway pressure = 0 cm H_2O. At FRC, the elastic recoil of the lungs tends to collapse the lungs. The tendency of the lungs to collapse is balanced exactly by the tendency of the chest wall to spring outward.
- The result of the opposing forces of the lungs and chest wall cause the intrapleural pressure (P_{IP}) to be negative (a vacuum). The P_{IP} is the pressure in the intrapleural space, which lies between the lungs and chest wall.

Clinical Correlation

If sufficient air is introduced into the intrapleural space, the P_{IP} becomes atmospheric (0 mm Hg), and the lungs and chest wall follow their normal tendencies: the lungs collapse and the chest wall expands. This is a **pneumothorax**.

► Surface Tension

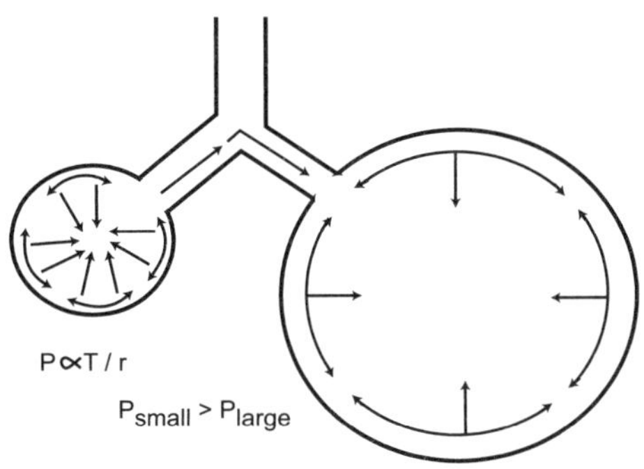

- The attractive forces between adjacent molecules of liquid are stronger than those between liquid and gas, creating a collapsing pressure.
- **Laplace's Law:** $P = \frac{2T}{r}$, where P = collapsing pressure
  T = surface tension
  r = radius of alveoli
- Large alveoli (↑r) have low collapsing pressures (easy to keep open).
- Small alveoli (↓r) have high collapsing pressures (difficult to keep open).
- **Surfactant** reduces surface tension (T). With ↓ surfactant (e.g., premature infants), smaller alveoli tend to collapse (**atelectasis**).
- **Surfactant**, produced by **type II alveolar cells**, ↑ **compliance.**

► Airway Resistance

Airflow	$Q = \frac{\Delta P}{R}$	where Q = airflow ΔP = pressure gradient R = airway resistance
Airway resistance	$R = \frac{8hl}{p r^4}$	where R = resistance η = viscosity of inspired gas l = airway length r = airway radius **Medium-sized bronchi** are the major sites of airway resistance (not the smaller airways because there are so many of them).
Changes in airway resistance	• **Bronchial smooth muscle:** – Parasympathetic nervous system → bronchoconstriction via M_3 muscarinic receptors (↑ resistance) – Sympathetic nervous system → bronchodilation via β_2 receptors (↓ resistance) • **Lung volume:** ↑ lung volume → ↓ resistance (greater radial traction on airways) ↓ lung volume → ↑ resistance • **Viscosity or density of inspired gas:** ↑ density → ↑ resistance (deep sea diving) ↓ density → ↓ resistance (breathing helium)	

► The Breathing Cycle

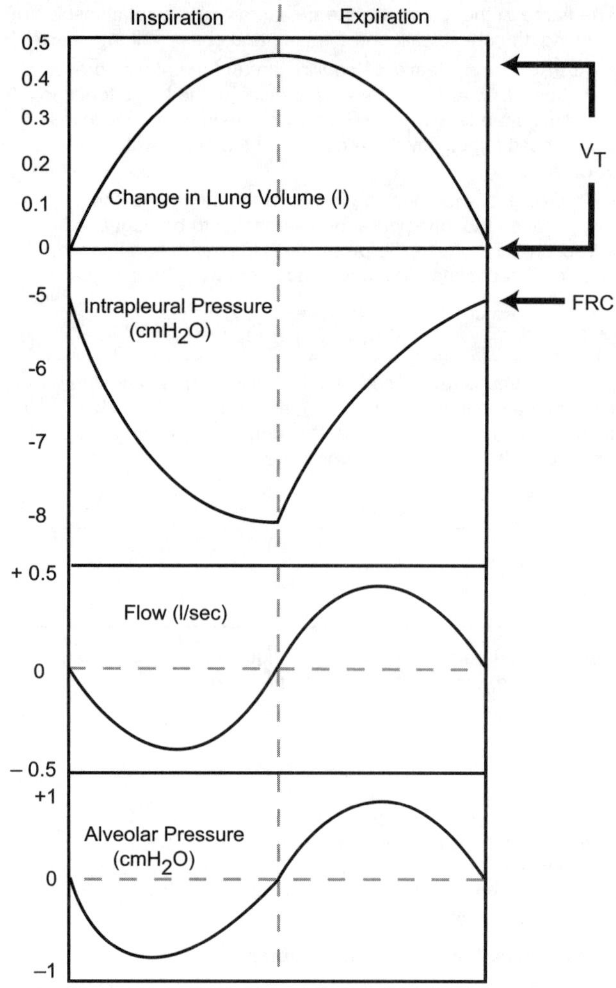

At rest (FRC): $P_A = P_{ATM} = 0$ mm Hg

Inspiration

1. Inspiratory muscles contract.
2. Thoracic volume ↑.
3. P_{IP} becomes more negative.
4. Lungs expand (also causes P_{IP} to be more negative because of ↑ elastic recoil).
5. P_A becomes negative.
6. Air flows in down pressure gradient ($P_{ATM} - P_A$).

Expiration

1. Muscles relax.
2. Thoracic volume ↓.
3. P_{IP} is less negative.
4. Lungs recoil inward (also causes P_{IP} to be less negative).
5. P_A becomes positive.
6. Air flows out down pressure gradient ($P_A - P_{ATM}$).

Clinical Correlation

Obstructive lung disease: a condition that causes an abnormal increase in R_{aw}. **Chronic obstructive pulmonary disease (COPD)** such as emphysema → destruction of elastic tissue → ↑ lung compliance → collapse of airways on expiration (**dynamic compression**). This occurs in normal individuals during a forced expiration but can occur during normal expiration in COPD. COPD patients learn to expire slowly and with pursed lips.

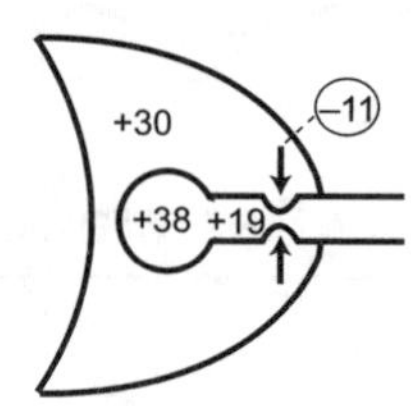

Definition of abbreviations: FRC, functional residual capacity; P_A, alveolar pressure; P_{ATM}, atmospheric pressure.

▶ Pulmonary Disease

Normal

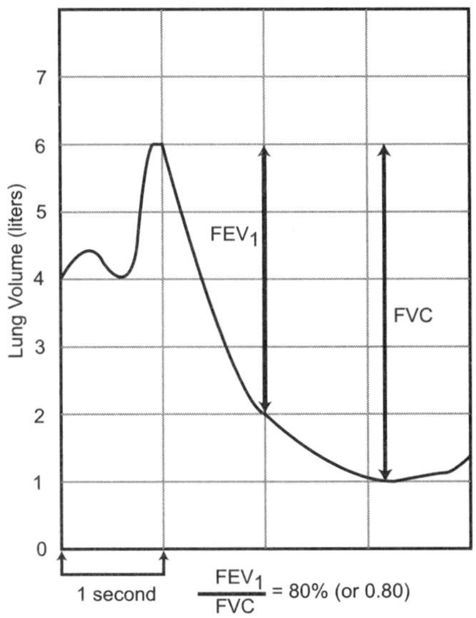

Obstructive Disease

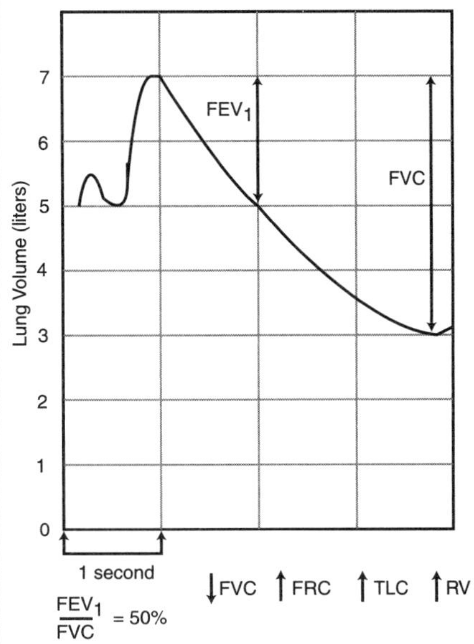

Restrictive Disease

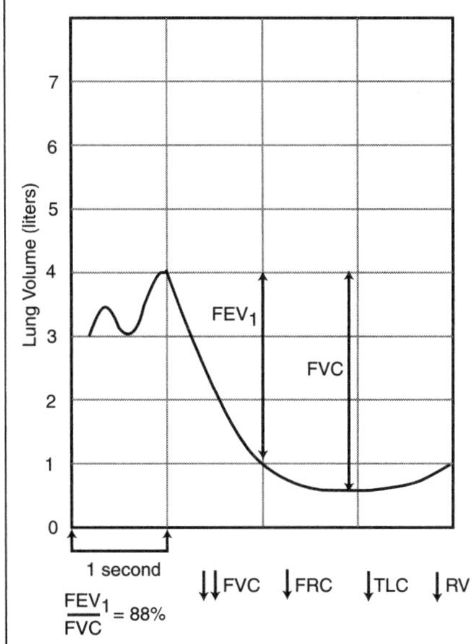

- **Forced vital capacity (FVC)** is the volume of air that can be expired with a maximal effort after a maximal inspiration.
- **Forced expiratory volume 1 (FEV_1)** is the volume of gas expired during the first second.

	TLC	RV	FRC	FVC	FEV_1	FEV_1/FVC	Most Diagnostic
Obstructive pattern	↑	↑↑	↑↑	NC or ↓	↓↓	↓↓	↓ FEV_1/FVC with ↑ TLC
Restrictive pattern	↓↓	↓	↓	↓↓	↓	NC or ↑	↓ FVC with ↓ TLC

Definition of abbreviation: NC, no change.

▶ Summary of Classic Lung Diseases

Disease	Pattern	Characteristics
Asthma	Obstructive	R_{aw} is ↑ and expiration is impaired. All measures of expiration are ↓ (FVC, FEV_1, FEV_1/FVC). Air is trapped →↑ FRC.
COPD	Obstructive	• Combination of **chronic bronchitis** and **emphysema** • There is ↑ **compliance**, and expiration is impaired. Air is trapped →↑ FRC. – **"Blue bloaters"** (mainly bronchitis): impaired alveolar ventilation → severe hypoxemia with cyanosis and ↑ $Paco_2$. They are blue and edematous from right heart failure. – **"Pink puffers"** (mainly emphysema): alveolar ventilation is maintained, so they have normal $Paco_2$ and only mild hypoxemia. They have a reddish complexion and breathe with pursed lips at an ↑ respiratory rate.
Fibrosis	Restrictive	• There is ↓ **compliance**, and inspiration is impaired. • **All lung volumes are decreased**, but because FEV_1 decreases less than FVC, FEV_1/FVC may be increased or normal.

Gas Exchange

► Partial Pressures of O_2 and CO_2

Dalton's Law of Partial Pressures: Partial pressure (p_{gas}) = total pressure (P_T) × fractional gas concentration (F_{gas})

Alveolar gas equation: $P_{AO_2} = P_{IO_2} - P_{CO_2}/R$

Alveolar ventilation equation: $\dot{V}_A = \dot{V}_{CO_2} \times K/P_{aCO_2}$; ($K = P_B - P_{H_2O} = 760 - 47 = 713$)

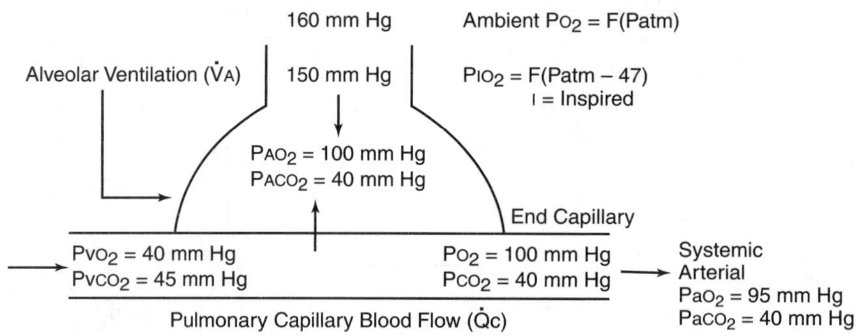

A = alveolar, a = systemic arterial

	Equation	O_2	CO_2
Dry inspired air (any altitude)	F_{gas}	0.21	0
Dry air at sea level	$P_{gas} = F_{gas} \times P_B$	0.21 (760) = 160	0
Inspired, humidified tracheal air (P_{IO_2})	$P_{gas} = F_{gas} \times (P_B - P_{H_2O})$	0.21 (760 – 47) = **150**	0
Alveolar air ($P_{A_{gas}}$)	**O_2**: $P_{AO_2} = P_{IO_2} - P_{ACO_2}/R$ **CO_2**: $\dot{V}_{CO_2}K/R$	150 – 40/0.8 = **100**	(280 mL/min × 713)/5,000 mL/min = **40**
Systemic arterial blood (Pa_{gas})	—	**100** (completely equilibrates with alveolar O_2 if no lung disease)	**40** (CO_2 is from pulmonary capillaries and equilibrates with alveolar gas)
Mixed venous blood ($P\bar{v}_{CO_2}$)	—	**40** (O_2 has diffused from arterial blood into tissues)	**45** (CO_2 has diffused from tissues to venous blood)

All pressures are expressed in mm Hg.

Definition of abbreviations: K, constant; P_{ACO_2}, partial pressure of alveolar carbon dioxide; P_{AO_2}, partial pressure of alveolar oxygen; P_B, barometric pressure; P_{H_2O}, water vapor pressure; P_{IO_2}, partial pressure of inspired oxygen; $\dot{V}_{CO_2}$, CO_2 production; R, respiratory exchange ratio.

▶ Diffusion

Fick's Law of Diffusion

- $\mathbf{V_{gas} \propto D(P_1 - P_2) \times A/T}$

  where V_{gas} = diffusion of gas, D = diffusion coefficient of a specific gas, A = surface area, T = thickness.

- A and T are physical factors that change mainly in disease.
- D of CO_2 >>> O_2

Time course in pulmonary capillary

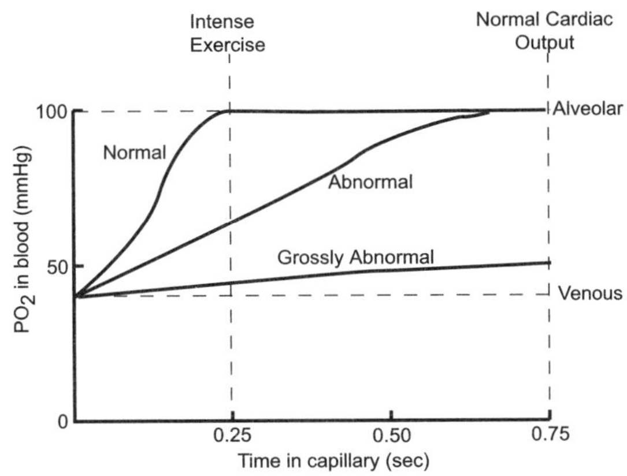

- A red blood cell remains in capillary for 0.75 seconds (s)
- Equilibrium is reached in 0.25 s in normal lung at resting state.
- Exercise reduces equilibration time, but there is still enough reserve for full equilibration of oxygen in a healthy individual.

Perfusion-Limited Gases	Diffusion-Limited Gases
Gases that **equilibrate** between the alveolar gas and pulmonary capillaries are **perfusion-limited**. The amount of gas transferred is **not dependent** on the properties of the blood-gas barrier. • $\mathbf{O_2}$ (under normal conditions) • $\mathbf{N_2O}$ (nitrous oxide) • $\mathbf{CO_2}$	Gases that **do not equilibrate** between the alveolar gas and the pulmonary capillaries are **diffusion-limited**. The amount of gas transferred **is dependent** on the properties of the blood-gas barrier. • $\mathbf{O_2}$: – Blood-gas barrier is thickened in **fibrosis**. – Surface area is ↓ in **emphysema**. – **Intense exercise** ↓ time for equilibration in pulmonary capillaries (can occur in normal lungs). – **Low O_2 gas mixture** (less partial pressure gradient, can occur in normal lungs) • **CO:** Binds so avidly to Hb, Paco does not ↑ much. Used to measure the **pulmonary diffusing capacity**.

▶ Oxygen Transport and the Hemoglobin–O_2 Dissociation Curve

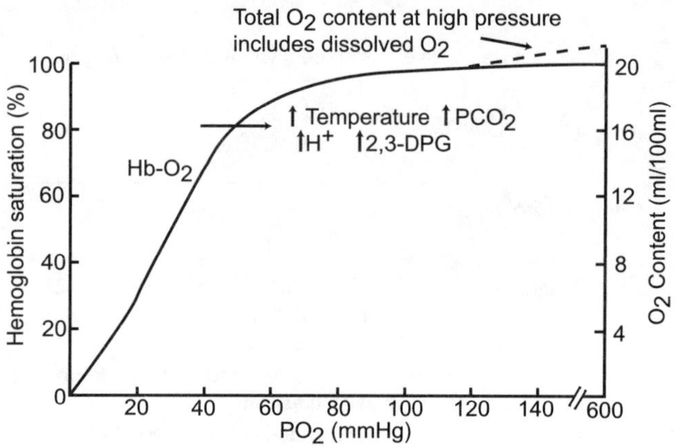

- Each hemoglobin (Hb) molecule has four subunits.
- Each subunit has a heme moiety with an iron in the ferrous state (Fe^{2+}), and two α and two β polypeptide chains.
- **O_2 capacity:** maximal amount of O_2 that can bind to Hb
- **O_2 content*:** Total O_2 in blood (bound + dissolved)
  = (O_2 capacity × % saturation) + dissolved O_2
  $= (1.39 \times \text{Hb} \times \frac{\text{Sat}}{100}) + 0.003\ P_{O2}$
- **Content** reflects O_2 bound to Hb (the amount of O_2 that is dissolved is trivial compared to bound).
- **Partial pressure** reflects dissolved O_2.

Key Pressures	Key Saturation %	Shift to Right (↑ P_{50})	Shift to Left (↓ P_{50})
Pa_{O_2} = 100 mm Hg	Almost 100% saturated	• **Facilitates unloading** • ↑ temperature, ↑ P_{CO_2}, ↓ pH, ↑ 2,3-DPG • Exercising muscle is hot, acidic, and hypercarbic	• **Facilitates loading** • ↓ temperature, ↓ P_{CO_2}, ↑ pH, ↓ 2,3-DPG • CO poisoning
$P\bar{v}_{O_2}$ = 40 mm Hg	75% saturated		
P_{50} = 27 mm Hg	50% saturated		

Definition of abbreviations: Hb, hemoglobin concentration; Sat, saturation; P_{50}, P_{O_2} at 50% saturation.
*1.39 mL of O_2 binds 1 g of Hb (some texts use 1.34 or 1.36).

▶ Additional Changes in the Hemoglobin–O_2 Dissociation Curve

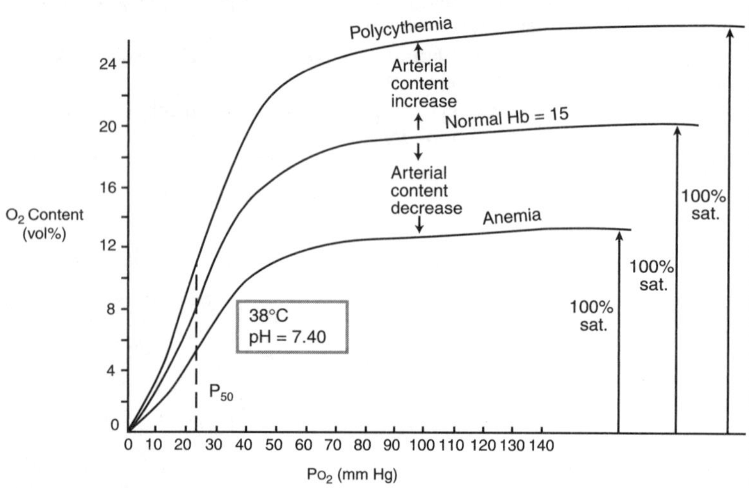

- **Polycythemia** and **anemia** change arterial **O_2 content**.
- Pa_{O_2} and P_{50} remain the same.

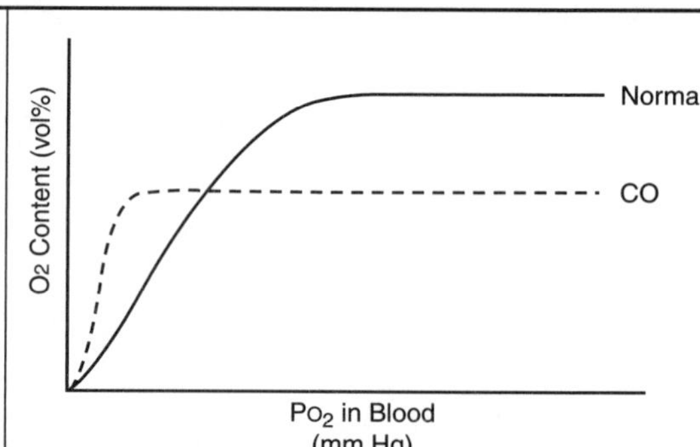

CO poisoning is dangerous for three reasons:

1. CO **left-shifts** the curve (↓ P_{50}), causing ↓ O_2 unloading in tissues.
2. CO has 240 times greater affinity for Hb as O_2, thus ↓ **the O_2 content** of blood.
3. CO inhibits cytochrome oxidase

► CO_2 Transport

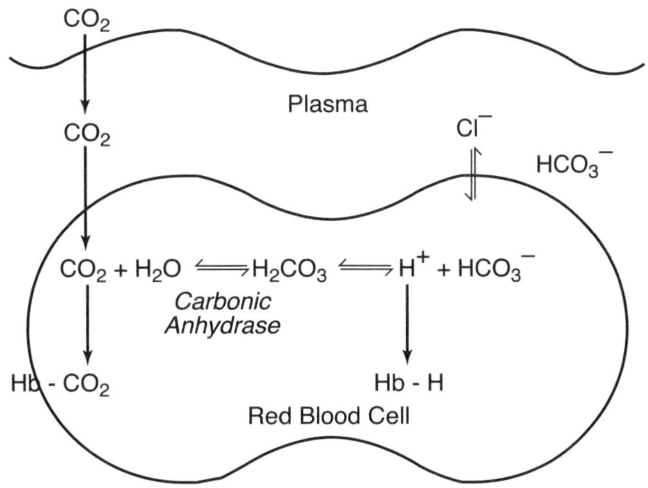

Forms of CO_2
Percentages reflect contribution in arterial blood.
1. **HCO_3^-** = 90%
2. Carbamino compounds (combination of CO_2 with proteins, especially Hb) = 5%
3. Dissolved CO_2 = 5%

► Pulmonary Blood Flow

Resistance (R)	Very low
Compliance	Very high
Pressures	Very low compared with systemic circulation
Effect of P_{AO_2}	• **Alveolar hypoxia → vasoconstriction.** • This is a local effect and the opposite of other organs, where hypoxia → vasodilation. • This directs blood away from hypoxic alveoli to better ventilated areas • This is also why fetal pulmonary vascular resistance is so high. Pulmonary resistance ↓ when the first breath oxygenates the alveoli, causing pulmonary blood flow to rise.
Gravity	Upright posture: greatest flow in base; lowest in apex
Filter	Removes small clots from circulation
Vasoactive substances	Converts angiotensin I → AII; inactivates bradykinin; removes prostaglandin E_2 and $F_{2\alpha}$ and leukotrienes

► Ventilation–Perfusion Relationships

$\dot{V}/\dot{Q}$: the ratio of alveolar ventilation ($\dot{V}$) to pulmonary blood flow ($\dot{Q}$).

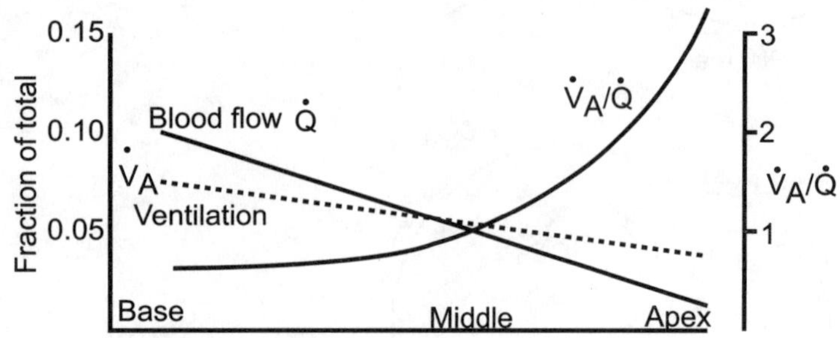

- **Blood flow** is lowest at the apex and highest at the base (gravity effect).
- **Ventilation** is lowest at the apex and highest at the base.
- The change in ventilation is not as great as blood flow, so the **$\dot{V}/\dot{Q}$ ratio** is highest at the apex and lowest at the base.

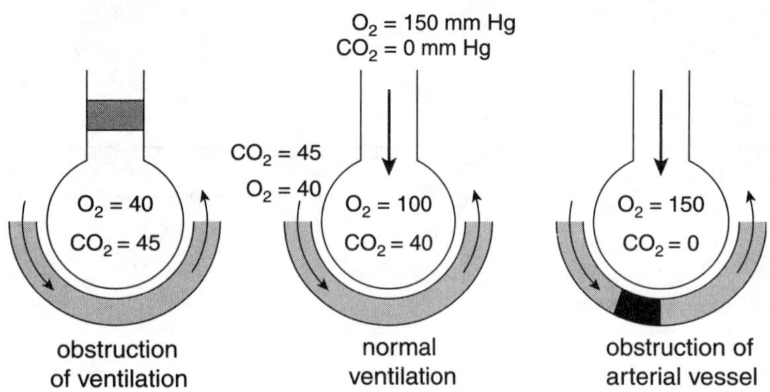

Changes in $\dot{V}/\dot{Q}$

A good way to remember the changes in partial pressures due to alterations in $\dot{V}/\dot{Q}$ is to think of the most extreme cases.

- If ventilation is 0 (airways blocked), $\dot{V}/\dot{Q}$ = 0 (a **shunt**). No gas exchange occurs and the P_{AO_2} and P_{ACO_2} are the same as mixed venous blood.
- If perfusion is 0 (embolism), $\dot{V}/\dot{Q} = \infty$ (**dead space**). No gas exchange occurs and P_{AO_2} and P_{ACO_2} are the same as inspired air.

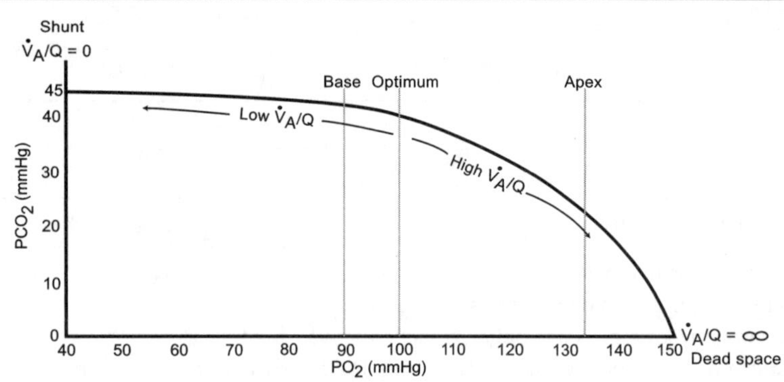

Summary of Changes

	Apex	Base
$\dot{V}_A$	↓↓	↑
$\dot{Q}$	↓↓↓	↑↑
$\dot{V}_A/\dot{Q}$	↑↑	↓
P_{O_2}	↑	↓
P_{CO_2}	↓	↑

▶ Disorders That Affect Arterial Oxygen Pressure or Content

	Notes	Pao_2	$Paco_2$	Cao_2	A-a*	Response to Supplemental O_2 ☠
Hypoventilation[1]	Drugs (e.g., opiates, barbiturates), head trauma, chest wall dysfunction	↓	↑	↓	NC	↑ Pao_2; ↑ Cao_2
↓ inspired pO_2	↑ altitude	↓	↓[2]	↓	NC	↑ Pao_2; ↑ Cao_2
Diffusion limitation[3]	PAO_2 and Pao_2 do not fully equilibrate	↓	NC[2]	↓	↑	↑ Pao_2; ↑ Cao_2
Shunt[4]	Venous blood mixes with arterial system, bypassing ventilated areas of lung	↓	NC[2]	↓	↑	Poor
$\dot{V}$/Q mismatch	Ventilation and perfusion are mismatched in the lung	↓	NC[2]	↓	↑	↑ Pao_2; ↑ Cao_2
CO poisoning	Exhaust fumes	NC	NC	↓	NC	↑ Pao_2; NC in Cao_2[5]
↓ [Hb]	Anemia	NC	NC	↓	NC	↑ Pao_2; NC in Cao_2[6]

Definition of abbreviation: NC, no change or minimal response.

*An increase in the A-a gradient indicates a problem with gas exchange.

☠ *Warning:* Supplemental O_2 in CNS depression and lung disease can shut off the hypoxic drive to ventilation and cause cessation of spontaneous breathing.

[1]Hypoventilation: ↓ $\dot{V}_A$, so ↑ $PACO_2$ → ↓ PAO_2 →↓ Pao_2 (As ↑ CO_2 diffuses into alveoli from blood, it displaces O_2.)

[2]Result of hypoxia-induced increase of ventilation

[3]Diffusion limitation causes disease (blood-gas barrier has less surface area or is thickened), ↓ transit time during intense exercise, exercise at high altitude

[4]Abnormal shunts (often congenital, e.g., Tetralogy of Fallot)

[5]Slow response of Cao_2 due to extremely high affinity of Hb for carbon monoxide

[6]Can only increase dissolved O_2 because Hb is saturated at normal Pao_2.

► Control of Ventilation

Brain Stem Respiratory Centers		
Medulla	Rhythm generator	**Inspiratory center:** generates breathing rhythm **Expiratory center:** not active during normal, passive expiration; involved in active expiration (e.g., exercise)
Pons	Regulates medulla	**Apneustic center:** stimulates prolonged inspiration **Pneumotaxic center:** terminates inspiration
Cortex	Conscious and emotional response	Lesions above the pons eliminate voluntary control, but basic breathing pattern remains intact.

► Chemoreceptors

	Central (Medulla) Chemoreceptors (Respond to Changes in pH of CSF)	Peripheral Chemoreceptors (Carotid and Aortic Bodies)
O_2	No response	• ↓ PaO_2 (<60 mm Hg) → stimulates chemoreceptors → increased ventilation. • *Note:* stimulated by changes in pressure, not O_2 content; thus, not stimulated by anemia.
CO_2	↑ **Pco_2** → stimulate chemoreceptors → ↑ **ventilation (via H^+)**	• ↑ $Paco_2$ → stimulation →↑ ventilation. • Central chemoreceptor response is most important during normal breathing.
H^+	↑ H^+ → stimulation ↑ ventilation detects H^+ in CSF; 80–95% of response to hypercapnia	• ↑ H^+ → stimulation → ↑ ventilation. • *Note:* Most of the response to metabolic acidosis is peripheral because fixed acids penetrate blood/brain barrier poorly.

Clinical Correlation

Patients with severe lung disease can have chronic CO_2 retention, and the pH of their CSF can return to normal despite their hypercapnia. Having lost their CO_2 stimulus to ventilate, their hypoxic ventilatory drive becomes very important. If these patients are given enriched O_2 to breathe to correct their hypoxemia, their primary ventilatory drive will be removed, which can cause severe depression of ventilation.

Note: Other receptors such as pulmonary stretch receptors, irritant receptors, and joint and muscle receptors also have roles in the regulation of ventilation.

► Response to High Altitude

Parameter	Response
P_AO_2	↓ (because P_B is ↓)
Pa_{O_2}	↓ (hypoxemia because P_AO_2 is ↓)
Respiratory rate	↑ (hypoxic stimulation of peripheral chemoreceptors)
$Paco_2$ and P_{ACO_2}	↓ (hyperventilation due to hypoxemia)
Arterial pH	↑ (because of respiratory alkalosis); later becomes normal (renal compensation)
[Hb]	↑ (polycythemia)
Hb % saturation	↓ (because ↓ Po_2)
Pulmonary vascular resistance	↑ (hypoxic vasoconstriction); this plus polycythemia lead to ↑ work and hypertrophy of right heart
[2,3-DPG]	↑
Hemoglobin-O_2 curve	Right-shift (because of ↑ 2,3-DPG)
Acute mountain sickness	Hypoxemia and alkalosis cause headache, fatigue, nausea, dizziness, palpitations, and insomnia. Treatment with acetazolamide can be therapeutic.
Chronic mountain sickness	Reduced exercise tolerance, fatigue, hypoxemia, polycythemia

Respiratory Pathology

► Ear, Nose, Throat, and Upper Respiratory System Infections

Type of Infection	Case Vignette/Key Clues	Diagnosis	Common Causative Agents	Pathogenesis	Treatment
Sinusitis	Sinus pain; low-grade fever	Gram ⊕ coccus, catalase ⊖	*Streptococcus pneumoniae*	Capsule, IgA protease	Penicillin
		Gram ⊖ rod, chocolate agar	*Haemophilus influenzae*	Capsule, IgA protease, endotoxin	Amoxicillin
		Gram ⊖ coccus	*Moraxella catarrhalis*	β-lactamase producer	Ceftriaxone
Oral cavitary disease	Sore mouth with thick, white coating that can be scraped off easily to reveal painful red base	Gram ⊕ yeast, germ tube test	*Candida albicans*	Overgrowth of normal flora, immunocompromised, overuse of antibiotics	Nystatin, miconazole
Sore throat	Inflamed tonsils/pharynx, abscesses; cervical lymphadenopathy, fever, ± stomach upset; ± sandpaper rash	Rapid antigen test; gram ⊕, catalase ⊖ coccus; β-hemolytic, bacitracin sensitive	*Streptococcus pyogenes*	Exotoxins A–C (superantigens)	Penicillin
	White papules with red base on posterior palate and pharynx, fever	Virus culture or PCR	Coxsackie A	Unknown	None
	Throat looks like *Streptococcus* with severe fatigue, lymphadenopathy, fever, ± rash	Heterophile ⊕ (Monospot test); mononucleosis; 70% lymphocytosis (Downey type II cells = CTLs)	Epstein-Barr virus	Infects B lymphocytes by attachment to CD21, causes ↑ CTLs	Supportive
	Low-grade fever with a 1–2 day gradual onset of membranous nasopharyngitis and/or obstructive laryngotracheitis; bull neck from lymphadenopathy; elevated BUN; abnormal ECG; little change in WBC; unvaccinated, dislodged membrane bleeds profusely	Gram ⊕ nonmotile rod, Loeffler medium, ELEK test	*Corynebacterium diphtheriae*	Diphtheria toxin inactivates eEF-2 in heart, nerves, epithelium; pseudomembrane → airway obstruction when dislodged	Penicillin, antitoxin
Common cold	Rhinitis, sneezing, coughing; seasonal peaks	Clinical	Rhinoviruses (summer–fall) Coronaviruses (winter–spring)	Virus attaches to ICAM-1 on respiratory epithelium	Supportive
Acute otitis media	Red, bulging tympanic membrane, fever 102–103°F; pain goes away if drum ruptures or if ear tubes are patent	Gram ⊕ coccus, catalase ⊖	*Streptococcus pneumoniae*	Capsule, IgA protease	Penicillin
		Gram ⊖ rod, chocolate agar	*H. influenzae* (nontypeable)	Capsule, IgA protease, endotoxin	Amoxicillin
		Gram ⊖ diplococcus	*Moraxella catarrhalis*	β-lactamase producer	Ceftriaxone

(Continued)

▶ Ear, Nose, Throat, and Upper Respiratory System Infections *(Cont'd.)*

Type of Infection	Case Vignette/Key Clues	Diagnosis	Common Causative Agents	Pathogenesis	Treatment
Otitis externa	Ear pain	Gram ⊕, catalase ⊕, coagulase ⊕	*Staphylococcus aureus*	Normal flora enter abrasions	β-lactamase-resistant penicillin
		Gram ⊕ yeast, germ tube test	*Candida albicans*	Normal flora enter abrasions	Nystatin, miconazole
		Gram ⊖ rod, urease ⊕, oxidase ⊖, swarming motility	*Proteus*	From water source	Susceptibility testing*
		Gram ⊖ rod, oxidase ⊕, blue-green pigments	*Pseudomonas aeruginosa*	From water source	Susceptibility testing*
Malignant otitis externa	Severe ear pain in diabetic; life-threatening	Gram ⊖ rod, oxidase ⊕, blue-green pigments, fruity odor	*Pseudomonas aeruginosa*	Capsule	Susceptibility testing*

Definition of abbreviations: CTLs, cytotoxic T lymphocytes.

*Because there is so much drug resistance in these genera, susceptibility testing is necessary.

▶ Middle Respiratory Tract Infections

Disease	Case Vignette/ Key Clues	Diagnosis	Common Causative Agents	Pathogenesis	Treatment
Epiglottitis	Inflamed epiglottis; patient often 2–3 years old and **unvaccinated**; **thumbprint** sign on lateral x-ray	Gram ⊖ rod, chocolate agar (requires hemin and NAD)	*Haemophilus influenzae*	Capsule (polyribitol phosphate) inhibits phagocytosis; IgA protease	Ceftriaxone
Croup	**Infant** with fever, sharp barking cough, inspiratory stridor, hoarse phonation; **steeple** sign on AP x-ray	Detect virus in respiratory washings	Parainfluenza virus (croup)	Viral cytolysis; multinucleated giant cells formed	Ribavirin
Laryngotracheitis, laryngotracheobronchitis	Hoarseness, burning retrosternal pain	Detect virus in respiratory washings	Parainfluenza virus	Viral cytolysis; multinucleated giant cells formed	Ribavirin
Bronchitis, bronchiolitis	Wheezy; **infant** or child ≤5 years old	Direct immunofluorescence for viral Ags	RSV	Fusion protein creates syncytia	Ribavirin
	>5 years old	Slow growth on Eaton medium, cold agglutinins	*Mycoplasma pneumoniae*, viruses	Release of O_2 radicals causes necrosis of epithelium	Symptomatic

Definition of abbreviations: Ag, antigens; NAD, nicotinamide adenine dinucleotide; RSV, respiratory syncytial virus.

▶ Pneumonia

Lobar pneumonia and bronchopneumonia—acute inflammation and consolidation (solidification) of the lung due to an extracellular bacterial agent. Lobar affects entire lobe (opacification = consolidation on x-ray); bronchopneumonia (patchy consolidation around bronchioles on x-ray). Associated with high fever and productive cough.

Interstitial (atypical) pneumonia causes interstitial pneumonitis without consolidation and can be due to viral agents (influenza virus; parainfluenza; RSV, especially in young children; adenovirus; CMV, especially in immunocompromised; varicella), *Mycoplasma pneumoniae, and Pneumocytis jiroveci.*

Clinical:

- Fever and chills
- Cough (may be productive)
- Tachypnea
- Pleuritic chest pain
- Decreased breath sounds, rales, and dullness to percussion
- Elevated WBC count with a left shift

Type of Infection	Case Vignette/ Key Clues	Diagnosis	Most Common Causative Agents	Pathogenesis	Treatment
Pneumonia—typical	Adults (including alcoholics), **rust-colored sputum** Lobar pneumonia or less commonly, bronchopneumonia	Gram ⊕ diplococcus, α hemolytic, catalase ⊖ lysed by bile, inhibited by Optochin	*Streptococcus pneumoniae, Haemophilus influenzae* (much less common)	Capsule antiphagocytic IgA protease	Third-generation cephalosporin, azithromycin
	Neutropenic patients, burn patients, CGD, CF	Gram ⊖ rod, oxidase ⊕, blue-green pigments	*Pseudomonas aeruginosa*	Opportunist	Sensitivity testing required
	Foul-smelling sputum, aspiration possible	Culture of sputum	Anaerobes, mixed infection *(Bacteroides, Fusobacterium, Peptococcus)*	Aspiration of vomitus → enzyme damage → anaerobic foci	Empiric antibiotic therapy (amoxicillin/ clavulanate, gentamicin)
	Alcoholic with aspiration, facultative anaerobic, gram ⊖ bacterium with huge capsule, **currant jelly sputum**	Gram ⊖ rod, lactose fermenting, oxidase ⊖	*Klebsiella pneumoniae*	Capsule protects against phagocytosis	Susceptibility testing necessary
Pneumonia—atypical	Poorly nourished, unvaccinated baby/ child; giant cell pneumonia with hemorrhagic rash, Koplik spots	Serology	Measles: malnourishment ↑ risk of pneumonia and blindness	Cytolysis in lymph nodes, skin, mucosa Syncytia → giant cell pneumonia	Supportive
	Pneumonia teens/ young adults; bad hacking, dry cough "walking pneumonia"	Serology, cold agglutinins	*Mycoplasma pneumoniae* (most common cause of pneumonia in school-age children)	Adhesin causes adhesion to mucus; oxygen radicals cause necrosis of epithelium	Doxycycline, azithromycin

(Continued)

► Pneumonia (*Cont'd.*)

Type of Infection	Case Vignette/ Key Clues	Diagnosis	Most Common Causative Agents	Pathogenesis	Treatment
Pneumonia—atypical (*cont'd.*)	Air-conditioning exposure, common showers, especially >50 years, heavy smoker, drinker	Direct fluorescent antibody	*Legionella* spp.	Intracellular in macrophages	Macrolide
	Bird exposure ± hepatitis	Direct fluorescent antibody, intracytoplasmic inclusions	*Chlamydophilia psittaci*	Obligate intracellular	Tetracycline, erythromycin
	AIDS patients with staccato cough; **"ground glass"** x-ray; biopsy: honeycomb exudate with silver staining cysts; premature infants	Silver-staining cysts in alveolar lavage	*Pneumocystis jiroveci (carinii)*	Attaches to type I pneumocytes, causes excess replication of type II pneumocytes	Trimethoprim sulfamethoxazole
	Primary influenza pneumonia Secondary (bacterial)	Virus culture	Influenza virus	Cytolysis in respiratory tract; cytokines contribute; secondary infections common	Oseltamivar, zanamivar
Acute pneumonia or chronic cough with weight loss, night sweats	Over 55 years, HIV ⊕, or immigrant from developing country	Auramine-rhodamine stain of sputum acid-fast bacilli	*Mycobacterium tuberculosis*	Facultative intracellular parasite → cell-mediated immunity and DTH	Multidrug therapy
	Dusty environment with bird or bat fecal contamination (Missouri chicken farmers, Ohio river)	Intracellular yeast cells in sputum	*Histoplasma capsulatum*	Facultative intracellular	Amphotericin B
	Desert sand S.W. United States	Endospores in spherules in tissues	*Coccidioides immitis*	Acute, chronic lung infection, dissemination	Amphotericin B
	Rotting, contaminated wood, same endemic focus as *Histoplasma* and east coast states	Broad-based budding yeast cells in sputum or skin	*Blastomyces dermatitidis*	Acute, chronic lung infection, dissemination	Ketoconazole
Sudden acute respiratory syndromes	Travel to Far East, Toronto, winter, early spring	Serology, virus, isolation	SARS agent	Replication in cells of upper respiratory tree	None
	"Four Corners" region (CO, UT, NM, AZ), spring, inhalation rodent urine	Serology, virus, isolation	Hantavirus (Sin Nombre)	Virus disseminates to CNS, liver, kidneys, endothelium	Ribavirin

Definition of abbreviations: CGD, chronic granulomatous disease; CMV, cytomegalovirus; CF, cystic fibrosis; DTH, delayed-type hypersensitivity; RSV, respiratory syncytial virus.

▶ Granulomatous Diseases

Tuberculosis

Causes **caseating granulomas** containing acid-fast mycobacteria; transmission is by inhalation of aerosolized bacilli; increasing incidence in the U.S., secondary to AIDS

- Primary tuberculosis (initial exposure) can produce a **Ghon complex**, characterized by a subpleural caseous granuloma above or below the lobar fissure, accompanied by hilar lymph node granulomas.
- Secondary tuberculosis (reactivation or reinfection) tends to involve the **lung apex**.
- Progressive pulmonary tuberculosis can take the forms of cavitary tuberculosis, miliary pulmonary tuberculosis, and tuberculous bronchopneumonia. Miliary tuberculosis can also spread to involve other body sites.

Clinical: fevers and night sweats, weight loss, cough, hemoptysis, positive skin test (PPD)

Sarcoidosis

Sarcoidosis is a granulomatous disease of unknown etiology; affects females > males, ages 20–60; most common in African American women. **Noncaseating granulomas** occur in any organ of the body; hilar and mediastinal adenopathy are typical.

Clinical: Cough, shortness of breath, fatigue, malaise, skin lesions, eye irritation or pain, fever/night sweats

Labs: ↑ serum **angiotensin-converting enzyme** (ACE)
Schaumann bodies: laminated calcifications
Asteroid bodies: stellate giant-cell cytoplasmic inclusions

▶ Obstructive Lung Disease

Increased resistance to airflow secondary to obstruction of airways

Chronic obstructive pulmonary disease (COPD) includes chronic bronchitis, emphysema, asthma, and bronchiectasis.

Disease	Characteristics	Clinical Findings
Chronic bronchitis	• Persistent cough and copious **sputum production for at least 3 months** each year in 2 consecutive years • Highly **associated with smoking** (90%)	• Cough, sputum production, dyspnea, frequent infections • Hypoxia, cyanosis, weight gain
Emphysema	• Associated with destruction of alveolar septa, resulting in enlarged air spaces and a loss of elastic recoil, and producing overinflated, enlarged lungs • Thought to be due to protease/antiprotease imbalance *Gross:* • **Overinflated, enlarged lungs** • Enlarged, grossly visible air spaces • Formation of apical blebs and bullae (centriacinar type)	• Progressive dyspnea • Pursing of lips and **use of accessory muscles** to breathe • **Barrel chest** • Weight loss
Centriacinar (centrilobular) emphysema	• **Proximal respiratory bronchioles** involved • Most common type (95%) • **Associated with smoking** • Worst in apical segments of upper lobes	
Panacinar (panlobular) emphysema	• **Entire acinus involved**; distal alveoli spared • Less common • **Alpha-1-antitrypsin deficiency** • *Distribution:* entire lung; worse in bases of lower lobes	
Asthma	• Due to hyperreactive airways, resulting in episodic **bronchospasm**, producing **wheezing**, severe **dyspnea**, and coughing. • Inflammation, edema, hypertrophy of mucous glands with **goblet cell hyperplasia** and **mucus plugs** are characteristic findings. • Hypertrophy of bronchial wall smooth muscle, thickened basement membranes	

(Continued)

▶ Obstructive Lung Disease *(Cont'd.)*

Extrinsic asthma	• **Type I hypersensitivity** reaction • **Allergic (atopic)**—most common type • Childhood and young adults; ⊕ **family history** • Allergens: pollen, dust, food, molds, animal dander, etc. • Occupational exposure: fumes, gases, and chemicals
Intrinsic asthma	• Unknown mechanism • **Respiratory infections** (usually viral) • **Stress** • **Exercise** • **Cold** temperatures • Drug induced (**aspirin**)
Bronchiectasis	• An abnormal permanent airway dilatation due to **chronic necrotizing infection** • Most patients have underlying lung disease, such as bronchial obstruction, necrotizing pneumonias, **cystic fibrosis**, or **Kartagener syndrome**.

▶ Drugs for Asthma

Class	Agents	Mechanism	Comments
		Bronchodilators	
β_2 agonists	Albuterol Terbutaline Metaproterenol Salmeterol Formoterol	Stimulate β_2 receptors → ↑ cAMP → smooth muscle relaxation	• Generally have the advantage of **minimal cardiac side effects** • Most often used as **inhalants** • Salmeterol and formoterol are **long-acting** agents, so are useful for prophylaxis • Cause skeletal muscle **tremors**; some **CV** side effects (tachycardia, arrhythmias) can still occur
Non-selective β agonists	Epinephrine (α_1,α_2,β_1,β_2) Isoproterenol (β_1, β_2)	Stimulate β_2 receptors → ↑ cAMP → smooth muscle relaxation	• Not used as much as the β_2 agonists • Epinephrine is used for **acute** asthma attacks and for **anaphylaxis**
Muscarinic antagonists	Ipratropium Tiotropium	Block muscarinic receptors, inhibiting vagally induced bronchoconstriction	• Used as an inhalant; there are minimal systemic side effects • Used in asthma and COPD • β_2 agonists are generally preferred for acute bronchospasm • These are useful in **COPD** because it decreases bronchial secretions and has fewer CV side effects • Tiotropium is longer-acting
Methylxanthines	Theophylline	Inhibit PDE; block adenosine receptors	• Available orally • Major use is for asthma (although β_2 agonists are first-line)
		Leukotriene Antagonists	
Leukotriene antagonists	Zafirlukast Montelukast	Block LTD_4 (and LTE_4) leukotriene receptors	• Orally active; not used for acute asthma episodes • Prevents exercise-, antigen-, and aspirin-induced asthma
5-lipoxygenase inhibitors	Zileuton	Block leukotriene synthesis	
		Anti-inflammatory Agents	
Corticosteroids	Beclomethasone Prednisone, prednisolone Others	Inhibit phospholipase A_2 → ↓ arachidonic acid synthesis	• ↓ inflammation and edema • Used orally and inhaled • IV use in status asthmaticus
Release inhibitors	Cromolyn Nedocromil	Inhibit mast cell degranulation	• Can prevent allergy-induced bronchoconstriction • Available as nasal spray, oral, eye drops

▶ Restrictive Lung Disease

(Decreased Lung Volumes and Capacities)

Examples
Chest wall disorders: obesity, kyphoscoliosis, polio, etc. **Intrinsic lung disease:** Adult respiratory distress syndrome (ARDS) Neonatal respiratory distress syndrome (NRDS) Pneumoconioses (silicosis, asbestosis, "black lung" disease from coal dust) Sarcoidosis Idiopathic pulmonary fibrosis (Hamman-Rich syndrome) Goodpasture syndrome Wegener granulomatosis Eosinophilic granuloma Collagen-vascular diseases Hypersensitivity pneumonitis Drug exposure

▶ Respiratory Distress Syndromes

Adult Respiratory Distress Syndrome (ARDS)

- Diffuse damage to the alveolar epithelium and capillaries, resulting in progressive respiratory failure unresponsive to oxygen therapy
- **Causes:** shock, sepsis, trauma, gastric aspiration, radiation, oxygen toxicity, drugs, pulmonary infections, and many others
- **Clinical presentation:** dyspnea, tachypnea, hypoxemia, cyanosis, and use of accessory respiratory muscles
  - X-ray: **bilateral lung opacity** ("white out")
  - Gross: heavy, **stiff, noncompliant lungs**
  - Micro:
    - Interstitial and intra-alveolar edema
    - Interstitial inflammation
    - Loss of type I pneumocytes
    - **Hyaline membrane formation**
  - Overall mortality 50%

Neonatal Respiratory Distress Syndrome (NRDS)

Also known as **hyaline membrane disease of newborns**. Causes respiratory distress within hours of birth and is seen in infants with **deficiency of surfactant** secondary to prematurity (gestational age of <28 weeks has a 60% incidence), maternal diabetes, multiple births, or C-section delivery

- Clinical presentation: often normal at birth, but within a few hours develop increasing respiratory effort, tachypnea, nasal flaring, use of accessory muscle of respiration, an expiratory grunt, cyanosis
- X-ray: "**ground-glass**" reticulogranular densities
- Labs: lecithin: sphingomyelin ratio <2
- Micro: atelectasis and **hyaline membrane formation**
- Treatment: surfactant replacement and oxygen
- Complications of oxygen treatment in newborns:
  - **Bronchopulmonary dysplasia**
  - **Retrolental fibroplasia** (retinopathy of prematurity)
- **Prevention:** delay labor and corticosteroids to mature the lung

▶ Tumors of the Lung and Pleura

Bronchogenic carcinoma is the leading cause of cancer deaths among both men and women.

Major Risk Factors

- **Cigarette smoking**
- Occupational exposures (asbestosis, uranium mining, radiation)
- Air pollution

Histologic Types

Adenocarcinoma, bronchioloalveolar carcinoma, squamous cell carcinoma, small cell carcinoma, and large cell carcinoma

- Oncogenes
  - **L-*myc*:** small cell carcinomas
  - **K-*ras*:** adenocarcinomas
- Tumor suppressor genes
  - **p53** and the retinoblastoma gene

Complications

- **Spread to hilar, bronchial, tracheal, or mediastinal nodes** in 50% of cases
- **Superior vena cava syndrome** (obstruction of SVC by tumor)
- Esophageal obstruction
- **Recurrent laryngeal nerve** involvement (hoarseness)
- **Phrenic nerve** damage, causing diaphragmatic paralysis
- Extrathoracic metastasis to adrenal, liver, brain, and bone
- **Pancoast tumor:** compression of cervical sympathetic plexus, leading to ipsilateral **Horner syndrome** (miosis, ptosis, anhidrosis)

Type of Cancer/ (Percentage of Total)	Association with Smoking; Sex Preference	Location	Pathology
Adenocarcinoma/35% **Bronchioloalveolar carcinoma** (5%)—subset of adenocarcinoma	**Less strongly related;** female > male; most common lung cancer in nonsmokers	**Peripheral**, may occur in scars; can have associated pleural involvement	Forms glands and may produce mucin
Squamous cell/30%	**Strongly related;** male > female	**Central**	• Invasive nests of squamous cells, intercellular bridges (desmosomes); keratin production ("**squamous pearls**") • Hyperparathyroidism secondary to increased secretion of parathyroid related peptide
Small cell (oat cell) carcinoma/20%	**Strongly related;** male > female	**Central**	• Very aggressive; micro: small round cells • Frequently associated with paraneoplastic syndromes, including production of ACTH (Cushing syndrome), ADH, and parathyroid related peptide
Large cell/10%	—	—	Large anaplastic cells without evidence of differentiation
Carcinoid/<5%	—	Bronchial	May produce carcinoid syndrome

▶ Diseases of the Pleura

Pleural effusion	• Accumulation of **fluid in the pleural cavity**; may be a transudate or exudate • Chylous fluid in pleural space secondary to obstruction of thoracic duct (usually by tumor) = chylothorax
Pneumothorax	• **Air in the pleural cavity**, often due to penetrating chest wall injuries • *Spontaneous pneumothorax:* young adults with rupture of emphysematous blebs • *Tension pneumothorax:* life-threatening shift of thoracic organs across midline • Clinical: ↓ breath sounds, hyperresonance, tracheal shift to opposite side
Mesothelioma	• Highly malignant tumor of pleura (and peritoneum) • Pleural mesothelioma is associated with **asbestos exposure** in 90% of cases (**bronchogenic carcinoma** also strongly associated with asbestos exposure)

▶ Pulmonary Vascular Disorders

Pulmonary edema	Fluid accumulation within the lungs that can be due to many causes, including left-sided heart failure, mitral valve stenosis, fluid overload, nephrotic syndrome, liver disease, infections, drugs, shock, and radiation
Pulmonary emboli	Mostly arise from **deep vein thrombosis** in the leg (also arise from pelvic veins) and may be asymptomatic, cause pulmonary infarction, or cause sudden death; severity related to size of embolus and other comorbid conditions
Pulmonary hypertension	Pulmonary hypertension is increased artery pressure, usually due to increased vascular resistance or blood flow; can be idiopathic or related to underlying COPD, interstitial disease, pulmonary emboli, mitral stenosis, left heart failure, and congenital heart disease with left-to-right shunt

The Renal and Urinary System

Chapter 4

Renal Embryology and Anatomy

► Development of the Kidney and Ureter (Mesoderm)

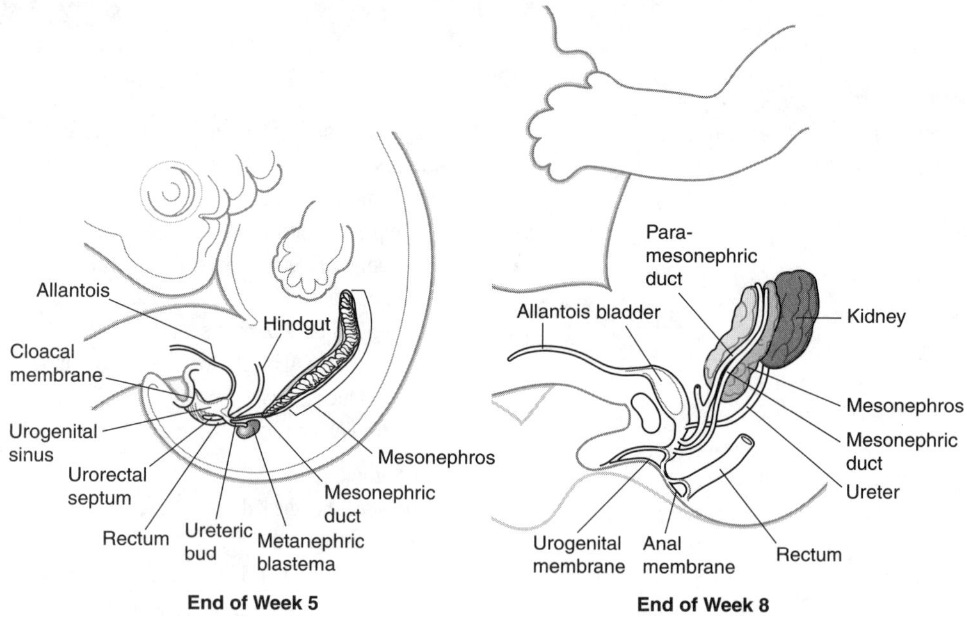

The **ureteric bud** penetrates the **metanephric mass**, which condenses around the diverticulum to form the metanephrogenic blastema. The **bud** dilates to form the **renal pelvis**, which subsequently splits into the cranial and caudal **major calyces**, which form the **minor calyces**. One to 3 million collecting tubules develop from the minor calyces, forming the renal pyramids.

Penetration of collecting tubules into the metanephric mass induces cells of the tissue cap to form nephrons, or excretory units.

- The **proximal nephron forms Bowman capsule**, whereas the **distal nephron connects to a collecting tubule**.
- Lengthening of the excretory tubule gives rise to the **proximal convoluted tubule**, the **loop of Henle**, and the **distal convoluted tubule**.

The kidneys develop in the pelvis but appear to ascend into the abdomen as a result of fetal growth of the lumbar and sacral regions. With their ascent, the ureters elongate, and the kidneys become vascularized by lateral splanchnic arteries, which arise from the abdominal aorta.

► Development of the Bladder and Urethra (Endoderm)

Bladder

- The **urorectal septum** divides the cloaca into the **anorectal canal** and the **urogenital sinus** by Week 7. The upper and largest part of the urogenital sinus becomes the **urinary bladder**, which is initially continuous with the **allantois**. As the lumen of the allantois becomes obliterated, a fibrous cord, the **urachus**, connects the apex of the bladder to the umbilicus. In the adult, this structure becomes the **median umbilical ligament**.
- The **mucosa** of the trigone of the bladder is initially formed from mesodermal tissue, which is replaced by **endodermal epithelium**. The smooth muscle of the bladder is derived from splanchnic mesoderm.

Urethra

- The **male urethra** is anatomically divided into three portions: **prostatic**, **membranous**, and **spongy** (penile). The **prostatic urethra, membranous urethra, and proximal penile urethra** develop from the narrow portion of the **urogenital sinus** below the urinary bladder. The **distal spongy urethra** is derived from the **ectodermal cells** of the glans penis.
- The **female urethra** is derived entirely from the **urogenital sinus** (endoderm).

▶ Congenital Abnormalities

Renal agenesis	Failure of one or both kidneys to develop because of early degeneration of the ureteric bud. Unilateral genesis is fairly common; bilateral agenesis is fatal (associated with oligohydramnios, and the fetus may have **Potter sequence**: clubbed feet, pulmonary hypoplasia, and craniofacial anomalies).
Pelvic and horseshoe kidney	Pelvic kidney is caused by a failure of one kidney to ascend. **Horseshoe kidney** (usually **normal renal function**, predisposition to calculi) is a fusion of both kidneys at their ends and failure of the fused kidney to ascend.
Double ureter	Caused by the early splitting of the ureteric bud or the development of two separate buds.
Patent urachus	**Failure of the allantois to be obliterated**. It causes urachal fistulas or sinuses. In male children with congenital valvular obstruction of the prostatic urethra or in older men with enlarged prostates, a patent urachus **may cause drainage of urine through the umbilicus**.

▶ Gross Anatomy of the Kidney

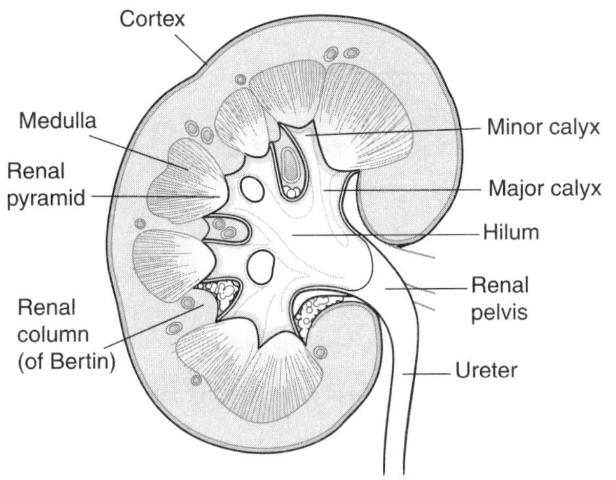

The kidney is divided into three major regions:

Hilum

Located medially and is the point of entrance and exit for the renal artery and vein, and ureter

Cortex

Forms the outer zone of the kidney, as well as several renal columns, which penetrate the entire depth of the kidney

Medulla

Appears as a series of medullary pyramids. The apex of each pyramid directs the urinary stream into a minor calyx, which then travels to the major calyx, through the renal pelvis, and into the ureter

Relation of the Kidneys to the Posterior Abdominal Wall

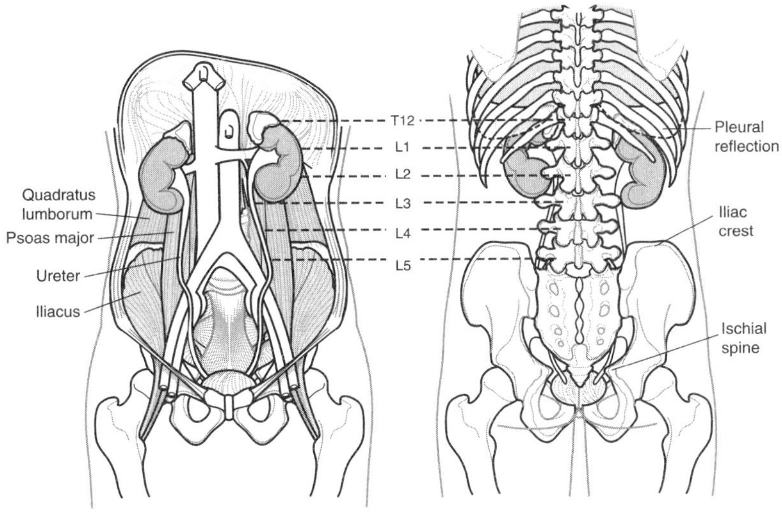

Clinical Correlation

Blockage by Renal Calculi

The most common sites of ureteral constriction susceptible to blockage by renal calculi are:

- where the renal pelvis joins the ureter
- where the ureter crosses the pelvic inlet
- where the ureter enters the wall of the urinary bladder

Renal Physiology

► Basic Functions of the Kidneys

Fluid balance	Maintain normal extracellular (ECF) and intracellular (ICF) fluid volumes
Electrolytes	Balance excretion with intake to maintain normal plasma concentrations
Wastes	Excrete metabolic wastes (nitrogenous products, acids, toxins, etc.)
Fuels	Reabsorb metabolic fuels (glucose, lactate, amino acids, etc.)
Blood pressure	Regulate ECF volume for the long-term control of blood pressure
Acid–base	Regulate absorption and excretion of H^+ and HCO_3^- to control acid–base balance

► Fluid Balance: Estimation of Fluid Volumes

Basic Concepts

Body fluid compartments: TBW = ICF + ECF   ECF = plasma + ISF   TBW = ICF + (plasma + ISF)

Estimating body fluid volumes:
(must assume normal hydration)

TBW in Liters = 0.6 × weight in kg
ICF = 0.4 × weight
ECF = 0.2 × weight

Measuring body fluid volumes (indicator dilution principle):

V = Q/C, where V = body fluid volume, Q = quantity of indicator administered, C = concentration of indicator after dilution in body fluid compartment

Indicators: must disperse evenly in compartment, must disperse only in compartment of interest, and cannot be metabolized or excreted (no indicator is perfect)

TBW indicators: D_2O, ^3H_2O, antipyrine ($C_{11}H_{12}N_2O$)
ECF indicators: ^{22}Na, inulin, mannitol
PV indicators: ^{125}I-albumin, Evans blue dye, ^{51}Cr-red blood cells

Osmolarity vs. molarity: Ionic substances dissociate, covalently bonded substances do not, therefore:
- 100 mM glucose = 100 mOsm/L
- 100 mM NaCl = 200 mOsm/L

Osmolarity of ECF always = osmolarity of ICF: Estimate by 2× plasma [Na^+]

All water and solutes pass through ECF: Evaluate changes in ECF first, then ICF

ICF volume is controlled by ECF osmolarity:
- ECF volume does not control ICF volume
- Water enters/leaves ICF to keep osmolarity of ICF = ECF

Definition of abbreviations: ECF, extracellular fluid; ICF, intracellular fluid; ISF, interstitial fluid; PV, plasma volume; TBW, total body water.

► Normal Values
(Body weight = 100 kg, 300 mOsm/L)

	ECF	ICF	TBW
Volume (liters)	20	40	60
Osmolarity (mOsm/L)	300	300	300
Solute mass in compartment (mOsm)	6,000	12,000	18,000

► Fluid and Electrolyte Abnormalities

Diarrhea

- Weight loss = 4 kg (assume all weight loss is fluid loss)
- Solutes lost from ECF
- Isoosmotic loss: osmolarity remains at 300 mOsm/L; calculate TBW, ECF, ICF

	ECF	ICF	TBW
Volume (liters)	V = 4,800/300 = 16	ICF = TBW – ECF 56 – 16 = 40	60 – 4 = 56
Osmolarity (mOsm/L)	300	300	300
Solute mass in compartment (mOsm)	6,000 – (300 × 4) = 4,800	12,000	56 × 300 = 16,800

Conclusion: Isoosmotic volume gain or loss only changes ECF volume; ICF volume is unchanged.

Sweating

- Weight loss = 8 kg (assume all weight loss is fluid loss)
- Solutes lost from ECF
- Loss of hypoosmotic fluid, osmolarity = 330 mOsm/L; calculate TBW, ECF, ICF

	ECF	ICF	TBW
Volume (liters)	V = 5,160/330 = 15.6	ICF = TBW – ECF 52 – 15.6 = 36.4	60 – 8 = 52
Osmolarity (mOsm/L)	330	330	330
Solute mass in compartment (mOsm)	6,000 – 840 = 5,160	12,000	52 × 330 = 17,160 = loss of 840 from ECF

Conclusion: ECF loss of water and solutes, but ↑ osmolarity → ↓ ICF volume due to water shift.

Drink 3 L Pure Water

- Weight gain = 3 kg
- No solutes lost or gained
- Gain of hypoosmotic fluid; calculate new osmolarity, TBW, ECF, ICF

	ECF	ICF	TBW
Volume (liters)	V = 6,000/285.7 = 21	V = 12,000/285.7 = 42	60 + 3 = 63
Osmolarity (mOsm/L)	285.7	285.7	18,000/63 = 285.7
Solute mass in compartment (mOsm)	21 × 285.7 = 6,000	42 × 285.7 = 12,000	63 × 285.7 = 18,000

Conclusion: Addition of pure water ↓ osmolarity, causing proportionate increases in ICF and ECF volumes.

► Processes in the Formation of Urine

Filtration	• Glomerular capillaries—same forces as described in cardiovascular section • Glomerular filtration rate **(GFR)**
Secretion (S)	Active transport of solutes from plasma (via interstitial fluid) into tubular fluid
Reabsorption (R)	Passive or active movement of solutes and water from tubular fluid back into capillaries
Excretion of X (E_x)	• Result of the balance of filtration, secretion, and reabsorption • $\mathbf{E_x = \dot{V} \times [X]_{urine}}$; $\dot{V}$ = urine flow; $[X]_{urine}$ = urinary concentration of X
Filtered load (F)	• $\mathbf{F = GFR \times [solute]_{plasma}}$ • Solute fraction bound to plasma protein does not filter
Mass balance	**E = F + S – R**
Transport	$F_x > E_x$ = net reabsorption of X; $F_x < E_x$ = net secretion of X

► Examples Using Mass Balance to Evaluate Renal Processing of a Solute

Data	Calculations	Conclusions
• GFR = 100 mL/min • $[Subst.]_{plasma}$ = 1 µg/mL • $\dot{V}$ = 2 mL/min • $[Subst.]_{urine}$ = 75 µg/mL	F = 100 × 1 = 100 µg/min E = 2 × 75 = 150 µg/min	Subst. must be secreted because the amount excreted is > the amount filtered. S ≈ 50 µg/min*
• GFR = 100 mL/min • $[Subst.]_{plasma}$ = 3 µg/mL • $\dot{V}$ = 1 mL/min • $[Subst.]_{urine}$ = 100 µg/mL	F = 100 × 3 = 300 µg/min E = 1 × 100 = 100 µg/min	Subst. must be reabsorbed because the amount filtered is > the amount excreted. R ≈ 200 µg/min†
• GFR = 100 mL/min • $[Subst.]_{plasma}$ = 2 µg/mL • $\dot{V}$ = 4 mL/min • $[Subst.]_{urine}$ = 50 µg/mL	F = 100 × 2 = 200 µg/min E = 4 × 50 = 200 µg/min	Subst. is neither secreted nor reabsorbed because the amount excreted = the amount filtered.¶

Definition of abbreviation: Subst., substance.

*Assumes no reabsorption

†Assumes no secretion

¶Still possible that S = R, but this is unlikely.

► Clearance and Its Applications

Definition	Volume of plasma from which a substance is removed (cleared) per unit time
Concept	Relates the excretion of a substance to its concentration in plasma
Calculation	$C_s = (U_s \times \dot{V})/P_s$ where, C_s = clearance of substance, U_s = urine concentration of substance, $\dot{V}$ = urine flow, P_s = plasma concentration of substance
Application: GFR	• **Inulin clearance** can be used to calculate **GFR**. • Rationale: inulin is filtered, but is neither secreted nor reabsorbed. Therefore, Clearance of inulin = $(U_{[inulin]} \times \dot{V})/P_{[inulin]}$ = GFR • **Creatinine clearance** is the best clinical measure of GFR because it is produced continually by the body and is freely filtered but not reabsorbed. Creatinine is partially secreted, but its clearance is still a reasonable clinical estimate of GFR.
Application: **Renal plasma flow (RPF)** **Renal blood flow (RBF)**	**Para-aminohippuric acid (PAH)** is filtered and secreted; at low doses it is almost completely cleared from blood flowing through the kidneys during a single pass. Therefore, PAH clearance = RPF. However, PAH clearance is a measure of *plasma* flow rather than *blood* flow. Renal blood flow (RBF) can be calculated as follows: **RBF = RPF / (1 – hematocrit)**, using hematocrit as decimal proportion, e.g., 0.40
Application: **Free water clearance (C_{H_2O})**	• C_{H_2O} is not a true clearance. It is the volume of water that would have to be added to or removed from urine to make the urine isoosmotic to plasma. • C_{H_2O} is the difference between water excretion (urine flow) and osmolar clearance. Thus: $C_{H_2O} = \dot{V} - C_{osm} = \dot{V} - (U_{osm} \times \dot{V})/P_{osm}$ • **Positive C_{H_2O}:** Urine is hypotonic, ADH is low, “free water” has been removed from body, and plasma osmolarity is being increased. • **Negative C_{H_2O}:** Urine is hypertonic, ADH is high, water is being conserved, and plasma osmolarity is being decreased. • Use C_{H_2O} to evaluate whether urine osmolarity is appropriate. If P_{osm} is elevated, C_{H_2O} should be negative to compensate; if P_{osm} is low, C_{H_2O} should be positive.

Definition of abbreviation: ADH, antidiuretic hormone.

▶ Structure of the Nephron
(Approximately 1 million nephrons/kidney)

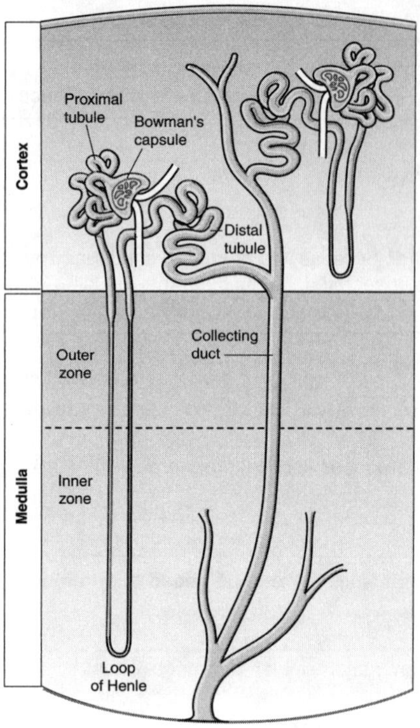

Sequence of Fluid Flow in a Nephron	
Structure	**Basic Function**
Bowman capsule	Formation of filtrate
Proximal tubule (PT)	Reabsorption of H_2O, solutes; some secretion
Descending thin loop of Henle (DTL)	Reabsorption of H_2O, no solute transport
Ascending thin loop of Henle (ATL)	Reabsorption of solutes, not water
Thick ascending loop of Henle (TAL)	Reabsorption of solutes, not water
Early distal tubule (EDT)	Reabsorption of solutes; special sensory region
Late distal tubule (LDT); cortical collecting duct (CCD)	Reabsorption of solutes and water; regulation of acid–base status
Medullary collecting duct (MCD)	Reabsorption of H_2O; final control of urine volume and osmolarity

▶ Association of Blood Vessels With the Nephron

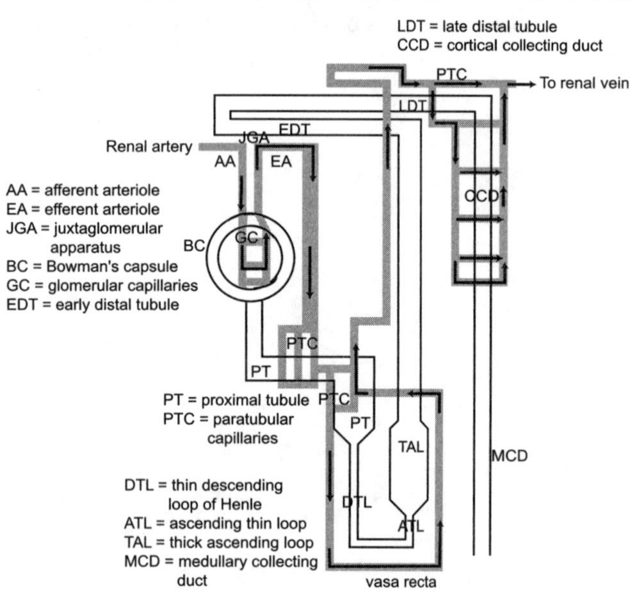

Each tubular segment has a blood supply that allows exchange of water and/or solute.

Sequence of Blood Flow in Nephrons	
Blood Vessel	**Tubular Segment**
Afferent arteriole	No exchange
Glomerular capillaries	Bowman capsule
Efferent arteriole	No exchange
Peritubular capillaries	Sequence: proximal tubule → loop of Henle → distal tubule → collecting duct
Vasa recta: specialized portion of peritubular capillaries that perfuse medulla 1–2% of blood flow	Loop of Henle, collecting duct

▶ The Juxtaglomerular Apparatus (JGA)

The **juxtaglomerular apparatus** includes the site of **filtration** (Bowman capsule [BC] and glomerular capillaries), as well as the arterioles and macula densa tubule cells found at the end of the thick ascending limb. Macula densa cells sense tubular fluid NaCl and contribute to **autoregulation** and regulation of **renin secretion**.

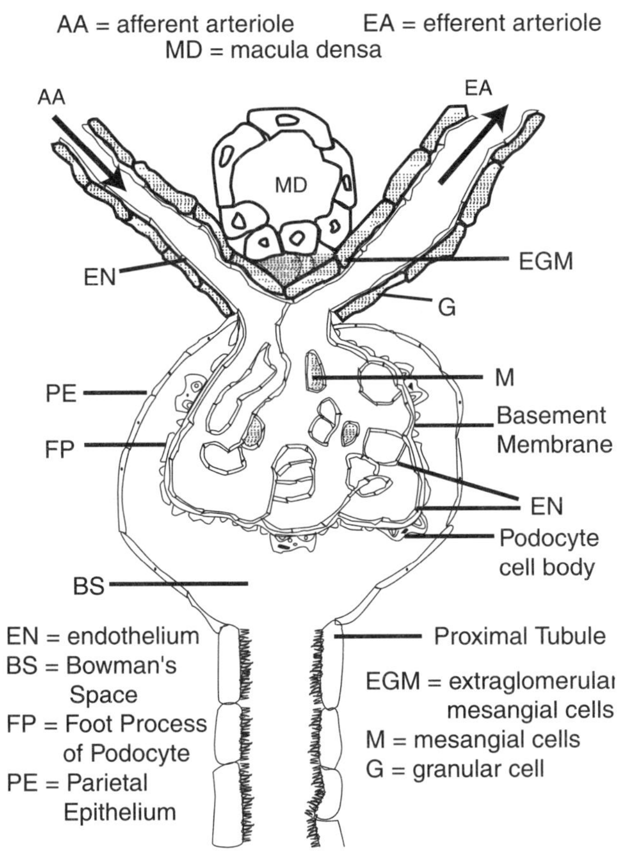

Filtration	
Bowman capsule	A pouch wrapped around capillaries
Podocytes	Specialized cells of BC, which help prevent protein filtration
Glomerular capillaries (GC)	Fenestrated, which allows rapid filtration of water and small solutes, but prevents protein filtration
Filtration = GFR = $K_f[(P_{GC} - P_{BC}) - (\varpi_{GC} - \varpi_{BC})]$ (same forces as discussed in CV)	
K_f	Filtration coefficient is high for H_2O, electrolytes, small solutes
P_{GC}	Remains high along GC due to very low GC resistance, favoring filtration
P_{BC}	Remains low unless urinary tract obstruction is present
π_{GC}	Rises along GC due to high filtration, until filtration ceases in distal capillary; reduced with low plasma protein
π_{BC}	≈ zero normally, proteinuria increases it
Filtration Fraction = GFR/RPF	

Ranges from 15–30%, usually ≈20%

- Nonrenal capillary filtration fraction ≈1–2%
- Nonrenal P_{cap} falls along capillary due to capillary resistance, so filtration only occurs at proximal end and reabsorption occurs distally.

▶ Autoregulation of GFR and RBF

An isolated change in renal perfusion pressure between 75 and 175 mm Hg will not change RBF or GFR significantly because **autoregulation** maintains RBF at a constant level by adjusting afferent and efferent arteriolar resistances. Autoregulation occurs via a **myogenic response** and **tubuloglomerular feedback**.

Mechanisms of Autoregulation	
Myogenic	↑ arterial pressure stretches vessel wall, which ↑ calcium movement into smooth muscle cells, causing them to contract.
Tubuloglomerular feedback (TGF)	↓ arterial pressure causes GFR to ↓, which in turn ↓ delivery of NaCl to macula densa. This results in an ↑ in efferent arteriolar resistance and a ↓ in afferent arteriolar resistance, both of which ↑ GFR to a normal level. The ↑ in efferent arteriolar resistance occurs in response to ↑ levels of angiotensin II.

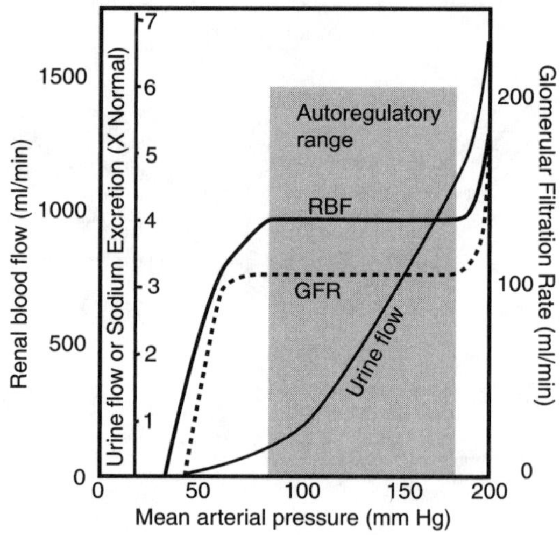

Autoregulatory range	Between approximately 75–175 mm Hg mean arterial pressure (MAP)
Renal shutdown	Lower than 50 mm Hg MAP; both GFR and RBF are very low; kidney shuts down

▶ Regulation of Filtration (GFR and RBF)

Vessel	Constriction			Dilation		
	P_{cap}	GFR	RBF	P_{cap}	GFR	RBF
Afferent arteriole	↓	↓	↓	↑	↑	↑
Efferent arteriole	↑	↑	↓	↓	↓	↑

▶ Tubular Function: Reabsorption and Secretion

Active Facilitated Transporters Display Maximum Transport (T_{max}) Rates	
Transport maximum	T_{max} = mass of solute per time transported *when carriers saturated*
Limited carrier population	Transport mediated by these carriers is saturable under pathophysiologic conditions, e.g., glucose transporters
Reabsorption < T_{max}	None of solute in urine until filtered load > T_{max}
Secretion < T_{max}	All of solute delivered in plasma appears in urine until delivery > T_{max}
Interpretation	Reduced T_{max} for glucose indicates reduced number of functioning nephrons

Estimation of T_{max} by Graphical Interpretation

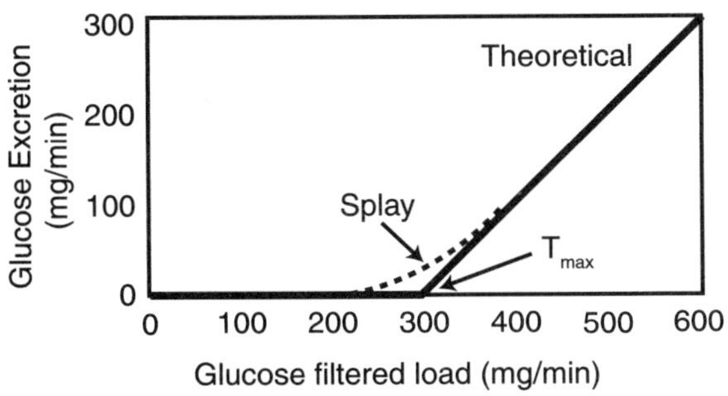

The *solid line* represents the theoretical relationship between glucose filtered load (FL) and glucose excretion (E). Actually, some glucose appears in the urine below the T_{max} due to competition for binding sites. When the filtered load > T_{max}, E = FL – T_{max}.

Select a point on linear portion:

Reabsorption = excretion – filtered load

T_{max} = 300 mg/min reabsorption

$FL_{glucose}$ = 500 mg/min; $E_{glucose}$ = 200 mg/min

$R_{glucose}$ = 200 mg/min – 500 mg/min = –300 mg/min

Therefore, $R_{glucose}$ = T_{max}, and carriers are saturated

Proximal Tubule

First Half of the Proximal Tubule

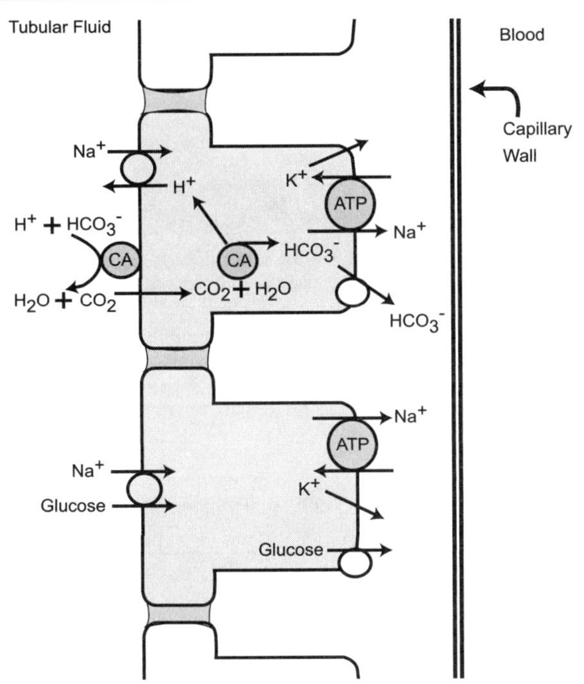

1) $NaHCO_3^-$ reabsorption is depicted at the *top of the diagram.*
2) The Na^+-glucose symporter is depicted in the *bottom cell*; other symporters reabsorb amino acids, lactate, and phosphate.

Second Half of the Proximal Tubule

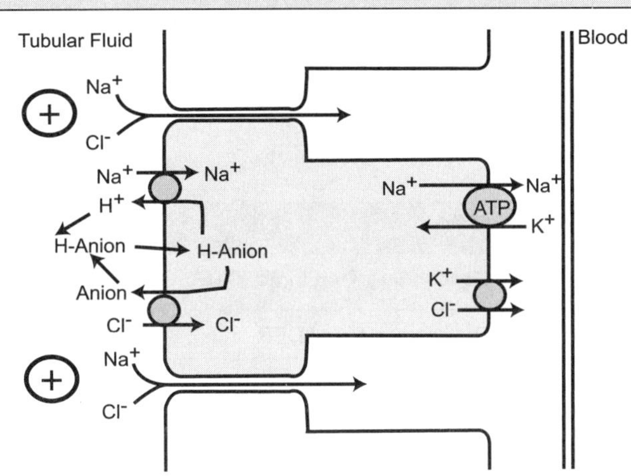

The processes in the left figure continue on in the second half of the proximal tubule and others are added:

3) Secondary active NaCl reabsorption is mediated by the parallel operation of the Na^+/H^+ antiport and Cl^-/anion antiport (e.g., OH^-, formate, oxalate, sulfate). H^+ plus anion associate into the neutral acid in the tubular fluid and diffuse passively into the cell, where they dissociate again to move through the antiports.
4) Water follows non-Cl^- solute reabsorption in the first half of the PT and increases tubular fluid [Cl^-]. Passive Cl^- diffusion pulls Na^+ electrically after it, but creates a small negative electrical potential in the tubular lumen.

(Continued)

Proximal Tubule *(Cont'd.)*		
Substance	**Action**	**Mechanism**
Water	67% reabsorbed	• Simple diffusion; filtration forces favor reabsorption • Solute reabsorption creates osmotic gradient, water follows it; paracellular and transcellular • Cell membranes permeable to water
Na^+	67% reabsorbed	• Na^+/K^+-ATPase in the basolateral membrane creates an electrochemical gradient; secondary active transport, luminal (apical) surface; co- and countertransport • Simple diffusion, paracellular
Glucose, lactate, amino acids, phosphate	≈100% reabsorbed	• Secondary active transport at the luminal (apical) surface; cotransport with Na^+; Na^+ electrochemical gradient provides the power • Transport maximum processes (*see* below)
H^+	Secreted	Primary ATPase and secondary active antiport with Na^+
HCO_3^-	≈100% reabsorbed	Reabsorbed as CO_2 at the apical surface; facilitated diffusion and exchange with Cl^- on basolateral surface; carbonic anhydrase located at the apical surface and intracellularly
Cl^-	≈67% reabsorbed	• Transcellular: at the apical surface, exchange with anions; at the basolateral surface, facilitated diffusion and symport with K^+ • Paracellular, simple diffusion
Ca^{2+}	≈70% reabsorbed	80% of proximal tubule reabsorption paracellular; 20% transcellular
Organic cations, anions	Mainly secreted	Various mechanisms

Loop of Henle: Overview			
	Descending Thin Limb (DTL)	**Ascending Thin Limb (ATL)**	**Thick Ascending Limb (TAL)**
H_2O	Reabsorbs 15% of GFR	Impermeable	Impermeable
Solutes	Diffuse into tubule	Slight active reabsorption	Reabsorbs 25% FL of NaCl, K^+; 20% FL of Ca^{2+}; 50–60% FL of Mg^{2+}
Tubular fluid volume	Decreases	No change	No change
Tubular fluid osmolarity	Increases; DTL is called the "concentrating segment"	Decreases	Decreases below normal plasma; TAL is called the "diluting segment"

Definition of abbreviation: FL, filtered load.

Thick Ascending Loop of Henle

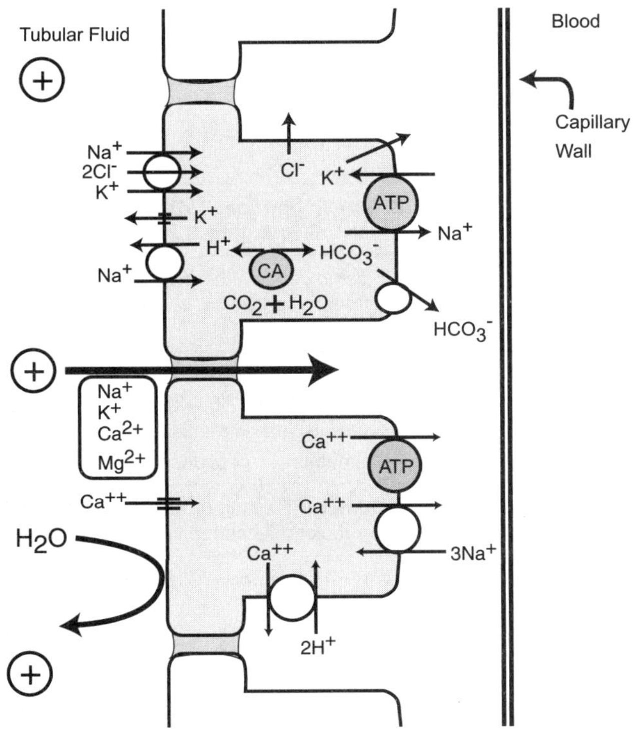

Mechanisms of Solute Transport, Thick Ascending Loop of Henle	
Na^+	**Reabsorption:** • Symport with Cl^- and K^+ • Antiport with H^+ • Paracellular due to electrical force
K^+	**Reabsorption:** • Paracellular reabsorption (electrical force) • Symport with Na^+ and Cl^-
Ca^{2+}	**Reabsorption:** • Paracellular (electrical force) • Transcellular, apical surface, simple diffusion • Basolateral Ca^{2+}-ATPase, Na^+-Ca^{2+} exchange • $2H^+/Ca^{2+}$ ATPase antiport; parathyroid hormone stimulates
Mg^{2+}	**Reabsorption:** • Paracellular (electrical force) • Transcellular, active transport
H^+	**Secretion:** • Na^+/H^+ exchange, NH_4^+
"Diluting segment": reabsorption of solutes without reabsorption of water produces hyperosmotic interstitium of medulla; needed for descending loop water reabsorption and collecting duct ability to regulate water reabsorption	

Distal Tubule and Collecting Duct Overview

	Tubular Fluid Volume	Tubular Fluid Osmolarity	Tubular Fluid Solutes
Delivered from TAL	≈15% of GFR	Hypotonic at ≈1/2 P_{OSM}	• ≈10% FL of NaCl, K^+, and Ca^{2+} • ≈5% FL of HCO_3^-
Early distal convoluted tubule (EDT)	No H_2O reabsorbed	Hypotonic at **≈1/3** $\mathbf{P_{OSM}}$	• Reabsorb ≈5% FL of NaCl via **apical Na^+-Cl^- symporter** (NCC) in secondary active transport inhibited by **thiazide** diuretics • Reabsorb ≈10% FL of Ca^{2+} via secondary active transport stimulated by **parathyroid hormone (PTH)** and indirectly by **thiazide** diuretics
Late distal tubule (LTD) and cortical collecting duct (CCD)	H_2O reabsorption regulated by **antidiuretic hormone (ADH)**	Varies primarily with H_2O reabsorption	• Reabsorb ≈4% of FL of NaCl via active transport regulated by **aldosterone** • Reabsorb ≈5% FL of HCO_3^- via active transport regulated by **aldosterone** • Secretion of K^+ determines total excretion; active secretion regulated by **aldosterone**
Medullary collecting duct (MCD)	H_2O reabsorption regulated by **ADH**	Varies primarily with H_2O reabsorption	Reabsorb ≈60% of FL of urea passively via transporter regulated by **ADH**; urea reabsorption is needed for medullary osmolarity

Definition of abbreviation: FL, filtered load.
*Some refer to the LDT as the connecting tubule.

► Renal Regulation of Excretion of Water and Solutes

Overview				
Steady-State Balance (maintained by renal regulation of excretion)		**Fractional E = (Excreted)/(Filtered)**		**Major Regulators of Renal Excretion**
		Range	**Typical**	
Water	Volume liquid drunk/day = E_{H_2O}	0.5–14%	≈1%	**Antidiuretic hormone (ADH)** acting on LDT and **collecting duct**
Solute	Osmols generated as water soluble wastes = $E_{osmoles}$		≈1.5%	Major osmoles excreted are salts, acids, and nitrogenous wastes; excrete ≈600–900 mOsm/day
NaCl	Amount NaCl eaten/day = E_{NaCl}	0.1–5%	≈0.5–1%	• **Aldosterone** acting on LDT and **CCD**; renal **SNS** tone acting on **PT** • **Angiotensin II** on multiple segments • Atrial natriuretic peptide, etc.
K^+	Amount K^+ eaten/day $\approx E_{K^+}$	1–80%	≈15%	• **Aldosterone** acting on LDT and **CCD**; other factors described later
Ca^{2+}	Amount Ca^{2+} absorbed from GI/day = $E_{Ca^{2+}}$	0.1–3%	≈1%	**Parathyroid hormone** (PTH) acting on **DCT**
HCO_3^-	• *New* HCO_3^- added to blood/day = net acid excretion (NAE) = $(E_{ammonium})$+ $(E_{H_2PO_4^-})$ – $(E_{bicarbonate})$ • NAE determines $[HCO_3^-]_{plasma}$	HCO_3^- $H_2PO_4^-$	≈0% ≈20%	**Aldosterone** acting on LDT and **CCD**; plasma pH and other factors described later
Urea	Amount generated/day = E_{urea}	20% – 80%	≈40%	Synthesis depends on protein metabolism; regulated by **ADH** acting on medullary **collecting duct**

Definition of abbreviations: CCD, cortical collecting duct.

Regulation of Urine Osmolarity and Urine Flow: Antidiuretic Hormone (ADH)

Collecting Duct

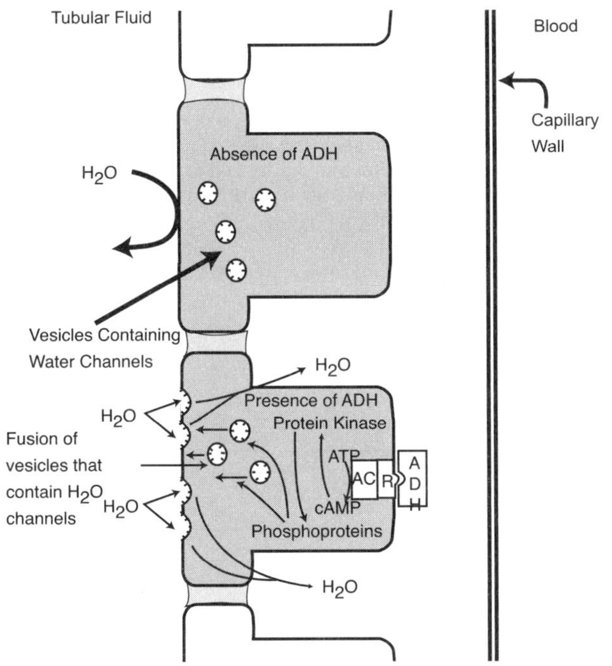

The ADH-receptor complex on the basolateral membrane activates adenylate cyclase. cAMP activates a kinase that phosphorylates proteins involved in movement of vesicles and fusion with the membrane. The resulting channels allow diffusion of water across the apical membrane.

Effect of Plasma ADH on Urine Osmolarity, Urine Flow, and Total Solute Excretion

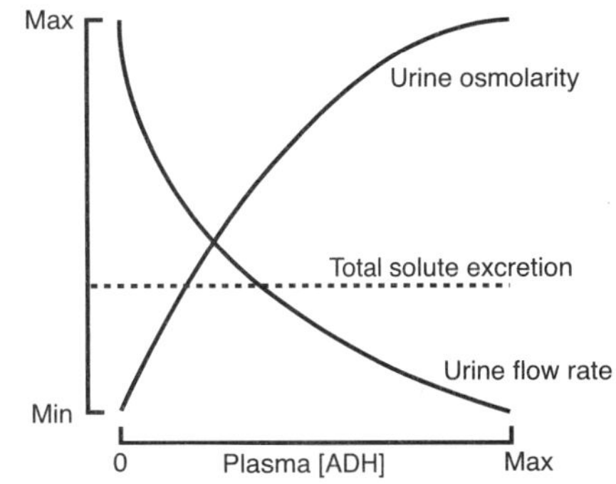

Urine Osmolarity Versus Urine Flow

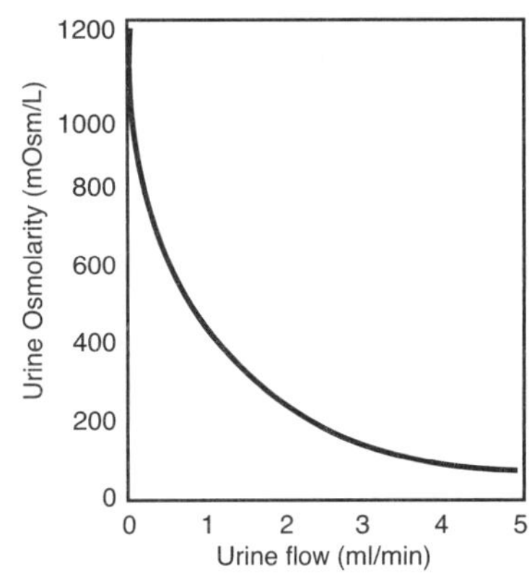

In the normal system, urine flow and osmolarity have an inverse relationship.

Loop of Henle and the Countercurrent Mechanism Antidiuresis (Presence of ADH)

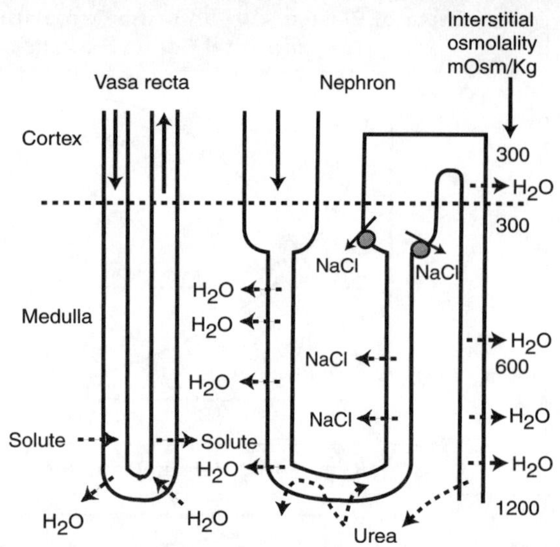

In the presence of ADH, the collecting duct is permeable to water. Because of the high osmolarity of the medulla, water is reabsorbed, so the urine volume is small and the urine concentration is the same as the medulla (hyperosmotic).

Vasa recta	• Only 1–2% of renal blood flow • Reabsorbed solutes "trapped" in medulla
Balance of solutes and water	• In total loop, more solute than H_2O reabsorbed • Produces hyperosmotic interstitium of medulla
Descending thin loop	• Fluid enters isoosmotic with normal plasma • H_2O reabsorption → ↓volume with ↑ osmolarity
Ascending loop	• Solute reabsorption only, not H_2O → hypoosmotic tubular fluid • Accumulation of solutes in interstitium of medulla
Collecting duct	• With ADH, collecting duct permeable to H_2O and urea • As duct passes through hyperosmotic interstitium, reabsorption of H_2O → small volume of concentrated urine • Negative CH_2O; dilutes plasma

Loop of Henle and the Countercurrent Mechanism
Water-Induced Diuresis (Absence of ADH)

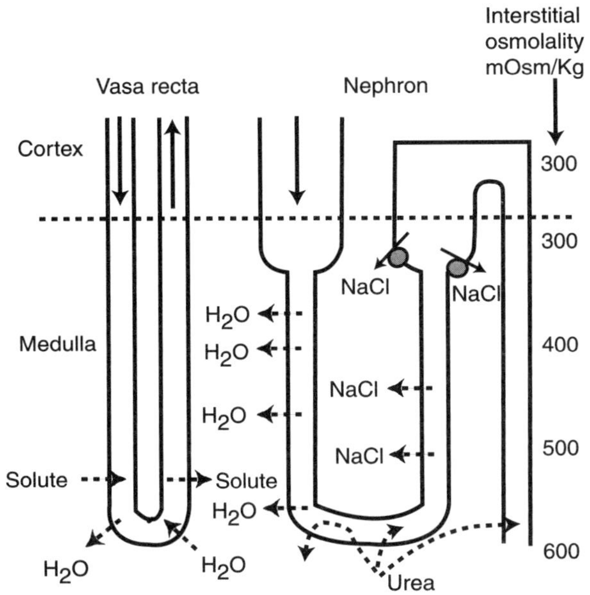

In the absence of ADH, the collecting duct is impermeable to water, so urine flow is high and the urine is dilute. Note that medullary osmolality is also lower than when ADH is present.

Vasa recta	• ↑ blood flow with lower-than-normal osmolarity • Washes out solutes, medullary osmolarity reduced
Balance of solutes and water	Medullary osmolarity still higher than normal plasma, but not as high as during antidiuresis
Descending thin loop	Less H_2O is reabsorbed because the medulla is not as concentrated as during antidiuresis
Ascending loop	Solute reabsorption continues, but a significant portion of solutes that are reabsorbed are washed into the vasa recta
Collecting duct	• Without ADH, the collecting duct is impermeable to H_2O and urea • No H_2O reabsorption because tubular fluid passes through medulla • ↑ urine flow,↓ urine osmolarity • Positive CH_2O; acts to concentrate plasma

Regulation of Plasma Osmolarity by ADH

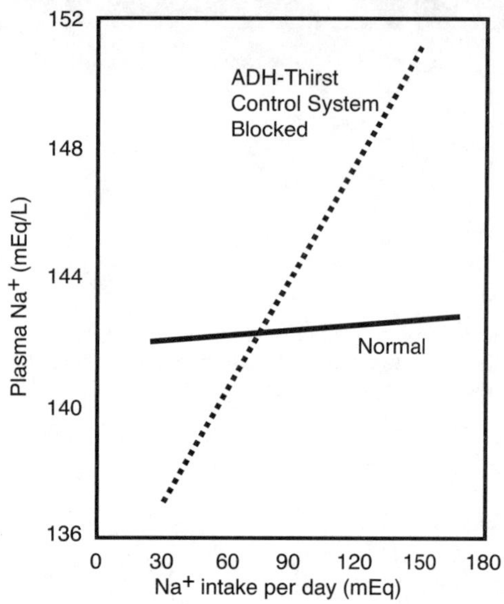

Normal function of the control system for ADH secretion and water consumption prevents large changes of plasma sodium concentration. Loss of this system causes plasma sodium concentration to increase in proportion to sodium intake.

ADH secretion is increased by elevated plasma sodium or osmolarity and decreased by high blood volume or high pressure. This acts as a negative feedback system to control plasma osmolarity. (See **Antidiuretic Hormone and Control of Osmolarity and Volume** in the Endocrine section.)

Calculation of Plasma Osmolality (mOsm/kg solution)
Plasma osmolality = 2 (plasma [Na^+]) + [glucose mg/dL]/18 + [urea mg/dL]/2.8
Example: sodium = 145 mEq/L, glucose = 180 mg/dL, urea = 28 mg/dL Plasma osmolality = 290 + 10 + 10 = 310 mOsm/kg However: plasma Na^+ dominates control of ADH because of its osmotic effect; urea and glucose usually irrelevant. *Note:* glucose may be important part of **urine** osmolality (especially in diabetes); when present, it causes osmotic diuresis.

Control Signals for Na^+ and H_2O Excretion

System	Action	Segment/Site
Renal sympathetic nerves	↓ GFR	Afferent arteriole constriction
	↑ NaCl reabsorption	Proximal, TAL, DT, CD → ↑ H_2O reabsorption (except TAL, due to impermeability of water)
Renin–angiotensin II–aldosterone	Angio II → ↑ NaCl reabsorption	Proximal → ↑ H_2O reabsorption
	Aldosterone →↑ NaCl reabsorption	TAL, DT, CD →↑ H_2O reabsorption (except TAL, due to impermeability of water)
Atrial natriuretic peptide (ANP)	↑ GFR	Glomerulus
	↓ renin, angio II, aldosterone	JGA and adrenal cortex
	↓ NaCl and H_2O reabsorption	CD (urodilatin* assists)
	↓ ADH secretion and actions	Posterior pituitary and CD
ADH	↑ permeability to H_2O	CD → ↑ H_2O reabsorption → ↓ urine flow and ↑ urine osmolarity

*Urodilatin is a peptide produced by DT and CD when blood pressure/volume increase. Very potent inhibition of NaCl and water reabsorption, but only local action; it does not circulate.

Disorders of Solute and Water Regulation						
Disorder	**ECF Volume**	**$[Na^+]_{plasma}$**	**Blood Pressure**	**Urine Volume and Osmolarity**	**Arterial pH**	**$[K^+]_{plasma}$**
Diabetes insipidus*	↓	↑	↔ or ↓	↑ volume ↓ osmolarity	↑	↓ (↑ aldosterone and alkalosis)
SIADH	↑	↓	↑ or ↔	↓ volume ↑ osmolarity	↓	↑ (but negative balance)
Aldosterone deficiency (primary)	↓	↓	↓	↑ volume ↑ osmolarity	↓	↑ positive balance
Aldosterone excess (primary)	↑	↑	↑	↓ volume ↓ osmolarity	↑	↓ negative balance
Polydipsia	↑	↓	↔	↑ volume ↓ osmolarity	↓	↑ balance variable
Water deprivation (dehydration)	↓	↑	↓	↓ volume ↑ osmolarity	↑	↑, ↓, ↔ depends on multiple factors

Definition of abbreviation: SIADH, syndrome of inappropriate (excessive) ADH secretion.

*ADH deficiency is called primary, central, or neurogenic; ↓ renal response to ADH is nephrogenic. Distinguish by response to administration of ADH; ↑ urine osmolarity in response to ADH injection indicates primary.

Osmotic Diuresis	
Cause	**Effect**
Excessive solute in tubular fluid	Decrease reabsorption of H_2O
Diabetic ketoacidosis	• Glucose and ketones in urine → polyuria, K^+ wasting • Na^+ loss → hyponatremia
Starvation and alcoholic ketoacidosis	Ketonuria → polyuria, K^+ wasting, hyponatremia
Osmotic diuretics (mannitol, carbonic anhydrase inhibitors)	Inhibit proximal tubule H_2O reabsorption → diuresis, K^+ wasting (due to ↑ flow)
Loop diuretics (furosemide) and distal tubule diuretics (thiazides)	Inhibit NaCl reabsorption →↑ tubular solutes → diuresis and K^+ wasting

Causes of Increased Potassium Excretion		
Tubular Flow and K^+ Secretion	**Factor**	**Mechanism**
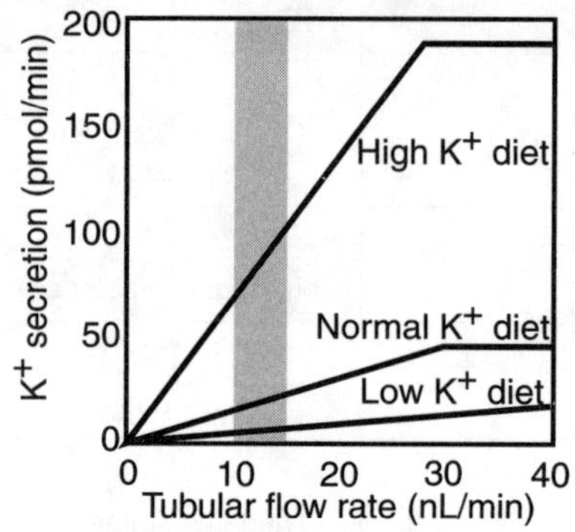	↑ Tubular flow	Washes K^+ out of tubular cells
	↑ Tubular load of Na^+	Stimulates DT Na^+ pump →↑ tubular cells K^+
	↑ Plasma K^+	↑ FL and →↑ aldosterone →↑ K^+ secretion
	Aldosterone on DT	↑ Apical permeability K^+ ↑ Na^+ pump →↑ DT cell K^+ →↑ K^+ secretion
	Metabolic alkalosis	↑ Tubular cell K^+ →↑ secretion of K^+
• *Shaded bar*: normal flow range • High flow → high secretion • Flow is not a normal control mechanism; changes are pathologic.	Chronic metabolic acidosis	Osmotic diuresis and ↑ aldosterone

Effects of Volume Expansion and Contraction on K^+ Secretion	
Volume Expansion	**Volume Contraction**
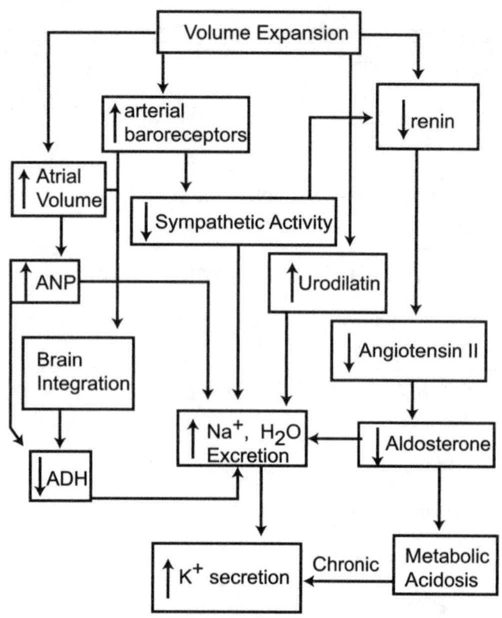	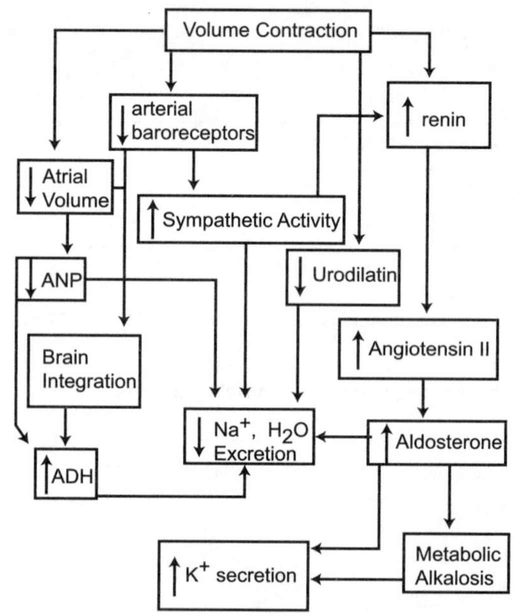

Volume expansion causes acidosis due to responses that ↓ reabsorption of bicarbonate in proximal tubule and ↓ aldosterone. Volume contraction causes alkalosis due to ↑ proximal tubular reabsorption of bicarbonate and ↑ aldosterone. Both can cause K^+ wasting because metabolic alkalosis and chronic metabolic acidosis both ↑ K^+ secretion in distal tubule and collecting duct.

Effects of Metabolic Alkalosis and Acidosis on K^+ Excretion

Metabolic Alkalosis

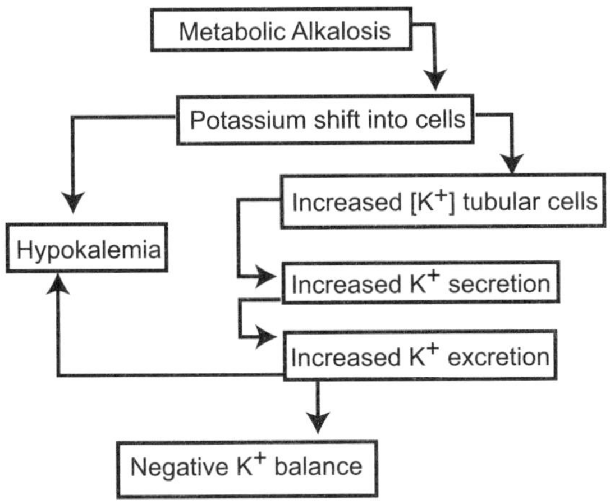

Both acute and chronic metabolic alkalosis cause hypokalemia with a negative potassium balance.

Metabolic Acidosis

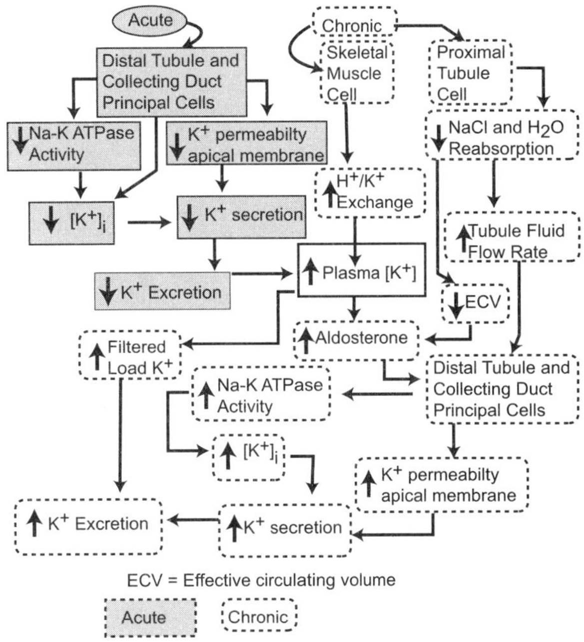

Acute (<24 hours) and chronic metabolic acidosis **both** increase extracellular [K^+]. However, acute decreases K^+ excretion, but chronic increases K^+ excretion.*

*Elevated aldosterone is the key to the reversal of the effect of acidosis on K^+ excretion. Also, increased cellular H^+ causes efflux of K^+ from cells; low cellular H^+ causes influx. Acidosis impairs metabolism; thus, ↓ solute reabsorption causes osmotic diuresis.

▶ Renal Mechanisms for Acid/Base Regulation

Fundamental Principles	
Tubular cell pH	• If a cell is acidotic, it will secrete acid. • If a cell is alkalotic, it will ↓ reabsorption of bicarbonate or secrete it.
Fluid volume	If ECV is decreased, ↑ Na^+ reabsorption will be accompanied by ↑ bicarbonate reabsorption.
Overall role of kidneys	This is the only significant mechanism for excretion of nonvolatile, metabolic acids.
Response time	Requires 24–72 hours for maximal compensatory response
Net acid excretion (NAE)	There is no net excretion of newly formed acid unless all bicarbonate is reabsorbed. $NAE = \dot{V} \times [NH_4+] + \dot{V} \times [H_2PO_4^-] - \dot{V} \times [HCO_3^-]$
Free H^+ excretion	Trivial amount even at most acidic urine pH ≅ 4.4
NH_4^+ excretion	Largest quantity of excreted acid; metabolized from glutamine; "nontitratable acid"
$H_2PO_4^-$ excretion	Second largest quantity; "titratable acid"
NH_4^+ secretion	NH_4^+ secreted in the proximal tubule is reabsorbed in TAL and added to interstitium; it is then taken up by DT and CD cells and secreted.

Tubular Handling of Bicarbonate

Proximal Tubule Reabsorption of Bicarbonate Ion	Intercalated Cells of the Collecting Duct: Reabsorption and Secretion

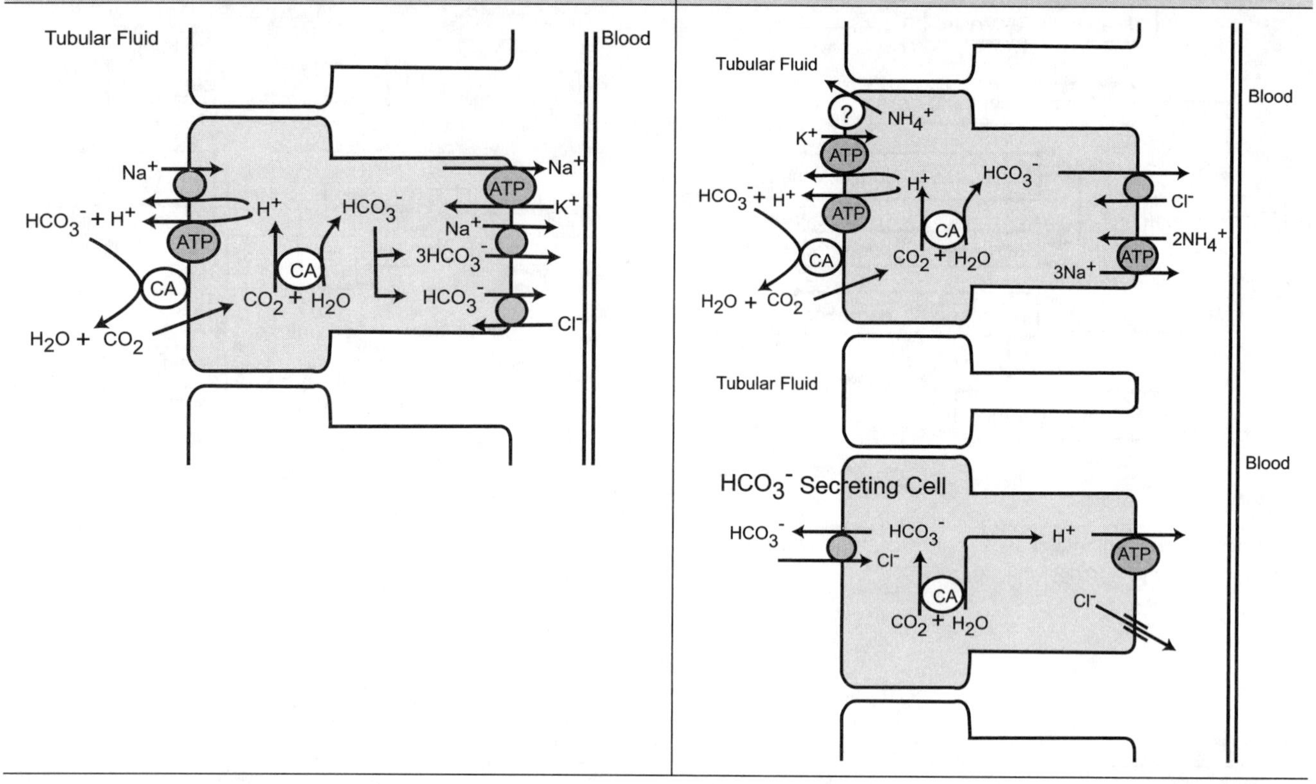

Tubular Handling of Ammonia

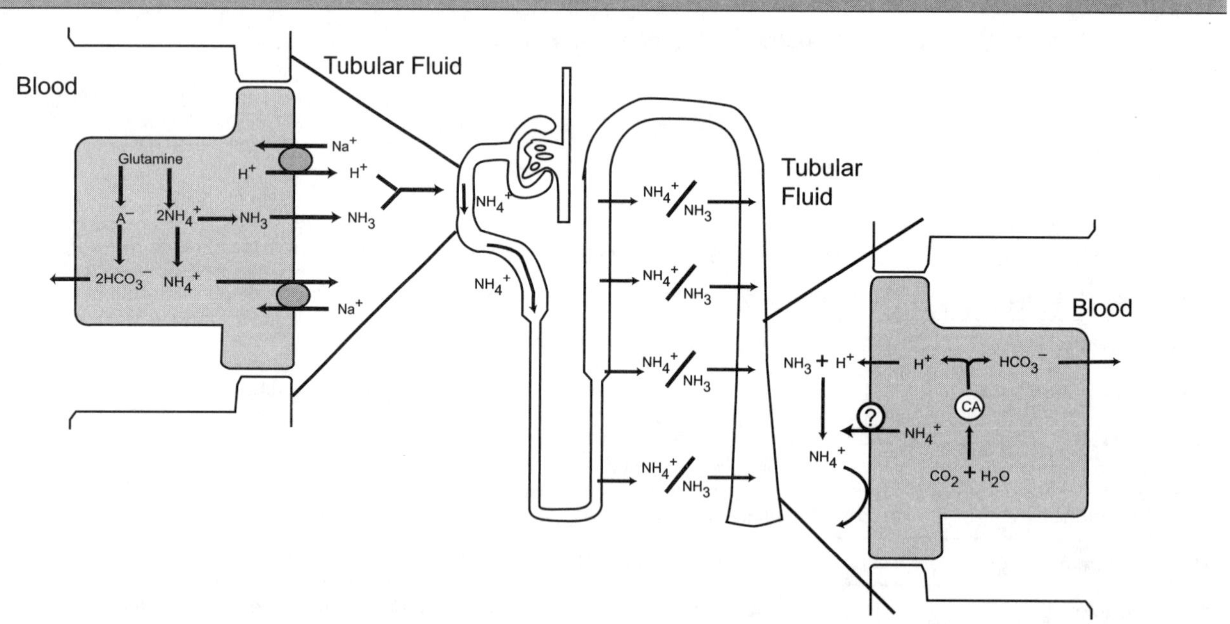

NH_4^+ can substitute for K^+ in the sodium pump. Apical secretion may be by substitution for H^+ in the H^+-K^+ exchanger or the H^+-ATPase. Production of NH_4^+ adds HCO_3^- to blood.

▶ Integrated Control of Cardiac Output and Arterial Blood Pressure

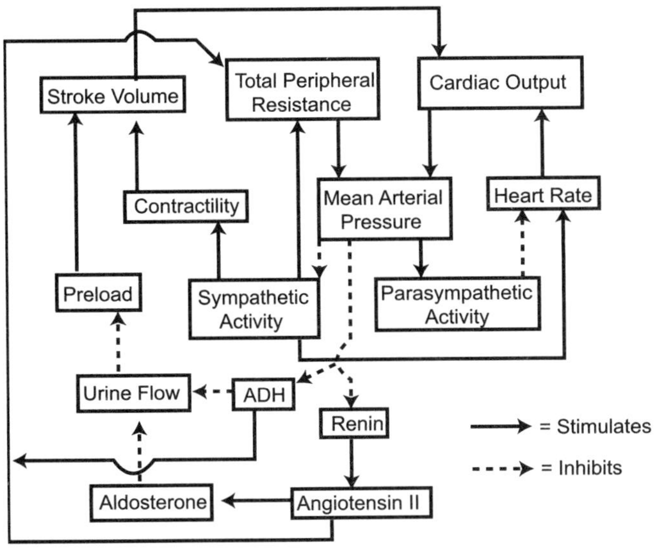

Notes on Use of Feedback Diagram
• Many intermediate steps omitted. • ADH (vasopressin) also vasoconstricts. • Diagram merges elements of cardiovascular and endocrine physiology. • For applications, make the most direct connection; e.g., hemorrhage: begin at reduced preload →↓ stroke volume, and so on. For an understanding of ACE inhibition, begin at ↓ angiotensin II.

▶ Acid/Base and Its Regulation

Fundamental Principles	
Carbonic anhydrase reaction	Produces strong acid and weak base → acidic solution
Respiratory contribution	Determined by arterial Pco_2: ↑ Pco_2 → acidosis; ↓ Pco_2 → alkalosis
Metabolic contribution	Determined by arterial HCO_3^-: ↑ HCO_3^- → alkalosis ; ↓ HCO_3^- → acidosis
Simple disorder	One disorder with or without compensation
Mixed or combined disorder	Two simultaneous disorders
Compensation	• A response that tends to correct pH: compensation is never perfect. • Fully compensated means that the mechanism has come as close as possible to restoring normal pH.
Normal arterial blood gas	pH = 7.40; Pco_2 = 40 mm Hg; Po_2 = 83 – 100 mm Hg; HCO_3^- = 24 mEq/L
Henderson-Hasselbalch Eq.	Several forms; they show relationship between pH, Pco_2, and HCO_3^-.

The Carbonic Anhydrase Reaction	Henderson-Hasselbalch Equation
$CO_2 + H_2O \overset{CA}{\rightleftharpoons} H_2CO_3 \rightleftharpoons H^+ + HCO_3^-$ CA, carbonic anhydrase	$pH = 6.1 \log \frac{[HCO_3^-]}{0.03\ Pco_2}$ • ↑ Pco_2 → ↓ pH • ↑ HCO_3^- → ↑ pH

Examples of Calculations	
Pco_2 = 60 mm Hg; HCO_3^- = 18 mEq/L	pH = 6.1 + log (18/1.8) = 6.1 + log 10 = 6.1 + 1 = 7.1
Pco_2 = 40 mm Hg; HCO_3^- = 24 mEq/L	pH = 6.1 + log (24/1.2) = 6.1 + log 20 = 6.1 + 1.3 = 7.4
Pco_2 = 20 mm Hg; HCO_3^- = 24 mEq/L	pH = 6.1 + log (24/0.6) = 6.1 + log 40 = 6.10 + 1.60 = 7.70
Pco_2 = 60 mm Hg; HCO_3^- = 36 mEq/L	pH = 6.1 + log (36/1.8) = 6.1 + log 20 = 6.1 + 1.3 = 7.4
Note: pH is normal, but this is not normal acid/base status; both PCO_2 and HCO_3^- are abnormal.	

Fundamental Mechanisms to Control pH	
Buffers	Fast, seconds: ECF bicarbonate (largest), phosphate, and proteins
Respiratory	Ventilation response fast, within a few minutes: change P_{CO_2} by changing ventilation. • ↑ ventilation →↓ P_{CO_2} → alkalosis • ↓ ventilation →↑ P_{CO_2} → acidosis
Renal	• Slow; 24–72 hours; powerful: major mechanism to excrete nonvolatile acids. • Change in renal acid excretion and HCO_3^- production is called a metabolic response.
Primary disorders	• Primary disorder ventilation = respiratory acid/base disorder • Primary disorder excess production of acid, ↓ renal excretion of acid, or loss of bicarbonate in urine or feces = metabolic disorder

The Davenport Diagram

- Above the base buffer line, there is excess metabolic base (a positive base excess).
- Below it, there is excess metabolic acid (negative base excess).
- Read pH perpendicular to the *x*-axis; HCO_3^- perpendicular to the *y*-axis, but P_{CO_2} along the curves.

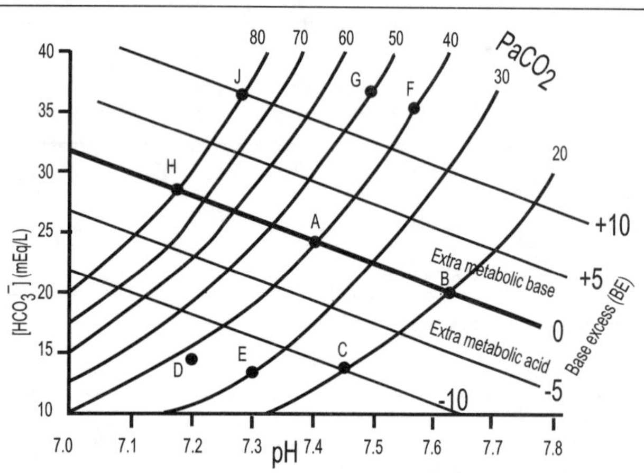

Point	Interpretation
A	Normal acid/base status
B	Uncompensated respiratory alkalosis
C	Respiratory alkalosis with compensatory metabolic acidosis
D	Uncompensated metabolic acidosis
E	Metabolic acidosis with compensatory respiratory alkalosis
F	Uncompensated metabolic alkalosis
G	Metabolic alkalosis with compensatory respiratory acidosis
H	Uncompensated respiratory acidosis
J	Respiratory acidosis with compensatory metabolic alkalosis

Patient Examples

Predicted bicarbonate concentration with changes of PCO_2

PCO_2 (mm Hg)	80	60	40	20
HCO_3^- (mEq/L)	29	27	24	21

Draw a vertical line through the PCO_2 to get the predicted HCO_3^-

PCO_2 (mm Hg)	80	60	40	20
HCO_3^- (mEq/L)	29	27	24	21

A patient has PCO_2 = 60 mm Hg and $[HCO_3^-]$ = 28 mEq/L
Has metabolism changed?
No: the bicarbonate is almost exactly as expected from the PCO_2

PCO_2 (mm Hg)	80	60	40	20
HCO_3^- (mEq/L)	29	27	24	21

A patient has PCO_2 = 80 mm Hg and $[HCO_3^-]$ = 35 mEq/L
What is the predicted bicarbonate? 29 mEq/L
Is there more or less bicarbonate than predicted? More
Has metabolism changed? Yes, there is excess bicarbonate.
What is the metabolic contribution? Alkalosis

Simple Acid–Base Disorders

Type of Disorder	pH	$Paco_2$	HCO_3^-
Metabolic acidosis	↓	↓*	↓
Metabolic alkalosis	↑	↑*	↑
Respiratory acidosis	↓	↑	↑*
Respiratory alkalosis	↑	↓	↓*

*Change due to compensation

A Step-by-Step Approach to Diagnosis of Simple Disorders

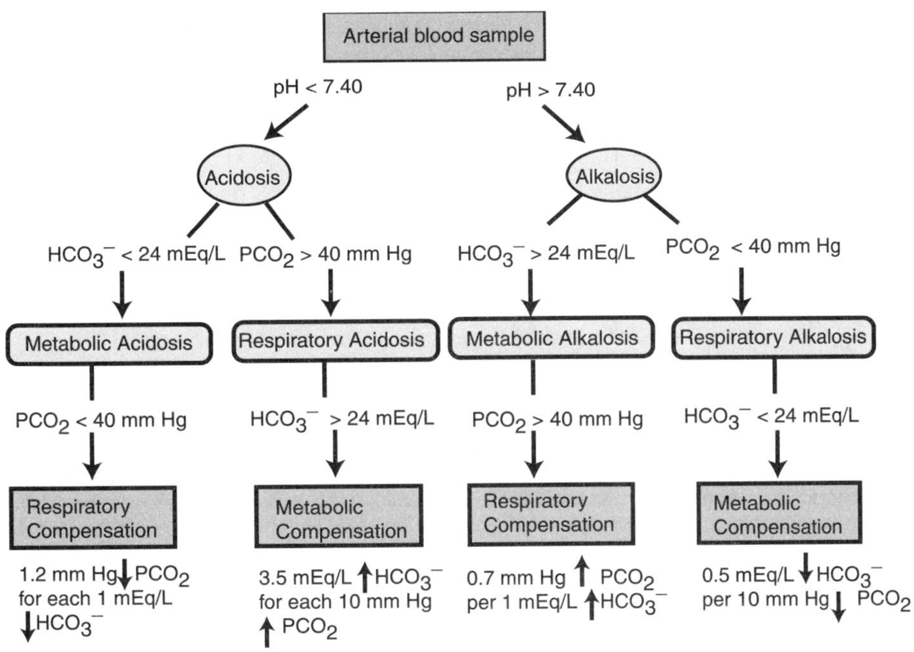

1. What is the pH? Acidotic or alkalotic?
2. What is the respiratory contribution? Acidosis, alkalosis, or no change?
3. What is the metabolic contribution? Acidosis, alkalosis, or no change?
4. What causes the acid–base disorder? *Ans:* the factor (respiratory or metabolic) that would produce the abnormal pH.
5. Is there compensation? Did the other factor change in the direction that would help offset the disorder?

Use of the Plasma Anion Gap (PAG)	
Use	To determine whether the cause of a metabolic acidosis is due to ↑ concentration of nonvolatile acid
Discriminates	Whether the primary disorder is loss of bicarbonate in urine or feces
Principle	Cations = anions in plasma, if all were measured; commonly measure Na^+, Cl^-, and HCO_3^-; metabolic acids are not measured. So there is a gap between cations and anions as measured.
Calculation	$PAG = [Na^+] - ([Cl^-] + [HCO_3^-])$; normal = 12 ± 2
Interpretation ↑ PAG	Excess molecules of acid, e.g., diabetic ketoacidosis, aspirin, lactic acidosis, etc.
Non-anion gap acidosis (normal PAG)	Acidosis due to loss of bicarbonate in urine or diarrhea results in hyperchloremic acidosis; kidneys reabsorb excess Cl^- in replacement for bicarbonate

Urinary Anion Gap (UAG)	
Principle	Hard to measure NH_4^+ in urine, but it is the major form of acid excreted Cations = anions in urine, if all are measured
Ions measured	Na^+, K^+, Cl^-: anions > cations because did not measure NH_4^+
UAG calculation	$UAG = [Na^+] + [K^+] - [Cl^-]$
Interpretation of negative	Kidneys are excreting acid
Interpretation of positive	Kidneys are excreting base
In acidosis	UAG should be negative if kidneys are compensating appropriately
In alkalosis	UAG should be positive if kidneys are compensating appropriately

Sample case:

Arterial: pH = 7.15, Pa_{CO_2} = 30 mm Hg, $[HCO_3^-]$ = 10 mEq/L, Cl^- = 100 mEq/L, Na^+ = 145 mEq/L

Urine: Na^+ = 100 mEq/L, K^+ = 90 mEq/L, Cl^- = 140 mEq/L

Diagnosis: metabolic acidosis with respiratory compensation; PAG = 35; therefore, grossly excessive acid in the body. Diagnosis is either non-renal metabolic acidosis or renal failure with low GFR (e.g., uremia). UAG is only reliable for measuring urine acid excretion in normal anion gap metabolic acidosis, such as to discriminate renal tubular acidosis (RTA) vs. non-renal causes. Avoid in high PAG acidosis.

Renal Pathology

► Cystic Disease of the Kidney

Childhood polycystic disease	• Rare **autosomal recessive** disease, presenting in infancy with renal (and often hepatic) cysts and progressive renal failure • *Gross:* bilaterally enlarged kidneys with smooth surfaces. *Cut section:* sponge-like appearance with multiple small cysts in the cortex and medulla
Adult polycystic disease	• **Autosomal dominant**, usually have normal renal function until middle age • Present with renal insufficiency, hematuria, flank pain, and hypertension • *Extrarenal manifestations:* liver cysts, **circle of Willis berry aneurysms**, mitral valve prolapse • *Gross:* marked bilateral enlargement with large cysts bulging through the surface • *Micro:* cysts involve <10% of nephrons
Simple cysts	Common, can be single or multiple; have little clinical significance
Medullary sponge kidney	• Multiple **cystic dilatations of collecting ducts in medulla** • Most are asymptomatic
Acquired cystic disease	• Multiple cortical and medullary cysts may result from **prolonged renal dialysis** • ↑ risk for development into renal cell carcinoma

► Glomerular Diseases

Type	Clinical Presentation	Mechanism	Light Microscopy	Electron Microscopy	Immuno-fluorescence
Poststreptococcal glomerulonephritis (acute proliferative)	Nephritis; **elevated ASO**; low complement; children > adults Usually recover completely; occasionally progress to RPGN	Immunologic (type III hyper-sensitivity)	Polymorpho-nuclear neutrophil leukocyte infiltration; proliferation	**Subepithelial humps**	**Granular pattern**; GBM and mesangium contain IgG and C3
Minimal change disease (lipid nephrosis)	**Nephrotic syndrome; children > adults** Usually normal renal function; may respond to steroids	Unknown	Normal	No deposits; **loss of epithelial foot processes**	Negative
Membranous glomerulonephritis	**Nephrotic syndrome; adults > children** May respond to steroids	Immunologic	Capillary wall thickening	**Subepithelial spikes**; loss of epithelial foot processes	Granular pattern of IgG and C3
Membranoproliferative glomerulonephritis	Variable: mild proteinuria, mixed nephritic/nephrotic, or frank nephrotic syndrome Poor response to steroids	*Type I:* immune complex and both classic and alternate complement pathways *Type II:* immune complex and alternate complement pathway	Basement membrane thick and split; mesangial proliferation	*Type I:* **sub-endothelial deposits** *Type II:* **dense deposit disease**	*Type I:* IgG and C3, C1q, and C4 *Type II:* C3 (IgG, C1q, and C4 usually absent) "C3 nephritic factor"
Focal segmental glomerulosclerosis	Nephrotic syndrome (most common cause in adults) Poor prognosis; rarely responds to steroids	Immunologic; aggressive variant of lipoid nephrosis; **IV drug use; HIV nephropathy**	Focal and segmental sclerosis and hyalinization	Epithelial damage; loss of foot processes	IgM and C3 focal deposits

Definition of abbreviations: ASO, antistreptolysin O.

(Continued)

► Glomerular Diseases (*Cont'd.*)

Type	Clinical Presentation	Mechanism	Light Microscopy	Electron Microscopy	Immuno-fluorescence
Goodpasture syndrome	RPGN + pulmonary hemorrhage Often poor prognosis; may respond to steroids, plasmapheresis, cytotoxic agents	**Anti-GBM antibodies** (type II hyper-sensitivity)	**Crescents**; mesangial proliferation in early cases	GBM disruption; no deposits	**Linear IgG and C3**
Idiopathic RPGN	RPGN; may follow flu-like syndrome Extremely poor prognosis	Immunologic	**Crescents**	Variable, ± deposits; all have GBM ruptures	Granular or linear
Focal proliferative glomerulonephritis	Primary focal glomerulonephritis or part of multisystem disease; may be subclinical or present with hematuria, proteinuria, nephrotic syndrome Variable prognosis	Immunologic	Proliferation limited to certain segments of particular glomeruli	Variable; may show mesangial deposits	Variable; may show mesangial deposits
IgA nephropathy (Berger disease)	Variable: recurrent hematuria, mild proteinuria, nephrotic syndrome; children and young adults Usually slowly progressive course	Unknown	Variable: normal or segmental/ mesangial proliferation or crescentic	Mesangial deposits	**Mesangial IgA deposition**
Diabetic glomerulopathy	Microscopic proteinuria; or can eventually cause nephrotic syndrome Prognosis variable, depends on diabetic control	Nonenzymatic glycosylation causes glomerular basement membrane thickening and mesangial matrix expansion	Capillary basement membrane thickening; diffuse and nodular glomerular sclerosis (Kimmelstiel-Wilson)	Thickened glomerular basement membrane and well-demarcated, roughly round nodules in the glomeruli	Not really helpful; may show non-specific immunoglobulin G deposition along the basement membrane
Chronic glomerulonephritis	Chronic renal failure; may follow a variety of acute glomerulopathies Poor prognosis	Variable	**Hyalinized glomeruli**	Not specific	Negative or granular
Amyloidosis	Nephrotic syndrome Prognosis variable, depends in underlying condition	Amyloid deposition, often accompanying diseases e.g., multiple myeloma, chronic infections, tuberculosis, and rheumatoid arthritis	Eosinophilic amorphous deposits in glomeruli and interstitium that show apple-green birefringence when stained with Congo Red	Fibrillar depositions of amyloid material	Immuno-fluorescence is not usually helpful
Alport syndrome	Hematuria, proteinuria, which slowly progress to renal failure; **deafness**; ocular disorders Renal failure common by age 50	**X-linked** disorder of collagen	Segmental and focal glomerulo-sclerosis, tubular atrophy, interstitial fibrosis, chronic inflammation	**Thickening** (sometimes thinning) and **splitting the basement membrane**	**Immuno-fluorescence for individual chains of type IV collagen** can be diagnostic

Definition of abbreviations: ASLO, antistreptolysin O; GBM, glomerular basement membrane; RPGN, rapidly progressive glomerulonephritis.

► Tubular Diseases of the Kidney

Acute Tubular Necrosis (ATN)	**Most common cause of acute renal failure**; associated with reversible injury to the tubular epithelium; excellent prognosis if patient survives disease responsible for the ATN
Ischemic ATN	• **Most common cause of ATN** • ↓ blood flow caused by severe renal vasoconstriction, hypotension, or shock
Nephrotoxic ATN	Caused by heavy metals such as mercury, drugs, and myoglobin
Four Phases of ATN	
Initial phase	*36 hours*: after precipitating event occurs
Oliguric phase	*10 days:* ↓ urine output; uremia, fluid overload, and hyperkalemia may occur
Diuretic phase	*2–3 weeks:* gradual ↑ in urine volume (up to 3 L/day); hypokalemia, electrolyte imbalances, and infection may occur
Recovery phase	*3 weeks:* improved concentrating ability, restoration of tubular function; normalization of BUN and creatinine

► Tubulointerstitial Diseases of the Kidney

Pyelonephritis	• Infection of the renal pelvis, tubules, and interstitium • **Ascending infection is the most common route** with organisms from the patient's fecal flora; hematogenous infection is much less common. • Etiologic agents usually gram-negative bacilli (e.g., *E. coli*, *Proteus,* and *Klebsiella*). *E. coli* pili mediate adherence, motility aids movement against flow of urine. *Proteus* (urease, alkaline urine, struvite stones), *Klebsiella* (large capsule)
Acute pyelonephritis	• Risk factors: urinary obstruction, vesicoureteral reflux, pregnancy, instrumentation, diabetes mellitus • Under 40 more common in women (shorter urethra); over 40, ↑ incidence in men due to benign prostatic hypertrophy • **Symptoms:** fever, malaise, dysuria, frequency, urgency, and costovertebral angle (CVA) tenderness. **Fever, CVA tenderness,** and **WBC casts** distinguish pyelonephritis from cystitis. • **Urine:** many WBCs and WBC casts • **Gross:** scattered yellow microabscesses on the renal surface • **Micro:** foci of interstitial suppurative necrosis and tubular necrosis • Blunting of the calyces may be seen on intravenous pyelogram
Chronic pyelonephritis	• **Reflux nephropathy** most common cause • Interstitial parenchymal scarring deforms the calyces and pelvis • **Symptoms:** onset can be insidious or acute; present with renal failure and hypertension • **Gross:** irregular scarring and deformed calyces with overlying corticomedullary scarring • **Micro:** chronic inflammation with tubular atrophy • Pyelogram diagnostic
Acute allergic interstitial nephritis	• **Hypersensitivity reaction** to infection or drugs (e.g., NSAIDs, penicillin, methicillin) • Leads to interstitial edema with a mononuclear infiltrate • Presents 2 weeks after exposure with hematuria, pyuria, eosinophilia, and azotemia
Analgesic nephritis	Interstitial nephritis and renal papillary necrosis, induced by large doses of analgesics
Gouty nephropathy	• **Urate crystals** in tubules, inducing tophus formation and a chronic inflammatory reaction • *Note:* Urate crystals appear as **birefringent**, **needle-shaped crystals** on light microscopy.
Acute urate nephropathy	• Precipitation of crystals in the collecting ducts, causing obstruction • Seen in **lymphoma and leukemia**, especially after chemotherapy
Multiple myeloma	**Bence-Jones proteins** are directly toxic to tubular epithelium
Diffuse cortical necrosis	• Generalized infarction of both kidneys; preferentially involves the renal cortex • Seen in settings of obstetric catastrophes (abruptio placentae) and shock • Mechanism thought to be a combination of vasospasm and DIC

▶ Vascular Diseases of the Kidney

Ischemia	• Caused by embolization of mural thrombi usually left side of heart or aorta • **Gross:** sharply demarcated, wedge-shaped pale regions, which undergo necrosis with subsequent scarring • **Symptoms:** infarcts may be asymptomatic or may cause pain, hematuria, and hypertension
Renal vein thrombosis	• Thrombosis of one or both renal veins may occur • Associated with the nephrotic syndrome, particularly membranous glomerulonephritis • Renal cell carcinoma may also provoke renal vein thrombosis as a result of direct invasion by tumor • Presents with hematuria, flank pain, and renal failure • **Gross:** kidney enlarged • **Micro:** hemorrhagic infarction of renal tissue

▶ Urolithiasis

- Affects 6% of the population; men > women
- Renal colic may occur if small stones pass into the ureter, where they may also cause hematuria and urinary obstruction and predispose to infection

Calcium stones	• **75% of stones**; most patients have hypercalciuria without hypercalcemia • Calcium stones are **radiopaque**; they are the only ones that can be seen on x-ray
Magnesium-ammonium phosphate stones	• 15% of stones; occur after infection by urease-producing bacteria, such as ***Proteus*** • Urine becomes alkaline, resulting in precipitation of **magnesium-ammonium phosphate salts**; may form large stones (e.g., **staghorn calculi**)
Uric acid stones	Seen in **gout**, **leukemia**, and in patients with acidic urine
Cystine stones	• Very rare • Associated with an autosomal recessive amino acid transport disorder, leading to **cystinuria** • Most stones are unilateral and formed in calyx, pelvis, bladder

▶ Obstructive Uropathy and Hydronephrosis

Hydronephrosis	• Multiple etiologies, including stones, benign prostatic hypertrophy, pregnancy, neurogenic bladder, tumor, inflammation, and posterior urethral valves • Persistence of glomerular filtration despite urinary obstruction, causing dilation of calyces and pelvis. High pressure in the collecting system causes atrophy and ischemia. • **Gross:** dilatation of the pelvis and calyces with blunting of renal pyramids • **Symptoms:** – *Unilateral:* may remain asymptomatic as the kidney atrophies – *Bilateral incomplete:* loses concentrating ability, causing urinary frequency, polyuria and nocturia – *Bilateral complete:* causes anuria, uremia, and death if untreated

▶ Tumors of the Kidney

	Benign
Cortical adenomas	• Common finding at autopsy • **Gross:** yellow, encapsulated cortical nodules • **Micro:** may be identical to renal cell carcinoma, distinguished by size
Angiomyolipomas	• Hamartomas, composed of fat, smooth muscle, and blood vessels • Particularly common in patients with tuberous sclerosis
	Malignant
Renal cell carcinomas	• 90% of all renal cancers in adults; seen in ages 50–70 with no sex predilection • Moderate association with smoking and a familial predisposition • Occurs in 2/3 of patients with von Hippel-Lindau disease • **Symptoms:** "classic" triad of hematuria, palpable mass, and costovertebral pain (10% of cases); hematuria in middle-aged patient should raise concern • **Gross:** most common in the upper pole; usually solitary, with areas of necrosis and hemorrhage; often invades the renal vein and extends into the vena cava and heart • **Micro:** polygonal clear cells with abundant clear cytoplasm • **Genetics:** often associated with loss of function of VHL gene and activation of the MET oncogene • Paraneoplastic syndrome: polycythemia, hypercalcemia, Cushing syndrome, etc. • High incidence of metastasis on initial presentation • 5-year survival depends on stage, especially poor (25–50%) if tumor extends into the renal vein
Wilms tumor (nephroblastoma)	• Common childhood malignancy with peak incidence at age 2 • **Symptoms**: abdominal mass and hypertension, nausea, hematuria, intestinal obstruction • May be associated with other congenital anomalies • **Gross**: very large, demarcated masses; most are unilateral, but may be bilateral if familial • **Micro:** embryonic glomerular and tubular structures surrounded by mesenchymal spindle cells • 90% survival rate when patients are treated with surgery, chemotherapy, radiotherapy
Transitional cell carcinoma	• Can involve the epithelium of the renal pelvis • Histology similar to transitional cell carcinoma of the bladder, but is less common • Can present with hematuria

▶ Anomalies of the Ureters

Double ureters	• Form when two same-sided ureters join at some point before the junction to the bladder or enter the bladder separately • Associated with double renal pelvises or an abnormally large kidney
	Ureteral Obstruction in Hydroureter and Hydronephrosis
Internal obstruction	• **Renal calculi** are most common cause; usually impact at the ureteropelvic junction, entrance to the bladder, and where they cross iliac vessels • Other causes: strictures, tumors
External obstruction	• Pelvic tumors may compress or invade the ureteral wall; sclerosing retroperitonitis, a fibrosis of retroperitoneal structures, can cause obstruction. • Pregnancy may cause obstruction and may also cause dilation (secondary to progesterone).

► Pathology of the Bladder

Diverticula	• **Pouch-like evaginations** of the bladder wall • Occur in older men and women and may lead to urinary stasis and therefore infection
Exstrophy of bladder	• Caused by **absence of the anterior musculature** of the bladder and abdominal wall; developmental failure of downgrowth of mesoderm over the anterior bladder • Site of severe chronic infections, with ↑ incidence of adenocarcinoma
Patent urachus	• Fistula that **connects the bladder with the umbilicus** • Isolated persistence of the central urachus termed a urachal cyst • Carcinomas may develop in these cysts
Infectious cystitis	• Cystitis causes frequency, urgency, dysuria, and suprapubic pain • **Causative organisms:** *E. coli, Staphylococcus saprophyticus* (associated with intercourse), *Proteus, Klebsiella* (esp. in diabetics), *Pseudomonas (*capsule is antiphagocytic, exotoxin A inhibits EF-2, esp. in patients with structural abnormalities and antibiotic usage)*, Enterococcus* (esp. in males with prostate problems) • No WBC casts in urine (as compared with pyelonephritis) • Systemic signs, such as fever and chills, are also uncommon with lower urinary tract infections; CVA tenderness usually absent
Hemorrhagic cystitis	Marked mucosal hemorrhage secondary to viruses, radiation, or chemotherapy (**cyclophosphamide**, protect with **mesna**)
Cystitis emphysematosa	• Submucosal gas bubbles • Occurs mostly in diabetics
Bladder obstruction	• **Men:** benign prostatic hyperplasia or carcinoma most common cause • **Women:** cystocele of the bladder most common cause • **Gross:** thickening, hypertrophy, and trabeculation of the smooth muscle bladder wall
Carcinoma of the bladder	• **Transitional cell carcinoma:** 90% of primary bladder neoplasms • **Risk factors: Smoking,** occupational exposure **(e.g., naphthylamine),** infection with *Schistosoma haematobium* **(more commonly associated with squamous cell carcinoma)** • 3% of all cancer deaths in the United States - peak incidence between 40 and 60 years of age. • Usually presents with painless hematuria, may also cause dysuria, urgency, frequency, hydronephrosis, and pyelonephritis. • **Prognosis:** Determined by grade and stage at the time of diagnosis; high incidence of recurrence at multiple locations.

The Gastrointestinal System

Chapter 5

Embryology of the Gastrointestinal System

► Development of the Gastrointestinal Tract

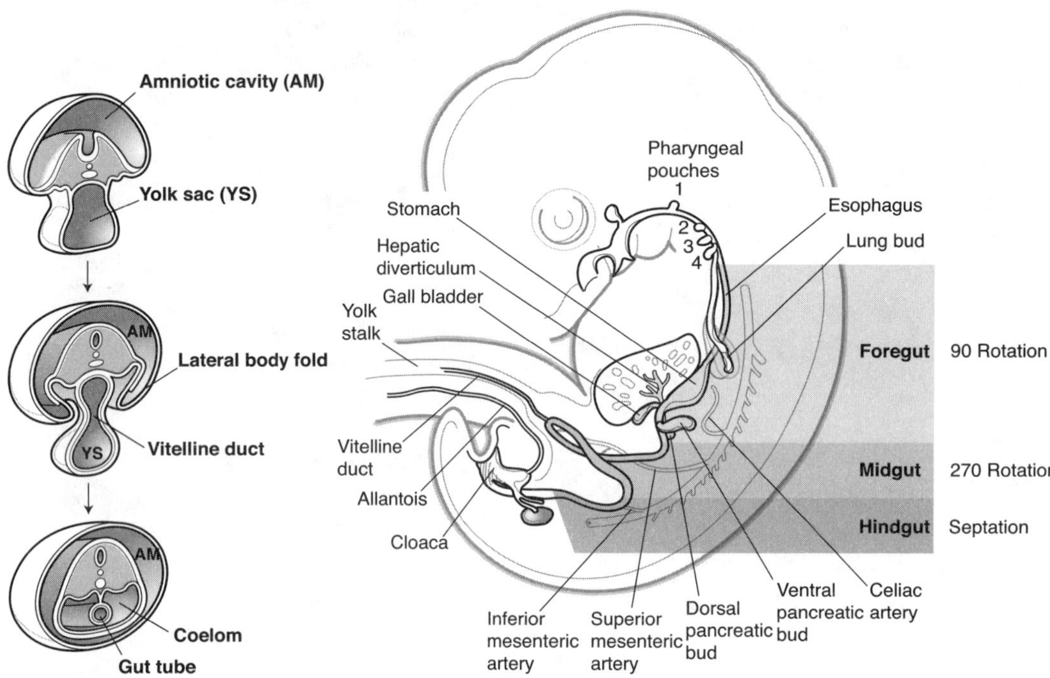

The **primitive gut tube** is formed by incorporation of the yolk sac into the embryo during cranial–caudal and lateral folding.

- The epithelial lining and glands of the mucosa are derived from **endoderm**. The epithelial lining of the gut tube proliferates rapidly and obliterates the lumen, followed by recanalization.
- The lamina propria, muscularis mucosa, submucosa, muscularis externa, and adventitia/serosa are derived from **mesoderm**.

The primitive gut tube is divided into the **foregut**, **midgut**, and **hindgut**, each supplied by a specific artery, each receiving a slightly different autonomic innervation, and each having slightly different relationships to a mesentery.

► Adult Structures Derived from Each of the Three Divisions of the Primitive Gut Tube

Foregut	Midgut	Hindgut
Artery: celiac **Parasympathetic innervation:** vagus nerves **Sympathetic innervation:** greater splanchnic nerves, T5–T9*	**Artery:** superior mesenteric **Parasympathetic innervation:** vagus nerves **Sympathetic innervation:** lesser and lowest splanchnic nerves, T9–T12*	**Artery:** inferior mesenteric **Parasympathetic innervation:** pelvic splanchnic nerves **Sympathetic innervation:** lumbar splanchnic nerves L1–L2*
Foregut Derivatives	**Midgut Derivatives**	**Hindgut Derivatives**
Esophagus Stomach Duodenum (first and second parts) Liver Pancreas Biliary apparatus Gall bladder Pharyngeal pouches† Lungs† Thyroid† Spleen‡	Duodenum (second, third, and fourth parts) Jejunum Ileum Cecum Appendix Ascending colon Transverse colon (proximal two thirds)	Transverse colon (distal third) Descending colon Sigmoid colon Rectum Anal canal (above pectinate line)

***Referred pain**—stimulation of visceral pain fibers that innervate a gastrointestinal structure results in a dull, aching, poorly localized pain that is referred over the T5 through L1 dermatomes. The **sites of referred pain** generally correspond to the spinal cord segments that provide the sympathetic innervation to the affected gastrointestinal structure.

†Derivatives of endoderm, but not supplied by the celiac artery or innervated as above.

‡Spleen is not a foregut derivative, but is supplied by the celiac artery.

Gastrointestinal Histology

► Layers of the Digestive Tract

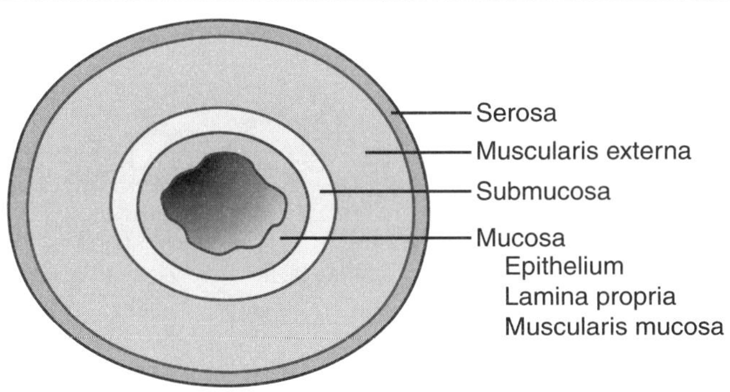

***Submucosal plexus** (Meissner plexus):* a collection of ganglia and interneurons of the enteric nervous system (ENS), predominantly responsible for regulating epithelial function and some circular smooth muscle function

***Myenteric plexus** (Auerbach plexus):* a collection of ganglia and interneurons of the enteric nervous system (ENS), predominantly responsible for regulating longitudinal and some circular smooth muscle function

Note that the first third of esophageal muscle is skeletal, the middle third is mixed skeletal and smooth, and the final third is smooth muscle. Also, the stomach smooth muscle contains an oblique layer between the submucosa and circular layer of smooth muscle.

► Histology of Specific Regions

Region	Major Characteristics	Mucosal Cell Types at Surface	Function of Surface Mucosal Cells
Esophagus	• Nonkeratinized stratified squamous epithelium • Skeletal muscle in muscularis externa (upper 1/3) • Smooth muscle (lower 1/3)	—	—
Stomach (body and fundus)	*Rugae:* shallow pits; deep glands	Mucous cells	Secrete mucus; form protective layer against acid; tight junctions between these cells probably contribute to the acid barrier of the epithelium.
		Chief cells	Secrete pepsinogen and lipase precursor
		Parietal cells	Secrete HCl and intrinsic factor
		Enteroendocrine (EE) cells	Secrete a variety of peptide hormones
Pylorus	Deep pits; shallow branched glands	Mucous cells	Same as above
		Parietal cells	Same as above
		EE cells	High concentration of gastrin
Small intestine	Villi, plicae, and crypts	Columnar absorptive cells	Contain numerous microvilli that greatly increase the luminal surface area, facilitating absorption
Duodenum	Brunner glands, which discharge alkaline secretion	Goblet cells	Secrete acid glycoproteins that protect mucosal linings
		Paneth cells	Contains granules that contain lysozyme. May play a role in regulating intestinal flora
		EE cells	High concentration of cells that secrete cholecystokinin and secretin
Jejunum	Villi, well developed plica, crypts	Same cell types as found in the duodenal epithelium	Same as above
Ileum	Aggregations of lymph nodules called Peyer patches	M cells found over lymphatic nodules and Peyer patches	Endocytose and transport antigen from the lumen to lymphoid cells
Large intestine	Lacks villi, crypts	Mainly mucus-secreting and absorptive cells	Transports Na^+ (actively) and water (passively) out of lumen

Gross Anatomy

▶ Abdominal Viscera

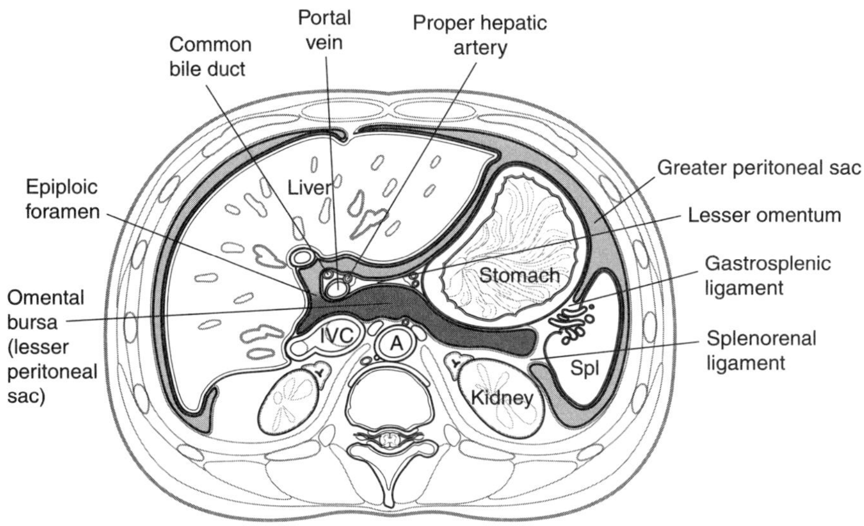

Viscera are classified as:

- **Peritoneal organs**—have a mesentery and are almost completely enclosed in peritoneum. These organs are mobile.
- **Retroperitoneal organs**—are partially covered with peritoneum and are immobile or fixed organs.

This figure is a cross-section of the abdomen that shows the greater and lesser peritoneal sacs and associated abdominal viscera.

Major Peritoneal Organs (suspended by a mesentery)	**Major Secondary Retroperitoneal Organs** (lost a mesentery during development)	**Major Primary Retroperitoneal Organs** (never had a mesentery)
Stomach	Midgut duodenum	Kidneys
Liver and gallbladder	Head, neck, and body of pancreas	Adrenal glands
Spleen	Ascending colon	Ureter
Foregut duodenum	Descending colon	Aorta
Tail of pancreas	Upper rectum	Inferior vena cava
Jejunum		Lower rectum
Ileum		Anal canal
Appendix		
Transverse colon		

▶ The Abdominal Aorta and Celiac Circulation

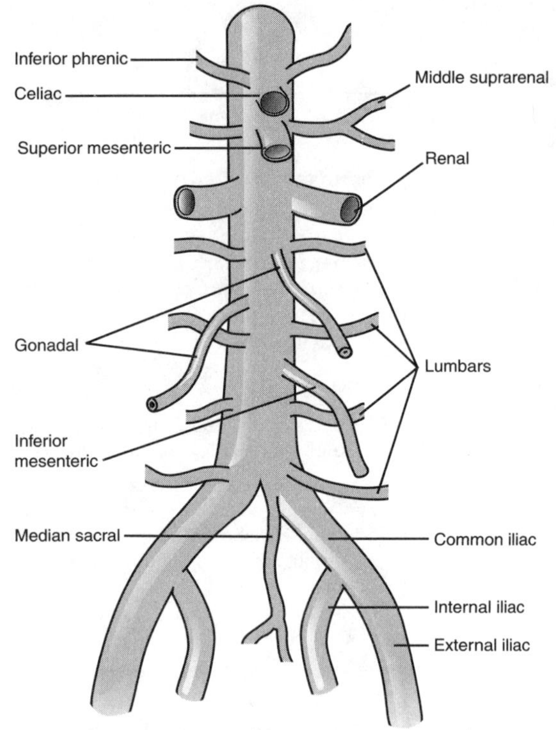

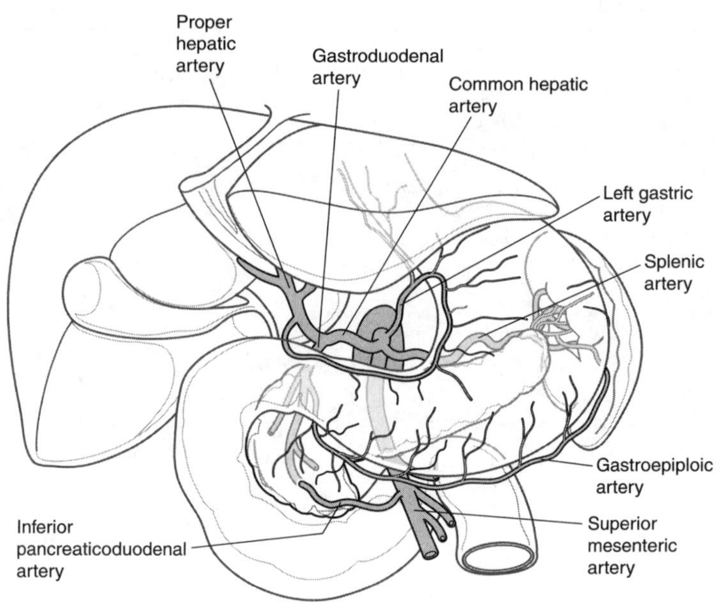

Clinical Correlations

In an **occlusion of the celiac artery** at its origin from the abdominal aorta, collateral circulation may develop in the **head of the pancreas** by way of anastomoses between the **pancreaticoduodenal branches of both the superior mesenteric** and the gastroduodenal arteries.

Branches of the **celiac circulation** may be subject to **erosion** if an ulcer penetrates the posterior wall of the stomach or the posterior wall of the duodenum.

- The **splenic artery** may be subject to erosion by a penetrating ulcer of the **posterior wall** of the stomach.
- The **left gastric artery** may be subject to erosion by a penetrating ulcer of the **lesser curvature** of the stomach.
- The **gastroduodenal artery** may be subject to erosion by a penetrating ulcer of the **posterior wall** of the first part of the duodenum.

Patients with a penetrating ulcer may have **pain referred to the shoulder**, which occurs when air escapes through the ulcer and stimulates the peritoneum covering the inferior aspect of the diaphragm. The contents of a **penetrating ulcer** of the posterior wall of the stomach or the duodenum may enter the **omental bursa**.

Hematemesis may result from bleeding into the lumen of the esophagus, stomach, or duodenum proximal to the ligament of Treitz. Hematemesis is commonly caused by a duodenal ulcer, a gastric ulcer, or esophageal varices.

▶ Superior and Inferior Mesenteric Arteries

Superior Mesenteric Artery Distribution	Inferior Mesenteric Artery Distribution
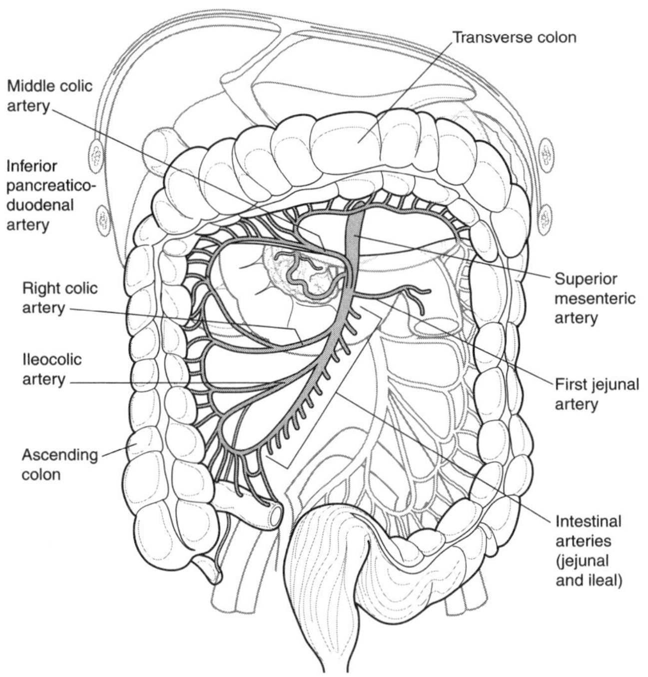	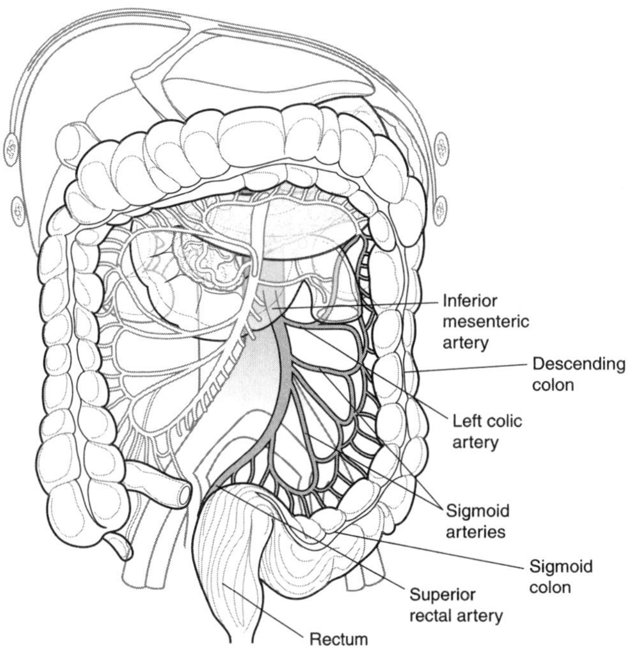

Clinical Correlation

- Common sites of **ischemic bowel infarction** are in the transverse colon near the splenic flexure and in the rectum.
- **Infarction of the transverse colon** occurs between the distal parts of the middle colic branches of the superior mesenteric and left colic branches of the inferior mesenteric arteries.
- **Infarction of the rectum** occurs between the distal parts of the superior rectal branches of the inferior mesenteric artery and the middle rectal branches of the internal iliac artery.

► Hepatic Portal Circulation

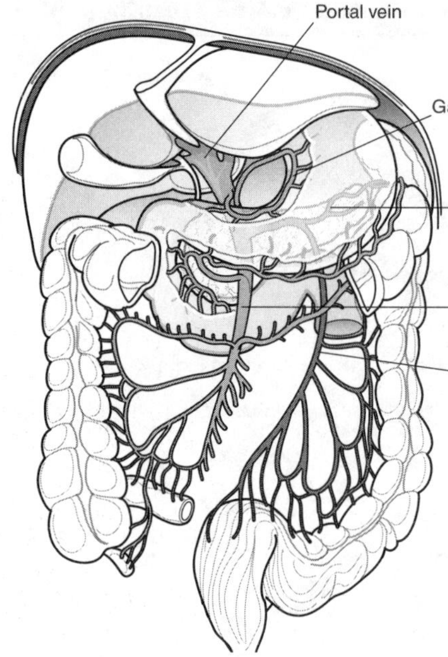

Clinical Correlation

Patients with cirrhosis of the liver may develop **portal hypertension**, in which venous blood from gastrointestinal structures, which normally enters the liver by way of the portal vein, is forced to flow in the retrograde direction in tributaries of the portal vein.

Retrograde flow forces portal venous blood into tributaries of the superior or inferior vena cava; **portacaval anastomoses** are established at these sites, permitting portal venous blood to bypass the liver.

Sites of Anastomoses	Portal	Caval	Clinical Signs
1. Umbilicus	Paraumbilical veins	Superficial veins of the anterior abdominal wall	Caput medusa
2. Rectum	Superior rectal veins (inferior mesenteric vein)	Middle and inferior rectal veins (internal iliac vein)	Internal hemorrhoids
3. Esophagus	Gastric veins	Veins of the lower esophagus, which drain into the azygos system	Esophageal varices
4. Retroperitoneal organs	Tributaries of the superior and inferior mesenteric veins	Veins of the posterior abdominal wall	Not clinically relevant

► Inferior Vena Cava (IVC) and Tributaries

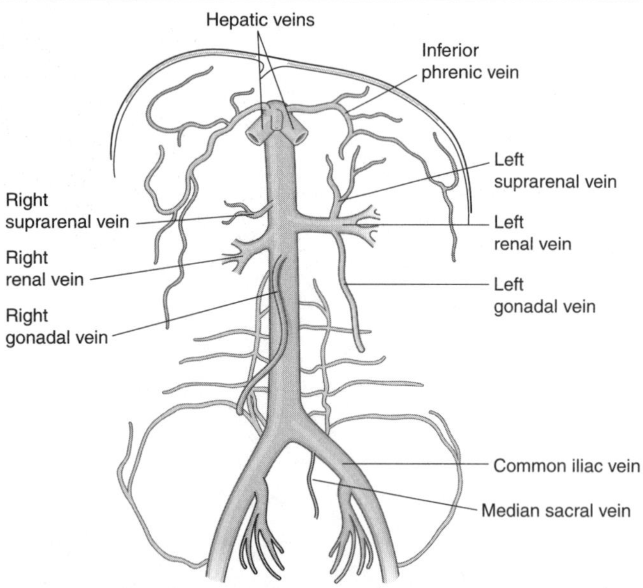

The **inferior vena cava** is formed at about the level of the L5 vertebra by the union of the common iliac veins. It ascends just to the right of the midline.

On the right, the renal, adrenal, and gonadal veins drain directly into the inferior vena cava.

On the left, only the **left renal vein** drains directly into the inferior vena cava; the left gonadal and the left adrenal veins drain into the left renal vein. The left renal vein crosses the anterior aspect of the aorta just inferior to the origin of the superior mesenteric artery.

Clinical Correlation

The **left renal vein may be compressed** by an **aneurysm of the superior mesenteric artery** as the vein crosses anterior to the aorta. Patients with compression of the left renal vein may have renal and adrenal hypertension on the left, and, in males, a varicocele on the left.

► Cross-Sectional Anatomy

Abdomen: CT, T_{11}	Abdomen: CT, L_1
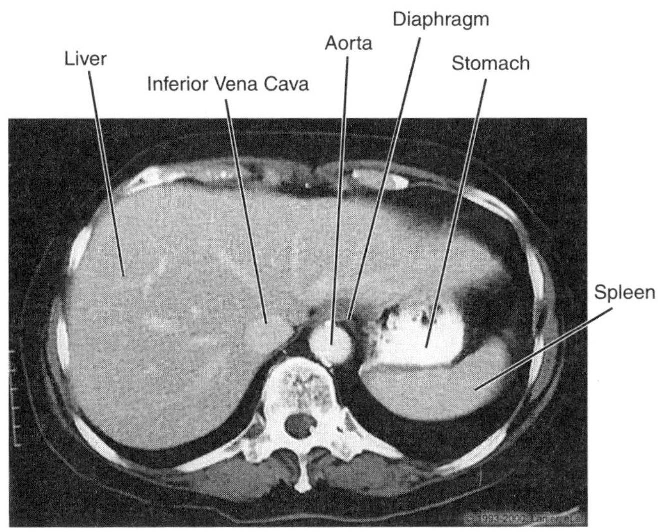	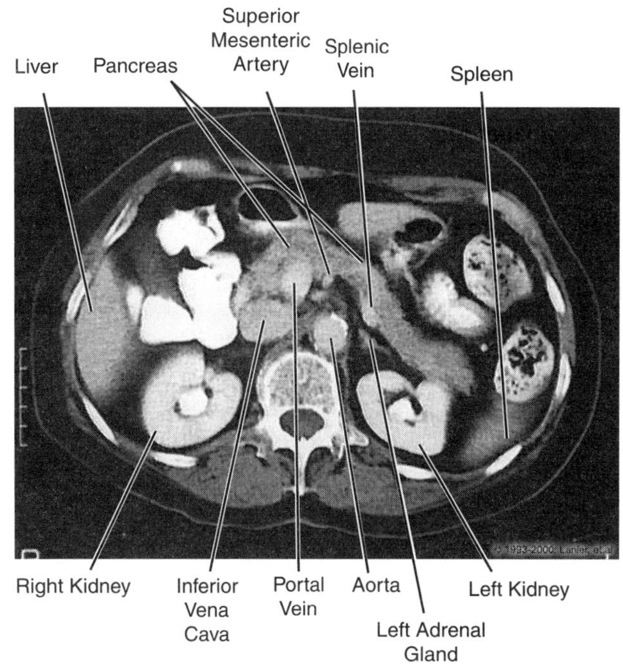

Abdomen: CT, L_2	Abdomen: CT, S_1
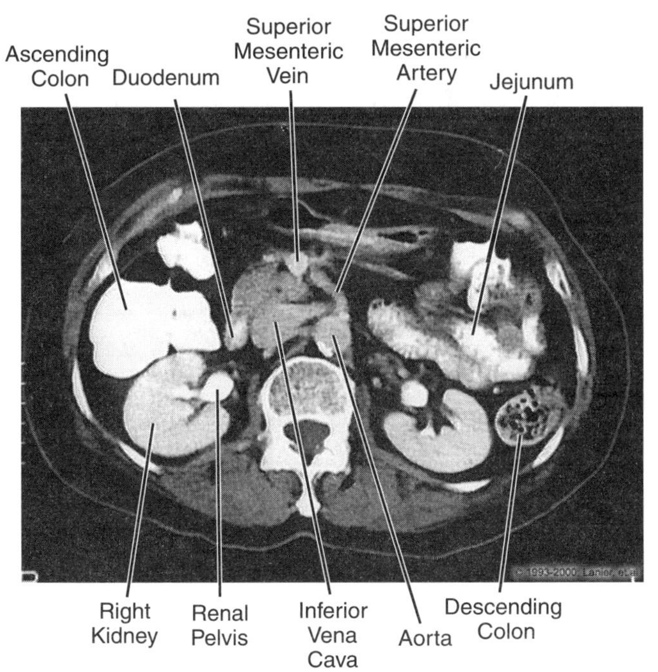	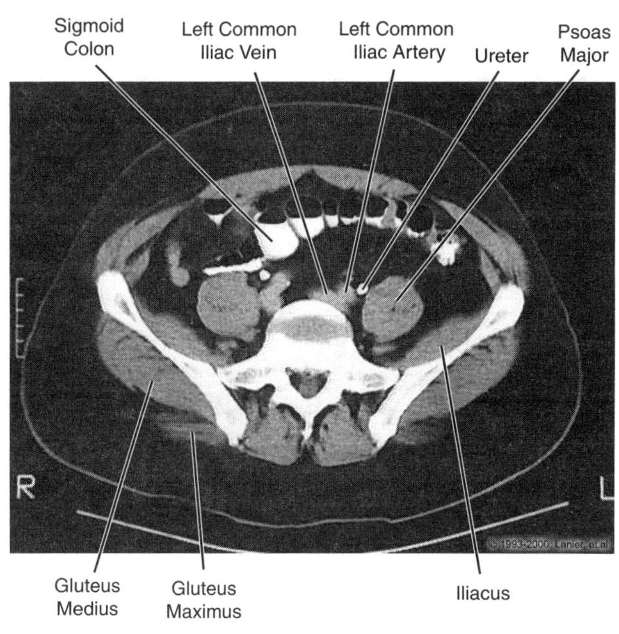

Gastrointestinal Physiology

▶ Appetite

Appetite is primarily regulated by two regions of the hypothalamus: a feeding center and a satiety center. Normally, the feeding center is active, but is transiently inhibited by the satiety center.

Hypothalamus			
	Location	**Stimulation**	**Destruction**
Feeding center	Lateral hypothalamic area	Feeding	Anorexia
Satiety center	Ventromedial nucleus of hypothalamus	Cessation of feeding	Hypothalamic obesity syndrome

Hormones That May Affect Appetite	
Cholecystokinin (CCK)	• Released from I-cells in the mucosa of the small intestine • CCK-A receptors are in the periphery • CCK-B receptors are in the brain—both reduce appetite when stimulated
Calcitonin	• Released mainly from the thyroid gland • Has also been reported to decrease appetite by an unknown mechanism
Ghrelin	• ↑ levels provoke hunger • Levels rise during fasting
Leptin	• Promotes satiety • Levels ↑ after meals and ↓ with fasting

Mechanical Distention

- Distention of the alimentary tract inhibits appetite, whereas the contractions of an empty stomach stimulate it.
- Some satiety is derived from mastication and swallowing alone.

Miscellaneous

Other factors that help to determine appetite and body weight include body levels of fat and genetic factors.

▶ Saliva

Salivary glands Submandibular Parotid Sublingual	• Produce approximately 1.5 L/day of saliva • The presence of food in the mouth, the taste, smell, sight, or thought of food, or the stimulation of vagal afferents at the distal end of the esophagus increase the production of saliva.	
Functions	• Initial triglyceride digestion (lingual lipase) • Initial starch digestion (α-amylase) • Lubrication	
Composition	**Ions:** HCO_3^- 3× [plasma]; K^+ 7 × [plasma]; Na^+ 0.1 × [plasma]; Cl^- 0.15 × [plasma] **Enzymes:** α-amylase, lingual lipase **Hypotonic** **pH:** 7–8 **Flow rate:** alters the composition **Antibacterial:** lysozyme, lactoferrin, defensins, IgA	
Regulation	**Parasympathetic**	↑ synthesis and secretion of **watery** saliva via muscarinic receptor stimulation (anticholinergics → dry mouth)
	Sympathetic	↑ synthesis and secretion of **viscous** saliva via β-adrenergic receptor stimulation

▶ Swallowing

Swallowing is a reflex action coordinated in the **swallowing center** in the medulla. Afferents are carried by the glossopharyngeal (CN IX) and vagus (CN X) nerves. Food is moved to the esophagus by the movement of tongue (hypoglossal nerve, CN XII) and the palatal and pharyngeal muscles (CNs IX and X).

1. **Initiation of swallowing** occurs voluntarily when the mouth is closed on a bolus of food and the tongue propels it from the oral cavity into the pharynx.
2. **Involuntary contraction** of the **pharynx** advances the bolus into the esophagus.
3. Automatic **closure of the glottis** during swallowing inhibits breathing and prevents aspiration.
4. Relaxation of the **upper esophageal sphincter (UES)** allows food to enter the esophagus.
5. **Peristaltic contraction of the esophagus** propels food toward the **lower esophageal sphincter (LES)**, the muscle at the gastroesophageal junction.
6. The LES is tonically contracted, relaxing on swallowing. **Relaxation of the LES** is mediated via the vagus nerve; **VIP** (vasoactive inhibitory peptide) is the major neurotransmitter causing LES relaxation.

Clinical Correlation	
Achalasia	**Pathologic inability of the LES to relax** during swallowing. Food accumulates in the esophagus, sometimes causing **megaesophagus**.
Gastric reflux	**LES tone** is low, allowing acid reflux into the esophagus; can lead to gastroesophageal reflux disease (**GERD**).

▶ The Stomach

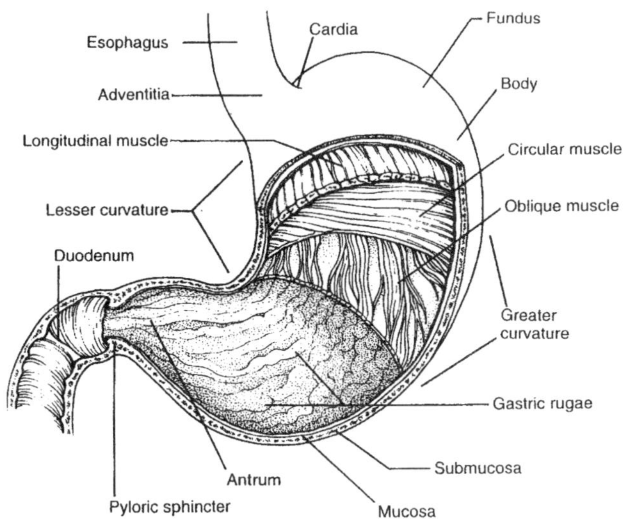

- The stomach has **three layers of smooth muscle**: longitudinal (outer, for peristalsis), circular (for mixing), and oblique (inner).
- The stomach is composed of the **fundus**, **body**, and **antrum**.
- **Receptive relaxation** mediated by VIP occurs in the fundus. As the stomach fills, a vagovagal-mediated receptive relaxation occurs, allowing storage.
- The bolus of swallowed food received by the stomach is further macerated and mixed with HCl, mucus, and pepsin. The food **(chyme)** is then discharged at a controlled rate into the duodenum. Only a small amount of chemical digestion actually occurs in the stomach.

Gastric Motility

- A pacemaker within the greater curvature produces a **basal electric rhythm (BER)** of 3 to 5 waves/min.
- The **magnitude** of the gastric contractions are **increased by parasympathetic** and **decreased by sympathetic stimulation**.
- **Migrating motor complexes (MMC)** are propulsive contractions initiated during fasting that begin in the stomach and move undigested material from the stomach and small intestine into the colon. They repeat every 90 to 120 minutes and are mediated by **motilin**. This housekeeping function lowers the bacterial count in the gut.

Gastric Emptying

- The **pylorus** is continuous with the circular muscle layer and acts as a "valve" to control gastric emptying.
- The contractions of the stomach (peristalsis) propel chyme through the pylorus at a regulated rate.
- Pyloric sphincter contraction at the time of antral contraction limits the movement of chyme into the duodenum and promotes mixing by forceful regurgitation of antral contents back into the fundus (**retropulsion**).
- **Gastric emptying is delayed by:**
  - **Fat/protein in the duodenum stimulating CCK release**, which increases gastric distensibility
  - **H^+ in the duodenum** via neural reflexes
  - Stomach contents that are hypertonic or hypotonic

Definition of abbreviation: VIP, vasoactive intestinal peptide.

▶ The Small Intestine

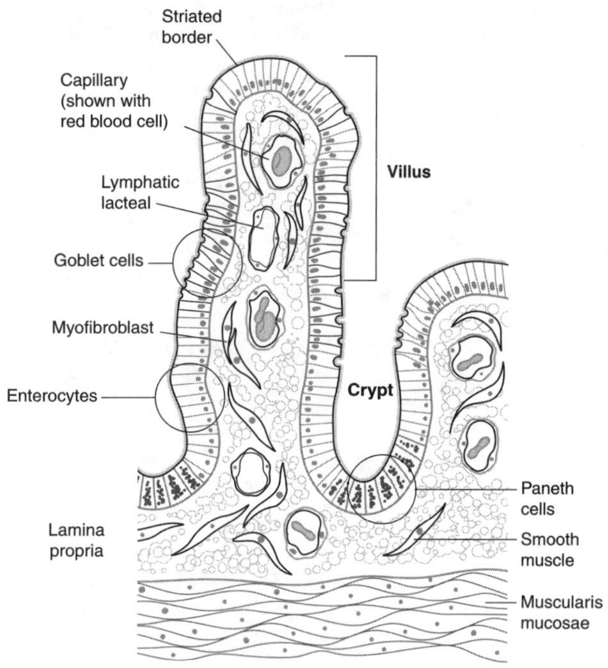

- The small intestine participates in the **digestion and absorption** of nutrients. It has specialized villi on the epithelial surface to aid in this function.
- The **duodenum** is the proximal pyloric end of the small intestine. Distal to the duodenum is the **jejunum**, and then the **ileum.**
- In the small intestine, the chyme from the stomach is **mixed** with mucosal cell secretions, exocrine pancreatic juice, and bile.
- **Mucus production** occurs in surface epithelial cells throughout the gastrointestinal tract, **Brunner glands** in the duodenum, and **goblet cells** in the mucosa throughout the intestine.
- **Mucus functions** include lubrication of the gastrointestinal tract, binding bacteria, and trapping immunoglobulins where they have access to pathogens.
- The **rate of mucus** secretion is increased by cholinergic stimulation, chemical irritation, and physical irritation.

Clinical Correlate

Any compromise of the mucous protection can lead to significant damage and irritation of the gastrointestinal tract, leading to gastritis, duodenitis, or even peptic ulcer disease.

Intestinal Motility

- **Small bowel slow waves** move caudally in the circular smooth muscle. The rate slows from approximately 12/min in the jejunum to approximately 9/min in the ileum.
- **Segmentation contractions** are ring-like contractions that **mix intestinal contents**. They occur at random "nodes" along the intestine. These relax, and then new nodes are formed at the former internodes. This action moves the chyme back and forth, increasing mucosal exposure to the chyme.
- **Peristalsis** is a reflex response initiated by stretching of the lumen of the gut. There is contraction of muscle at the oral end and relaxation of muscle at the caudal end, thus **propelling the contents caudally**. Although peristalsis is modulated by autonomic input, it can occur even in isolated loops of small bowel with no extrinsic innervation.
  - The intrinsic control system senses stretch with calcitonin gene-related polypeptide neurons (CGRP).
  - The contractile wave is initiated by acetylcholine (ACh) and substance P.
  - The relaxation caudal to the stimulus is initiated by nitric oxide (NO) and VIP.
- **Parasympathetic stimulation ↑ contractions** and **sympathetic stimulation ↓ contractions.**
- The **gastroileal reflex** is caused by food in the stomach, which stimulates peristalsis in the ileum and relaxes the ileocecal valve. This delivers intestinal contents to the large intestine.
- Small intestinal **secretions** are generally **alkaline**, serving to neutralize the acidic nature of the chyme entering from the pylorus.

Clinical Correlation

Peristalsis is activated by the **parasympathetic system**. For those suffering from decreased intestinal motility manifesting as constipation (paralytic ileus, diabetic gastroparesis), dopaminergic and cholinergic agents are often used (e.g., metoclopramide).

▶ The Large Intestine (Colon)

General Features
• The colon is larger in diameter and shorter in length than is the small intestine. Fecal material moves from the **cecum**, through the colon (**ascending**, **transverse**, **descending**, and **sigmoid colons**), rectum, and anal canal. • Three longitudinal bands of muscle, the **teniae coli**, constitute the outer layer. Because the colon is longer than these bands, pouching occurs, creating **haustra** between the teniae and giving the colon its characteristic "caterpillar" appearance. • The mucosa has **no villi**, and mucus is secreted by short, inward-projecting colonic glands. • Abundant lymphoid follicles are found in the cecum and appendix and more sparsely elsewhere. • The major functions of the colon are **reabsorption of fluid and electrolytes** and **temporary storage of feces**.

Colonic Motility
• **Peristaltic waves** briefly open the normally closed ileocecal valve, passing a small amount of chyme into the cecum. Peristalsis also advances the chyme in the colon. Slow waves, approximately 2/min, are initiated at the ileocecal valve and increase to approximately 6/min at the sigmoid colon. • **Segmentation contractions** mix the contents of the colon back and forth. • **Mass movement contractions** are found only in the colon. Constriction of long lengths of colon propels large amounts of chyme distally toward the anus. Mass movements propel feces into the rectum. Distention of the rectum with feces initiates the **defecation reflex**.

Absorption
The mucosa of the colon has great absorptive capability. **Na^+ is actively transported with water following**, and **K^+ and HCO_3^- are secreted into the colon**.

Defecation	
Feces	Contains undigested plant fibers, bacteria, inorganic matter, and water. Nondietary material (e.g., sloughed-off mucosa) constitutes a large portion of the feces. In normal feces, 30% of the solids may be bacteria. Bacteria synthesize **vitamin K**, B-complex vitamins, and folic acid, split urea to NH_3, and produce small organic acids from unabsorbed fat and carbohydrate.
Defecation	Rectal distention with feces activates intrinsic and cord reflexes that cause relaxation of the internal anal sphincter (smooth muscle) and produce the urge to defecate. If the external anal sphincter (skeletal muscle innervated by the **pudendal nerve**) is then voluntarily relaxed, and intra-abdominal pressure is increased via the **Valsalva maneuver**, defecation occurs. If the external sphincter is held contracted, the urge to defecate temporarily diminishes.
Gastrocolic reflex	Distention of the stomach by food **increases the frequency of mass movements** and produces the urge to defecate. This reflex is mediated by **parasympathetic** nerves.

▶ Vomiting

Vomiting occurs in three phases: **nausea**, **retching**, and **vomiting**.

- **Nausea**—hypersalivation, decreased gastric tone, increased duodenal and proximal jejunal tone → reflux of contents into stomach
- **Retching**—Gastric contents travel to the esophagus. Retching occurs if upper esophageal sphincter (UES) remains closed.
- **Vomiting**—If pressure increases enough to open the UES, vomiting occurs; vomiting can be triggered by oropharyngeal stimulation, gastric overdistention and gastroparesis, vestibular stimulation, or input from the **chemoreceptor trigger zone**, located in the **area postrema** in the floor of the fourth ventricle, which stimulates the medullary vomiting center.

► Antiemetics

Drug Class	Agents	Comments
$5HT_3$ antagonists	**Ondansetron** Granisetron, dolasetron	May act in chemoreceptor trigger zone and in peripheral sites
DA antagonists	**Phenothiazine**, metoclopramide*	Block D_2 receptors in chemoreceptor trigger zone
Cannabinoids	**Dronabinol**	Active ingredient in marijuana

► Emetics

Ipecac	• Locally irritates the GI tract and stimulates the chemoreceptor trigger zone • If emesis does not occur in 15-20 min, lavage must be used to remove ipecac
Apomorphine	• Dopamine-receptor agonist that stimulates the chemoreceptor trigger zone • Vomiting should occur within 5 min

*Also a prokinetic agent

► Gastrointestinal Hormones

Gastrointestinal hormones are released into the systemic circulation after physiologic stimulation (e.g., by food in gut), can exert their effects independent of the nervous system when administered exogenously, and have been chemically identified and synthesized. The five gastrointestinal hormones include **secretin**, **gastrin**, **cholecystokinin (CCK), gastric inhibitory peptide (GIP)**, and **motilin**.

Hormone	Source	Stimulus	Actions
Gastrin*, ‡	**G cells** of gastric antrum	• **Small peptides, amino acids, Ca^{2+}** in lumen of stomach • Vagus (via **GRP**) • **Stomach distension** • **Inhibited by: H^+** in lumen of antrum	• ↑ **HCl secretion by parietal cells** • **Trophic effects on GI mucosa** • ↑ pepsinogen secretion by chief cells • ↑ histamine secretion by ECL cells
CCK*	**I cells** of duodenum and jejunum	• **Fatty acids, monoglycerides** • **Small peptides and amino acids**	• **Stimulates gallbladder contraction** and **relaxes sphincter of Oddi** • ↑ **pancreatic enzyme secretion** • Augments secretin-induced stimulation of pancreatic HCO_3^- • **Inhibits gastric emptying** • Trophic effect on exocrine pancreas/gallbladder
Secretin†	**S cells** of duodenum	• ↓ **pH** in duodenal lumen • **Fatty acids** in duodenal lumen	• ↑ **pancreatic HCO_3^- secretion** (neutralizes H^+) • Trophic effect on exocrine pancreas • ↑ **bile production** • ↓ **gastric H^+ secretion**
GIP†	K cells of duodenum and jejunum	**Glucose, fatty acids, amino acids**	• ↑ **insulin release** • ↓ **gastric H^+ secretion**
Motilin	Enterochromaffin cells in duodenum and jejunum	Absence of food for >2 hours	Initiates MMC motility pattern in stomach and small intestine

(Continued)

▶ Gastrointestinal Hormones *(Cont'd.)*

Paracrines/ Neurocrines	Source	Stimulus	Actions
Somatostatin	D cells throughout GI tract	↓ pH in lumen	• ↓ gallbladder contraction, pancreatic secretion • ↓ gastric acid and pepsinogen secretion • ↓ small intestinal fluid secretion • ↓ ACh release from the myenteric plexus and decreases motility • ↓ α-cell release of glucagon, and β-cell release of insulin in pancreatic islet cells
Histamine	Enterochromaffin cells	• Gastrin • ACh	↑ **gastric acid secretion** (directly, and potentiates gastrin and vagal stimulation)
VIP[†, ¶]	Neurons in GI tract	• Vagal stimulation • Intestinal distention	• **Relaxation of intestinal smooth muscle, including sphincters** • ↑ **Pancreatic HCO_3^- secretion** • **Stimulates intestinal secretion of electrolytes and H_2O**
GRP	Vagal nerve endings	Cephalic stimulation, gastric distension	**Stimulates gastrin release** from G cells
Pancreatic polypeptide	F cells of pancreas, small intestine	Protein, fat, glucose in lumen	↓ pancreatic secretion
Enteroglucagon	L cells of intestine	—	• ↓ gastric, pancreatic secretions • ↑ insulin release

Definition of abbreviations: ECL, enterochromaffin-like cells; GIP, gastric inhibitory peptide; GRP, gastrin-releasing peptide.
*Member of gastrin-CCK family
†Member of secretin-glucagon family

Clinical Correlates:

‡**Zollinger-Ellison syndrome (gastrinoma)**—non-β islet-cell pancreatic tumor that produces gastrin, leading to ↑ in gastric acid secretion and development of peptic ulcer disease

¶**VIPoma**—tumor of non-α, non-β islet cells of the pancreas that secretes VIP, causing watery diarrhea

► Gastric Secretions

Secretion Product	Cell Type	Region of Stomach	Stimulus for Secretion	Inhibitors of Secretion	Action of Secretory Product
HCl	Parietal (oxyntic) cells	Body/fundus	• Gastrin • ACh (from vagus) • Histamine	• **Low pH** inhibits (by inhibiting gastrin) • Prostaglandins • Chyme in duodenum (via GIP and secretin)	• Kills pathogens • Activates pepsinogen to pepsin
Intrinsic factor					Necessary for **vitamin B_{12}** absorption by the ileum; forms complex with vitamin B_{12}
Pepsinogen (zymogen, precursor of **pepsin**)	Chief cells	Body/fundus	• ACh (from vagus) • Gastrin • HCl	H^+ (via somatostatin)	• Converted to pepsin by ↓ pH and pepsin (autocatalytic) • **Digests up to 20% of proteins**
Gastrin	G cells	Antrum	• Small peptides/aa • Vagus (via GRP) • Stomach distention	H^+ (via somatostatin)	• ↑ **HCl secretion (parietal cells)** • ↑ pepsinogen secretion (chief cells) • ↑ histamine secretion by ECL cells
Mucus	Mucous cells	Entire stomach	ACh (from vagus)		Forms gel on mucosa to protect mucosa from HCl and pepsin; traps HCO_3^- to help neutralize acid

Definition of abbreviations: aa, amino acids; ECL, enterochromaffin-like cells.

► Mechanism of Gastric H^+ Secretion

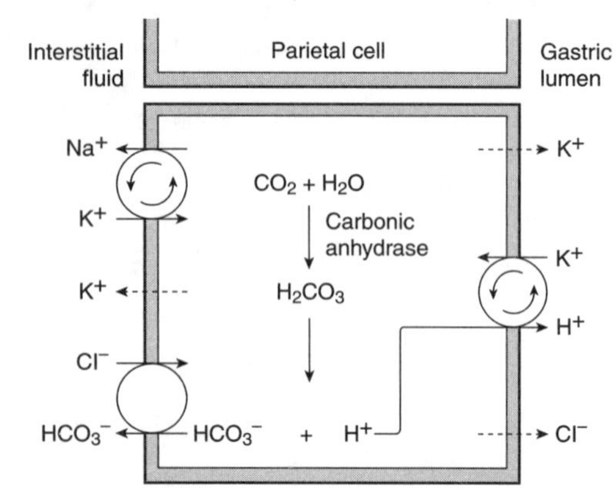

- In the parietal cell, CO_2 and H_2O are converted by carbonic anhydrase to H^+ and HCO_3^-.
- H^+ is secreted into the lumen of the stomach by H^+-K^+ pump (**H^+/K^+–ATPase**). Cl^- is secreted with H^+.
- HCO_3^- is absorbed into the bloodstream in exchange for Cl^-.
- After a meal, enough H^+ may be secreted to raise the pH of systemic blood and turn the urine alkaline **("alkaline tide")**.

The three primary triggers of H^+ secretion are:

- **ACh** (from vagus), via the M_3 muscarinic receptor
- **Histamine**, via the H_2 histamine receptor
- **Gastrin**, via unidentified receptor

▶ Drugs for Peptic Ulcer Disease

Drug Class	Agents	Comments
Antacids	Magnesium hydroxide, aluminum hydroxide, calcium carbonate	*Magnesium:* **laxative** effect *Aluminum hydroxide:* **constipating** effect
H_2 antagonists	**Cimetidine**, ranitidine, famotidine, nizatidine	• Useful in PUD, GERD, Zollinger-Ellison syndrome, but not as effective as proton pump inhibitors • **Cimetidine inhibits hepatic drug metabolizing enzymes** and has **antiandrogen effects**
Proton pump inhibitors	**Omeprazole,** lansoprazole, esomeprazole, pantoprazole, rabeprazole	• Irreversibly **inactivate H^+/K^+-ATPase**, thus blocking H^+ secretion. • Work very well—useful in PUD, Zollinger-Ellison syndrome, and GERD
Mucosal protective agents	**Sucralfate**	Polymerizes in the stomach and forms protective coating over ulcer beds.
	Misoprostol	PGE_1 derivative used for peptic ulcers caused by NSAIDs
Antibiotics	Macrolides, metronidazole, tetracyclines (various combinations)	To treat ***H. pylori***

Definition of abbreviations: GERD, gastroesophageal reflux disorder; PGE_1, prostaglandin E_1; NSAIDs, nonsteroidal antiinflammatory drugs; PUD, peptic ulcer disease.

▶ Phases of Gastric Secretion

Cephalic phase	The smell, sight, thought, or chewing of food can increase gastric secretion via parasympathetic (vagal) pathways. Responsible for approximately 30% of acid secreted.
Gastric phase	Food in the stomach ↑ secretion. The greatest effects occur with proteins and peptides, leading to **gastrin** release (alcohol and caffeine also exert a strong effect). Gastric distention initiates vagovagal reflexes. Accounts for approximately 60% of acid secreted.
Intestinal phase	Protein digestion products in the duodenum stimulate duodenal gastrin secretion. In addition, absorbed amino acids act to stimulate H^+ secretion by parietal cells. The intestinal phase accounts for less than 10% of the gastric secretory response to a meal.

► Pancreatic Secretions

The exocrine secretions of the pancreas are produced by the **acinar cells**, which contain numerous enzyme-containing granules in their cytoplasm, and by the **ductal cells**, which secrete HCO_3^-. The secretions reach the duodenum via the **pancreatic duct**.

Bicarbonate (HCO_3^-)

- HCO_3^- in the duodenum **neutralizes HCl in chyme** entering from the stomach. This also deactivates pepsin.
- When H^+ enters the duodenum, S cells secrete **secretin**, which acts on pancreatic ductal cells to increase HCO_3^- production.
- HCO_3^- is produced by the action of **carbonic anhydrase** on CO_2 and H_2O in the pancreatic ductal cells. HCO_3^- is secreted into the lumen of the duct in exchange for Cl^-.

Pancreatic enzymes

- Approximately 15 enzymes are produced by the pancreas, which are responsible for **digesting proteins, carbohydrates, lipids, and nucleic acids**.
- When small peptides, amino acids, and fatty acids enter the duodenum, **CCK** is released by I cells, stimulating pancreatic enzyme secretion.
- **ACh** (via vagovagal reflexes) also stimulates enzyme secretion and potentiates the action of secretin.
- **Protection of pancreatic acinar cells against self-digestion:**
  - **Proteolytic enzymes are secreted as inactive precursors**, which are activated in the gut lumen. For example, the duodenal brush border enzyme, **enterokinase**, converts trypsinogen to the active enzyme, trypsin. Trypsin then catalyzes the formation of more trypsin and activates chymotrypsinogen, procarboxypeptidase, and prophospholipases A and B. Ribonucleases, amylase, and lipase do not exist as proenzymes.
  - Produce **enzyme inhibitors** to inactivate trace amounts of active enzyme formed within.

Enzyme	Reaction Catalyzed
Proteases:	
Trypsin	Proteins → peptides
Chymotrypsin	Proteins → peptides
Carboxypeptidase	Peptides → amino acids
Polysaccharidase:	
Amylase	Starch and glycogen → maltose, maltotriose, and α-limit dextrins
Lipases:	
Phospholipases A and B	Phospholipids → phosphate, fatty acids, and glycerol
Esterases	Cholesterol esters → free cholesterol and fatty acids
Triacylglycerol lipases	Triglycerides → fatty acids and monoglycerides
Nucleases:	
Ribonuclease	RNA → ribonucleotides
Deoxyribonuclease	DNA → deoxyribonucleotides

▶ Hepatic Excretion

Physiologic roles	• Excretion of **bilirubin**, **cholesterol**, drugs, and **toxins** • Promotion of **intestinal lipid absorption** • Delivery of **IgA** to small intestine
Components of bile	• Bile—composed of **bile salts, phospholipids, cholesterol, bilirubin (bile pigments), water, and electrolytes**

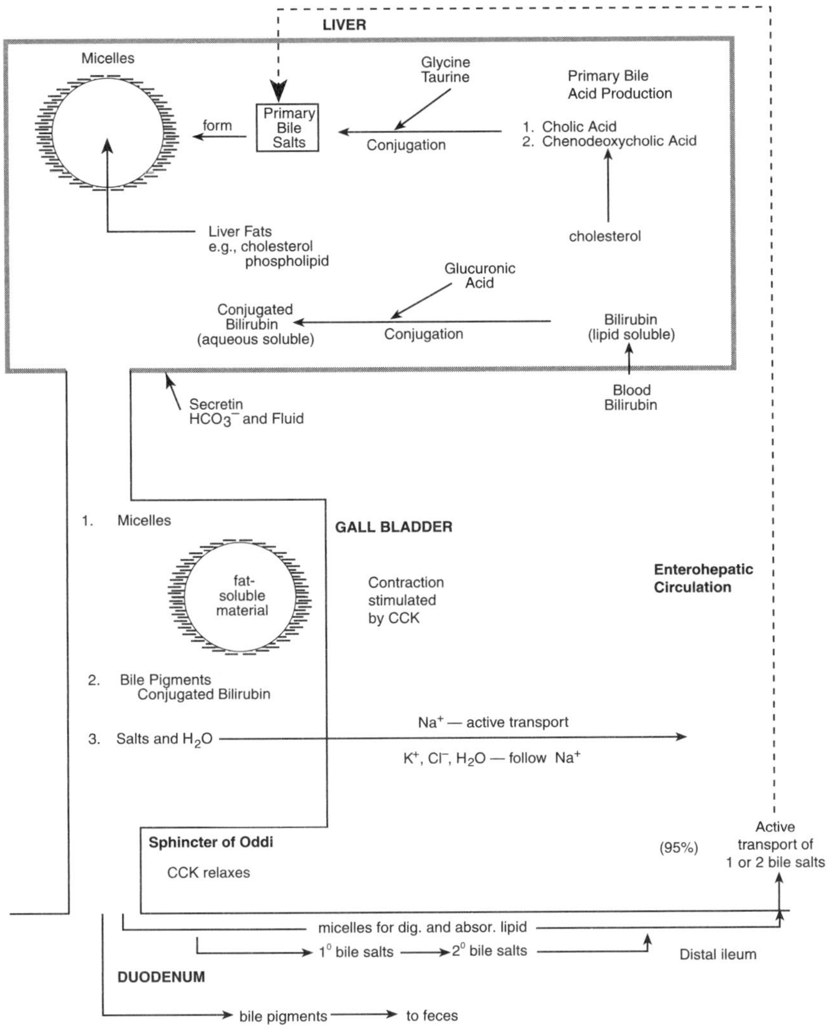

Formation of Bile

- Bile, produced by hepatocytes, drains into **hepatic ducts** and is stored in the **gallbladder** for later release.
- **Primary bile acids** (cholic and chenodeoxycholic acids) are made from cholesterol in the liver. **Secondary bile acids** (deoxycholic and lithocholic) are products of bacterial metabolism of primary bile acids in the gut.
- All bile acids must be conjugated with **glycine** or **taurine** to form their **bile salt** before being secreted into bile.
- Above a **critical micellar concentration**, bile salts form **micelles**. Electrolytes and H_2O are also added to the bile.

Micelles

- Micelles are water soluble-spheres with a lipid-soluble interior.
- Micelles are vital in the digestion, transport, and absorption of lipid-soluble substances from the duodenum to the distal ileum, where bile salts are actively reabsorbed and recycled (**enterohepatic circulation**).
- A lack of reabsorbing mechanisms or distal ileal disease can lead to deficiency of bile salts. This can lead to malabsorption, gallstones, and **steatorrhea**.

Gallbladder

- The gallbladder concentrates and stores bile for release during meals.
- During the interdigestive period, the **sphincter of Oddi** is closed and the gallbladder is relaxed, allowing it to fill with bile.
- Bile is **concentrated** in the gallbladder by water and electrolyte absorption.
- Small peptides and fatty acids in the duodenum cause **CCK** secretion, which causes **gallbladder contraction** and **relaxation of the sphincter of Oddi**. ACh also aids in this process.

(*Continued*)

► Hepatic Excretion *(Cont'd.)*

Bilirubin	• Bilirubin is a product of **heme metabolism**. • It is taken up by hepatocytes and **conjugated with glucuronic acid** prior to secretion into bile. This gives bile a golden yellow color. In the large intestine, bilirubin is deconjugated and metabolized by bacteria to form **urobilinogens** (colorless). Some of the urobilinogens are reabsorbed; most of the reabsorbed urobilinogens are secreted into bile, with the remainder excreted in the urine. • Most urobilinogen remains in the gut and is further reduced to pigmented compounds (stercobilins and urobilins) and excreted in feces. **Stercobilins** give a brown color to feces. • **Jaundice** (yellowing of the skin and whites of the eyes) is a result of **elevated bilirubin**.
Regulation of bile secretion	• **Secretin** stimulates the secretion of bile **high in HCO_3^- content** from the biliary ductules, but does not alter bile salt output. • Secretion of bile salts by hepatocytes is directly proportional to hepatic portal vein concentration of bile salts.

► Digestion and Absorption

- Carbohydrates, lipids, and proteins are digested and absorbed in the small intestine.
- The brush border of the small intestine increases surface area, greatly facilitating absorption of nutrients.

Carbohydrate digestion	Must be converted to **monosaccharides** in order to be absorbed
	Mouth
	• **Salivary amylase** normally hydrolyzes approximately 10 to 20% of ingested starch. • It **hydrolyzes** only **α-(1:4)-glycosidic linkages** to maltose, maltotriose, and α-limit dextrins.
	Intestine
	• **Pancreatic amylase** is found in the highest concentration in the duodenal lumen, where it rapidly hydrolyzes starch to oligosaccharides, maltose, maltotriose, and α-limit dextrins. • **Maltase**, **α-dextrinase, lactase**, **sucrase**, and **isomaltase** are found in the **brush border**, with the highest concentrations in the mid-jejunum and proximal ileum. – **α-dextrinase:** cleaves terminal α-1,4 bonds, producing free glucose – **Lactase:** converts lactose to glucose and galactose – **Sucrase:** converts sucrose to glucose and fructose – **Maltase:** converts maltose and maltotriose to 2 and 3 glucose units, respectively. • The monosaccharide end products (**glucose**, **galactose**, and **fructose**) are readily absorbed from the small intestine, primarily in the jejunum.
	Clinical Correlation
	• **Lactase deficiency** causes an inability to digest lactose into glucose and galactose. • *Consequence:* ↑ osmotic load, giving rise to **osmotic diarrhea** and **flatulence**. • Very common in African Americans, Asians, and Mediterraneans, and to a lesser degree, in Europeans/Americans.
Carbohydrate absorption	**Luminal Membrane**
	• **Glucose and galactose** compete for transport across the brush border by a **Na^+-dependent coporter (SGLT-1)**. Na^+ moves down its gradient into the enterocyte and the sugars move up their concentration gradients into the enterocyte (secondarily active). A Na^+-K^+ ATPase in the basolateral membrane helps maintain the Na^+ gradient (by keeping intracellular Na^+ low). • **Fructose:** facilitated diffusion (down its concentration gradient) via GLUT-5 transporter
	Basolateral Membrane
	Glucose, galactose, and **fructose** are transported across the basolateral membrane via facilitated diffusion (GLUT-2 transporter).

(*Continued*)

► Digestion and Absorption (*Cont'd.*)

Lipid digestion	**Stomach** • Fatty materials are **pulverized** to decrease particle size and increase surface area. • **CCK** slows gastric emptying to allow enough time for digestion and absorption in the small intestine. **Small Intestine** • **Bile acid micelles** emulsify fat. • **Pancreatic lipases** digest fat. • Fats are hydrolyzed by pancreatic lipases to **free fatty acids**, **monoacylglycerols**, and other lipids (e.g., **cholesterol**, and **fat-soluble vitamins A, D, E, K**), which collect in micelles.
Lipid absorption	• **Micelles** carry products of fat digestion in the aqueous fluid of the gut lumen to the brush border, where they can diffuse into the enterocyte. • Enterocytes **re-esterify the fatty acids** to form triacylglycerols, phospholipids, and cholesteryl esters, which are incorporated with **apoproteins** into **chylomicrons**. • Chylomicrons are **released by exocytosis** into the intercellular spaces, where they **enter the lacteals** of the lymphatic system. They then enter the venous circulation via the **thoracic duct**. • Glycerol diffuses into portal blood and is either oxidized for energy or stored as glycogen. • **Triacylglycerols** with **medium- and short-chain fatty acids** are hydrolyzed quickly and do not require micelle formation for absorption. They undergo little re-esterification and are absorbed directly into the portal venous system. **Clinical Correlation** **Abetalipoproteinemia** results from a deficiency of apoprotein B, causing an inability to transport chylomicrons out of intestinal cells.
Protein digestion	**Stomach** **Pepsin** begins protein digestion in the stomach. It functions best at pH 2 and is irreversibly deactivated above pH 5; therefore, it will be inactivated in the duodenum. Pepsin is not an essential enzyme. **Small Intestine** Protein digestion continues with **pancreatic proteases** (trypsin, chymotrypsin, elastase, carboxypeptidases A and B) activated by brush border peptidases. These are essential enzymes.
Protein absorption	**Luminal Membrane** • Protein products can be absorbed as **amino acids**, **dipeptides**, and **tripeptides**. • Amino acids are absorbed via **Na^+-dependent amino acid cotransport**. Many different transport systems have been identified, e.g., carriers for neutral, basic, acidic, and imino amino acids. • Dipeptides and tripeptides are absorbed via an **H^+-dependent cotransport** mechanism. **Basal Membrane** • Dipeptides and tripeptides are hydrolyzed to amino acids intracellularly. • Amino acids are transported to the blood by facilitated diffusion. **Clinical Correlation** **Hartnup disease** is a disorder in which neutral amino acids cannot be absorbed.
Water and electrolyte absorption	The absorption of water and electrolytes occurs mainly in the **small intestine**. Approximately 5–10 liters of fluid must be absorbed daily (intake and secretion), with 80–90% being absorbed in the small intestine at a maximal rate of 700 mL/h.

(Continued)

► Digestion and Absorption *(Cont'd.)*

NaCl	• In the **proximal intestine**, there is **Na^+-H^+ exchange**, **Na^+-glucose or Na^+-amino acid cotransport**, **Na^+-Cl^- cotransport,** and **passive diffusion** through Na^+ channels. • In the colon, passive diffusion through Na^+ channels is more important and is stimulated by **aldosterone**. • **Cl^-** is absorbed via Na^+-Cl^- cotransport, Cl^--HCO_3^- exchange, and passive diffusion.
K^+	• K^+ absorption occurs in the small intestine by passive diffusion. • K^+ is secreted in the colon (stimulated by aldosterone).
Ca^{2+}	• Absorption in the small intestine is via a vitamin D-dependent carrier. • Vitamin D deficiency → ↓ Ca^{2+} absorption → **osteomalacia** (adults) and **rickets** (children).
H_2O	• Secondary to solute absorption • Isoosmotic absorption in gallbladder and small intestine; permeability is lower in colon.
Iron	• Absorbed as **free Fe^{2+}** or as **heme** iron, primarily in the duodenum • **Fe^{2+}** is bound to transferrin in the blood.
Vitamins	• **Fat-soluble (A, D, E, K)**—incorporated into micelles and absorbed • **Water soluble**—usually via Na^+-dependent cotransporters • **Vitamin B_{12}**—absorption occurs in ileum and is transported while bound to intrinsic factor; ↓ intrinsic factor (gastrectomy) → **pernicious anemia**
H_2O, electrolyte secretion	Secretion occurs in **crypts**. **Cl^-** is the main ion secreted, via cAMP-regulated channels in the luminal membrane. **Clinical Correlation** **Cholera toxin** stimulates adenylate cyclase → ↑ cAMP → open Cl^- channels; Na^+ and H_2O follow → secretory diarrhea.

Gastrointestinal Pathology

► Lesions of the Oral Cavity

Leukoplakia	• White plaques on oral mucosa, produced by hyperkeratosis of the epithelium • 10% have epithelial dysplasia, a precancerous lesion • *Predisposing factors:* smoking, smokeless tobacco, alcohol abuse, chronic friction, and irritants
Erythroplakia	• Flat, smooth, and red. • Significant numbers of atypical epithelial cells • High risk of malignant transformation
Hairy leukoplakia	• Wrinkled patches on side of tongue • Epstein-Barr virus associated • No malignant transformation
Lichen planus	White reticulate lesions on the buccal mucosa and tongue
Tumors of the Oral Cavity	
Benign tumors	Hemangiomas, hamartomas, fibromas, lipomas, adenomas, papillomas, neurofibromas, and nevi
Malignant tumors	• **Squamous carcinoma** most common. Peak incidence from ages 40–70 years. • Associated with tobacco and alcohol use, particularly when used together • **Lower lip** most common site, but may affect floor of mouth and tongue

► Esophageal Pathology

Achalasia	• **Lack of relaxation of the LES** secondary to loss of myenteric plexus • *Most common ages:* 30–50. • *Symptoms:* dysphagia, regurgitation, aspiration, chest pain • Can be idiopathic, secondary to Chagas disease (*Trypanosoma cruzi*), or malignancy
Barrett esophagus	• Gastric or intestinal **columnar epithelium** replaces normal squamous epithelium • Occurs with chronic insult, usually reflux (**increases risk of adenocarcinoma** 30–40 times)
Boerhaave syndrome	• Violent retching causes potentially fatal esophageal rupture
Diverticula	• Sac-like protrusions of one or more layers of the pharyngeal or esophageal wall • **Zenker diverticula:** – Occur at the junction of the pharynx and esophagus in elderly men – *Symptoms:* dysphagia and regurgitation of undigested food soon after ingestion • **Traction diverticula:** true diverticula in mid-esophagus; usually asymptomatic
Esophageal carcinoma	• Most are **adenocarcinomas** occurring after 50 and have male:female ratio of 4:1 • Incidence higher in northern Iran, Central Asia • Associated with smoking, alcohol, nitrosamines, achalasia, Barrett esophagus, and vitamin A deficiency • Presents with dysphagia (first to solids) • Liver and lung most common sites of metastasis; poor prognosis
Esophageal strictures	• Narrowing of the esophagus, often as a result of fibrosis after severe inflammation. Caused by reflux, Herpes virus, Cytomegalovirus, *Candida,* chemical burns (e.g., lye ingestion). • Carcinoma should be ruled out
Esophageal varices	• Dilated tortuous vessels of the esophageal venous plexus resulting from **portal hypertension** • Esophageal varices are prone to **bleeding**; may be life-threatening

(Continued)

▶ Esophageal Pathology *(Cont'd.)*

Esophagitis	• Most common cause is reflux; other causes include infections (Herpes virus, Cytomegalovirus, *Candida*) and eosinophilic esophagitis	
Hernia	**Sliding**	90% of cases, gastroesophageal junction above diaphragm, associated with **reflux**
	Paraesophageal	Gastric cardia above diaphragm, gastroesophageal junction remains in the abdomen; herniated organ at risk for strangulation and infarction
Mallory-Weiss tears	Occur at gastroesophageal junction secondary to recurrent **forceful vomiting**, usually seen in **alcoholics**	
Schatzki rings	Mucosal rings at the squamocolumnar junction below the aortic arch	
Tracheoesophageal fistula	• Usually esophageal blind pouch with a fistula between the lower segment of the esophagus and trachea • Associated with congenital heart disease and other gastrointestinal malformations	
Webs	• Mucosal folds in the upper esophagus above the aortic arch • **Plummer-Vinson syndrome:** dysphagia, glossitis, iron-deficiency anemia, and esophageal webs	

Definition of abbreviation: LES, lower esophageal sphincter.

▶ Stomach Pathology

Acute gastritis (erosive)	Can be caused by alcohol, aspirin, smoking, shock, steroids, and uremia Patients experience heartburn, epigastric pain, nausea, vomiting, and hematemesis
Chronic gastritis	
Fundal (type A)	Autoimmune; associated with **pernicious anemia**, achlorhydria, and intrinsic factor deficiency
Antral (type B)	Caused by ***Helicobacter pylori*** and is most common form of chronic gastritis in U.S.
Carcinoma	• *Risk factors:* genetic predisposition, diet, hypochlorhydria, pernicious anemia, and nitrosamines • Usually asymptomatic until late, then presents with anorexia, weight loss, anemia, epigastric pain. Virchow node (left supraclavicular lymph node) common site of metastasis • *Pathology:* 50% arise in the antrum and pylorus • *Linitis plastica:* infiltrating gastric carcinoma with a diffuse fibrous response • *Histology:* signet ring cells characteristic of gastric carcinoma
Hypertrophic gastropathy	• **Menetrier disease:** markedly thickened rugae due to hyperplastic superficial mucus glands with atrophy of deeper glands • **Hypertrophic-hypersecretory gastropathy:** hyperplasia of parietal and chief cells in gastric glands • **Excessive gastrin secretion (e.g., gastrinoma, Zollinger-Ellison syndrome):** produces gastric gland hyperplasia. Risk of peptic ulcer disease.
Peptic ulcers	• *Common locations:* proximal duodenum, stomach, and esophagus • ***H. pylori*** infection important etiologic factor. Modification of acid secretion coupled with antibiotic therapy that eradicates *H. pylori* is apparently curative in most patients. • *Symptoms:* episodic epigastric pain; *complications:* hemorrhage, perforation • Duodenal ulcers do not become malignant. Gastric ulcers only rarely • *Stress ulcers:* burns → Curling ulcers; CNS trauma → Cushing ulcers
Pyloric stenosis	• Congenital hypertrophy of pyloric muscle • *Classic case:* firstborn boy, presenting with **projectile vomiting** 3–4 weeks after birth; associated with a palpable **"olive" mass** in epigastric region • *Treatment:* surgical

► Small Intestine Pathology

Celiac sprue	• Allergic reaction to the **gliadin** component of gluten; genetic predisposition • Predisposes to neoplasm, especially lymphoma • *Pathology:* atrophy of villi in the jejunum; affects only **proximal** small bowel
Congenital anomalies	• **Meckel diverticulum:** persistent omphalomesenteric vitelline duct. Located near ileocecal valve. May contain ectopic gastric, pancreatic, or endometrial tissue, which may produce ulceration • **Vitelline fistula:** direct connection between the intestinal lumen and the outside of the body at the umbilicus due to persistence of the vitelline duct. Associated with drainage of meconium from the umbilicus • Atresia: congenital absence of a region of bowel (e.g., **duodenal atresia**); polyhydramnios, obstruction, and bile-stained vomiting in neonate • Stenosis: narrowing that may cause obstruction • **Omphalocele:** when the midgut loop fails to return to the abdominal cavity, forming a light gray shiny sac at the base of the umbilical cord filled with loops of small intestine • **Gastroschisis:** A failure of the lateral body folds to fuse causes extrusion of the intestines through a open defect in the abdominal wall that is usually to the right of the umbilicus; unlike omphalocele, the intestines are exposed to the open air rather than being covered with a membrane.
Hernias	• Cause 15% of small intestinal obstruction, most commonly at the inguinal and femoral canals • **Inguinal hernias** – **Indirect inguinal hernia:** the intestinal loop goes through the internal (deep) inguinal ring, external (superficial) inguinal ring, and into the scrotum. Much more common in males; may present in infancy if there is a failure of the processus vaginalis to close. – **Direct inguinal hernia:** the intestinal loop protrudes through the inguinal (Hesselbach's) triangle to cause a bulge in the abdominal wall medial to the inferior epigastric artery. Hesselbach's triangle is defined by the inferior epigastric artery, the lateral border of the rectus abdominus, and the inguinal ligament. The typical patient is an older man, and the hernia is covered by the external spermatic fascia. • **Femoral hernia:** the intestinal loop protrudes below the inguinal ligament through the femoral canal below and lateral to the pubic tubercle. More common in women. This type of hernia is particularly likely to produce a dangerous bowel incarceration. • **Diaphragmatic hernia:** infants with defective development of pleuroperitoneal membrane may have intestines and other abdominal structures herniated into the thorax; potentially fatal because of impairment of lung expansion
Ischemic bowel disease	• Thrombosis or embolism of the **superior mesenteric artery** accounts for approximately 50% of cases; venous thrombosis for 25% of cases • Internal hernias can strangulate entrapped loops of bowel • Usually after age 60 and presents with abdominal pain, nausea, and vomiting
Intussusception	• Telescoping of one segment of bowel into another • More common in infants and children; may be reduced with a diagnostic barium enema • In adults, lead point usually an intraluminal mass; usually requires surgery
Lymphoma	• Usually non-Hodgkin, large cell, diffuse type • In immunosuppressed patients, the incidence of primary lymphomas of small intestine is increasing. • **MALToma:** often follicular and follow a more benign course; associated with *H. pylori* infection; may regress after antibiotic therapy.
Necrotizing enterocolitis	• Life-threatening acute, necrotizing inflammation of the small and large intestines • Usually in premature or low birth weight neonates • Peak incidence when babies start oral foods at 2 to 4 days, but can occur any time in first three months of life • If surgical treatment is required, it may cause short bowel syndrome
Tropical sprue	• Unknown etiology; high incidence in the tropics; especially Vietnam, Puerto Rico • *Pathology:* similar to changes in celiac disease, but affects **entire** length of small bowel
Volvulus	• Twisting of the bowel about its mesenteric base; may cause obstruction and infarction • May be associated with malrotation of the midgut • Typical patient is elderly
Whipple disease	• Rare, periodic acid-Schiff (PAS)–positive **macrophages in the lamina propria** of intestines • Caused by small bacilli ***(Tropheryma whippelii)***; more common in men (10:1)

▶ Appendix Pathology

Appendicitis	• The vermiform appendix may become inflamed as a result of either an obstruction by stool, which forms a **fecalith** (common in adults), or **hyperplasia** of its lymphatic tissue (common in children). • An inflamed appendix may stimulate visceral pain fibers, which course back in the lesser splanchnic nerves and result in colicky pain referred over the umbilical region.

▶ Large Intestine Pathology

Angiodysplasia	• Dilated tortuous vessels of the right colon → lower gastrointestinal bleeding in elderly • Highest incidence in the cecum
Diverticular disease	• Multiple outpouchings of colon present in 30–50% of adults; higher incidence with ↑ age • Presents with pain and fever
Hirschsprung disease	• **Absence of ganglion cells** of Meissner and Auerbach plexus in distal colon • Produces markedly distended colon, proximal to aganglionic portion • **Failure to pass meconium**, with constipation, vomiting, and abdominal distention
Imperforate anus	Failure of perforation of the membrane that separates endodermal hindgut from ectodermal anal dimple
Polyps	
Tubular adenomas	• Pedunculated polyps; 75% of adenomatous polyps • Sporadic or familial; average age of onset is 60; most occur in left colon • Cancer occurs in approximately 4% of patients
Villous adenomas	• Largest, least common polyps; usually sessile • **1/3 cancerous**
Tubulovillous adenomas	• Combined tubular and villous elements • **Increased villous elements →↑ likelihood of malignant transformation**
Polyposis Syndromes	
Peutz-Jeghers syndrome	• **Autosomal dominant**; involves entire gastrointestinal tract; **melanin pigmentation** of the buccal mucosa • Polyps—**hamartomas**; not premalignant
Turcot syndrome	Colonic polyps associated with brain tumors
Familial multiple polyposis	• **Autosomal dominant**; appearance of polyps during adolescence • Start in rectosigmoid area and spread to cover entire colon • **Virtually all patients develop cancers**; prophylactic total colectomy recommended
Gardner syndrome	• Colonic polyps associated with **desmoid tumors** • **Risk of colon cancer nearly 100%**
Malignant Tumors	
Adenocarcinoma	• **98% of all colonic cancers;** third most common tumor in both women and men; peak incidence in 60s • *Symptoms:* rectal bleeding, change in bowel habits, weakness, malaise, and weight loss • Tumor spreads by direct extension and **metastasis to nodes, liver, lungs, bones** • **Carcinoembryonic antigen (CEA) tumor marker** helps to monitor tumor recurrence after surgery • 75% of tumors in rectum, sigmoid colon • **Left-sided lesions:** annular constriction, infiltration of the wall, **obstruction** • **Right-sided lesions:** often bulky, polypoid, protuberant masses; **rarely obstruct** because fecal stream is liquid on right side
Squamous cell carcinoma	• Occur in anal region, associated with **papilloma viruses** • Incidence rising in homosexual men with AIDS

▶ Inflammatory Bowel Disease: Crohn Disease Versus Ulcerative Colitis

	Crohn Disease	Ulcerative Colitis
Most common site	Terminal ileum	Rectum
Distribution	Mouth to anus	Rectum → colon; "backwash" ileitis
Spread	Discontinuous/"skip"	Continuous
Gross features	Focal ulceration with intervening normal mucosa, linear fissures, cobblestone appearance, thickened bowel wall, "creeping fat"	Extensive ulceration, pseudopolyps
Micro	Noncaseating granulomas	Crypt abscesses
Inflammation	Transmural	Limited to mucosa and submucosa
Complications	Strictures, "string sign" on barium studies, obstruction, abscesses, fistulas, sinus tracts	Toxic megacolon
Genetic association	Family history of any type of inflammatory bowel disease is associated with increased risk.	
Extraintestinal manifestations	Less common	Common (e.g., arthritis, spondylitis [HLA B27 positive], primary sclerosing cholangitis, erythema nodosum, pyoderma gangrenosum)
Cancer risk	Slight 1–3%	5–25%

▶ Exocrine Pancreas

Acute hemorrhagic pancreatitis	• Diffuse necrosis of the pancreas by release of activated enzymes • Most often associated with **alcoholism** and **biliary tract disease** • *Symptoms:* sudden onset of acute, continuous, and intense abdominal pain, often radiating to back; accompanied by nausea, vomiting, and fever → frequently results in shock • *Lab values:* **high amylase**, **high lipase** (elevated after 3–4 days), leukocytosis • *Gross:* gray areas of enzymatic destruction, white areas of fat necrosis, red areas of hemorrhage
Chronic pancreatitis	• Remitting and relapsing episodes of mild pancreatitis → progressive pancreatic damage • X-rays reveal **calcifications** in pancreas • Chronic pancreatitis may result in **pseudocyst formation**, **diabetes**, steatorrhea
Pseudocysts	• Possible sequelae of pancreatitis or trauma • Up to 10 cm in diameter with a fibrous capsule; no epithelial lining or direct communication with ducts
Carcinoma	• *Risk factors:* smoking, high-fat diet, chemical exposure • Commonly develop in **head of the pancreas**, may result in compression of bile duct and main pancreatic duct → obstructive jaundice • **Asymptomatic until late** in course, then weight loss, abdominal pain (classically, epigastric pain radiating to back), jaundice, weakness, anorexia; **Trousseau syndrome (migratory thrombophlebitis)** often seen • Very poor prognosis
Cystic fibrosis	• Autosomal recessive; ***CFTR*** (cystic fibrosis transmembrane conductance regulator protein) gene located on chromosome 7; **Δ508** is a common mutation • **Defective chloride channel**: secretion of very thick mucus and **high sodium and chloride levels in sweat** • 10% present with **meconium ileus** (most present during first year with steatorrhea, **pulmonary infections**, and obstructive pulmonary disease) • ***Pseudomonas aeruginosa*** is most common etiologic agent; **blue-green sputum** • Median survival age 37; mortality most often due to pulmonary infections
Annular pancreas	Occurs when the ventral and dorsal pancreatic buds form a ring around the duodenum → obstruction of the duodenum

► Congenital Hepatic Diseases

Extrahepatic biliary atresia	• Incomplete recanalization → cholestasis, cirrhosis, portal hypertension • **Within first weeks of life:** jaundice, dark urine, light stools, hepatosplenomegaly
Intrahepatic biliary atresia	• Diminished number of bile ducts; sometimes associated with **α-1-antitrypsin deficiency** • **Presents in infancy** with cholestasis, pruritus, growth retardation, ↑ serum lipids • Icterus visible when serum bilirubin exceeds 2 mg/dL (true in any case of jaundice)
Conjugated hyperbilirubinemia	• **Dubin-Johnson syndrome:** benign conjugated hyperbilirubinemia due to impaired transport; liver grossly **black** • **Rotor syndrome:** asymptomatic, similar to Dubin-Johnson, but the liver **not pigmented**
Unconjugated hyperbilirubinemia	• Can be due to hemolysis, diffuse hepatocellular damage, enzymatic defect • **Gilbert syndrome:** autosomal recessive disease; deficiency of glucuronyl transferase; benign • **Crigler-Najjar syndrome:** – *Type 1:* autosomal recessive with **complete absence of glucuronyl transferase**, marked unconjugated hyperbilirubinemia, severe kernicterus, death – *Type 2:* autosomal dominant with **mild deficiency of glucuronyl transferase**; no kernicterus

► Common Patterns of Liver Disease Presentation

Cholestasis	• Impaired excretion of conjugated bilirubin; can have chalky stool • *Intrahepatic:* viral hepatitis, cirrhosis, drug toxicity • *Extrahepatic:* gallstones, carcinoma of bile ducts, ampulla of Vater or head of pancreas
Hepatic failure	Causes jaundice, encephalopathy, renal failure, palmar erythema, spider angiomas, gynecomastia, testicular atrophy, prolonged prothrombin time, hypoalbuminemia
Chronic passive congestion	• Associated with **right heart failure** • *Pathology:* congestion of central veins and centrilobular hepatic sinusoids (known as **"nutmeg liver"**)

► Acquired Hepatic Diseases

Disease	Form	Features
Alcoholic liver disease		• Three major forms: 1) **fatty liver**, 2) **alcoholic hepatitis**, 3) **alcoholic cirrhosis**
	Fatty liver	• Yellow, greasy liver • Accumulation of lipids within hepatocytes • Potentially reversible
	Alcoholic hepatitis	• Alcoholic hepatitis usually associated with fatty change; occasionally seen with cirrhosis • Results from a heavy drinking binge • *Note:* **Mallory bodies** may be seen, but may also be seen in Wilson disease, hepatocellular carcinoma, and primary biliary cirrhosis • AST/ALT > 2.0 indicates alcoholic liver disease
	Cirrhosis	• Third leading cause of death in the 25- to 65-year-old age group • *Leading etiologies:* **alcoholism** and **hepatitis C**
Alpha-1-antitrypsin deficiency		• Autosomal recessive; characterized by deficiency of a protease inhibitor • Results in **pulmonary emphysema** and **hepatic damage (cirrhosis)**
Budd-Chiari syndrome		• Congestive liver disease secondary to thrombosis of the inferior vena cava or hepatic veins • Causes "nutmeg liver" (also seen in right heart failure) with centrilobular congestion and necrosis • May develop rapidly or slowly; more likely to be fatal if it develops rapidly
Hemochromatosis		• **Primary** form **autosomal recessive** inheritance; **secondary** form usually **related to multiple blood transfusions** • Deposits of iron in the liver, pancreas, heart, adrenal, skin **"bronze diabetes"** • *Also seen:* cardiac arrhythmias, gonadal insufficiency, arthropathy • High incidence of hepatocellular carcinoma
Portal hypertension		• **Intrahepatic:** most common cause and usually secondary to cirrhosis of the liver; *other causes:* schistosomiasis, sarcoid • **Posthepatic:** right-sided heart failure, Budd-Chiari syndrome • **Prehepatic:** portal vein obstruction • *Clinical:* ascites, portosystemic shunts that form hemorrhoids, **esophageal varices**, periumbilical varices (**caput medusae**), **encephalopathy**, splenomegaly • *Additionally,* impaired estrogen metabolism: **gynecomastia**, gonadal atrophy, amenorrhea in females, **spider angiomata**, palmar erythema
Primary biliary cirrhosis		• Autoimmune etiology; causes sclerosing cholangitis, cholangiolitis • Associated with other autoimmune diseases; **primarily affects middle-aged women** • Presents with fatigue and pruritus; elevated alkaline phosphatase • **Antimitochondrial antibody** in over 90% of patients
Secondary biliary cirrhosis		• Longstanding large bile duct obstruction, stasis of bile, inflammation, secondary infection, and scarring • Usually presents with jaundice
Reye syndrome		• Usually affects children between 6 months and 15 years of age • Characterized by **fatty change in the liver, edematous encephalopathy** • *Etiology:* unclear; **frequently preceded by a mild upper respiratory infection**, **varicella**, **influenza** A or B infection • Also associated with **aspirin** administration at levels not ordinarily toxic
Sclerosing cholangitis		• Chronic fibrosing inflammatory disease of the extrahepatic and larger intrahepatic bile ducts • Associated with inflammatory bowel disease; predisposition for cholangiocarcinoma
Wilson disease (hepatolenticular degeneration)		• **Autosomal recessive—inadequate excretion of copper** • *Clinical:* rarely manifests before age 6, then presents with weakness, **jaundice**, fever, angiomas, and eventually **portal hypertension**; ***CNS*** *manifestations:* **tremor**, **rigidity**, disorders of affect and thought • *Labs:* **low serum ceruloplasmin**; ↑ urinary copper excretion • *Pathology:* macronodular cirrhosis, degenerative changes in the lenticular nuclei of brain, pathognomonic **Kayser-Fleischer rings**, a deposition of copper in Descemet membrane of the corneal limbus

▶ Hepatic Tumors

Liver cell adenoma (benign)	• ↑ incidence with **anabolic steroid** and **oral contraceptive use** • Forms a mass, which may be mistaken for carcinoma, or may rupture (especially during pregnancy)
Nodular hyperplasia (benign)	• Appears as solitary nodule that often has a fibrous capsule and bile ductules • Stellate fibrous core usually present • Nodular regenerative hyperplasia—multiple nodules composed of normal hepatocytes with loss of normal architecture
Cholangiocarcinomas	• 10% of primary liver neoplasms; **associated with primary sclerosing cholangitis** • In developing countries, also associated with **infection with *Clonorchis sinensis*** (liver fluke) • *Clinical:* weight loss, jaundice, pruritus • 50% metastasize to lungs, bones, adrenals, and brain, exhibiting both hematogenous and lymphatic spread
Hepatoblastoma	• Rare, malignant neoplasm of children • Hepatomegaly, vomiting, diarrhea, weight loss, elevated serum levels of AFP
Hepatocellular carcinoma	• **90% of primary liver neoplasms; strongly associated with cirrhosis, HCV and HBV** infections • *Clinical:* tender hepatomegaly, ascites, weight loss, fever, polycythemia, hypoglycemia • **Alpha-fetoprotein is present in 50–90%** of patients' serum (AFP also found with other forms of liver disease, pregnancy, fetal neural tube defects, germ-cell carcinomas of the ovaries and testes) • Death due to gastrointestinal bleed and liver failure; generally, metastases first occur in lungs

▶ Hepatic Infections

Acute viral hepatitis	• Can be icteric or anicteric • *Symptoms:* malaise, anorexia, fever, nausea, upper abdominal pain, hepatomegaly • *Labs:* elevated transaminases
Chronic hepatitis	• 5–10% of HBV infections and **well over 50% of HCV**; *other etiologies:* drug toxicity, Wilson disease, alcohol, α-1-antitrypsin deficiency, autoimmune hepatitis • *Histology:* chronic inflammation with hepatocyte destruction, cirrhosis, liver failure
Fulminant hepatitis	• **Massive hepatic necrosis** and progressive hepatic dysfunction; mortality of 25–90% • *Etiologies:* HBV, HCV, delta virus (HDV) superinfection, HEV, chloroform, carbon tetrachloride, certain mushrooms, acetaminophen overdose • *Pathology:* progressive shrinkage of liver as parenchyma is destroyed
Liver abscesses	Pyogenic: • *E. coli, Klebsiella, Streptococcus, Staphylococcus*; ascending cholangitis most common cause • Seeding of liver due to bacteremia another potential cause Parasitic: • *Entamoeba histolytica:* especially in men over age 40 following intestinal disease; thick, brown abscess fluid • *Ascaris lumbricoides:* can cause blockage of bile ducts, eosinophilia, verminous abscesses
Parasitic infections	• **Schistosomiasis:** splenomegaly, portal hypertension, ascites • **Amebiasis:** *Entamoeba histolytica*, bloody diarrhea, pain, fever, jaundice, hepatomegaly

Definition of abbreviations: HBV, hepatitis B virus; HCV, hepatitis C virus.

▶ Characteristics of Viral Hepatitides

	Hepatitis A	Hepatitis B	Hepatitis C	Hepatitis D	Hepatitis E
Nucleic acid	RNA (Picornavirus)	DNA (Hepadnavirus)	RNA (Flavivirus)	RNA	RNA (Hepevirus)
Characteristics	• 50% seropositivity in people >50 • *Clinical disease:* mild or asymptomatic; rare after childhood	• Worldwide carrier rate 300 million • 300,000 new infections/year in U.S.	• 150,000 new cases/year in U.S. • **Most important cause of transfusion-related hepatitis**	• Replication defective • **Dependent on HBV coinfection** for multiplication	**Fulminant** hepatitis 0.3–3%; **20% in pregnant women**
Transmission	• **Fecal-oral**, raw shellfish (concentrate virus) • Not shed in semen, saliva, urine • Shed in stool 2 weeks before onset of jaundice and 1 week after	• **Parenteral**, close personal contact • Transfusion • Dialysis • Needle-sticks • IV drug use • Male homosexual activity	• **Parenteral**, close personal contact • **Route of transmission undetermined in 40–50%** of cases	**Parenteral**, close personal contact	• **Waterborne** • Young adults
Incubation	2–6 weeks	4–26 weeks	2–26 weeks	4–7 weeks in superinfection	2–8 weeks
Carrier state	**None**	1% blood donors	1%	1–10% in drug addicts	Unknown
Progression to chronic hepatitis	None	5–10% acute infections, 90% in infants	**>80%**	• <5% in coinfection* • 80% superinfection†	None
Increased risk of hepatocellular carcinoma	No	**Yes**	**Yes**	**Yes**, same as for B	Unknown, although not likely
Diagnosis	IgM against HAV	• **HBcAb is the 1st antibody, HBsAg indicates current infection** • **HBeAg indicates infectivity**	ELISA for HCV Abs	Ab to Delta Agent plus HBsAg	ELISA for HEV Abs

*Coinfection: hepatitis B and delta agent acquired at the same time
†Superinfection: delta agent acquired during chronic hepatitis B infection

▶ Serology of Hepatitis B Infection

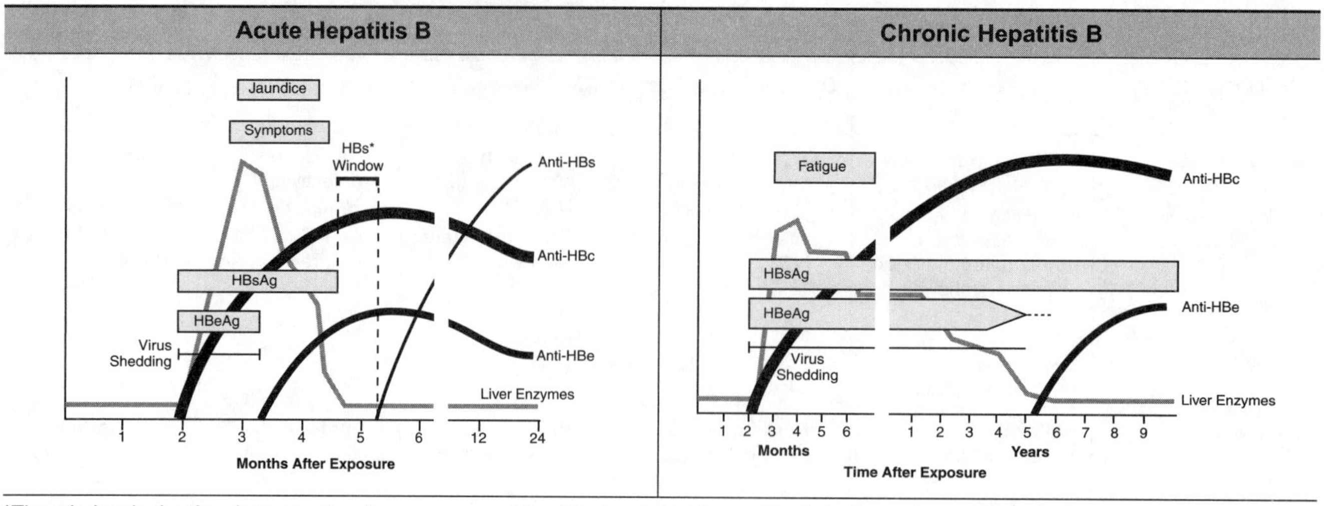

*The window is the time between the disappearance of the HBsAg and before antibody to the surface antigen is detected.

▶ Biliary Disease

Cholelithiasis (gallstones)	• 20% of women and 8% of men in U.S.; rare before age 20, but seen in 25% of persons >60 years • Most stones remain in gallbladder and are asymptomatic • Famous **“4 Fs”: fat, female, fertile (multiparous), older than 40 years** **Three Types of Stones** **Cholesterol Stones** Pure cholesterol stones are radiolucent, solitary, 1–5 cm (diameter), yellow, more common in Northern Europeans **Pigment Stones** • Small, black, multiple, and radiolucent; high incidence in Asians • Associated with **hemolytic disease**, e.g., hereditary spherocytosis • Cholelithiasis occurs in the young; think of hereditary spherocytosis, sickle cell disease, or other chronic hemolytic process **Mixed Stones** • 80% of all stones and **associated with chronic cholecystitis** • Composed of cholesterol and calcium bilirubinate
Carcinoma of gallbladder	• Disease asymptomatic until late • *Symptoms:* dull abdominal pain, mass, weight loss, anorexia • *Pathology:* typically involves fundus and neck; 90% differentiated or undifferentiated adenocarcinomas • Poor prognosis, with 3% 5-year survival rate • *Risk factors:* cholelithiasis and cholecystitis (in up to 90% of patients), porcelain gallbladder (due to calcium deposition in gallbladder wall); occurs predominantly in elderly
Carcinoma of bile ducts (cholangiocarcinoma)	• Not associated with gallstones • Men are affected more frequently; usually elderly • *Symptoms:* obstructive jaundice • *Risk factors:* chronic inflammation, infections, (e.g., liver flukes), ulcerative colitis

Gastrointestinal Microbiology

► Microbial Diarrhea: Organisms Causing Inflammatory Diarrhea/Dysentery

(Invasive Organisms Eliciting Blood, Pus In Stool, Fever)

Organism	Most Common Sources	Common Age Group Infected	Incubation Period	Pathogenesis/ Vignette Clues	Diagnosis	Treatment
Campylobacter jejuni	**Poultry, domestic animals, water**	All	3–5 days	**Invades epithelium**, RBC and WBC in stools (most common bacterial diarrhea in U.S.)	Oxidase ⊕, gram ⊖, curved rod, seagull-wings shape; grows at 42°C; microaerophile	• Treatment for severe cases only • Erythromycin for invasive disease
***Salmonella* spp.**	**Poultry, domestic animals,** water	All	8–48 hours	Penetrates to lamina propria of ileocecal region → **PMN response and prostaglandin synthesis, which stimulates** cAMP	Gram ⊖, motile rods; encapsulated, oxidase ⊖	• Severe cases only • Sensitivity testing required
***Shigella* spp.**	Water, no animal reservoirs, fecal-oral transmission	All	1–7 days	**Shallow mucosal ulcerations and dysentery; septicemia rare**	Gram ⊖ rod; nonlactose fermenting; nonmotile	• Severe cases only • Fluoroquinolones, trimethoprim-sulfamethoxazole
Yersinia enterocolitica	Milk, wild and **domestic animals,** fecal-oral	All	2–7 days	Cold-climate **pseudoappendicitis**; heat-stable enterotoxin; arthritis may occur	Gram ⊖ , motile rod; nonencapsulated, oxidase ⊖; urease ⊕; bipolar staining; best growth at 25°C	• Severe cases only • Aminoglycosides, trimethoprim-sulfamethoxazole
Clostridium difficile	Associated with **antibiotic use**	Pt. on antibiotics	NA	Pt. on antibiotic (clindamycin)	Gram ⊕ rod; anaerobic spore former	Switch antibiotic; metronidazole
Enteroinvasive *E. coli*	Food, water, fecal-oral	Adults	2–3 days	Similar to *Shigella*	Gram ⊖ rod; motile, lactose fermenter; serotyping compares O, H, K antigens	Sensitivity testing required
Entamoeba histolytica	Food, water, fecal-oral	All	2–4 weeks	Trophozoites invade colon; **flask-like lesions, extraintestinal abscesses (liver)**; travelers to Mexico	Motile trophozoites or quadrinucleate cysts	Metronidazole

Definition of abbreviation: Pt., patient.

► Microbial Diarrhea: Organisms Causing Noninflammatory Diarrhea

(Noninvasive Organisms: No Blood, Pus In Stool)

Organism	Most Common Sources	Common Age Group Infected	Incubation Period	Pathogenesis/ Vignette Clues	Diagnosis	Treatment
Rotaviruses	Day care, water, fecal-oral	**Infants** and toddlers	1–3 days	Microvilli of small intestine blunted; dehydration	Diagnosis by exclusion: dsRNA naked, double-shelled, icosahedral (Reovirus family)	Supportive
Norwalk virus Norovirus (Norwalk-like)	Water, food, fecal-oral	**Older kids and adults**	18–48 hours	Blunting of microvilli; "cruise ship" diarrhea	Diagnosis by exclusion: ⊕ ssRNA, naked, icosahedral (Calicivirus family)	Supportive
Adenovirus 40/41	Nosocomial	Young kids, immunocompromised	7–8 days	Death of enteric cells causes diarrhea	Diagnosis by exclusion: naked, dsDNA, icosahedral	No specific therapy
Clostridium perfringens	**Beef, poultry, gravies**, Mexican food	All	8–24 hours	**Enterotoxin**	Anaerobic, gram ⊕ rods, spore-forming, Nagler reaction	Not indicated
Vibrio cholerae	Water, food, fecal-oral	All ages	9–72 hours	• Toxin stimulates adenylate cyclase • Rice water stools	Curved, gram ⊖ rod; oxidase ⊕; "shooting-star" motility	Oral rehydration therapy; tetracycline shortens symptoms
Vibrio parahaemolyticus	Raw or **undercooked shellfish**	Anyone eating raw shellfish	5–92 hours	Self-limited gastroenteritis mimicking cholera	Curved, gram ⊖ rod; oxidase ⊕; "shooting-star" mobility	Not indicated
Enterotoxigenic *E. coli* (ETEC)	Water, uncooked fruits and vegetables	All ages	12–72 hours	**Heat labile toxin (LT) stimulates adenylate cyclase**; stable toxin stimulates guanylate cyclase	Gram ⊖ rod; motile; lactose fermenter; serotyping compares O, H, K antigens	Sensitivity testing required
Enteropathogenic *E. coli* (EPEC)	Food, water, fecal-oral	Infants in developing countries	2–6 days	**Adherence to enterocytes through pili → damage to** adjoining microvilli	Gram ⊖ rod; motile; lactose fermenter; serotyping compares O, H, K antigens	Sensitivity testing required
Enterohemorrhagic *E. coli* (EHEC)	Food, fecal-oral (**hamburger**)	50% <10 years, all	3–5 days	**Verotoxin, which inhibits 60S ribosomal subunit, causes bloody diarrhea, no fever**	• Gram ⊖ rod; motile; lactose fermenter; serotyping compares O, H, K antigens • O157H7 most common • Does not ferment sorbitol	Antibiotics may increase risk of hemolytic-uremic syndrome

(Continued)

► Microbial Diarrhea: Organisms Causing Noninflammatory Diarrhea (CONT'D)
(Noninvasive Organisms: No Blood, Pus In Stool)

Organism	Most Common Sources	Common Age Group Infected	Incubation Period	Pathogenesis/ Vignette Clues	Diagnosis	Treatment
Giardia lamblia	Water, day care, camping, beavers, dogs, etc.	All, children	5–25 days	Cysts ingested; trophozoites; **multiply and attach to small intestinal villi by sucking disk**, cause fat malabsorption → steatorrhea	Flagellated binucleate trophozoites; "falling-leaf" motility; quadrinucleate cysts	Metronidazole
Cryptosporidium parvum	Day care, fecal-oral, animals, homosexuals	Children, AIDS patients	2–4 weeks	Parasites intracellular in brush border	Acid-fast oocytes in stool	Nitazoxanide, puromycin, azithromycin in immunocompromised

► Diarrhea by Intoxication

Organism	Most Common Sources	Common Age Group Infected	Incubation Period	Pathogenesis/ Vignette Clues	Symptoms	Diagnosis	Treatment
Staphylococcus aureus	Ham, potato salad, cream pastries	All	**1–6 hours**	Heat-stable enterotoxin is produced in food (contamination by food handler with skin lesions); food sits at room temperature	Abdominal cramps, vomiting, diarrhea; sweating and headache may occur; no fever	Symptoms, time of onset, food source	Recovery without treatment
***Bacillus cereus:* emetic form**	**Fried rice**	All	**<6 hours**	Heat-stable toxin causes vomiting	Vomiting 1–6 hours; diarrhea 18 hours	Symptoms, time of onset, food source	Recovery without treatment
Bacillus cereus: diarrheal form	Meat, vegetables	All	>6 hours	Heat-labile toxin causes diarrhea (similar to *E. coli* LT)	Nausea, abdominal cramps, diarrhea	Symptoms, time of onset, food source	Recovery without treatment
Clostridium perfringens	Meat, vegetables	All	18–24 hours	Enterotoxin	Nausea, abdominal cramps, diarrhea	Symptoms, time of onset, food source	Recovery without treatment

Definition of abbreviation: LT, labile toxin.

The Endocrine System

Chapter 6

Endocrine System

▶ General Characteristics of Hormones

	Peptides and Proteins (Water Soluble)	Steroids and Thyroid Hormones (Lipid Soluble)
Receptors	Membrane surface	Cytoplasm and/or nucleus
Mechanism	Second messenger	mRNA transcription
Storage	Yes	No (except thyroid as thyroglobulin)
Plasma protein binding	No (except somatomedins)	Yes; acts as pool and prolongs effective half-life
Synthesis	Rough endoplasmic reticulum	Smooth endoplasmic reticulum

Hypothalamus and Pituitary Overview

▶ Hypothalamus-Anterior Pituitary System

Hypothalamus and Anterior Pituitary Vascular System

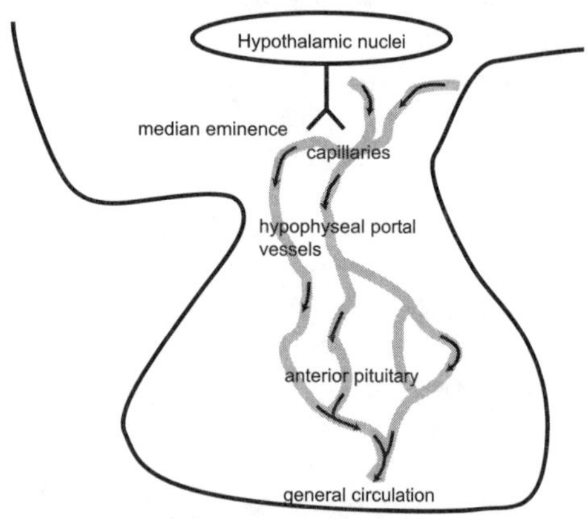

General Characteristics of the Pituitary

	Anterior Pituitary	Posterior Pituitary
Tissue	Glandular	Neuronal
Vascular	Indirect (portal via hypothalamus)	Direct
Control	Neurohormones	Neural
Hormones secreted	TSH, ACTH, LH FSH, GH, prolactin	ADH Oxytocin

Occlusion or lesion of pituitary stalk reduces secretion of all anterior and posterior pituitary hormones, *except* prolactin, which is controlled by inhibitory effects of dopamine.

Hypothalamus	Anterior Pituitary	Peripheral Target
Thyrotropin-releasing hormone (TRH)	Increases secretion of **thyroid-stimulating hormone (TSH)**	TSH stimulates synthesis and secretion of thyroid hormones; hypertrophy of thyroid gland
Corticotropin-releasing hormone (CRH)	Increases secretion of **adrenocorticotropic hormone (ACTH)**	ACTH stimulates synthesis and secretion of cortisol; hypertrophy of adrenal cortex
Gonadotropin-releasing hormone (GnRH)	Increases secretion of **luteinizing hormone (LH)** and **follicle-stimulating hormone (FSH)**	• LH stimulates gonadal steroids • FSH stimulates follicular development (females) and spermatogenesis (males)
Growth hormone–releasing hormone (GHRH) (the dominant control of GH)	Increases secretion of **growth hormone (GH)**	GH actions: causes liver to produce somatomedins; metabolic and growth effects other tissues
Somatostatin (also known as growth hormone–inhibiting hormone [GHIH])	Inhibits secretion of **GH**	—
Prolactin-inhibiting factor (dopamine [PIH])	Inhibits secretion of **prolactin**	Prolactin stimulates lactation and inhibits GnRH, LH, and FSH

▶ Anterior Pituitary Hyperfunction

Hyperprolactinemia	• Elevated serum prolactin associated with prolactinoma (chromophobic); **most common pituitary tumor** • Women: amenorrhea and galactorrhea; men: galactorrhea and infertility • **Treatment:** dopamine agonists (e.g., pergolide, bromocriptine)	
Excess GH	**Gigantism**	• Results from excess GH secretion **before fusion of growth plates** • Excessive skeletal growth may result in heights close to 9 feet • Eosinophilic granuloma
	Acromegaly	• Results from excess GH secretion **after fusion of growth plates** • Circumferential deposition of bones—enlargement of the hands and feet with frontal bossing • Classic case—hat does not fit anymore
Cushing disease	• ACTH-secreting tumors in the anterior pituitary (compare with Cushing syndrome); rarely cause mass effect (see page 373)	
Pathology	• May be micro- or macroadenomas; generally, if active compound is released, lesion is noticed when small • Large lesions can cause mass effect on the optic chiasm; very large masses (10 cm) may invade surrounding structures	

▶ Pituitary Hypofunction

Anterior pituitary hypofunction	• **Sheehan syndrome:** postpartum hemorrhagic infarction of pituitary associated with excessive bleeding; presents as failure to lactate • **Empty sella syndrome:** atrophy of the pituitary; sella is enlarged on skull x-ray and may mimic neoplasm	
Posterior pituitary hypofunction	**Diabetes insipidus (DI)**	• Insufficient or absent antidiuretic hormone • *Clinical:* polydipsia, polyuria, **hypotonic urine, high serum osmolality, hypernatremia** • Central DI responds to exogenous ADH (desmopressin) therapy; nephrogenic DI does not
Posterior pituitary hyperfunction	• **Syndrome of inappropriate ADH secretion (SIADH):** as name suggests, inappropriate, excessive ADH secretion unrelated to serum osmolality • *Causes:* May be paraneoplastic (**small cell lung cancer**), CNS damage, drugs, or infections (TB) • *Clinical:* fluid retention, weight gain, and lethargy, **low serum osmolality, hypertonic urine, hyponatremia**	

Definition of abbreviation: GH, growth hormone.

Adrenal Gland

► Adrenal Hormones

Adrenal Gland: Cortex and Medulla

The Adrenal Gland

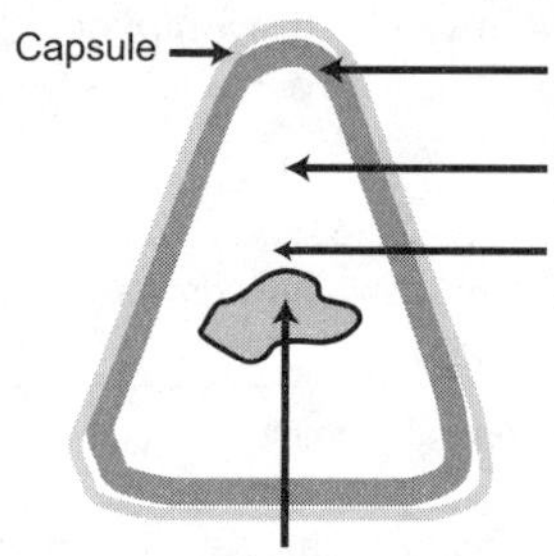

Region	Hormones	Control system
Zona Glomerulosa	Aldosterone	Angiotensin II, $[K^+]_{plasma}$
Zona Fasciculata	Cortisol	ACTH
Zona Reticularis	Androgens	ACTH (LH has no effect here)

Medulla, produces epinephrine, controlled by sympathetic nervous system

Control of Cortisol

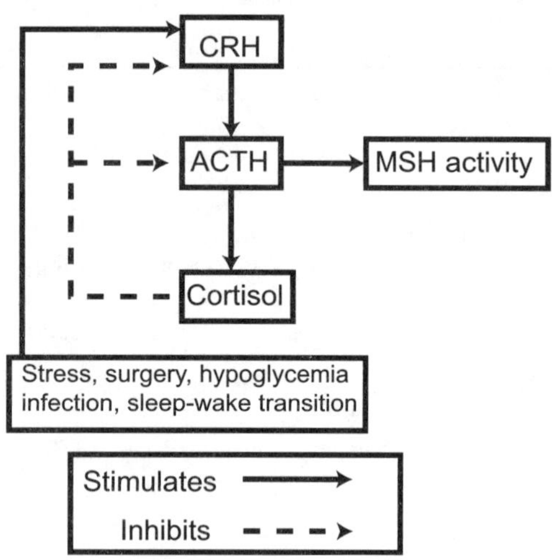

Actions of Cortisol

Carbohydrates	• Inhibits response to insulin • Promotes liver gluconeogenesis from amino acids • Inhibits cellular glucose uptake and utilization of glucose for energy • Raises blood glucose
Fats	Promotes lipolysis (permissive for catecholamines and glucagons) and release of fatty acids and glycerol into blood
Proteins	Promotes protein catabolism to provide substrates of gluconeogenesis
Vascular	• Increases response to catecholamines • Cortisol deficiency → hypotension

Note: Fragments of ACTH precursor proopiomelanocortin (POMC) are also released and have biologic effects, notably melanocyte-stimulating hormone (MSH) activity.

▶ Cushing Syndrome

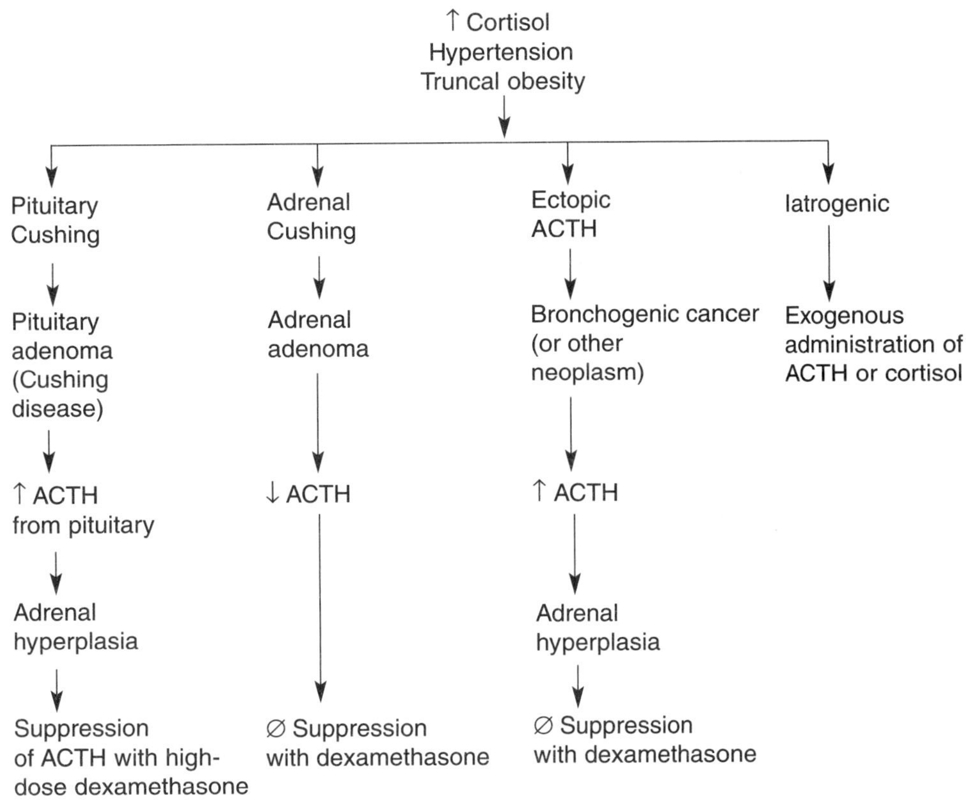

Cushing (pituitary)	↑ cortisol ↑ ACTH
Cushing (adrenal)	↑ cortisol ↓ ACTH ↑ aldosterone (often)

Clinical
Truncal obesity, buffalo hump, moon facies, facial plethora, hirsutism, menstrual disorders, hypertension, muscle weakness, back pain (osteoporosis), striae, acne, psychological disorders, bruising

▶ Differential Diagnosis of Cortisol Excess and Deficiency Based on Feedback Control

Disorder	Plasma Cortisol	Plasma CRH	Plasma ACTH	Hyperpigmentation
Primary (adrenal) excess	↑	↓	↓	No
Primary deficiency	↓	↑	↑	Yes
Secondary (pituitary) excess	↑	↓	↑	Yes
Secondary deficiency	↓	↑	↓	No
Steroid administration (synthetics other than cortisol)	↓ (but symptoms of excess)	↓	↓	No

► Aldosterone

Actions of Aldosterone

	Renal	Effects
Na^+	Reabsorption	↑ total body Na^+
K^+	Secretion	↓ plasma $[K^+]$
H^+	Secretion	Metabolic alkalosis
HCO_3^-	Production	Metabolic alkalosis
H_2O	Reabsorption	Volume expansion

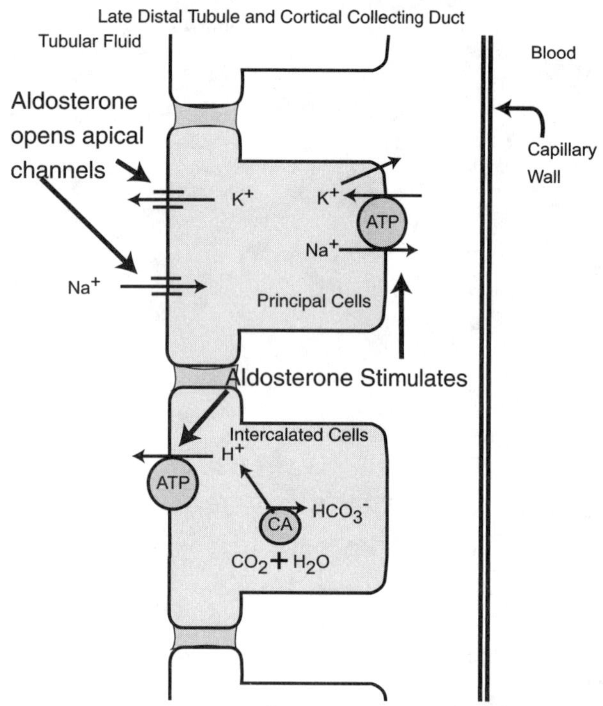

Control of Aldosterone

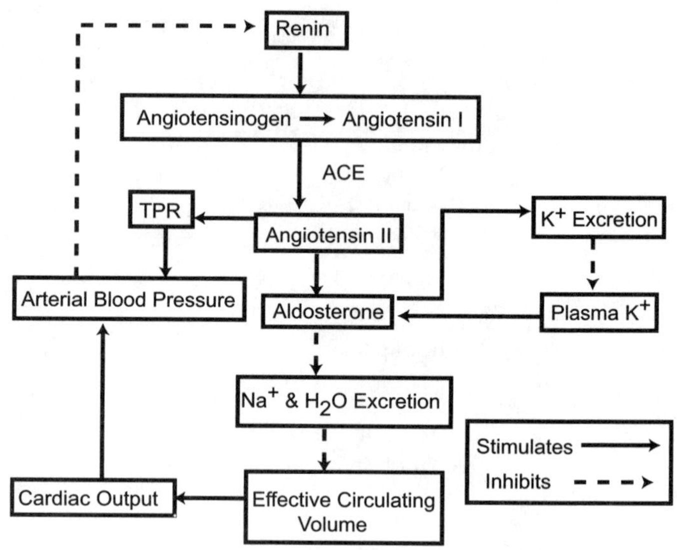

Aldosterone promotes isoosmotic **reabsorption of sodium and water**. It also causes **secretion of acid** into urine and addition of bicarbonate to blood.

Definition of abbreviations: ACE, angiotensin-converting enzyme; CA, carbonic anhydrase; TPR, total peripheral resistance.

► Long-Term Control of Blood Pressure by Renin-Angiotensin-Aldosterone

Event	Effects	Compensation
Volume expansion Saline infusion Polydipsia	↑ preload, cardiac output, and BP	• ↓ renin →↓ AII and ALD • ↓ AII, ↓ ALD →↓ Na^+ and H_2O reabsorption →↑ urine flow →↓ EFV →↓ preload and cardiac output →↓ BP to normal
Volume loss Hemorrhage Dehydration	↓ preload, cardiac output, and BP	↑ renin →↑ AII and ALD →↑ Na^+ and H_2O reabsorption → ↓ urine flow →↑ EFV →↑ preload and cardiac output toward normal →↑ BP to normal
Heart failure	↓ cardiac output and BP	↑ renin →↑ AII and ALD → ↑ Na^+ and H_2O reabsorption →↓ urine flow →↑ EFV →↑ preload and cardiac output toward normal

Definition of abbreviations: AII, angiotensin II; ALD, aldosterone; BP, blood pressure; EFV, extracellular fluid volume.

▶ Hyperaldosteronism

Primary hyperaldosteronism (Conn syndrome)	• ↑ aldosterone secretion • Adrenal adenoma most common cause • **Clinical:** diastolic hypertension, weakness, fatigue, polyuria, polydipsia, headache, no edema • **Lab values: hypokalemia, low renin levels, metabolic alkalosis, hypernatremia**, failure to suppress aldosterone with salt loading • **Pathology:** single well-circumscribed adenoma with lipid-laden clear cells
Secondary hyperaldosteronism	• Etiologies: congestive heart failure, decreased renal blood flow (increased renin), renin-producing neoplasms, and Bartter syndrome (juxtaglomerular cell hyperplasia, hyperreninemia, hyperaldosteronism) • **Clinical:** Same as for primary, but edema may be present • **Lab values: high renin levels, hypernatremia, hypokalemia**

▶ Steroid Synthetic Pathways Most Commonly Involved in Pathology

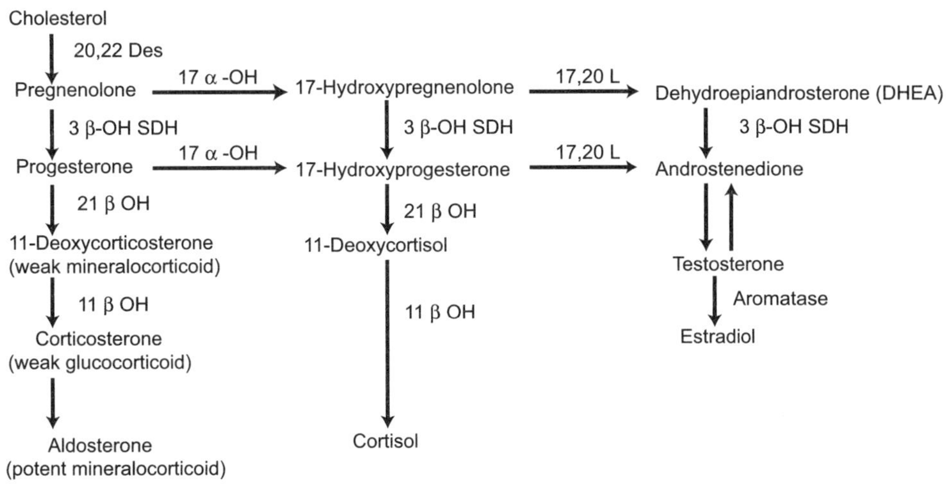

20,22 Des (20,22 Desmolase)
3 β-OH SDH (3 β-Hydroxysteroid Dehydrogenase)
21 β OH (21 β-Hydroxylase)
17 α -OH (17 α-Hydroxylase)
17,20 L (17,20 Lyase)
11 β OH (11 β-Hydroxylase)

Simplified scheme for understanding enzyme deficiencies; a vertical cut (e.g., 17 α -OH deficiency) all products to the right are deficient (cortisol, androgens) and products to the left are in excess (mineralocorticoids); a horizontal cut (e.g., 11 β OH) all products above are excess (11-Deoxycorticosterone, 11-Deoxycortisol, androgens) and below are deficient (Aldosterone, Cortisol).

Congenital Adrenal Hyperplasia	• Usually due to a congenital enzyme deficiency characterized by **cortisol deficiency and enlargement of adrenal glands** • The 3 most common forms **all cause virilism** and are called **adrenogenital syndromes**: – **Partial 21-hydroxylase deficiency:** normal aldosterone function and impaired cortisol production. – **Salt-losing syndrome: near total 21-hydroxylase deficiency** and aldosterone deficiency; infants present with vomiting, dehydration, hyponatremia, hyperkalemia – **11-hydroxylase deficiency:** leads to excessive androgen production and buildup of 11-deoxycorticosterone (a weak mineralocorticoid, which, in excess, has a strong mineralocorticoid effect), causing virilization, hypertension, hypokalemia

► Congenital Enzyme Deficiency Syndromes

Enzyme Deficiency	Glucocorticoids	Mineralocorticoids	Androgens	Other Effects
20,22 desmolase	↓	↓	↓	Lethal if complete
3 β-OH SDH	↓	↓	↑ DHEA	• Masculinization of females in utero • Incomplete precocious puberty (males) • Adrenal hyperplasia • Hyponatremia and hypovolemia
21 β-OH	↓	↓	↑	• Masculinization of females in utero • Incomplete precocious puberty (males) • Adrenal hyperplasia • Hyponatremia and hypovolemia
11 β-OH	↓	↓ aldosterone ↑↑↑ DOC*	↑	• Mineralocorticoid excess (DOC) • Hypervolemia and hypernatremia • Sexual effects as above
17 α-OH	↓	↓ aldosterone ↑↑↑ DOC*	↓↓	• DOC excess • Absent secondary sexual aspects both sexes • Amenorrhea
17, 20 L	Normal	Normal	↓↓	• Absent secondary sexual aspects both sexes • Amenorrhea

*11-deoxycorticosterone, a weak mineralocorticoid that causes symptoms of mineralocorticoid overload when excessive amounts are secreted

► Adrenal Cortical Hypofunction

Acute adrenocortical insufficiency	• Rapid withdrawal of exogenous steroids in patients with chronic adrenal suppression • Adrenal apoplexy seen in **Waterhouse-Friderichsen syndrome** (adrenal hemorrhage associated with meningococcal septicemia)
Primary adrenocortical insufficiency (Addison disease)	• Etiology: most common cause autoimmune adrenalitis; other causes: tuberculosis, other infections, iatrogenic, metastases, adrenal hemorrhage, pituitary insufficiency • For clinically apparent insufficiency, 90% of the adrenal gland must be nonfunctional • **Clinical:** weakness, weight loss, anorexia, nausea, vomiting, hypotension, skin pigmentation, hypoglycemia with prolonged fasting, inability to tolerate stress, abdominal pain • **Lab values:** hyponatremia, hypochloremia, hyperkalemia, metabolic acidosis; ACTH levels high, cortisol and ALD levels low • **Pathology:** bilateral atrophied adrenal glands • ACTH and MSH share amino acid sequences; in cases of high ACTH → skin pigmentation
Secondary (pituitary) adrenocortical insufficiency	• **Etiology:** metastases, irradiation, infection, infarction, affecting the hypophysial-pituitary axis • Results in decreased ACTH (less skin pigmentation)
Hypoaldosteronism	Hyponatremia, hypovolemia, hypotension, metabolic acidosis, hyperkalemia
Primary	• ↓ aldosterone, ↑ renin and AII
Secondary	• ↓ aldosterone, ↓ renin and AII, ↓ total peripheral resistance

Definition of abbreviations: AII, angiotensin II; ACTH, adrenocorticotropic hormone; ALD, aldosterone; MSH, melanocyte-stimulating hormone.

▶ Adrenal Cortical Neoplasms

Adrenal adenomas	• Mostly asymptomatic and not steroid-producing • Steroid-producing adenomas may produce Conn syndrome, Cushing syndrome, or virilization in women • **Pathology:** small and unilateral nodule, yellow-orange on cut section, poorly encapsulated
Adrenal carcinomas	• Relatively rare and usually very malignant • Greater than 90% are steroid-producing • Pathology: tumors often large and yellow with areas of hemorrhage and necrosis

▶ Adrenal Medulla

Tissue	Hormones	Control	Actions
Neural, chromaffin	Epinephrine (80%) Norepinephrine (20%)	Sympathetic nervous system	Glycogenolysis, lipolysis, ↑ blood glucose, ↑ metabolic rate (requires cortisol and thyroid)

Disorders of Adrenal Medulla	
Pheochromocytoma	• Neoplasm of **neural crest-derived chromaffin cells** that secrete catecholamines (norepinephrine and epinephrine) → hypertension • Highest incidence in children and adults age 30–50 • **Clinical:** paroxysmal or constant hypertension is most classic symptom; also, sweating, headache, arrhythmias, palpitations • **Lab values:** elevated urinary homovanillic acid (HVA) and vanillylmandelic acid (VMA) • **The Rule of 10s for pheochromocytoma:** – 10% extra-adrenal – 10% bilateral – 10% malignant – 10% affect children – 10% familial
Neuroblastoma	• **Most common malignant extracranial solid tumor of childhood** • Occurs most frequently in the adrenal medulla, but may arise in sympathetic chain • Amplification of the **N-*myc*** oncogene—more copies = more aggressive • **Clinical:** tumors grow rapidly, metastasize widely (especially to bone); prognosis in younger patients (less than 1 year old) better than for older children • **Pathology:** lobulated with areas of necrosis, hemorrhage, calcification • **Microscopic appearance:** rosette pattern of small cells

▶ Treatment for Adrenocortical Disease

Class	Mechanism	Indications
Glucocorticoids (hydrocortisone)	Replacement therapy	For adrenocortical insufficiency (Addison disease, acute adrenal insufficiency from other causes)
Mineralocorticoids (fludrocortisone)	Replacement therapy	For chronic treatment of Addison disease in patients requiring mineralocorticoids
Glucocorticoid synthesis inhibitors (aminoglutethimide metyrapone ketoconazole)	Inhibits glucocorticoid synthesis via different mechanisms	To suppress adrenocortical steroid production in variety of disorders, e.g., Cushing disease, Cushingoid states, congenital adrenal hyperplasia

▶ Antidiuretic Hormone and Control of Osmolarity and Volume

Normal function of antidiuretic hormone (ADH, vasopressin): prevents changes of plasma osmolarity, restores normal blood volume and blood pressure, ↑ **permeability of renal collecting duct to water,** ↑ **reabsorption of water, causes** ↓ **urine flow, and** ↑ **urine osmolarity**

ADH Control of Plasma Osmolarity and ECF Volume	Release of ADH from the Pituitary
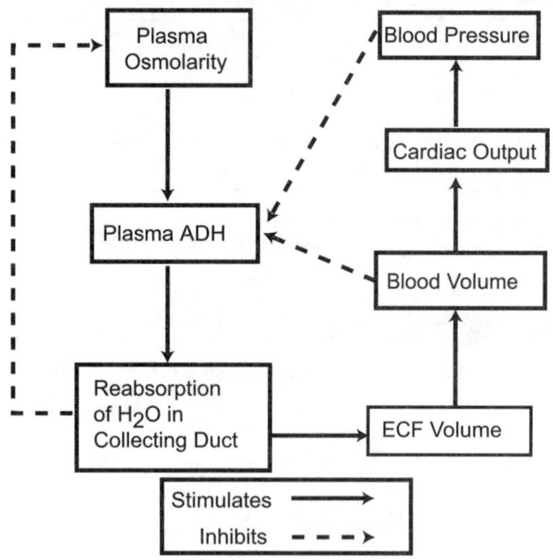	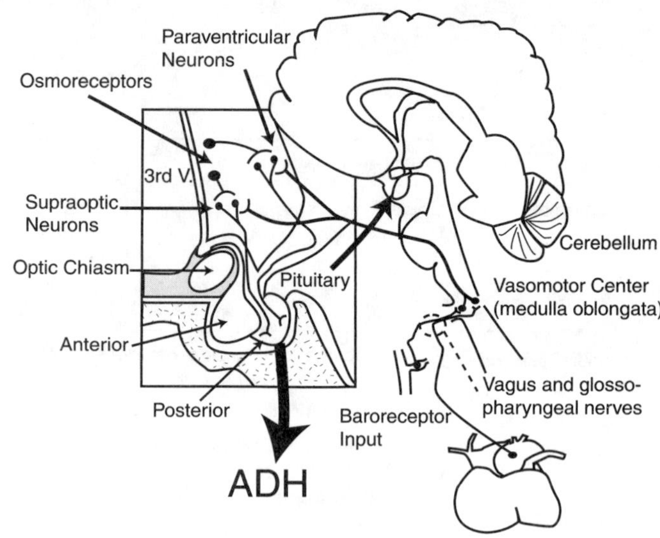

Secretion of ADH by neurons with cell bodies located in the **supraoptic and paraventricular nuclei** of the hypothalamus is **under the control of osmoreceptors and baroreceptors.** The osmoreceptors are in the AV3V region and are influenced by blood osmolarity. Atrial stretch receptors (detecting blood volume) are the largest cardiovascular influence, and arterial baroreceptors, including the carotid sinus (moderate effect) and the aortic arch (minor effect), are processed in medullary centers that regulate cardiovascular function, such as the nucleus tractus solitarius (NTS). The NTS sends efferents to the ADH-secreting neurons. The axon terminals of these neurons are in the posterior pituitary and release the hormone into the blood. Normally, osmolarity dominates control of ADH secretion; extreme changes of blood volume or cardiac output can overrride osmolarity.

▶ Disorders of Antidiuretic Hormone (Vasopressin)

Diabetes insipidus ↓ ADH (central, neurogenic) ↓ response (nephrogenic)	• Hypovolemia, hypernatremia, metabolic alkalosis, tendency toward hypotension, large volume of dilute urine (distinguishes from dehydration) • Distinguish central versus nephrogenic by testing response to ADH injection (nephrogenic → no response; central → response = concentration of urine)
Dehydration (water deprived) ↑ ADH to compensate	Hypovolemia, hypernatremia, metabolic alkalosis, tendency toward hypotension, small volume of concentrated urine (distinguishes from diabetes insipidus)
Syndrome of inappropriate ADH (SIADH; ↑ ADH)	Hypervolemia, hyponatremia, metabolic acidosis, small volume of concentrated urine (distinguishes from polydipsia)
Primary polydipsia	Hypervolemia, hyponatremia, large volume of dilute urine

▶ Atrial Natriuretic Peptide

Secretion	• Secreted by **heart (right atrium)** • Stimulated by **stretch (blood volume)**
Actions	• ↑ renal sodium excretion due to ↑ GFR and ↓ reabsorption of sodium (late distal tubule and collecting duct) • ↓ reabsorption of water due to ↓ reabsorption of sodium • Inhibits response to ADH
Clinical	• No known disorder caused by deficiency • Elevated levels have clinical use as index of the severity of congestive heart failure

Pancreas

▶ Endocrine Pancreas

Hormones of the Islets of Langerhans

Hormone	Control of Secretion	Target Tissues	Actions
Insulin (β cells)	• Glucose, amino acids • Effect of glucose via ↑ ATP, closes ATP-dependent K^+ channels, producing depolarization and exocytosis of insulin • Gastric inhibitory peptide (GIP) stimulates release	Liver	↑ glucose uptake (enzymatic effect) ↑ glucose utilization ↑ triglyceride synthesis ↑ protein synthesis ↑ glycogen synthesis ↓ gluconeogenesis ↓ glycogenolysis ↓ lipolysis ↓ protein catabolism ↓ ureagenesis, ketogenesis ↓ **blood glucose concentration**
		Muscle	↑ glucose uptake (GLUT4 transport) ↑ glucose utilization ↑ protein synthesis ↓ glycogenolysis ↓ protein catabolism ↓ **blood glucose concentration**
		Adipose	↑ glucose uptake (GLUT4 transport) ↑ triglyceride synthesis (↑ lipoprotein lipase to ↑ uptake of fatty acids) ↓ lipolysis (↓ hormone-sensitive lipase) ↓ **blood glucose concentration**
Glucagon (α cells)	• Glucose inhibits • Hypoglycemia stimulates • Amino acids stimulate	Liver	↑ gluconeogenesis ↑ glycogenolysis ↑ lipolysis ↑ protein catabolism ↑ ureagenesis, ketogenesis ↑ **blood glucose concentration**
Somatostatin (δ cells)	Stimulated by glucose, amino acids, fatty acids	Pancreas, GI tract	Inhibits secretion of insulin and glucagon; role is disputed

▶ Integrated Control of Plasma Glucose by Insulin and Glucagon

Use the fact that a carbohydrate meal increases plasma glucose as a sample application. Tracking through the feedback diagram predicts effects on carbohydrate, fat, and protein metabolism.

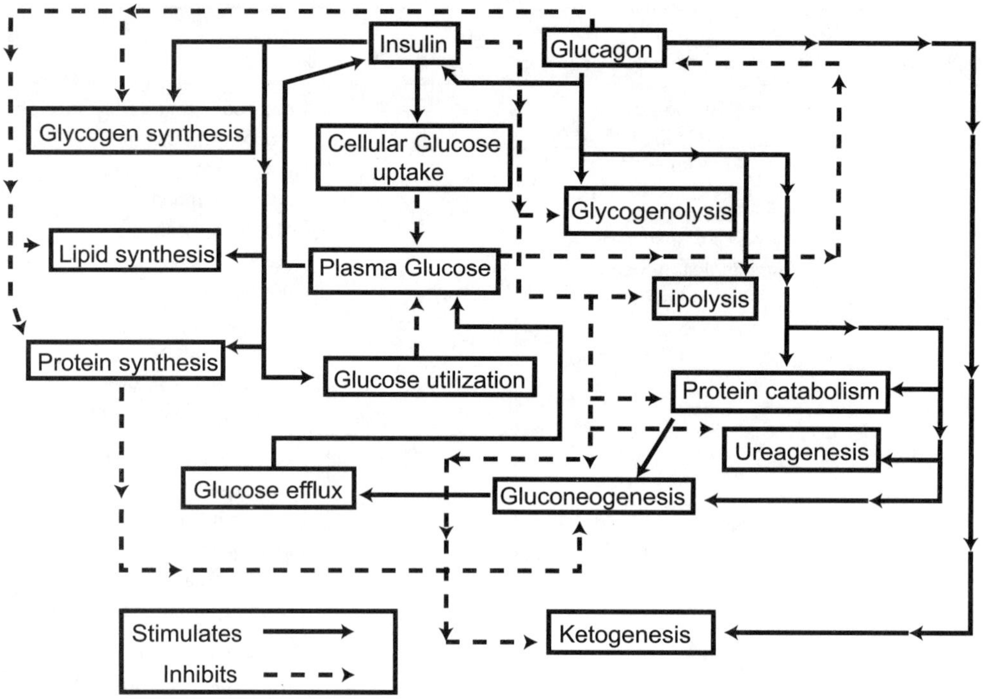

▶ Summary of Glucose Counter-Regulation

Hormone	Stimulus	Actions
Glucagon	• Fasting, hypoglycemia, stress • **Insulin/glucagon ratio is key to metabolism balance**	• Inhibits response to insulin (mainly in liver) • Promotes catabolism, gluconeogenesis, glycogenolysis
Cortisol	Stress, fasting, hypoglycemia	• Inhibits response to insulin • Reduces cellular glucose uptake • Permissive for lipolysis • Increases gluconeogenesis and protein catabolism • Inhibits cellular glucose uptake
Epinephrine	Stress, severe hypoglycemia	• Increases glycogenolysis and lipolysis
Growth hormone	Fasting, sleep, stress	• Inhibits cellular uptake of glucose • Stimulates lipolysis
Thyroid hormone	Cold, stress	• Permissive for epinephrine's effects • Required for production of GH

▶ Insulin-Related Pathophysiology

	Glucose	Insulin	C-peptide	Ketoacidosis	Other Features
Diabetes type 2	↑	↑ or ↔	↑ or ↔	Uncommon	Familial, often obese
Diabetes type 1	↑	↓	↓	Yes	Often islet antibodies
Insulinoma	↓	↑	↑	No	Tachycardia (epinephrine)
Insulin overdose	↓	↑	↓	No	Tachycardia (epinephrine)
Fasting hypoglycemia	↓	↑	↑	No	Insulin remains at postprandial level in fasting
Reactive hypoglycemia	↓	↑	↑	No	Excessive secretion with oral glucose tolerance test

▶ Disorders of the Endocrine Pancreas

Diabetes mellitus (DM) **Type 1**	• Often, abrupt onset with **ketoacidosis** • Marked, absolute insulin deficiency, resulting from **diminished β-cell mass** • Characterized by **low serum insulin** levels
Type 2	• Constitutes most cases of idiopathic diabetics, characterized by **peripheral insulin resistance** • Most patients have **central obesity**; onset of disease usually after age 40 • These patients are **not prone to ketoacidosis**
Acute metabolic complications of diabetes	• **Diabetic ketoacidosis** (DKA) may occur in type 1 diabetics, rarely in type 2 • Metabolic acidosis results from accumulation of ketones • High blood glucose → dehydration via an **osmotic diuresis** • Treatment with insulin normalizes the metabolism of carbohydrate, protein, fat • Fluids given to correct the dehydration • **Hyperosmolar nonketotic coma** in patients with mild type 2; blood glucose can be elevated; treatment similar to treatment of DKA
Late complications of diabetes	• Series of long-term complications, including **atherosclerosis** (leading to strokes, myocardial infarcts, gangrene), **nephropathy, neuropathy** (distal, symmetric polyneuropathy with "stocking-glove" distribution), **retinopathy** that may lead to blindness • Patients with DM are also at high-risk for: – ***Klebsiella pneumoniae*** – **Sinus mucormycosis** – **Malignant otitis externa (*Pseudomonas aeruginosa*)**
ß-cell tumors	• Insulinomas most commonly occur between ages of 30 and 60 • **Pathogenesis:** β-cell tumors produce hyperinsulinemia → hypoglycemia • **Clinical features:** patients experience episodes of altered sensorium (i.e., disorientation, dizziness, diaphoresis, nausea, tremulousness, coma), which are relieved by glucose intake • **Pathology:** most tumors solitary, well-encapsulated, well-differentiated adenomas of various sizes.; 10% are malignant carcinomas
Zollinger-Ellison syndrome	• Due to gastrinoma and often associated with **MEN type I** • **Pathogenesis:** tumors of pancreatic islet cells secrete gastrin → gastric hypersecretion of acid • **Clinical:** includes intractable peptic ulcer disease and severe diarrhea • **Pathology:** 60% malignant; most tumors located in pancreas (10% in duodenum)
MEN I	• Tumors of parathyroids, adrenal cortex, pituitary gland, pancreas • Associated with peptic ulcers and Zollinger-Ellison syndrome
MEN IIa	Tumors of adrenal medulla (pheochromocytoma), medullary carcinoma of thyroid, parathyroid hyperplasia or adenoma
MEN IIb/III	Medullary carcinoma of the thyroid, pheochromocytoma, and mucosal neuromas.

► Treatment of Diabetes

Insulin				
Classes	**Insulin Types**	**Onset (hours)**	**Peak (hours)**	**Duration (hours)**
Rapid-acting	Lispro, aspart, glulisine	0.25	0.5–1.5	3–5
Short-acting	Regular	0.5–1	2–4	5–8
Intermediate-acting	NPH	1–3	8	12–16
Long-acting	Glargine, detemir	1	No peak	20–26

Noninsulin Antidiabetic Agents		
Drug	**Mechanism**	**Notes**
Insulin secretagogues • **Sulfonylureas** – **First generation (tolbutamide, chlorpropamide)** – **Second generation (glipizide, glyburide, glimepiride)** • **Meglitinides (repaglinide, nateglinide)**	• Block K^+ channels → depolarization of pancreatic β cells → ↑ Ca^{2+} influx → insulin release	• Requires functional β cells • Repaglinide: faster onset and shorter duration than sulfonylureas; taken before meals to control postprandial glucose levels • Side effects: hypoglycemia, weight gain
Biguanides (metformin)	May ↑ tissue sensitivity to insulin and/or ↓ hepatic gluconeogenesis	• Does not require functional β cells • Will not cause hypoglycemia • Most serious side effect: lactic acidosis
Thiazolidinediones (rosiglitazone, pioglitazone)	• Bind nuclear peroxisome proliferator-activated receptor-γ (PPAR-γ receptor) • ↑ target tissue sensitivity to insulin, inhibits hepatic glucose output, ↑ glucose uptake	• Hypoglycemia rare • Weight gain, edema
α-Glucosidase inhibitors (acarbose, miglitol)	Inhibits intestinal brush border α-glucosidase →↓ glucose absorption →↓ postprandial glucose →↓ demand for insulin	• GI distress, flatulence, diarrhea
Drugs affecting glucagon-like peptide-1 (GLP-1) (exenatide*, sitagliptin)	• GPL-1, an incretin released from the small intestine in response to food, augments glucose-dependent insulin release, inhibits glucagon secretion, slows gastric emptying, and increases feelings of satiety • Exenatide: long-acting GLP-1 receptor agonist • Sitagliptin: oral DDP-4 inhibitor, prevents the breakdown of GLP-1	• Extenatide: nausea, hypoglycemia when combined with sulfonylureas • Sitagliptin: headache, URI, nasopharyngitis
Pramlintide*	Synthetic analog of amylin, which decreases glucagon release, slows gastric emptying, and promotes satiety	• Used in type 1 and type 2 DM • Hypoglycemia, GI disturbances

Hyperglycemic Drugs		
Glucagon	↑ hepatic glycogenolysis and gluconeogenesis, ↑ heart rate and force of contraction, relaxes smooth muscle	• Administered via intramuscular injection • Major side effect: hyperglycemia • Glucagon receptors stimulate adenylate cyclase and ↑ cAMP; this is basis for its use in beta-blocker overdose

* Exanatide and pramlintide are injectables, the rest are given orally

Definition of abbreviations: DDP-4, dipeptidyl peptidase 4; URI, upper respiratory infection

Endocrine Regulation of Calcium and Phosphate

▶ Overview of Hormonal Regulation of Calcium and Phosphate

Hormone	Site Produced	Stimuli to Secretion or Production	Effect on Plasma Free Ca^{2+}	Effect on Plasma Phosphate
Parathyroid Hormone (PTH)	Parathyroid gland	Low plasma Ca^{2+}	↑	↓
1,25-$(OH)_2$-vitamin D_3	Skin → liver → kidney	Sunlight, PTH, dietary intake	↑	↑
Calcitonin (not essential for control)	Parafollicular cells of thyroid	High plasma Ca^{2+}	↓	Little net effect

▶ Parathyroid Hormone

Effects on kidneys	• Calcium ↑ reabsorption • Phosphate ↓ reabsorption • Vitamin D ↑ production of active form 1,25 $(OH)_2$ vitamin D_3 from precursor 25-OH D_3 formed in liver
Effects on bone	• Receptors on osteo*blasts*, not on osteo*clasts* • Rapid mobilization of Ca^{2+} and phosphate from bone fluid • ↑ osteoclast activity via mediators released from osteoblasts • Causes bone resorption, release of Ca^{2+}, phosphate into plasma
Effects on GI tract	Indirectly stimulates Ca^{2+} and phosphate absorption in small intestine through its effect to produce active form of vitamin D_3

▶ Vitamin D (Calcitriol)

Effects on kidneys	↓ Ca^{2+} and phosphate excretion (by ↑ reabsorption of both)
Effects on bone	↑ resorption (with PTH); releases Ca^{2+} and phosphate into plasma (but normal growth and maintenance also requires both vitamin D and PTH)
Effects on GI tract	↑ Ca^{2+} and phosphate absorption in intestine, ↑ both in plasma

▶ Calcitonin

Effects on kidneys	↑ phosphate excretion; ↓ Ca^{2+} excretion (minor effect)
Effects on bone	↓ resorption; ↑ deposition; ↓ plasma Ca^{2+} (major effect)
Effects on GI tract	↑ Ca^{2+} and phosphate absorption in intestine (minor effect)

▶ Regulation of Calcium and Phosphate

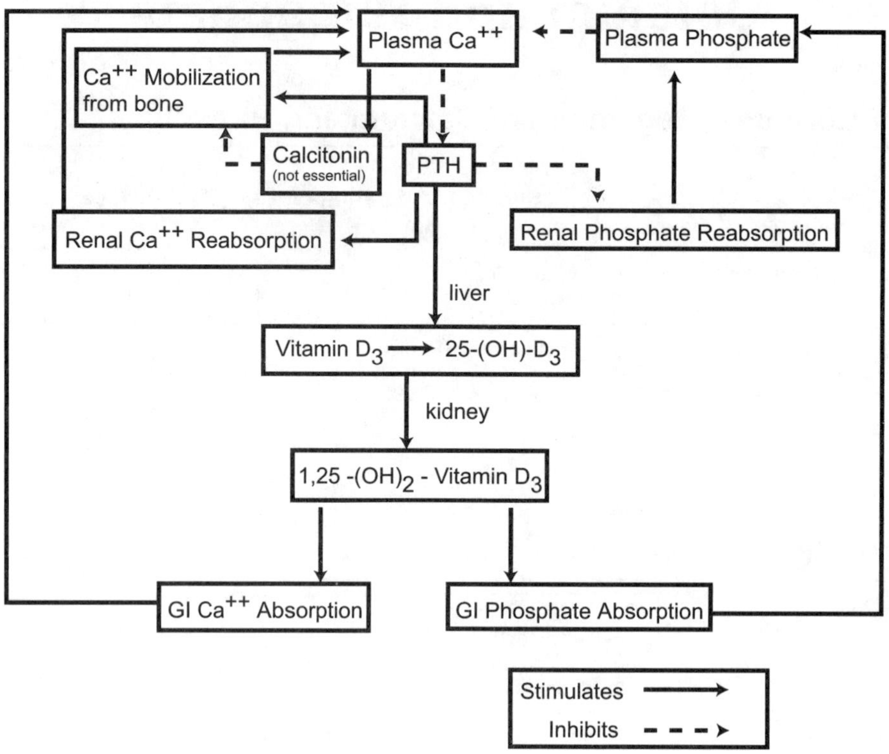

▶ Disorders of Calcium and Phosphate Regulation

	Plasma (Ca^{2+})	Plasma (Phosphate)	Effects on Bone
Primary hyperparathyroidism	↑	↓	Demineralization and osteopenia
Primary hypoparathyroidism	↓	↑	Malformation
Deficient vitamin D (secondary hyperparathyroidism)	↓	↓	• Osteomalacia in adults • Rickets in children
Excess vitamin D (secondary hypoparathyroidism)	↑	↑	Osteoporosis
Renal failure with high plasma phosphate (secondary hyperparathyroidism)	↓ (precipitation)	↑	Osteomalacia and osteosclerosis

Note: Clinical presentation of hypocalcemia often includes muscle spasms and tetany; hypercalcemia presents with weakness and flaccid paralysis.

► Pathophysiology of Calcium Homeostasis

Primary hyperparathyroidism	• Parathyroid adenoma is the most common cause; can see in MEN I and MEN IIa • **Clinical:** elevated serum calcium often asymptomatic • **Lab values: ↑ PTH and alkaline phosphatase, hypercalcemia, hypophosphatemia**
Osteitis fibrosa cystica (von Recklinghausen disease of bone)	• Occurs in **chronic primary hyperparathyroidism** • Cystic changes in bone occur due to osteoclastic resorption • Fibrous replacement of resorbed bone may lead to a non-neoplastic “brown tumor”
Secondary hyperparathyroidism	• Usually caused by **chronic renal failure** and decreased Ca^{2+} absorption, stimulating PTH • Hyperphosphatemia due to decreased phosphate excretion in renal failure causes hypocalcemia; this provokes increased PTH secretion. Treatment to lower plasma phosphate is often effective. • Vitamin D deficiency and malabsorption less common causes • May show soft tissue calcification and osteosclerosis • **Lab values: ↑ PTH and alkaline phosphatase, hypocalcemia, hyperphosphatemia**
Hypoparathyroidism	• Common causes are accidental removal during thyroidectomy, idiopathic, and DiGeorge syndrome • **Clinical:** irritability, anxiety, tetany, intracranial and lens calcifications • **Lab values: hypocalcemia, hyperphosphatemia**
Pseudohypoparathyroidism	• Autosomal dominant disorder, resulting in kidney unresponsive to circulating PTH • Skeletal abnormalities: short stature, shortened fourth and fifth carpals and metacarpals
Hypercalcemia	• **Mnemonic** “MISHAP”: Malignancy, Intoxication (vitamin D), Sarcoidosis, Hyperparathyroidism, Alkali syndrome (Milk-Alkali), and Paget disease • **Clinical:** renal stones, abdominal pain, drowsiness, metastatic calcification

► Drugs in Bone and Mineral Disorders

Drug	Mechanism	Notes
Bisphosphonates (alendronate, etidronate, pamidronate, risedronate)	↓ bone resorption	• Osteoporosis • Paget disease • Esophageal ulceration may occur

Thyroid

▶ Physiologic Actions of Thyroid Hormone

Metabolic rate	↑ metabolic rate: high O_2 consumption, mitochondrial growth, ↑ Na^+/K^+-ATPase activity, ↑ food intake, thermogenesis, sweating, ↑ ventilation
Energy substrates	Mobilization of carbohydrates, fat and protein; ↑ ureagenesis; ↓ muscle and adipose mass
Growth	Required after birth for normal brain development and bodily growth (protein anabolic)
Circulation	↑ cardiac output (linked to metabolism), ↑ β-adrenergic receptors on heart

▶ Control of Thyroid Hormone

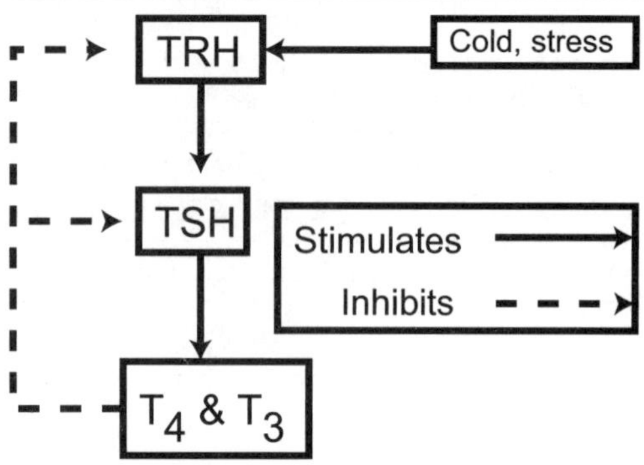

TRH = thyrotropin-releasing hormone (**hypothalamus**)

TSH = Thyroid-stimulating hormone (**anterior pituitary**); is also trophic (increases gland mass)

T_4 = thyroxine (tetraiodothyronine); 90% of production, but low biologic activity (**thyroid**)

T_3 = triiodothyronine; 10% of production, very potent (**thyroid**)

▶ Synthesis and Storage

Process	Mechanism	Result
Uptake of I^-	Active transport	↑ follicular cell iodide
Oxidation	Peroxidase	Produce oxidized iodine
Iodination	Peroxidase	Produces MIT and DIT within thyroglobulin
Coupling	Peroxidase	Links MITs and DITs to form T_4 and T_3
Exocytosis	Exocytosis into lumen	Storage of thyroglobulin

Definition of abbreviations: DIT, diiodotyrosine; MIT, monoiodotyrosine.

► Secretion

Process	Mechanism	Result
Transport	Endocytosis	Colloid taken up by follicular cells
Fusion	Lysosomes and colloid fuse	Incorporation in lysosomes
Proteolysis	Lysosomal enzymes	Cleave thyroglobulin into T_3, T_4, MITs, and DITs
Secretion	Simple diffusion	Lipid-soluble T_3 and T_4 diffuse into extracellular fluid to plasma
Deiodination	Deiodinase	Removes iodide from MITs and DITs to recycle it

► Regulation of Thyroid Activity

Transport	99% bound to thyroid binding globulin, 1% free; represents a pool to prevent rapid change of thyroid level
Peripheral Conversion	T_4 converted to more active T_3 by 5′-monodeiodinase or to inactive reverse T_3 by 5-monodeiodinase; occurs in most tissues giving local control of hormone action
Mechanism of action	Binding to nuclear receptors: T_4 has low affinity, T_3 has high affinity, so is responsible for most thyroid hormone effects
Degradation	Successive deiodination steps to thyronine, also sulfates and glucuronides

► Thyroid Disorders

Disorder	T_4	TSH	TRH	Gland Mass
Primary hypothyroidism	↓	↑	↑	↑, goiter possible
Pituitary hypothyroidism	↓	↓	↑	↓, due to low TSH
Hypothalamic hypothyroidism	↓	↓	↓	↓, due to low TSH
Iodine deficiency (prolonged, severe)	↓	↑	↑	↑, goiter likely
Pituitary hyperthyroidism	↑	↑	↓	↑, goiter possible
Primary hyperthyroidism (tumor)	↑	↓	↓	↓, due to low TSH
Graves disease (autoimmune production of thyroid-stimulating immunoglobulins [TSIs])	↑	↓	↓	↑, goiter possible

► Disorders of the Thyroid Gland

Hyperthyroidism	• Seen most often in Graves disease, toxic multinodular goiter, toxic adenoma • Clinical: tachycardia, cardiac palpitations (β-adrenergic effect), skin warm and flushed, ↑ body temperature, heat intolerance, hyperactivity, tremor, weight loss, osteoporosis, diarrhea and oligomenorrhea, eyes show a wide stare with lid lag; **exophthalmos** seen **only in Graves disease** • Thyrotoxic storm: severe hypermetabolic state with 25% fatality • **Lab values:** low TSH and elevated T_4; low TSH is most important • Note: in pregnancy, ↑ in TBG secondary to high estrogen levels elevates total serum T_4, but not free serum T_4
Graves disease	• Peaks in the third and fourth decades; more common in women; associated with other autoimmune diseases (including Hashimoto thyroiditis) • Type II non-cytotoxic hypersensitivity • Production of TSI and TGI bind and activate TSH receptors • **Pathology:** diffuse, moderate, symmetric enlargement of gland • **Microscopic appearance:** hypercellular with small follicles and little colloid
Hypothyroidism	• Clinical features depend on age group • Lab values: elevated TSH and low T_4
Infants	• Develop **cretinism**; major effects are on skeletal and CNS development; once apparent, syndrome is irreversible; neonatal screening for elevated TSH for early detection • **Clinical:** protuberant abdomen, wide-set eyes, dry rough skin, broad nose, delayed epiphyseal closure
Older children	Short stature, retarded linear growth (GH deficiency caused by thyroid hormone deficiency), delayed onset of puberty
Adults	• Lethargy, weakness, fatigue, decreased appetite, weight gain, cold intolerance, constipation • Myxedema: associated with severe hypothyroidism; periorbital puffiness, sparse hair, cardiac enlargement, pleural effusions, anemia
Hashimoto thyroiditis	• Chronic lymphocytic thyroiditis featuring goitrous thyroid gland enlargement • Autoimmune; may be autoantibodies to the TSH receptors, T_3 and T_4; **antimicrosomal antibodies** also seen • Type IV hypersensitivity • **Most common type of thyroiditis;** highest incidence in **middle aged females** • **Pathology:** painless goiter, gland enlarged and firm • **Microscopic appearance:** lymphocytic and plasma cell infiltrate with **Hürthle cells** (follicular cells with eosinophilic granular cytoplasm), evidence of cell-mediated cytolysis
Diffuse nontoxic goiter	Diffuse enlargement of gland in euthyroid patients; high incidence in certain geographic areas with iodine-deficient diets
de Quervain granulomatous subacute thyroiditis	• Self-limited disease; seen more often in females in the second to fifth decades • Follows **viral** syndrome, lasts several weeks with a **tender** gland • May initially have mild hyperthyroidism later, usually euthyroid
Riedel thyroiditis	• Rare, chronic thyroid disease, possibly of immune origin, that causes dense fibrosis of the thyroid gland leading to hypothyroidism • Presents with a hard, fixed, painless goiter • May be associated with idiopathic fibrosis in other sites such as the retroperitoneum
Thyroglossal duct cyst	• May communicate with skin or base of tongue • Remnant of incompletely descended midline thyroid tissue
Ectopic thyroid nests	Usually at the base of tongue; prior to removal, it must be documented that patient has other functioning thyroid tissue

Definition of abbreviations: GH, growth hormone; TBG, thyroid-binding globulin; TGI, thyroid growth immunoglobulin; TSI, thyroid-stimulating immunoglobulin; TSH, thyroid-stimulating hormone.

► Drugs for Thyroid Gland Disorders

Class	Mechanism	Comments/Agents
Hyperthyroidism Agents	These agents are used for short-term or long-term treatment of hyperthyroid states. The most common adverse effects are related to signs and symptoms of hypothyroidism.	
Thioamides	• Inhibit synthesis of thyroid hormones • They do *not* inactivate existing T_4 and T_3 • Propylthiouracil is able to inhibit peripheral conversion of T_4 to T_3	• **Examples: PTU, methimazole** • **Indications:** long-term hyperthyroid therapy, which may lead to disease remission and short-term treatment before thyroidectomy or radioactive iodine therapy • **Side effects:** skin rash (common), hematologic effects (rare)
Iodides	• Inhibit the release of T_4 and T_3 (primary) • Inhibit the biosynthesis of T_4 and T_3 and ↓ the size and vascularity of thyroid gland	• **Examples:** Lugol's solution (iodine and potassium iodide) and potassium iodide alone • **Indications:** preparation for thyroid surgery; treatment of thyrotoxic crisis and thyroid blocking in radiation emergency • **Note:** therapeutic effects can be seen for as long as 6 weeks
Beta-Blockers	Nonselective β-receptor blockers used for palpitations, anxiety, tremor, heat intolerance; partially inhibit peripheral conversion of T_4 to T_3	• **Examples: nadolol, propranolol** • Used to treat the signs and symptoms of hyperthyroidism
Radioactive Iodine [^{131}I]	Ablation of thyroid gland	• **Indications:** first-line therapy for Graves disease; treatment of choice for recurrent thyrotoxicosis in adults and elderly
Hypothyroidism Agents	These agents are used as thyroid replacement therapy. The most common adverse effects are related to signs and symptoms of hyperthyroidism.	
Thyroid Hormones	Acts by controlling DNA transcription and protein synthesis	**Examples:** synthetic T_4, synthetic T_3, or combination of synthetic T_4:T_3 in 4:1 ratio

Definition of abbreviation: PTU, propylthiouracil.

► Thyroid Neoplasms

Adenomas	• Follicular adenoma is most common; may cause pressure symptoms, pain, and rarely thyrotoxicosis • **Pathology:** usually small, well-encapsulated solitary lesions
Papillary carcinoma	• Most common thyroid carcinoma • Incidence higher in women • **Pathology:** papillary branching pattern; 40% have tumors containing psammoma bodies • Spread to local nodes is common; **hematogenous spread rare** • Resection curative in most cases
Follicular carcinoma	• More malignant than papillary cancer • **Pathology:** may be encapsulated, with penetration through the capsule; colloid sparse • Local invasion and pressure → dysphagia, dyspnea, hoarseness, cough • **Hematogenous metastasis to lungs or bones common**
Medullary carcinoma	• Arises from parafollicular C cells • Secretes calcitonin • May be associated with MEN IIa and IIb
Anaplastic carcinoma	• Rapid growing, aggressive with poor prognosis; affects older patients • **Pathology:** tumors usually bulky and invasive with undifferentiated anaplastic cells • **Clinical:** early, widespread metastasis and death within 2 years

Growth Hormone

▶ Control of Growth Hormone

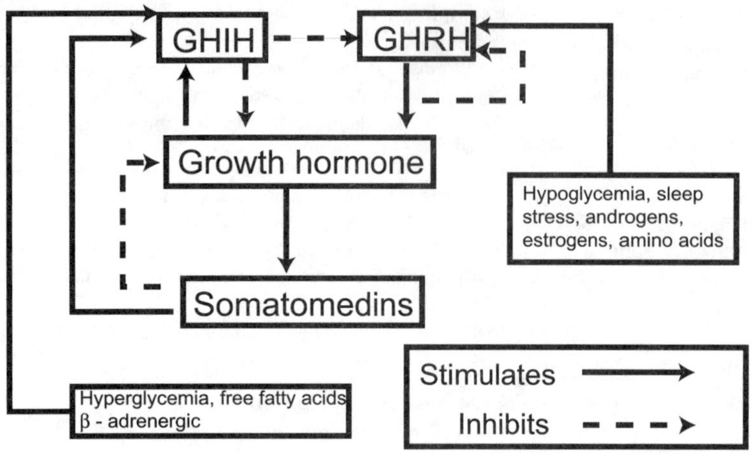

Secretion of GH

- Pulsatile, ↑ during sleep
- Moderate in childhood
- Increases at puberty
- Lower in adults
- Secretion requires thyroid hormone
- Increased by sex steroids

▶ Biologic Actions of Growth Hormone

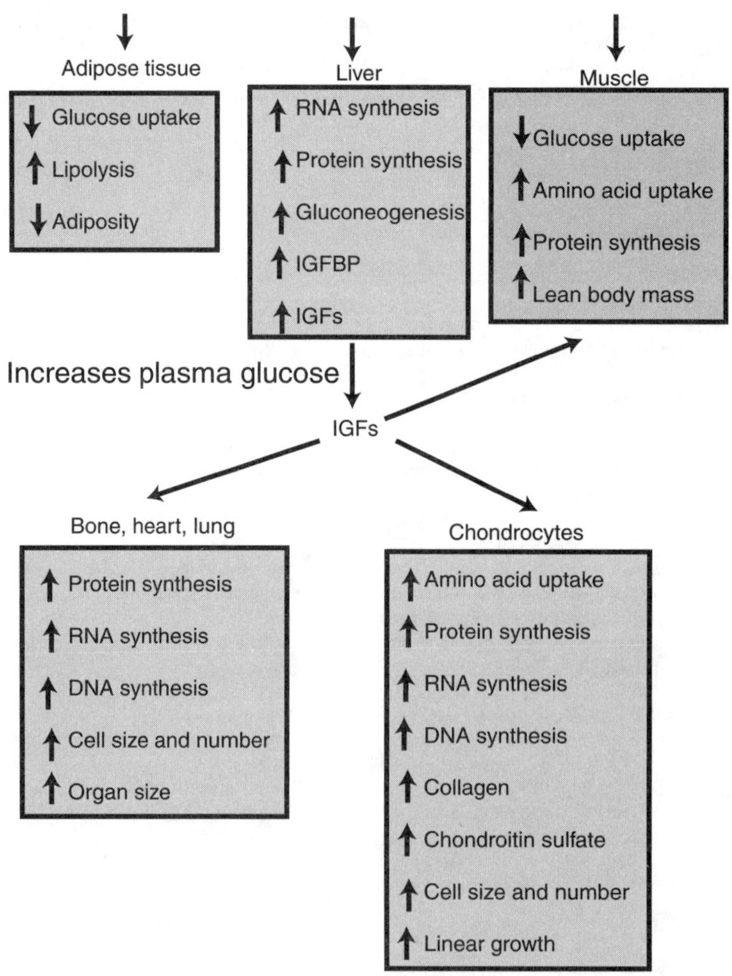

► Childhood Disorders

Dwarfism	• Caused by: – ↓ GH or ↓ liver production of IGF (Laron syndrome) – Defective GH receptors • Mental development normal • Reversible with GH treatment
Gigantism	• Caused by ↑ GH prior to epiphyseal closure • Increased height, increased body mass

Definition of abbreviation: GH, growth hormone; IGF, insulin-like growth factor.

► Adult Disorders of Growth Hormone

Acromegaly	↑ GH	• Enlargement of hands and feet • Protrusion of lower jaw, coarse facial features • ↑ lean body mass • ↓ body fat • ↑ size of visceral organs • Impaired cardiac function (related to mass) • Abnormal glucose tolerance with tendency to hyperglycemia
Deficiency	↓ GH	• Tendency to hypoglycemia when fasting • Susceptible to insulin-induced hypoglycemia • Significance of other effects disputed

Definition of abbreviation: GH, growth hormone.

► Treatment of Growth Hormone Disorders

Class	Mechanism	Comments/Agents
GH	Stimulation of linear/skeletal growth (pediatric patients only); potentiation of cell and organ growth; enhanced protein, carbohydrate and lipid metabolism	• **Somatropin** and **somatrem** (recombinant forms of human GH) • **Indications:** growth failure, Turner syndrome, cachexia, somatotropin deficiency
Octreotide	• Long-acting octapeptide that mimics somatostatin • Inhibits release of GH, glucagon, gastrin, thyrotropin, insulin	• **Indications:** acromegaly, carcinoid, glucagonoma, gastrinoma, other endocrine tumors

Definition of abbreviation: GH, growth hormone.

The Reproductive System

Chapter 7

Reproductive System

► Male and Female Development

Adult Female and Male Reproductive Structures Derived From Precursors of the Indifferent Embryo		
Adult Female	**Indifferent Embryo**	**Adult Male**
Ovary, follicles, rete ovarii	Gonads	Testes, seminiferous tubules, rete testes
Uterine tubes, uterus, cervix, and upper part of vagina	Paramesonephric ducts	Appendix of testes
Duct of Gartner	Mesonephric ducts	Epididymis, ductus deferens, seminal vesicle, ejaculatory duct
Clitoris	Phallus	Glans and body of penis
Labia minora	Urogenital folds	Ventral aspect of penis
Labia majora	Labioscrotal swellings	Scrotum

Congenital Reproductive Anomalies

Female Pseudointersexuality

- 46,XX genotype
- Have ovarian (but no testicular) tissue and masculinization of the female external genitalia
- Most common cause is **congenital adrenal hyperplasia**, a condition in which the fetus produces excess androgens

Male Pseudointersexuality

- 46,XY genotype
- Testicular (but no ovarian) tissue and stunted development of male external genitalia
- Most common cause is inadequate production of testosterone and müllerian-inhibiting factor (MIF) by the fetal testes; due to a 5α-reductase deficiency

5α-reductase 2 deficiency	• Caused by a mutation in the **5α-reductase 2 gene** that renders 5α-reductase 2 enzyme underactive in catalyzing the conversion of testosterone to dihydrotestosterone • *Clinical findings:* underdevelopment of the penis and scrotum (microphallus, hypospadias, and bifid scrotum) and prostate gland; epididymis, ductus deferens, seminal vesicle, and ejaculatory duct are normal • At puberty, they undergo virilization due to an increased **T:DHT ratio**
Complete androgen insensitivity (CAIS, or testicular feminization syndrome)	• Occurs when a fetus with a 46,XY genotype develops testes and female external genitalia with a rudimentary vagina; the uterus and uterine tubes are generally absent • Testes may be found in the labia majora and are surgically removed to circumvent malignant tumor formation • Individuals present as normal-appearing females, and their psychosocial orientation is female despite their genotype • Most common cause is a mutation in the **androgen receptor (AR) gene** that renders the AR inactive

▶ Male and Female Reproductive Anatomy

Male

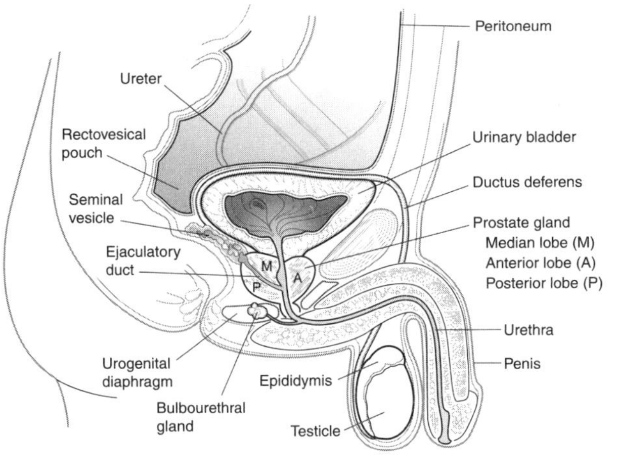

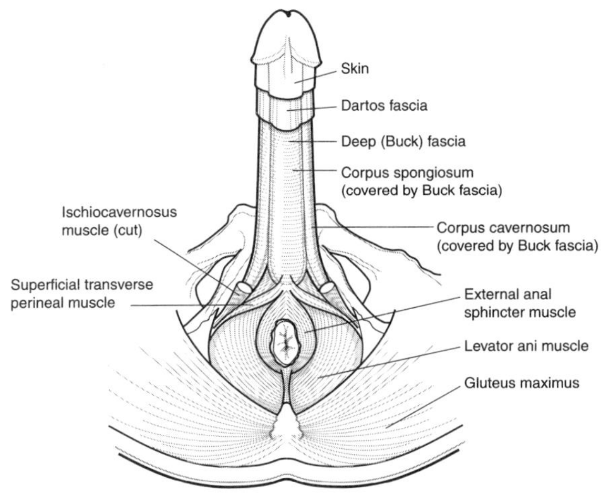

Female

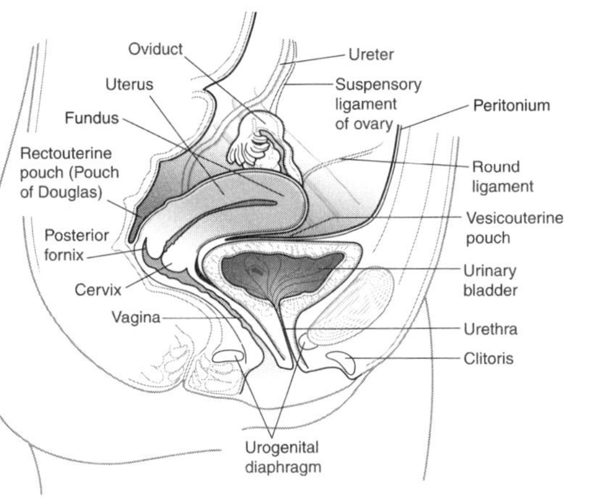

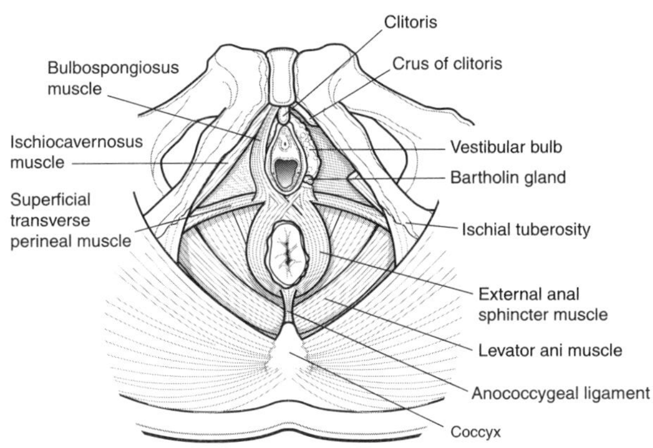

Pelvic Floor and Perineum

- The floor of the pelvis is formed by the **pelvic diaphragm** (two layers of fascia with a middle layer of skeletal muscle).
- The muscles forming the middle layer are the **levator ani** and **coccygeus**. The levator ani acts as a muscular sling for the rectum and marks the boundary between the rectum and anal canal.
- The region below the pelvic diaphragm is the **perineum**, which contains the **ischioanal fossa**, the fat-filled region below the pelvic diaphragm surrounding the anal canal.
- The **urogenital diaphragm** is in the perineum and extends between the two ischiopubic rami. The urogenital diaphragm (like the pelvic diaphragm) is composed of two layers of fascia with a middle layer of skeletal muscle.

(Continued)

► Male and Female Reproductive Anatomy (*Cont'd.*)

Perineal Pouches	
Deep perineal pouch (space)	The deep perineal pouch is the middle (muscle) layer of the urogenital diaphragm. It contains: • Sphincter urethrae muscle—serves as external sphincter of the urethra • Deep transverse perineal muscle • Bulbourethral (Cowper) gland (in the male only)—duct enters bulbar urethra
Superficial perineal pouch (space)	The superficial perineal pouch is the region below the urogenital diaphragm and is enclosed by the superficial perineal (Colles) fascia. It contains: • Crura of penis or clitoris—erectile tissue • Bulb of penis (in the male)—erectile tissue; contains urethra • Bulbs of vestibule (in the female)—erectile tissue; in lateral walls of vestibule • Ischiocavernosus muscle—skeletal muscle that covers crura of penis or clitoris • Bulbospongiosus muscle—skeletal muscle that covers bulb of penis or bulbs of vestibule • Greater vestibular (Bartholin) gland (in female only)—homologous to Cowper gland

Pelvic Innervation
The **pudendal nerve (S2, S3, S4 ventral rami) and its branches** innervate the skeletal muscles in the pelvic and urogenital diaphragms, the external anal sphincter and the sphincter urethrae, skeletal muscles in both perineal pouches, and the skin that overlies the perineum.

Male Reproductive System

► Male Reproductive Physiology

Penile Erection
Erection occurs in response to **parasympathetic** stimulation (pelvic splanchnic nerves). **Nitric oxide** is released, causing relaxation of the corpus cavernosum and corpus spongiosum, which allows blood to accumulate in the trabeculae of erectile tissue.

Ejaculation
• **Sympathetic** nervous system stimulation (lumbar splanchnic nerves) mediates movement of mature spermatozoa from the epididymis and vas deferens into the ejaculatory duct. • Accessory glands, such as the bulbourethral (Cowper) glands, prostate, and seminal vesicles, secrete fluids that aid in sperm survival and fertility. • **Somatic motor efferents** (pudendal nerve) that innervate the bulbospongiosus and ischiocavernous muscles at the base of the penis stimulate the rapid ejection of semen out the urethra during ejaculation. Peristaltic waves in the vas deferens aid in a more complete ejection of semen through the urethra.

Clinical Correlation
• Injury to the bulb of the penis may result in extravasation of urine from the urethra into the superficial perineal space. From this space, urine may pass into the scrotum, into the penis, and onto the anterior abdominal wall. • Accumulation of fluid in the scrotum, penis, and anterolateral abdominal wall is indicative of a laceration of either the membranous or penile urethra (deep to Scarpa fascia). This can be caused by trauma to the perineal region (saddle injury) or laceration of the urethra during catheterization.

▶ Agents for Erectile Dysfunction

Drug	Mechanism	Comments
Selective phosphodiesterase (PDE) 5 inhibitors **(sildenafil, vardenafil, tadalafil)**	Inhibits the enzyme phosphodiesterase (PDE) 5, which inactivates cGMP, leading to ↑ cGMP → vasodilation, more inflow of blood → better erection	PDE 5 inhibitors + **nitrates** (which ↑ cGMP production) → **severe hypotension**
Synthetic prostaglandin E_1 (PGE_1) agents **(alprostadil)**	↑ cAMP (via adenylate cyclase) → smooth muscle relaxation	Administered via transurethral or intracavernosal injection *Contraindications:* intercourse with pregnant women (can stimulate uterine contractions unless used with a condom); conditions that might predispose a patient to priapism (e.g., sickle cell anemia, multiple myeloma, leukemia)
Testosterone	Replacement/supplementation for males whose serum androgen concentrations are below normal	Used if diminished libido is a significant patient complaint

▶ Diseases of the Penis and Prostate

Noninfectious Disorders of the Penis	
Hypospadias and epispadias	With hypospadias, urethra opens onto the ventral surface of penis Often associated with a poorly developed penis that curves ventrally, known as **chordee** With epispadias, urethra opens onto dorsal surface; often associated with exstrophy of bladder Either of these malformations may cause infertility
Phimosis	Prepuce orifice too small to be retracted normally Interferes with hygiene; can also predispose to bacterial infections; if foreskin retracted over the glans, it may lead to urethral constriction → paraphimosis *Treatment:* circumcision
Penile carcinoma	
Bowen disease	Carcinoma in situ; can be associated with visceral malignancy Men >35 years; tends to involve shaft of the penis and scrotum *Gross:* thick, ulcerated plaque *Micro:* squamous cell carcinoma in situ
Squamous cell carcinoma	1% of cancers in men in the United States, usually age 40–70. Usually slow growing and non-painful; patients often delay seeking medical attention. Circumcision decreases the incidence. Human Papilloma virus (types 16 and 18) infection is closely associated. Gross: Plaque progressing to an ulcerated papule or fungating growth. Metastases can go to local lymph nodes.
Peyronie disease	Curved penis due to fibrosis of the tunica albuginea

(Continued)

▶ Diseases of the Penis and Prostate (*Cont'd.*)

Diseases of the Prostate	
Prostatic carcinoma	• Most common cancer in men; usually occurs after age 50, and the incidence increases with age • Associated with race (more common in African Americans than in Caucasians, relatively rare in Asians) • May present with urinary problems or a palpable mass on rectal examination • Prostate cancer more common than lung cancer, but lung cancer is bigger killer • Metastases may occur via the lymphatic or hematogenous route • Bone commonly involved with osteoblastic metastases, typically in the pelvis and lower vertebrae • Elevated PSA, together with an enlarged prostate on digital rectal exam, highly suggestive of carcinoma • Most patients present with advanced disease and have a 10-year survival rate of <30% • *Treatment:* surgery, radiation, and hormonal modalities (orchiectomy and androgen blockade).
Benign prostatic hyperplasia	• Formation of large nodules in the periurethral region (median lobe) of the prostate • May narrow the urethral canal to produce varying degrees of urinary obstruction and difficulty urinating • It is increasingly common after age 45; incidence increases steadily with age • Can follow an asymptomatic pattern, or can result in urinary symptoms and urinary retention
Prostatitis	
Acute	• Results from a bacterial infection of the prostate • Pathogens are often organisms that cause urinary tract infection • *Escherichia coli* most common • Bacteria spread by direct extension from the posterior urethra or the bladder; lymphatic or hematogenous spread can also occur
Chronic	• Common cause of recurrent urinary tract infections in men • Two types: bacterial and nonbacterial • Both forms may be asymptomatic or may present with lower back pain and urinary symptoms

▶ Antiandrogens

Drug	Mechanism	Clinical Uses
Flutamide	Androgen receptor antagonist	Prostate cancer
Spironolactone	Androgen receptor antagonist (also a potassium-sparing diuretic)	Hirsutism (also used for primary hyperaldosteronism, edema, hypertension)
Leuprolide	GnRH analog	Depot form is used for prostate cancer
Finasteride	5α-reductase inhibitor (prevents conversion of testosterone to DHT)	Benign prostatic hypertrophy (BPH), male pattern baldness
Ketoconazole	Inhibits steroid synthesis (also an antifungal agent)	Androgen receptor–positive prostate cancer

Definition of abbreviation: DHT, dihydrotestosterone.

▶ The Testes

Descent of the Testes	
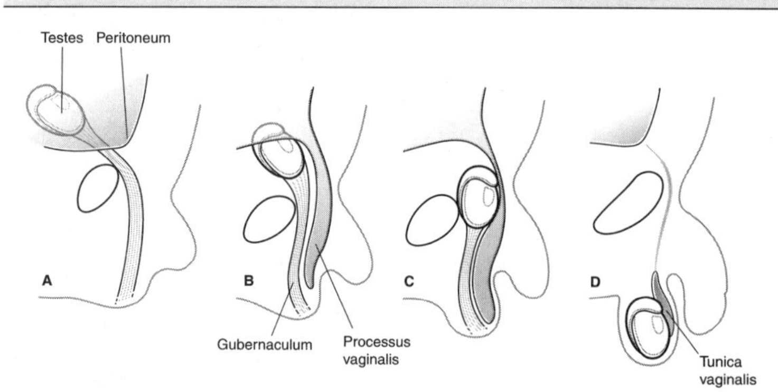	The **processus vaginalis** is an evagination of parietal peritoneum that descends through the inguinal canal during fetal life. The **tunica vaginalis** is a patent remnant of the processus vaginalis that covers the anterior and lateral parts of the testis. A **hydrocele** is an accumulation of serous fluid in the tunica vaginalis or in a persistent part of the processus vaginalis in the cord.

(Continued)

▶ The Testes (*Cont'd.*)

Normal Anatomy and Anatomic Abnormalities

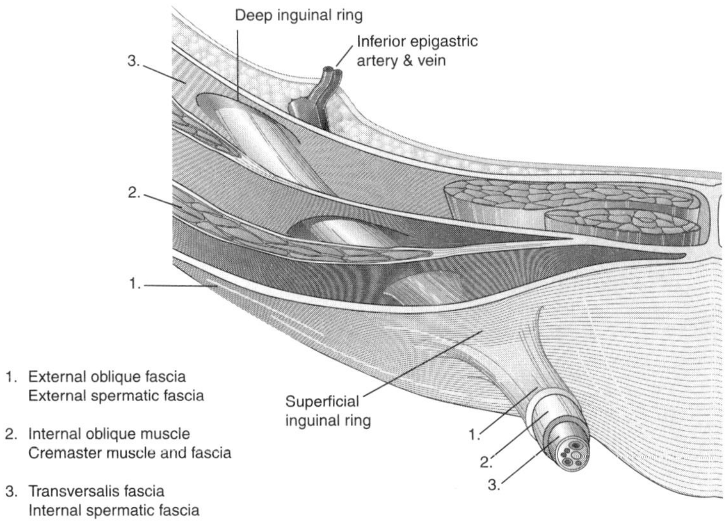

The **inguinal canal** is formed by four of the eight tissue layers of the anterior abdominal wall; outpocketings of three of these layers give rise to **spermatic fasciae**, which cover the testis and structures in the **spermatic cord**.

The spermatic cord contains the:

- **Ductus deferens**, which conveys sperm from the epididymis to the ejaculatory duct in the male pelvis
- **Testicular artery**, which arises from the abdominal aorta between the L2 and the L3 vertebrae
- **Artery to the ductus deferens**, which arises from a branch of the internal iliac artery
- **Pampiniform plexus of the testicular vein**
- **Right testicular vein**, which drains into the inferior vena cava
- **Left testicular vein**, which drains into the left renal vein.
- **Lymphatic vessels** that drain the testis. Testicular lymphatic vessels pass through the inguinal canal and drain directly to **lumbar nodes** in the posterior abdominal wall.

Cremasteric Reflex

The **cremasteric reflex** utilizes sensory and motor fibers in the ventral ramus of the L1 spinal nerve. Stroking the skin of the superior and medial thigh stimulates sensory fibers of the **ilioinguinal nerve**. **Motor fibers** from the genital branch of the **genitofemoral nerve** cause the cremaster muscle to contract, elevating the testis.

Abnormalities

Cryptorchidism	• Failure of normal descent of intra-abdominal testes into the scrotum • Most common location of a cryptorchid testis is in the inguinal canal • Unilateral or bilateral, more often on right side • Bilateral cryptorchidism can cause infertility • Maldescended testes are associated with a greatly increased incidence of testicular cancer, even once repositioned within scrotum
Torsion	• Precipitated by sudden movement, trauma, and congenital anomalies • Twisting of spermatic cord may compromise both arterial supply and venous drainage • Sudden onset of testicular pain and a loss of the cremasteric reflex are characteristic • If not surgically corrected early, may result in testicular infarction
Hydrocele	• Congenital hydrocele occurs when a small patency of the processus vaginalis remains so that peritoneal fluid can flow into the processus vaginalis; may occur later in life, often inflammatory causes (e.g., epididymitis) • Results in fluid-filled cyst near testes
Varicocele	• Results from dilatations of tributaries of the testicular vein in the pampiniform plexus • Varicosities of the pampiniform plexus are observed when the patient is standing and disappear when the patient is lying down
Spermatocele	• Retension cyst containing sperm in the rete testes or head of the epididymis

► Spermatogenesis

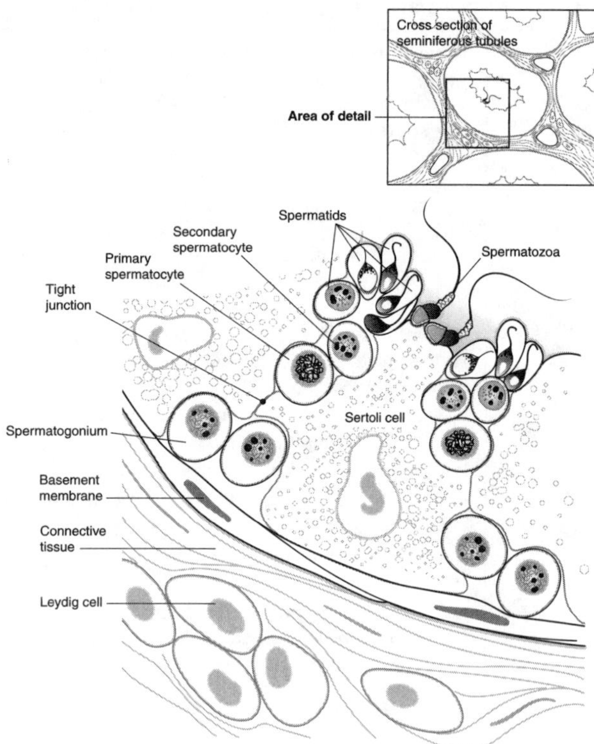

Spermatogenesis occurs in the seminiferous tubules between the **Sertoli cells**, which extend from the seminiferous tubule basement membrane to the lumen and are separated by tight junctions (blood–testis barrier) and germ cells in varying stages of spermatogenesis. The **blood–testis barrier** protects the spermatocytes and spermatids from the immune system

Three Stages of Spermatogenesis

1. **Spermatocytogenesis** begins at puberty adjacent to the basement membrane of the Sertoli cell. Spermatogonia first undergo spermatocytogenesis, during which mitosis divides the spermatogonia into spermatocytes.

2. **Meiosis** reduces the diploid spermatocytes into haploid spermatids.

3. **Spermiogenesis** is the maturation of spermatids into mature spermatozoa.

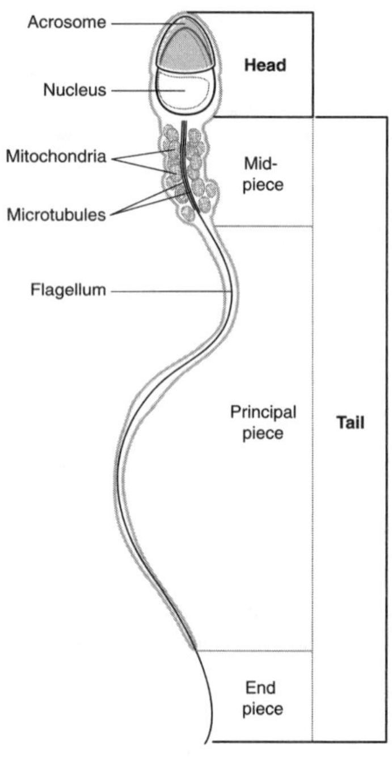

Spermatozoon

Spermiogenesis

During **spermiogenesis**, the spermatids undergo chromatin condensation and nuclear elongation, which forms the head of the spermatozoa.

The **acrosome**, a hydrolytic enzyme-containing region on the sperm cell head, also forms during this time.

The midpiece of the sperm has as a mitochondrial sheath that contains much of the ATP necessary for sperm movement. The **flagellum** contains an array of **9 + 2 microtubular pairs** linked by **dynein** for sperm motility. Patients with defective or absent dynein in **Kartagener syndrome** have reduced sperm motility, as well as reduced mucus clearance in the respiratory pathways, leading to bronchiectasis.

Once formed, spermatozoa detach from the Sertoli cells and combine with a fluid that aids in the movement of spermatozoa into the epididymis. In the epididymis, the fluid is reabsorbed, thereby concentrating sperm, and sperm interact with **forward motility factor**, a protein that aids in sperm motility. Ejaculated sperm must undergo **capacitation** in the uterus before fertilization can occur.

Fertilization

Fertilization is a three-step process:

1. **Acrosome reaction:** Sperm close to the corona radiata release hyaluronidase, which dissolves material between corona radiata cells, allowing sperm to reach the zona pellucida.
2. **Zonal reaction:** Sperm bind to a glycoprotein of the zona and release acrosin, which facilitates penetration of the zona by the sperm head.
3. **Cortical reaction:** The first sperm to penetrate the zona fuses with the plasma membrane of the ovum and induces a calcium-dependent release of cortical granules that prevents polyspermy.

▶ Hormonal Control of Steroidogenesis and Spermatogenesis

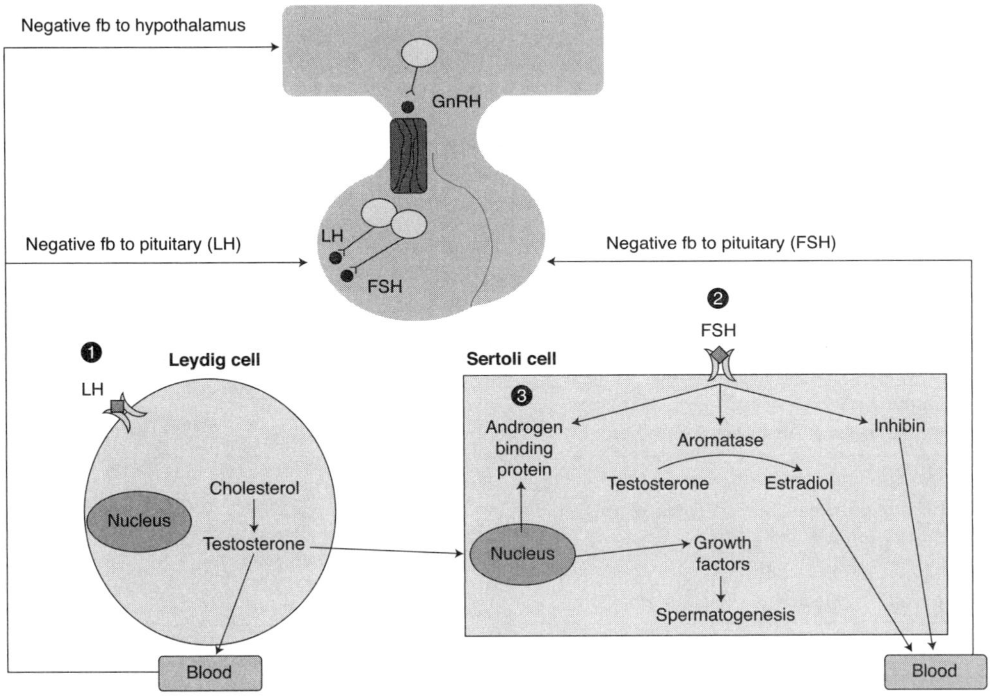

GnRH is synthesized in the **preoptic nucleus** and is released in a pulsatile manner into the hypophysial portal system. Binding of GnRH to its receptor on the anterior pituitary stimulates the release of LH and FSH.

Note: If the gonadotrophs are subjected to constant GnRH stimulation, the receptors will undergo downregulation.

❶ **LH** binds to the **Leydig cell** and stimulates the conversion of cholesterol into testosterone. Testosterone diffuses into blood and feeds back to inhibit hypothalamic GnRH and pituitary LH. Testosterone diffuses into the Sertoli cell and increases transcription of androgen-binding protein and growth factors that mediate spermatogenesis.

❷ **FSH** binds to the **Sertoli cell** and stimulates transcription of androgen-binding protein, the conversion of testosterone to estradiol, and the secretion of inhibin. Inhibin feeds back to inhibit further production of pituitary FSH.

❸ Sertoli cell-derived **androgen binding protein** provides an important reserve of testosterone in the testes. Because spermatogenesis is dependent on intratesticular testosterone rather than systemic testosterone, these reserves are important to normal spermatogenesis.

▶ Inflammatory Lesions

Mumps	• Orchitis develops in approximately 25% of patients over age 10, but is less common in patients under 10 • Rarely leads to sterility
Gonorrhea	• Neglected urethral gonococcal infection may spread to prostate, seminal vesicles, and epididymis, but rarely to testes
Syphilis	• Acquired or congenital syphilis may involve the testes • Two forms: gummas or a diffuse interstitial/lymphocytic plasma cell infiltrate • Can lead to sterility
Tuberculosis	• TB usually spreads from epididymis; this is almost always associated with foci of TB elsewhere

► Testicular Neoplasms

Germ Cell Tumors Most common malignancy in men 15 to 34 years of age	
Seminoma	• Rare in infants, incidence increases to a peak in the fourth decade • 10% are anaplastic seminomas; show nuclear atypia • *Prognosis:* with treatment; 5-year survival rate exceeds 90% • Highly radiosensitive; metastases rare
Embryonal carcinoma	• Most commonly in the 20–30-year-age group • Aggressive, present with testicular enlargement • 30% metastatic disease at time of diagnosis • Serum AFP: elevated • 5-year mortality rate 65% • Less radiosensitive than seminomas • Often metastasize to nodes, lungs, and liver • May require orchiectomy and chemotherapy
Choriocarcinoma	• Most common in men 15–25 years of age, highly malignant • May have gynecomastia or testicular enlargement • Elevated serum and urine hCG levels • Tends to disseminate hematogenously, invading lungs, liver, and brain • Treated with orchiectomy and chemotherapy
Yolk sac tumor	• Most common testicular tumor in children and infants, although rare overall in adults • Elevated alpha fetoprotein (AFP) • Very aggressive; exhibiting a 50% 5-year mortality rate
Teratoma	• Can occur at any age, but are most common in infants and children • Appears as a testicular mass • Exhibit a variety of tissues, such as nerve, muscle, cartilage, and hair • Benign behavior during childhood, malignant in adults • 2-year mortality is 30% • *Treatment:* orchiectomy, followed by chemotherapy and radiation
Non–Germ Cell Tumors	
Leydig cell tumor	• Usually unilateral • Can produce androgens or estrogens • *Children:* present with masculinization or feminization; *adults:* gynecomastia • Usually benign and only 10% are invasive; surgery may be curative
Sertoli cell	• Usually unilateral • Can produce small amounts of androgens or estrogens, usually not enough to cause endocrinologic changes • Present with testicular enlargement • Over 90% are benign
Lymphoma	• Lymphomas are the most common testicular cancer in elderly men • The tumors are rarely confined to the testes (often disseminated)

Note: Testicular neoplasms tend to metastasize to the **lumbar nodes**, whereas scrotal disease affects **superficial inguinal nodes**.

Female Reproductive System

▶ Hormonal Control of Steroidogenesis

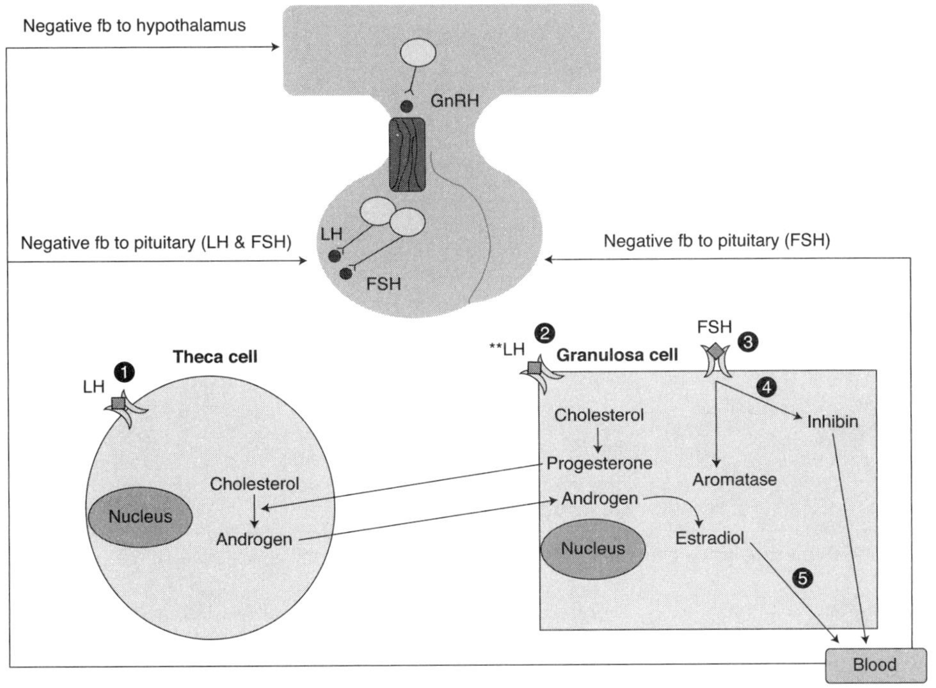

GnRH is synthesized in the **preoptic nucleus** and is released in a **pulsatile** manner into the hypophysial portal system. Binding of GnRH to its receptor on the anterior pituitary stimulates the release of LH and FSH.

Note: If the gonadotrophs are subjected to constant GnRH stimulation, the receptors will undergo downregulation.

1. **LH** binds receptors on **theca cells**, resulting in production of androstenedione or testosterone. Androgens produced by the theca cells enter the granulosa cells to be converted into estrogens.

2. **LH** also binds receptors on **granulosa cells** during the luteal phase and stimulates production of progesterone, which enters the theca cells. During the luteal phase, progesterone is required to maintain pregnancy if fertilization/implantation occur.

3. **FSH** binds receptors on **granulosa cells**, resulting in aromatization of androgens to estradiol and synthesis of new LH receptors on the granulosa cells. Estradiol can be released into the blood or can act locally to increase granulosa cell proliferation and sensitivity to FSH.

4. **FSH** also stimulates the production of **inhibin**, which negatively feeds back to inhibit further FSH secretion.

5. **Estradiol** secreted into the blood negatively feeds back to inhibit hypothalamic and pituitary secretion of GnRH, and LH and FSH, respectively. This action does not occur near the ovulatory period.

Definition of abbreviations: LH, luteinizing hormone; FSH, follicle-stimulating hormone; GnRH, gonadotropin-releasing hormone.

► Folliculogenesis and Ovulation

Follicular Development	Graafian follicle

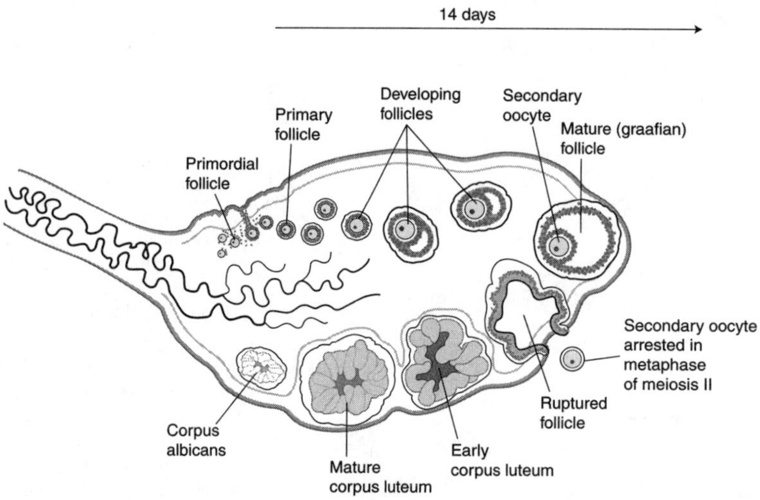

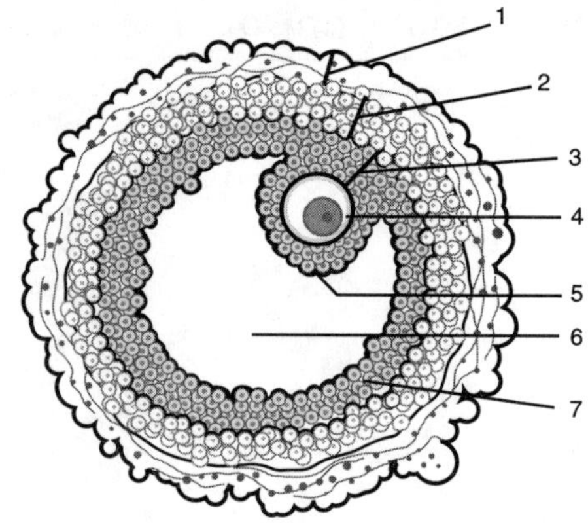

1. Theca externa
2. Theca interna
3. Cumulus oophorus
4. Zona pellucida
5. Corona radiata
6. Follicular antrum
7. Granulosa cells

Follicular Development

- At puberty, there are about 400,000 follicles present in the ovarian stroma, but only about 450 of these will develop (remaining follicles undergo atresia).
- The immature or **primordial follicle** (an oocyte surrounded by pregranulosa cells) is **arrested in prophase I of meiosis** until maturation.
- Starting at puberty, during each cycle, a primordial follicle becomes the **primary follicle** when the oocyte enlarges and the granulosa cells mature and proliferate. The granulosa cells secrete mucopolysaccharides, creating the **zona pellucida**, which protects the oocyte and provides an avenue for the oocyte to receive nutrients and chemical signals from the granulosa cells.
- As the follicle matures, additional granulosa cell layers are added and a layer of androgen-producing theca cells known as the **theca interna** surround the now **secondary follicle**. The secondary follicle continues to grow, and a fibrous theca externa surrounds the follicle. A follicular cavity (**antrum**) forms from granulosa cell secretions.
- The mature follicle, the **graafian follicle**, is now ready for ovulation. At the time of the LH surge, the oocyte resumes meiosis, **completes the first meiotic division, and is arrested in metaphase of meiosis II prior to ovulation**. Meiosis produces a nonfunctional first polar body, which degenerates, and a larger secondary haploid oocyte.
- If it is fertilized, the secondary oocyte completes meiosis II to form a **mature oocyte** and **polar body**.

Ovulation

- As the antral fluid increases, the pressure becomes greater until the follicle ruptures and the oocyte is extruded.
- Following ovulation, the theca cells enlarge and begin secreting estrogen and the granulosa cells enlarge and secrete progesterone. This new endocrine organ is called the **corpus luteum** and reaches maximal development about 7 days after ovulation.
- If fertilization does not occur, the corpus luteum degenerates.
- If fertilization does occur, the corpus luteum continues to grow for about 3 months and is maintained by **human chorionic gonadotropin (hCG)** from the embryo. Once the placenta is functional, the corpus luteum is no longer necessary to maintain pregnancy.

► Uterine Cycle

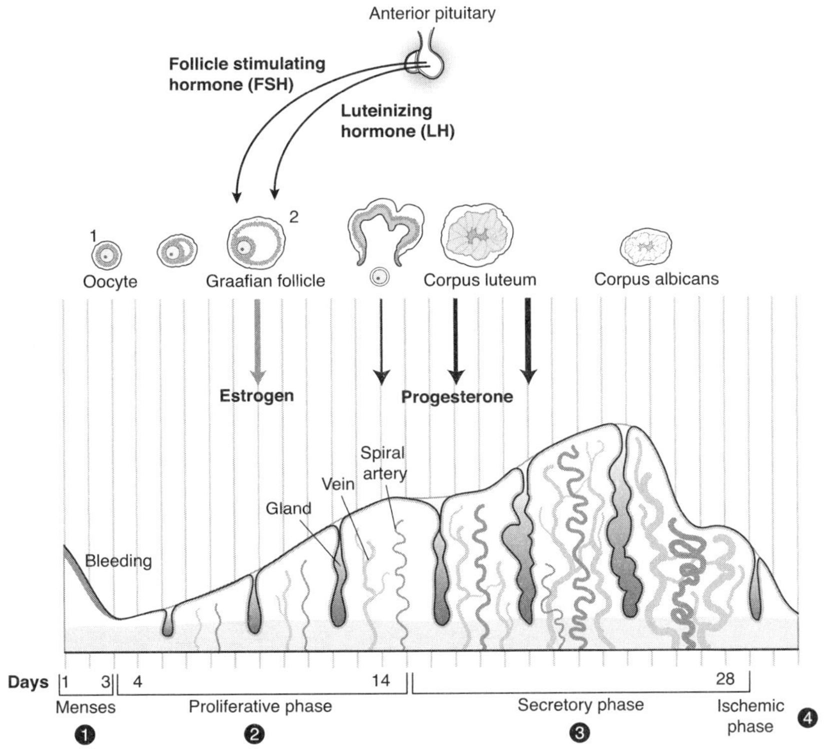

The **uterine cycle** can be divided into four phases:

1. **menstruation**
2. **proliferative phase**
3. **secretory phase**
4. **premenstruation**

As with the menstrual cycle, Day 1 of the uterine cycle begins at the onset of menses. This time period corresponds with the degeneration of the corpus luteum.

Proliferative Phase 2

- The **proliferative phase** follows menses, corresponding to the latter portion of the follicular phase of the menstrual cycle and ending near ovulation.
- During this time, elevated estrogen levels stimulate the **proliferation of endometrial cells**, an **increase in length and number of endometrial glands**, and **increased blood flow** to the uterus.
- The endometrium increases in thickness sixfold and becomes contractile. Estrogen also stimulates a marked increase in progesterone receptors in the endometrium to prepare it for fertilization. **Edema** develops in the uterus toward the end of the proliferative phase and continues to develop during the secretory phase.

Secretory Phase 3

- The **secretory phase** corresponds with the luteal phase of the menstrual cycle and is characterized by **endometrial cell hypertrophy, increased vascularity, and edema**.
- **Progesterone levels are elevated** during this phase and lead to a thick secretion consisting of glycoprotein, sugars, and amino acids. Like estrogen, progesterone increases cell proliferation and vascularization, but unlike estrogen, progesterone depresses uterine contractility.

Premenstrual Phase 4

- The **premenstrual phase** consists of constriction of arteries, causing ischemia and anoxia. The **superficial layer of the endometrium degenerates**, and blood and tissue appear in the uterine lumen.

► Menstrual Cycle

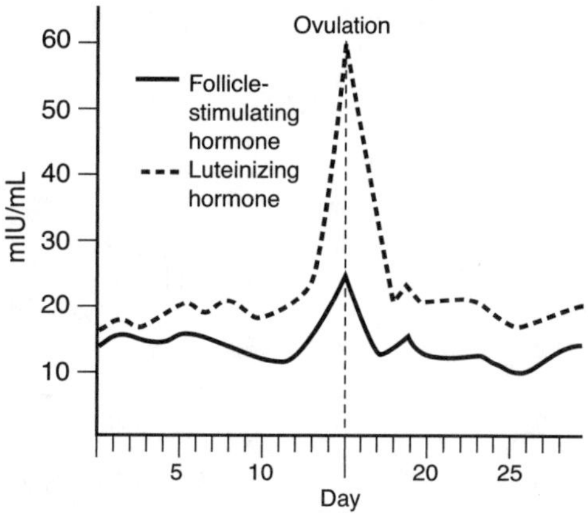

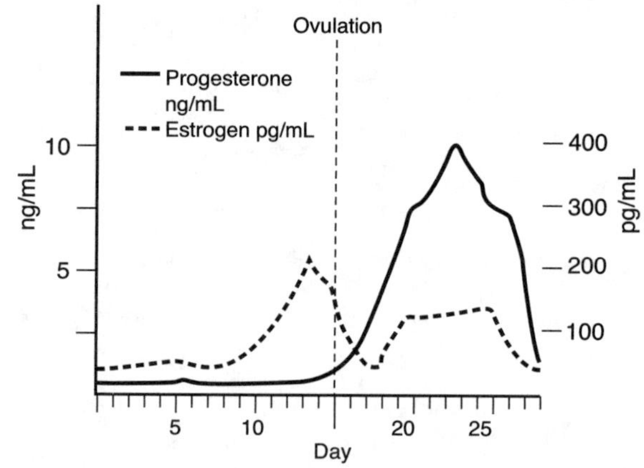

Overview

- There are **four phases** in the menstrual cycle: **menses**, **follicular phase**, **ovulation**, and **luteal phase**.
- The **average cycle length** is **28 days**, but can vary widely. The period from ovulation to the onset of menses is always 14 days, so any variation from 28 days occurs during the **follicular** phase.

Menses

- The onset of menses marks **Day 1** of the menstrual cycle and is triggered by a **decrease in estrogen** (decreased estrogen synthesis by granulosa cells and decreased LH) and **progesterone**. The decrease in estrogen and progesterone support for the endometrium results in tissue necrosis and arterial rupture, leading to sloughing of the superficial layer of the endometrium and bleeding.
- The elevated levels of progesterone in the luteal phase act to negatively feed back and decrease LH production. Also, luteal cells become less responsive to LH about 1 week following ovulation.

Follicular Phase

- The **follicular phase** begins on about **Day 5** of the menstrual cycle and lasts an average of 9 days.
- When progesterone and estrogen levels decrease, the negative feedback on the hypothalamus and pituitary is removed, allowing an **increase in the frequency of GnRH pulses**. This, in turn, **stimulates FSH secretion**, thereby stimulating follicular growth (and estrogen production from proliferating granulosa cells).
- One follicle will secrete more estradiol than the others and will become the **dominant follicle** while the others undergo atresia. **Estrogen** levels continue to increase until they reach a critical point, at which estrogen changes from **negative to positive feedback** to increase GnRH pulse frequency and LH and FSH secretion. This rapid rise in GnRH pulse frequency results in a surge of both LH and FSH.

Ovulation

- The **LH surge** and **high estrogen levels trigger ovulation** on about **Day 14** of the cycle.
- The **follicle ruptures about 24 to 36 hours after the LH surge**, during which the oocyte resumes meiosis and the first polar body is extruded.

Luteal Phase

- The **luteal phase** begins after ovulation around Day 14 and extends to about Day 28.
- During this time the follicular cells form the **corpus luteum** and secrete **high levels of progesterone** and a lower level of estrogen (even without LH stimulation). Progesterone negatively feeds back to slow the frequency of GnRH pulses, so LH and FSH levels remain low.
- In the absence of fertilization, the corpus luteum undergoes luteolysis, causing progesterone and estrogen levels to decrease until the hormonal support for the endometrial lining declines and the cells undergo apoptosis. Menses occurs and the cycle is back at the beginning.

▶ Fertilization

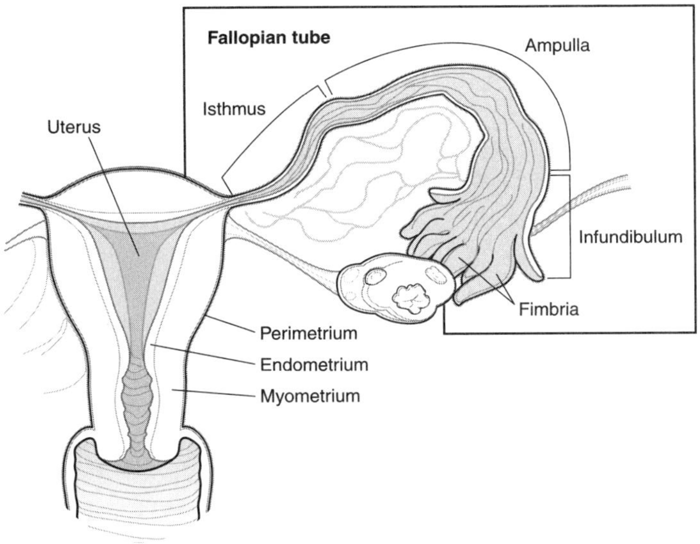

The ovulated oocyte is picked up from the intraperitoneal cavity by fimbria of the fallopian tube. Peristaltic contractions of the fallopian tube move the oocyte into the ampulla, where fertilization usually occurs 8 to 25 hours after ovulation.

Fertilization

- Semen ejaculated into the vagina quickly coagulates and **neutralizes** the **acidic vaginal fluids** to permit sperm survival. About 100,000 of the approximately 60 million sperm that enter the vagina will make it through the cervix. **Elevated estrogen** before ovulation **thins the cervical mucus**, allowing for easier transit of sperm to the uterus.
- Uterine fluid solubilizes the glycoproteins coating the sperm in a process called **capacitation**. Capacitation aids in fertilization by increasing energy metabolism, enhancing motility, and allowing the **acrosome reaction** that occurs at the zona pellucida. Sperm movement through the uterus is primarily accomplished by contraction of the female reproductive tract, primarily the uterus.

- Sperm are capable of fertilizing for as long as 72 hours after ejaculation. Once sperm reach the oocyte, they **bind to the zona pellucida** and **undergo the acrosome reaction**. This reaction releases hydrolytic enzymes stored in the acrosome cap, which dissolve the zona pellucida. Sperm motility is important to push the sperm head toward the oocyte. When the sperm reach the oocyte, the two membranes fuse and the contents of the sperm cell enter the oocyte. At this point, a **cortical reaction** occurs, during which the zona pellucida hardens and prevents additional sperm from entering the oocyte.
- Prior to fusing of the male and female pronucleus, the oocyte undergoes a second meiotic division, producing the second polar body and the female pronucleus. **The contents of the sperm form the male pronucleus, which fuses with the female pronucleus, forming the embryo**.

Early Embryogenesis

- The embryo remains in the ampulla several days, during which time rising levels of progesterone relax the uterine and fallopian tube musculature, making it easier for the embryo to pass into the uterus.
- The **embryo** usually **arrives in the uterus** by about the **third day following fertilization**, but **does not implant in the uterus for about 3 more days.** During the latter 3 days, the embryo develops a vascular system that aids in taking up nutrients it receives from uterine secretions.

► Implantation and Pregnancy

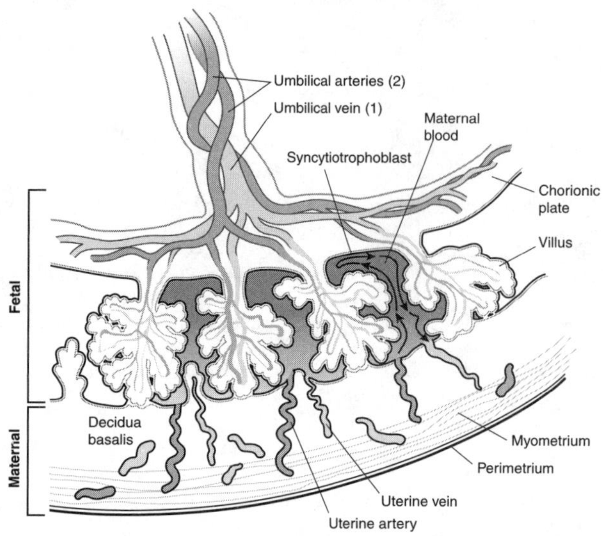

Implantation

At the time of implantation, the trophectoderm cells of the embryo contact the maternal epithelium, resulting in increased vascular permeability in the embryo, edema in the intracellular matrix, swelling of the stromal cells with addition of glycogen granules, and sprouting and ingrowth of capillaries. This reaction is called **decidualization** and prepares the decidua for the embryo. Within about 12 days after fertilization, the embryo is completely embedded in the decidua.

Between 8 to 12 days after fertilization, **human chorionic gonadotropin (hCG) is synthesized by the blastocyst** and is structurally and functionally similar to LH. It acts on the ovary to stimulate luteal growth and to suppress luteolysis.

Placenta

- The **placenta** allows for the exchange of nutrients and waste products between the maternal and fetal circulations. By about 5 weeks postfertilization, the placenta is developed and functional, although not fully mature.
- The placenta consists of **villi** from cell columns of chorionic **syncytiotrophoblast**, which have fetal blood vessels throughout. The villi branch and penetrate the maternal stroma, forming a mass of terminal villi that is separated from fetal capillaries by the thin layer of the villi.

Lactation

- During pregnancy, **estrogen and progesterone** stimulate the development of the mammary glands for **lactation** while preventing milk production.
- Following delivery, estrogen and progesterone levels decline and milk production is permitted.
- The production of milk requires **prolactin**, a hormone produced by the anterior pituitary. Prolactin is normally inhibited by hypothalamic dopamine, but suckling decreases dopamine release.
- The ejection of milk requires **oxytocin**, a hormone produced in the hypothalamus and released from the posterior pituitary. **Oxytocin is released in response to suckling or baby crying** and acts on the myoepithelial cells to stimulate contraction (milk let-down). Milk is then ejected from the nipple.

▶ Diseases of Pregnancy

Pregnancy-induced Hypertension	
Preeclampsia and eclampsia	**Preeclampsia:** Hypertension, proteinuria, and edema Symptoms can include headache, blurred vision, mental changes, facial and extremity edema, and abdominal pain Preeclampsia is common (>5% of pregnancies) from 20 weeks' gestation onward Can cause Hemolysis, Elevated Liver function tests, and Low Platelets (HELLP syndrome) Best treatment is delivery of fetus if possible; or manage with bed rest, salt restriction, IV magnesium sulfate, antihypertensives, and diazepam if needed for treatment and/or prevention of seizures. **Eclampsia** = Preeclampsia and **seizures** Rare because of aggressive management of preeclampsia
Placental Abnormalities	
Abruptio placentae	Placenta detaches prematurely from the endometrium, with risk of death for the fetus and DIC in the mother
Placenta previa	Placenta overlies the cervical os; the baby must be delivered by Caesarian section to prevent life-threatening maternal or fetal hemorrhage due to tearing of the placenta during delivery
Placenta accreta	Placenta implants directly in the myometrium rather than the endometrium; following delivery, hysterectomy is usually performed to be sure all of the placenta was removed
Amniotic Fluid Abnormalities	
Polyhydramnios	Very large amount of amniotic fluid; usually due to severe abnormalities in the fetus such as anencephaly, esophageal atresia, or duodenal atresia
Oligohydramnios	Very small amount of amniotic fluid; usually due to severe abnormalities in the fetus such as bilateral renal agenesis or posterior urethral valves (males) that prevent urination
Miscellaneous	
Ectopic pregnancy	Embryo lodges in an abnormal site (most commonly in a fallopian tube, but can also be on pelvic organs or in the abdomen) Typically because of fallopian tube pathology that prevents the egg from reaching the uterine cavity Risk of potentially fatal hemorrhage to the mother

▶ Infectous Agents That Cross the Placenta

(Mnemonic: TORCH)	Miscellaneous:
***T**oxoplasma*	*Listeria monocytogenes*
Other (Syphilis)	Parvovirus B19
Rubella	Coxsackie B
CMV	Polio
Herpes and **H**IV	

► Female Reproductive Pharmacology

Class	Mechanism	Comments/Agents
Contraception		
The most common methods of reversible contraception include oral contraceptives, long-acting injectable or implantable progestins, condoms, spermicides, withdrawal, diaphragm and intrauterine devices, and timely abstinence.		
Estrogens and progestins	Suppresses production of FSH and LH, which leads to inhibition of ovulation and alteration of cervical mucus and the endometrium.	• Commonly used estrogens: ethinyl estradiol and mestranol • Commonly used progestins: norgestrel, norethindrone, and medroxyprogesterone • Are available orally as monophasic, biphasic, and triphasic combinations; also available as progestin-only preparations • Are available in many other forms, including transdermal patches, vaginal rings, IUDs, and long-acting injections • Can cause nausea, breast tenderness, headache, depression, thromboembolism, and weight gain • Absolute contraindications include thrombophlebitis, thromboembolic disorders, cerebral vascular disease, coronary occlusion, known or suspected pregnancy, smokers over the age of 35; dramatically impaired liver function, and suspected breast cancer • Other uses: female hypogonadism, HRT, dysmenorrhea, uterine bleeding, and acne
Postcoital contraceptives	Prevents pregnancy if used within 72 hours of unprotected intercourse	Different types include estrogens alone, progestins alone, combination pills, mifepristone (RU486)
Intrauterine devices (IUD)	"Devices" that create a hostile environment in the endometrium through low-grade intrauterine inflammation and increased prostaglandin formation; therefore interfere with the implantation of the fertilized ovum	Examples: Copper-T 380 (IUD) and Progesterone T (IUD)
Hormone Replacement Therapy (HRT)		

- Used in the treatment of menopause, which is defined as a permanent cessation of menstruation secondary to a loss of ovarian follicular activity. HRT is used to prevent hot flashes, atrophic changes in the urogenital tract, and osteoporosis.
- When ERT is administered alone, it may induce endometrial growth and cancer; concomitant progesterone use prevents this. HRT has been associated with an increased breast cancer and stroke risk and is no longer as widely used.

(Continued)

► Female Reproductive Pharmacology *(Cont'd.)*

Class	Mechanism	Comments/Agents
Selective Estrogen Receptor Modulator (SERM) These drugs act as estrogen agonists, partial agonists, or antagonists, depending on the target tissue.		
Tamoxifen	• Estrogen antagonist in breast • Estrogen agonist in endometrium • Estrogen agonist in bone	• Used in hormone-responsive breast CA; reduces risk of breast CA in very high risk women • Increases risk of endometrial CA • Prevents osteoporosis in woman using it for breast CA • Causes hot flashes and increases risk of venous thrombosis
Raloxifene	• Partial estrogen agonist in bone • Estrogen antagonist in breast • Estrogen antagonist in uterus	• Prevents osteoporosis in postmenopausal women • Reduces risk of breast CA in very high risk women • No increased endometrial CA risk • Causes hot flashes and increases risk of venous thrombosis
Miscellaneous Agents		
Clomiphene	Fertility agent; nonsteroidal agent that selectively blocks estrogen receptors in the pituitary, reducing negative feedback mechanism and thereby increasing FSH and LH and stimulation of ovulation	Most common side effect: multiple birth pregnancy
Danazol	Inhibits ovarian steroid synthesis	Used in endometriosis and fibrocystic breast disease
Anastrozole **Exemestane**	Aromatase inhibitor (decrease in estrogen synthesis)	Used in breast CA in postmenopausal women
Mifepristone (RU 486)	Progesterone and glucocorticoid antagonist	Used as postcoital contraceptive and abortifacient
Dinoprostone	PGE_2 analog	Used to induce labor, causes cervical ripening and uterine contractions; also an abortifacient
Terbutaline	β_2 agonists	Relax uterus, have been used to suppress premature labor

Definition of abbreviations: CA, cancer; ERT, estrogen replacement therapy; FSH, follicle-stimulating hormone; HRT, hormone-replacement therapy; LH, luteinizing hormone.

Female Reproductive System Pathology

▶ Diseases of the Vulva

Disease	Description	Distribution	Etiology/Comments
Condyloma acuminatum	Verrucous, wartlike lesions Koilocytosis, acanthosis, hyperkeratosis, and parakeratosis	Vulva, perineum, vagina, and cervix	Associated with human papillomavirus (HPV) serotypes 6 and 11 Greatly increased risk of cervical carcinoma
Papillary hidradenoma	Benign tumor similar to an intraductal papilloma of the breast	Occur along the milk line	
Extramammary Paget disease of the vulva	Erythematous, crusted rash Intraepidermal malignant cells with pagetoid spread	Labia majora	Not associated with underlying tumor
***Candida* vulvovaginitis**	Erythema, thick white discharge	Vulva and vagina	Extremely common, especially in diabetics and after antibiotic use

Note: See also Sexually Transmitted Diseases, pages 419–421.

▶ Diseases of the Vagina

Vaginal Adenosis and Clear Cell Adenocarcinoma

- Rare in the general population, but greatly increased risk in females exposed to diethylstilbestrol (DES) in utero (1940–1970)
- Vaginal adenosis—benign condition thought to be a precursor of clear cell carcinoma

Embryonal Rhabdomyosarcoma (Sarcoma Botryoides)

- Rare tumor affecting female infants and young children (age <4)
- Polypoid, "grapelike," soft tissue mass protruding from the vagina
- Spindle-cell tumor, may show cross-striations, positive for desmin, indicating skeletal muscle origin

▶ Diseases of the Cervix/Fallopian Tubes

Disease	Description	Etiologies	Disease Manifestations	Clinical
Pelvic inflammatory disease	Ascending infection from cervix to endometrium, fallopian tubes, and pelvic cavity	***Neisseria gonorrhoeae*** (Gram ⊖ diplococcus) ***Chlamydia trachomatis*** (intracytoplasmic inclusions in mucosal cells)	Cervicitis, endometritis, salpingitis, peritonitis, pelvic abscess, perihepatitis (Fitz-Hugh-Curtis syndrome), chandelier sign *Complications:* tubo-ovarian abscess, tubal scarring, infertility, ectopic pregnancy, intestinal obstruction	• Vaginal discharge/ bleeding • Midline abdominal pain, bilateral lower abdominal and pelvic pain • Abdominal tenderness and peritoneal signs • Fever
Cervical carcinoma	Third most common malignant tumor of the female genital tract in United States; peak incidence in the 40s	Associated with early first intercourse, multiple sexual partners, infection by **HPV types 16, 18,** 31 and 33, smoking, and immunosuppression	**Begins as cervical intraepithelial neoplasia (CIN)** → carcinoma in situ → invasive squamous cell cancer	May be asymptomatic, or may have postcoital bleeding, dyspareunia, discharge Early detection possible with **Papanicolaou (Pap) smear – koilocytic cells**

▶ Diseases of the Uterus

Disease	Description	Location	Pathology	Clinical
Endometritis	Ascending infection from the cervix	Endometrium and decidua	*Ureaplasma*, *Peptostreptococcus*, *Gardnerella*, *Bacteroides*, Group B *Streptococcus*, *Chlamydia trachomatis*, *Actinomyces* (yellow, granular filaments on IUD)	Associated with pregnancy or abortions (acute) Associated with PID and intrauterine devices (IUDs) (chronic)
Endometriosis	• Presence of endometrial glands and stroma outside the uterus • Most commonly affects women of reproductive age	Ovary Ovarian and uterine ligaments Pouch of Douglas Serosa of bowel and bladder Peritoneal cavity	Red-brown serosal nodules **("powder burns")** Endometrioma: ovarian **"chocolate" cyst** Adenomyosis = endometrial glands in the myometrium	Chronic pelvic pain linked to menses Dysmenorrhea and dyspareunia Rectal pain and constipation Infertility
Leiomyoma	• **Benign smooth muscle tumor that grows in response to estrogen.** • Higher incidence in African Americans Malignant variant: leiomyosarcoma	May occur in subserosal, intramural, or submucosal locations in the myometrium	Well-circumscribed, rubbery, white-tan "whorled" masses Often multiple	Menorrhagia Abdominal mass Pelvic pain, back pain, or suprapubic discomfort Infertility
Leiomyosarcoma	Smooth muscle sarcoma of the uterus	Myometrium	**Gross:** Bulky tumor with necrosis and hemorrhage **Micro:** Malignant smooth muscle cells, often with nuclear pleomorphism and increased mitotic rate	Increased incidence in blacks Aggressive tumor that tends to recur May present with cervical bleeding
Endometrial adenocarcinoma	Most common malignant tumor of the female genital tract Most commonly affects postmenopausal women	Begins in endometrium and may invade myometrium	**Gross:** Tan polypoid endometrial mass Invasion of myometrium is prognostically important **Micro:** endometrioid adenocarcinoma (most common type)	Postmenopausal vaginal bleeding **Risk Factors:** **Early menarche and late menopause** **Nulliparity** Hypertension and diabetes Obesity **Chronic anovulation** **Estrogen-producing ovarian tumors, estrogen replacement therapy and tamoxifen** Endometrial hyperplasia Lynch syndrome (colon, endometrial, and ovarian cancers = HNPCC)

Definition of abbreviations: HNPCC, hereditary nonpolyposis colorectal cancer.

► Diseases of the Ovary

Disease	Presentation	Laboratory/Pathology	Etiology	Treatment
Polycystic ovary disease (Stein-Leventhal syndrome)	• Young, **obese**, **hirsute** females of reproductive age • Oligomenorrhea or secondary amenorrhea • **Infertility**	• **Elevated luteinizing hormone** (LH) • Low follicle stimulating hormone (FSH) • **Elevated testosterone** Bilaterally enlarged ovaries with multiple follicular cysts	Increased LH stimulation leads to increased androgen synthesis and anovulatory cycles	Oral contraceptives or medroxyprogesterone, metformin, surgical wedge resection
Epithelial Tumors				
Cystadenoma	Most common benign ovarian tumor Pathology: Unilocular cyst with simple serous or mucinous lining			
Cystadeno-carcinoma	Most common malignant ovarian tumor. Often asymptomatic until far advanced (presenting symptoms may be increased abdominal girth due to ascites, bowel or bladder problems) Can produce **pseudomyxoma peritonei**	CA-125- marker for cystadenocarcinoma of ovary. Used to monitor recurrence, measure response to therapy. Complex multiloculated cyst with solid areas • Serous (serous cystadenocarcinoma) or mucinous (mucinous cystadenocarcinoma) lining with tufting, papillary structures with **psammoma bodies** • Spreads by seeding pelvic cavity	**Genetic risk factors:** • BRCA-1: breast and ovarian cancers • Lynch syndrome	Surgery, antineoplastic drugs
Borderline tumor	Tumors of low malignant potential			
Brenner tumor	Rare tumor that resembles transitional carcinoma; can be benign or malignant			
Less common tumors	• Yolk sac tumor: may have structures resembling primitive glomeruli • Choriocarcinoma (see table below) and embryonal carcinoma: very aggressive tumors			
Germ Cell Tumors				
Teratoma	• Most are benign • Occur in younger women • Contain elements from **all three germ layers (ectoderm, mesoderm, endoderm)** • **Immature teratoma**- contains primitive cells **– higher malignant potential**	Ovarian cyst containing hair, teeth, and sebaceous material	May be due to abnormal differentiation of fetal germ cells that arise from the fetal yolk sac	Surgical
Dysgerminoma	• Malignant • Affects mainly young adults	Similar to seminoma in appearance	**Risk factors:** Turner syndrome, pseudohermaphroditism	Radiosensitive, so good prognosis

(Continued)

► Diseases of the Ovary (*Cont'd.*)

Sex Cord-Stromal Tumors	
Ovarian fibroma	Common tumor. Associated with Meigs syndrome = fibroma + ascites + pleural effusion
Granulosa cell tumor	Potentially malignant, **produces estrogen** and can produce precocious puberty, irregular menses, or dysfunctional uterine bleeding. Microscopic: made of polygonal tumor cells with formation of follicle-like structures **(Call-Exner bodies)** Complications: endometrial hyperplasia and cancer
Sertoli-Leydig cell tumor (androblastoma)	• Androgen producing tumor, presents with virilization

► Gestational Trophoblastic Disease

Hydatidiform Mole (Molar Pregnancy)—tumor of placental trophoblast		
Incidence	1:1,000 pregnancies	
Clinical	"Size greater than dates," vaginal bleeding, passage of edematous, grape-like tissue, elevated β-hCG, invasive moles invade myometrium	
Treatment	Curettage, follow β-hCG levels	
Types		
Complete mole	Results from fertilization of an ovum that lost all its chromosomal material; all chromosomal material is derived from sperm	90% 46,XX; 10% contain a Y chromosome
Partial mole	Results from fertilization of an ovum by two sperm, one 23,X and one 23,Y	Partial moles are triploid = 69, XXY (23,X [maternal] + 23X [one sperm] +23Y [the other sperm])
Choriocarcinoma	• **Malignant** germ cell tumor derived from trophoblast • Gross: necrotic and hemorrhagic mass • Micro: proliferation of cytotrophoblasts, intermediate trophoblasts, and syncytiotrophoblasts • Hematogenous spread to lungs, brain, liver, etc. • Responsive to chemotherapy	

► Partial Moles Versus Complete Moles

Properties	Partial Mole	Complete Mole
Ploidy	Triploid	Diploid
Number of chromosomes	69	46 (All paternal)
β-hCG	Elevated (+)	Elevated (+++)
Chorionic villi	Some are hydropic	All are hydropic
Trophoblast proliferation	Focal	Marked
Fetal tissue	Present	Absent
Invasive mole	10%	10%
Choriocarcinoma	Rare	2%

Breast Pathology

▶ Fibrocystic Disease

- Most common breast disorder, affecting approximately 10% of women; may be mistaken for CA
- Develops during reproductive life, distortion of the normal breast changes associated with the menstrual cycle
- Patients often have lumpy, tender breasts
- *Pathogenesis:* possibly due to high estrogen levels, coupled with progesterone deficiency
- *Pathology:* several morphologic patterns recognized

Fibrosis	• Women 35 to 49 years of age; not premalignant • *Gross:* dense, rubbery mass; usually unilateral, most often in the upper outer quadrant • *Histology:* increase in stromal connective tissue; cysts are rare
Cystic disease	• Women 45 to 55 years of age; not premalignant • *Gross:* serous cysts, firm to palpation, may be hemorrhagic; usually multifocal, often bilateral • *Histology:* cysts lined by cuboidal epithelium, may have papillary projections • May be an accompanying stromal lymphocytic infiltrate (chronic cystic mastitis)
Sclerosing adenosis	• Women 35 to 45 years of age; mild increased risk of CA • *Gross:* palpable, ill-defined, firm area most often in upper outer quadrant; usually unilateral. • *Histology:* glandular patterns of cells in a fibrous stroma; may be difficult to distinguish from cancer
Epithelial hyperplasia	• Women over 30 years of age, mild increased CA risk • *Gross:* variable with ill-defined masses • *Histology:* ductal epithelium is multilayered and produces glandular or papillary configurations • Atypical hyperplasia has a moderate risk of CA

▶ Tumors

Fibroadenoma	• Most common benign breast tumor • Single movable breast nodule, often in the upper outer quadrant; not fixed to skin • Occurs in reproductive years, generally before age 30, possibly related to increased estrogen sensitivity • May show menstrual variation and increased growth during pregnancy; postmenopausal regression usual • *Gross:* round and encapsulated with a gray-white cut surface • *Histology:* glandular epithelial-lined spaces with a fibroblastic stroma • Surgery required for definitive diagnosis
Phyllodes tumor (cystosarcoma phyllodes)	• Fibroadenoma-like tumors that have become large, cystic, and lobulated • Distinguished by the nature of the stromal component • Malignant fibrous, cartilaginous; bony elements may be present • *Gross:* irregular mass; often fungating or ulcerated • *Histology:* myxoid stroma with increased cellularity, anaplasia, and increased mitoses • Tumor initially localized but may spread later, usually to distant sites but not to local lymph nodes
Intraductal papilloma	• Most common in women 20–50 years of age; solitary lesion within a duct • May present with nipple discharge (serous or bloody), nipple retraction, or small subareolar mass • *Gross:* small, sessile or pedunculated, usually close to the nipple in major ducts • *Histology:* multiple papillae • Single intraductal papillomas may be benign, but multiple papillomas associated with an increased risk of CA

▶ Carcinoma of the Breast

General features	• Most common cause of CA in women • Lung CA causes more deaths • Rare in women under age 25 • Lifetime risk of breast CA for the average woman with no family history: 8 to 10%	
Risk factors	• Increasing age (40+ years) • Nulliparity • Family history • Early menarche • Late menopause	• Fibrocystic disease • Previous history of breast cancer • Obesity • High-fat diet
Clinical features	• 50% in the upper outer quadrant • Ninety percent arise in ductal epithelium • Slightly more common in the left breast; bilateral or sequential in 4% of cases • Breast mass usually discovered after self-examination or on routine physical	
Tumor suppressor genes: *BRCA1* and *BRCA2*	Mutated *BRCA1*— • Almost 100% lifetime risk for breast CA, often in the third and fourth decades of life • Also at increased risk for ovarian CA (men may be at increased risk for prostate CA) Mutated *BRCA2*— • Increased incidence of breast CA in both women and men • Smaller risk of ovarian CA compared with *BRCA 1*	
Invasion	• May grow into the thoracic fascia to become fixed to the chest wall • May extend into the skin, causing dimpling and retraction • May cause obstruction of subcutaneous lymphatics, causing an orange-peel consistency to skin called "peau d'orange" • May invade Cooper ligaments within ducts to cause nipple retraction	
Metastases	• Most breast CAs disseminate via lymphatic or hematogenous routes • Involve axillary, supraclavicular, and internal thoracic nodes • Can also involve nodes of the contralateral breast	

► Breast Carcinoma Types

Noninfiltrating intraductal carcinoma	• *Gross:* focus of increased consistency in breast tissue • *Histology:* typical duct epithelial cells proliferate and fill ducts, leading to ductal dilatation • Often called "comedocarcinomas" because cheesy, necrotic tumor tissue may be expressed from ducts. • Rarely have a papillary pattern
Infiltrating ductal carcinoma	• Most common breast CA • *Gross:* rock hard, usually 2 to 5 cm in diameter, foci of necrosis and calcification common (may be seen on mammography) • *Histology:* malignant duct epithelial cells appear in masses or ducts, invading the stroma • Fibrous reaction responsible for the hard, palpable mass
Paget disease of the breast	• Older women; poor prognosis • Form of intraductal carcinoma involving areolar skin and nipple • *Gross:* skin of the nipple and areola ulcerated and oozing • *Histology:* ductal carcinoma, as well as large, anaplastic, hyperchromatic "Paget cells"
Medullary carcinoma	• Better prognosis than infiltrating ductal carcinoma • *Gross:* fleshy masses, often 5 to 10 cm in diameter, little fibrous tissue, although foci of hemorrhage and necrosis common • *Histology:* sheets of large, pleomorphic cells with increased mitotic activity and a lymphocytic infiltrate
Colloid (mucinous) carcinoma	• Older women, slow growing, has a better prognosis than infiltrating ductal carcinoma • *Gross:* soft, large, gelatinous tumors • *Histology:* islands of tumor cells with copious mucin
Lobular carcinoma	• Multicentric; usually have estrogen receptors, arise from terminal ductules • *Gross:* rubbery and ill-defined (result of their multicentric nature) • *Histology:* tumor cells small and may be arranged in rings

► Fibrocystic Disease versus Breast Cancer

Fibrocystic Disease	Breast Cancer
• Often bilateral • May have multiple nodules • Menstrual variation • Cyclic pain and engorgement • May regress during pregnancy	• Often unilateral • Usually single nodule • No menstrual variation • No cyclic pain and engorgement • Does not regress during pregnancy

► Miscellaneous Breast Conditions

Acute mastitis	• Fissures in nipples during **early nursing** predispose to bacterial infection; usually unilateral with pus in ducts; necrosis may occur • Usual pathogens: *Staphylococcus aureus* and *Streptococcus* • Antibiotics and surgical drainage may be adequate therapy
Mammary duct ectasia (plasma cell mastitis)	• Occurs in fifth decade in multiparous women • Presents with pain, redness, and induration around the areola with thick secretions; usually unilateral • Skin fixation, nipple retraction, and axillary lymphadenopathy may occur—must be distinguished from malignancy
Gynecomastia	• Enlargement of the male breasts; most often unilateral, but may be bilateral • Secondary to Klinefelter syndrome, testicular tumors, puberty, or old age • Associated with hepatic cirrhosis (cirrhotic liver cannot degrade estrogens) • May be important signal that patient has high-estrogen state

Genitourinary System Disease

► Infections and Sexually Transmitted Diseases (STDs)

Type Infection	Case Vignette/ Key Clues	Most Common Causative Agent(s)	Pathogenesis	Diagnosis	Treatment
Urethritis	Gram ⊖ diplococci in PMNs in urethral exudate	*Neisseria gonorrhoeae*	Invasive; pili assist adherence; have antigenic variation; are antiphagocytic; IgA protease	Growth on Thayer-Martin agar, DNA probes	Ceftriaxone
	Culture ⊖, glycogen inclusion bodies in cytoplasm, tissue culture	*Chlamydia trachomatis*	Obligate intracellular in epithelial cells; CMI and DTH cause scarring	Tissue culture; glycogen-containing inclusion bodies in cytoplasm	Tetracyclines, macrolides
	Urease ⊕, no cell wall, ↑ urine pH, non-Gram staining	*Ureaplasma urealyticum*	Urease raises pH of urine → struvite stones	Not gram staining; diagnosed by exclusion, urinary pH	Tetracyclines, macrolides
	Flagellated protozoan with corkscrew motility	*Trichomonas vaginalis*	Unknown, PMN filtrate	Flagellated protozoan, corkscrew motility	Metronidazole
Cystitis	Painful urination, hematuria, fever,	*E. coli #1*, other gram ⊖ enterics	Pili, adhesins, motility, many are β hemolytic	Culture of urine ≥10^5 CFU/ml of gram ⊖ rods in urine	Fluoroquinolones, sulfonamide
	As above, in young, newly-sexually active female (honeymoon cystitis)	*Staphylococcus saprophyticus*	Sexual intercourse introduces normal flora organisms into urethra	Culture of urine, gram ⊕ cocci	Fluoroquinolones
	As above with increased urinary pH	*Proteus spp.*	Urease raises urinary pH, predisposes to struvite stones	Culture of urine, lactose non-fermenting gram ⊖ bacilli with swarming motility	Fluoroquinolones, TMP-SMX
Pyelonephritis	As above with flank pain and fever	*E. coli, Staphylococcus*	Strictures, urinary stasis allow colonization	Culture of urine	Fluoroquinolones, 3rd gen cephalosporin, ampicillin-sulbactam
Cervicitis	Friable, inflamed cervix with mucopurulent discharge	*Neisseria gonorrhoeae*	Invades mucosa, PMN infiltration, pili, IgA protease	Gram ⊖ diplococci, Thayer-Martin agar	Ceftriaxone
		Chlamydia trachomatis	Obligate intracellular, CMI and DTH → scarring	Tissue culture, cytoplasmic inclusions	Tetracyclines, macrolides
		Herpes simplex virus	Vesicular lesions, painful	dsDNA, nuclear envelope, icosahedral; Tzanck smear, intranuclear inclusions	Acyclovir, valacyclovir, famciclovir

(Continued)

► Infections and Sexually Transmitted Diseases (STDs; *Cont'd.*)

Type Infection	Case Vignette/ Key Clues	Most Common Causative Agent(s)	Pathogenesis	Diagnosis	Treatment
Vulvovaginitis	Adherent yellowish discharge, pH >5, fishy amine odor in KOH, clue cells, gram ⊖ cells dominate	Bacterial vaginosis	Overgrowth of *Gardnerella vaginalis*, anaerobes	Clue cells, gram ⊖ rods	Metronidazole
	Vulvovaginitis, pruritus, erythema, discharge with consistency of cottage cheese	*Candida* spp.	Antibiotic use → overgrowth, immunocompromised	Germ tube test, gram ⊕ yeasts in vaginal fluids	Nystatin, miconazole
	"Strawberry cervix," foamy, purulent discharge; many PMNs and motile trophozoites microscopically (corkscrew motility)	*Trichomonas vaginalis*	Vaginitis with discharge	Pear-shaped trophozoites with corkscrew motility	Metronidazole
Pelvic inflammatory disease	Adnexal tenderness, bleeding, dyspareunia, vaginal discharge, fever, chandelier sign, onset often follows menses	*Neisseria gonorrhoeae*	Pili and IgA protease production	Gram ⊖ diplococci in PMNs or culture on Thayer-Martin	Ceftriaxone + doxycycline (doxycycline given for presumed coinfection with *Chlamydia*)
		Chlamydia trachomatis	Intracellular in mucosal epithelia; causes type IV hypersensitivity damage	Tissue culture, intracytoplasmic inclusions in mucosal cells	Doxycycline, macrolides
Condyloma acuminatum (genital warts)	Lesions are papillary/wart-like, may be sessile or pedunculated, koilocytotic atypia is present, anogenital	Human papilloma virus (HPV; most common U.S. STD)	HPV proteins E6 and E7 inactivate cellular antioncogene Associated with cervical CA	dsDNA, naked, icosahedral, intranuclear inclusion bodies	Podophyllin, imiquimod
Genital herpes	Multiple, painful, vesicular, coalescing, recurring	Herpes simplex	Latent virus in sensory ganglia reactivates	Virus culture, intranuclear inclusions, syncytia (Tzanck smear), dsDNA enveloped (nuclear), icosahedral	Acyclovir, valacyclovir, famciclovir

(Continued)

▶ Infections and Sexually Transmitted Diseases (STDs; *Cont'd.*)

Type Infection	Case Vignette/ Key Clues	Most Common Causative Agent(s)	Pathogenesis	Diagnosis	Treatment
Syphilis **Primary**	Painless chancre forms on glans, penis (or vulva/ cervix) and heals within 1 to 3 months	*Treponema pallidum*	3-week incubation during which spirochetes spread throughout the body	Biopsy/scraping viewed with dark-field microscopy shows spirillar organisms	Penicillin, doxycycline is an alternative
Secondary	Local or generalized rash lasting 1 to 3 months, can involve the palms and soles		Develops 1 to 2 months after primary stage	Serology—VDRL ⊕ (nonspecific); FTA-ABS (specific)	
Tertiary	Affects central nervous system, heart, and skin; characteristic lesion is gumma, may be single or multiple; most common in the liver, testes, and bone		Develops in one-third of untreated patients; *neurosyphilis:* including meningovascular, tabes dorsalis, and general paresis; obliterative endarteritis of vasa vasorum of the aorta can lead thoracic aneurysm	Serology – FTA-Abs, non-specific tests may be negative	
Chancroid	Nonindurated, painful ulcer, suppurative with adenopathy; slow to heal	*Haemophilus ducreyi*	Unknown	Gram ⊖ rods, chocolate agar (requires NAD and hemin)	Cefotaxime, ceftriaxone
Lymphogranuloma venereum	Soft, painless papule heals, lymph nodes enlarge and develop fistulas, genital elephantiasis may develop	*Chlamydia trachomatis* serotypes L1–3	Obligate intracellular	Cell culture, glycogen-containing inclusions	Tetracyclines, erythromycin

Definition of abbreviations: CA, cancer; CMI, cell-mediated immunity; ds, double-stranded; DTH, delayed type hypersensitivity; PMNs, polymorphonuclear leukocytes.

The Musculoskeletal System, Skin, and Connective Tissue

Chapter 8

Structure, Function, and Pharmacology of Muscle

▶ Features of Skeletal, Cardiac, and Smooth Muscle

Characteristics	Skeletal	Cardiac	Smooth
Appearance	Striated, unbranched fibers Z lines Multinucleated	Striated, branched fibers Z lines Single nucleus	Nonstriated, fusiform fibers No Z lines; have dense bodies Single nucleus
T tubules	Form triadic contacts with SR at A-I junction	Form dyadic contacts with SR near Z line	Absent; have limited SR
Cell junctions	Absent	Junctional complexes between fibers (intercalated discs), including gap junctions	Gap junctions
Innervation	Each fiber innervated	Electrical syncytium	Electrical syncytium
Action potential			
Upstroke	Inward Na^+ current	• Inward Ca^{2+} current (SA node) • Inward Na^+ current (atria, ventricles, Purkinje fibers)	Inward Na^+ current
Plateau	No plateau	• No plateau (SA node) • Plateau present (atria, ventricles, Purkinje fibers)	No plateau
Excitation-contraction coupling	AP → T tubules → Ca^{2+} released from SR	• Inward Ca^{2+} current during plateau → Ca^{2+} release from SR • cAMP increases Ca^{2+} and force in myocytes	• AP → opens voltage-gated Ca^{2+} channels in sarcolemma; hormones and neurotransmitters → open IP_3-gated Ca^{2+} channels in SR • cAMP and cGMP inhibit smooth muscle contraction
Calcium binding	Troponin	Troponin	Calmodulin

Definition of abbreviations: AP, action potential; IP_3, inositol triphosphate; SR, sarcoplasmic reticulum.

▶ Skeletal Muscle Fiber Morphology and Function

Skeletal muscle connective tissue (*see* right):

Epimysium: dense connective tissue that surrounds the entire muscles

Perimysium: thin septa of connective tissue that extends inward from the epimysium and surrounds a bundle (fascicle) of muscle fibers

Endomysium: delicate connective tissue that surrounds each muscle fiber

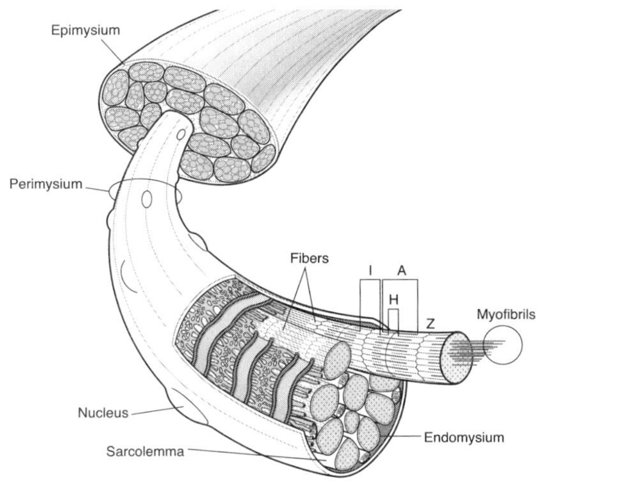

Subcellular components (*see* below):

Myofibrils: long, cylindrical bundles that fill the sarcoplasm of each fiber

Myofilaments: actin and **myosin**; are within each myofibril and organize into units called **sarcomeres**

During contraction:

A band: no change

H band: shortens

I band: shortens

Z lines: move closer together

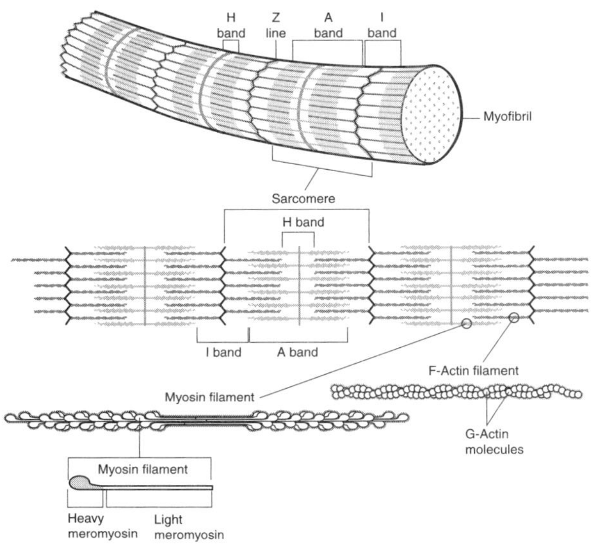

The Crossbridge Cycle

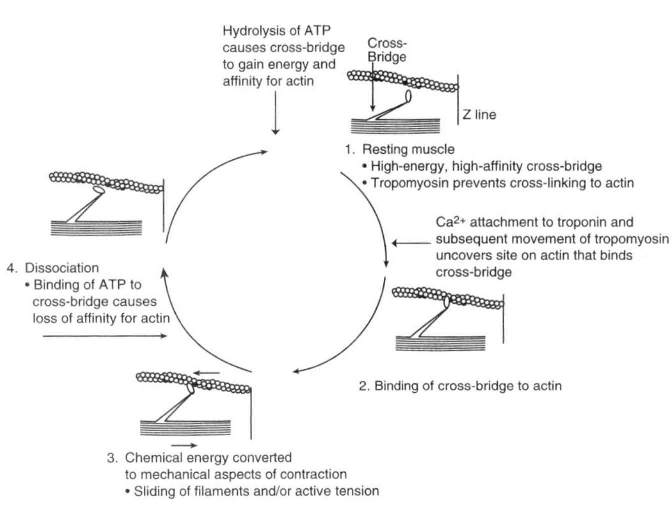

▶ Red versus White Skeletal Muscle Fibers

Red Fibers (Type I)	White Fibers (Type II)
Slow contraction	Fast contraction
$\downarrow$ ATPase activity	$\uparrow$ ATPase activity
$\uparrow$ Capacity for aerobic metabolism	$\uparrow$ Capacity for anaerobic glycolysis
$\uparrow$ Mitochondrial content	$\downarrow$ Mitochondrial content
$\uparrow$ Myoglobin (imparts red color)	$\downarrow$ Myoglobin
Best for slow, posture-maintaining muscles, e.g., back (think chicken drumstick/thigh)	Best for fast, short-termed, skilled motions, e.g., extraocular muscles of eye, sprinter's legs, hands (think chicken breast meat and wings)

▶ Smooth Muscle Function

Types of Smooth Muscle	
Multiunit	• Acts as individual motor unit • Little or no electrical coupling • Is densely innervated; contraction controlled by autonomic nervous system • In iris, ciliary muscle of lens, and vas deferens
Unitary (single unit)	• Extensive electrical coupling, allowing coordinated contraction • Has a resting tone; spontaneously active (slow waves), has pacemaker activity; activity is modulated by neurotransmitters and neurohormones • Found mainly in the walls of hollow viscera, e.g., GI tract, uterus, bladder, ureters
Vascular	• Has properties of both multiunit and single-unit smooth muscle

Smooth Muscle Contraction

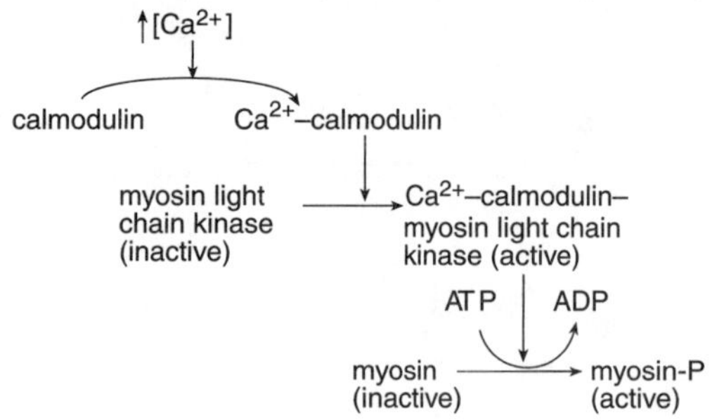

1. ↑ intracellular Ca^{2+}
2. Ca^{2+} binds calmodulin
3. Ca^{2+}-calmodulin binds to and activates **myosin light chain kinase (MLCK)**
4. Myosin is phosphorylated
5. Myosin-P binds actin and shortening occurs
6. Dephosphorylation of myosin → relaxation

Bridge to Pharmacology

α_1 and M_3 stimulation: ↑ IP_3 → ↑ intracellular Ca^{2+} → smooth muscle contraction

β_2 stimulation: ↑ cAMP → inhibits MLCK → smooth muscle relaxation

Head and Neck Embryology and Anatomy

▶ Skeletal Muscles Innervated by Cranial Nerves

Muscles Derived from a Pharyngeal Arch	Cranial Nerve	Muscles	Skeletal Elements (from neural crest)
First arch—mandibular (Mandibular hypoplasia is seen in **Treacher Collins syndrome** and in the **Robin sequence**. Both involve neural crest cells.)	**Trigeminal mandibular nerve (V3)**	Four muscles of mastication: • Masseter • Temporalis • Lateral pterygoid • Medial pterygoid Plus: • Digastric (anterior belly) • Mylohyoid • Tensor tympani • Tensor veli palatini	Mandibular process Maxillary process Malleus Incus
Second arch—hyoid	**Facial (VII)**	Muscles of facial expression: • Orbicularis oculi • Orbicularis oris • Buccinator and others Plus: • Digastric (posterior belly) • Stylohyoid • Stapedius	Hyoid (superior part) Styloid process Stapes
Third arch	**Glossopharyngeal (IX)**	Stylopharyngeus	Hyoid (inferior part)
Fourth arch	**Vagus (X) superior laryngeal (external branch)** **Vagus (X) pharyngeal branches**	Cricothyroid Levator veli palatini Uvular muscle Pharyngeal constrictors Salpingopharyngeus Palatoglossus Palatopharyngeus	Thyroid cartilage
Fifth arch	**Lost**	—	—
Sixth arch	**Vagus (X) recurrent laryngeal**	Lateral cricoarytenoid Posterior cricoarytenoid Transverse arytenoid Oblique arytenoid Thyroarytenoid (vocalis)	Cricoid, arytenoid, corniculate, cuneiform cartilages
Muscles of myotome origin	**Accessory (XI)**	Trapezius Sternocleidomastoid	
	Hypoglossal (XII)	Genioglossus Hyoglossus Styloglossus	
	Oculomotor (III)	Superior, inferior, and medial rectus; inferior oblique, levator palpebrae superioris	
	Trochlear (IV)	Superior oblique	
	Abducens (VI)	Lateral rectus	

▶ Pharyngeal Pouches

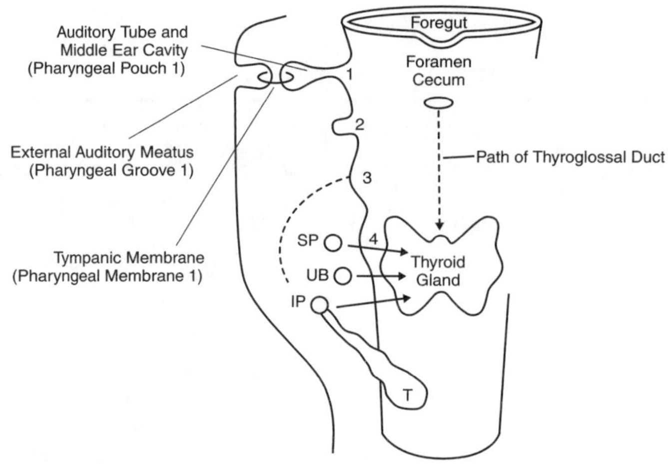

Adult Structures Derived from the Fetal Pharyngeal Pouches		
Pouch	**Adult Derivatives**	**Clinical Correlate**
1	Epithelial lining of auditory tube and middle ear cavity	The **DiGeorge sequence** occurs when pharyngeal pouches 3 and 4 fail to differentiate into the parathyroid glands and thymus. Patients have immunologic problems, hypocalcemia, and may have cardiovascular defects (persistent truncus arteriosus), abnormal ears, and micrognathia.
2	Epithelial lining of crypts of palatine tonsil	
3	Inferior parathyroid gland (IP) Thymus (T)	
4	Superior parathyroid gland (SP) Ultimobranchial body (UB)	

The thyroid gland does not develop in a pharyngeal pouch; it develops from midline endoderm of the oropharynx and migrates inferiorly along the path of thyroglossal duct. Neural crest cells migrate into the UB to form parafollicular C cells of the thyroid.

The external auditory meatus is the only postnatal remnant of a pharyngeal groove or cleft.

▶ Palate and Face Development

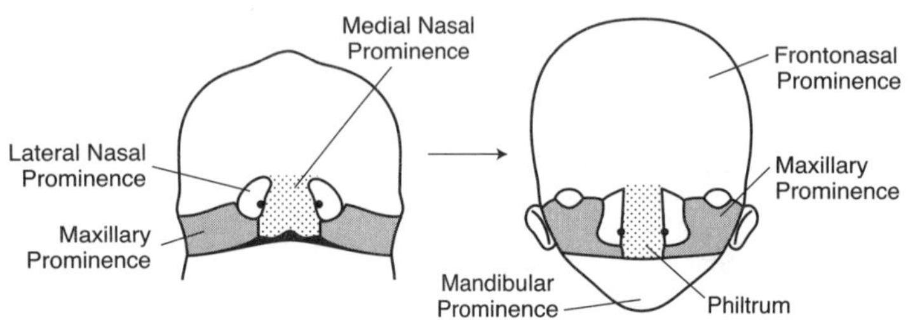

The **face** develops from the frontonasal prominence, the pair of maxillary prominences, and the pair of mandibular prominences.

The **intermaxillary segment** forms when the two medial nasal prominences fuse together at the midline and → the **philtrum of the lip**, **four incisor teeth**, and the **primary palate** of the adult.

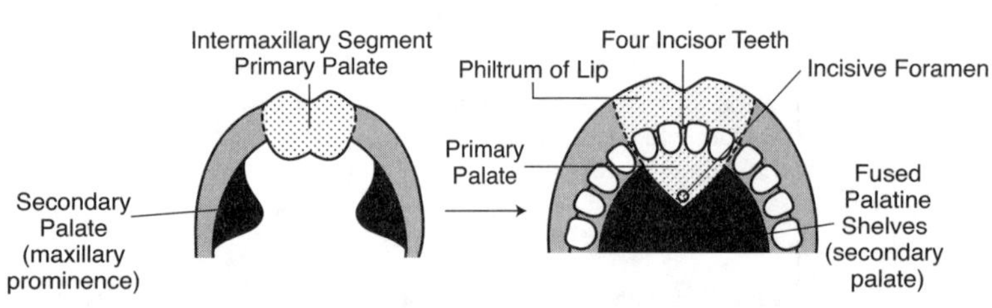

The **secondary palate** forms from palatine shelves, which fuse in the midline, posterior to the incisive foramen.

The primary and secondary palates fuse at the **incisive foramen** to form the definitive palate.

Clinical Correlation
Cleft lip occurs when the maxillary prominence fails to fuse with the medial nasal prominence.
Cleft palate occurs when the palatine shelves fail to fuse with each other or the primary palate.

► Cavernous Sinuses

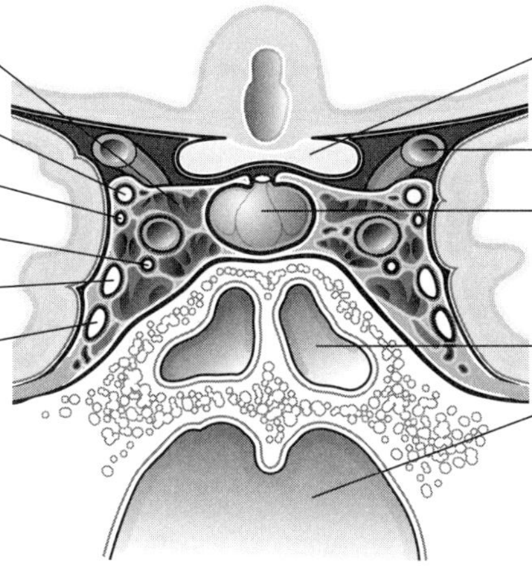

The cavernous sinuses are located on either side of the body of the sphenoid bone. Each sinus receives blood from some of the cerebral veins, ophthalmic veins, and the sphenoparietal sinus. Each cavernous sinus drains into a transverse sinus via the superior petrosal sinus and into the internal jugular vein via the inferior petrosal sinus.

Cavernous Sinus Thrombosis

Infection can spread from veins of the face into the cavernous sinuses, producing a thrombosis that may involve the cranial nerves that course through the cavernous sinuses. Cranial nerves III, IV, and VI and the ophthalmic and maxillary divisions of CN V, as well as the internal carotid artery and its periarterial plexus of postganglionic sympathetic fibers, traverse the cavernous sinuses. All of these cranial nerves course in the lateral wall of each sinus, except for CN VI, which courses through the middle of the sinus. Initially, patients have an internal strabismus. Later, all eye movements are affected, along with with altered sensation in skin of the upper face and scalp.

Upper Extremities and Back

▶ Brachial Plexus

The **brachial plexus** is formed by an intermingling of ventral rami from the C5 through T1 spinal nerves.

The ventral rami of the brachial plexus exhibit a proximal to distal gradient of innervation. Nerves that contain fibers from the superior rami of the plexus (C5 and C6) innervate proximal muscles in the upper limb (shoulder muscles). Nerves that contain fibers from the inferior rami of the plexus (C8 and T1) innervate distal muscles (hand muscles).

Five major nerves arise from the brachial plexus: the **musculocutaneous, median**, and **ulnar** nerves contain anterior division fibers and innervate muscles in the anterior arm, anterior forearm, and hand that act mainly as flexors. The **axillary** and **radial** nerves contain posterior division fibers, and innervate muscles in the posterior arm and posterior forearm that act mainly as extensors.

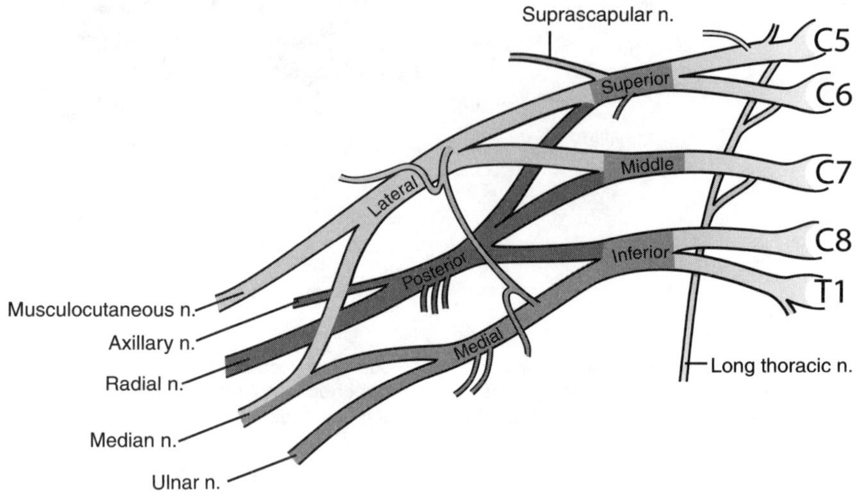

▶ Lesions of Roots of the Brachial Plexus

Lesioned Root	C5	C6	C7	C8	T1
Dermatome paresthesia	Lateral border of upper arm	Lateral forearm to thumb	Over triceps, midforearm, middle finger	Medial forearm to little finger	Medial arm to elbow
Muscles affected	Deltoid Rotator cuff Serratus anterior Biceps Brachioradialis	Biceps Brachioradialis Brachialis Supinator	Latissimus dorsi Pectoralis major Triceps Wrist extensors	Finger flexors Wrist flexors Hand muscles	Hand muscles
Reflex test	—	Biceps tendon	Triceps tendon	—	—
Causes of lesions	Upper trunk compression	Upper trunk compression	Cervical spondylosis Herniation of C6/C7 disk	Lower trunk compression	Lower trunk compression

► Upper and Lower Brachial Plexus Lesions

Upper (C5 and C6) Brachial Plexus Lesion: Erb-Duchenne Palsy
• Usually occurs when the head and shoulder are forcibly separated (e.g., accident, birth injury, or herniation of disk) • Trauma will damage **C5** and **C6** roots of the upper trunk • Primarily affects the **axillary, suprascapular,** and **musculocutaneous nerves** with loss of function of the intrinsic muscles of the shoulder and muscles of the anterior arm • Arm is medially rotated and adducted at the shoulder: loss of **axillary** and **suprascapular** nerves. The unopposed latissimus dorsi and pectoralis muscles pull the limb into adduction at the shoulder • The forearm is extended and pronated: loss of **musculocutaneous** nerve • **Sign is "waiter's tip"** • Sensory loss on lateral forearm to base of thumb: loss of musculocutaneous nerve
Lower (C8 and T1) Brachial Plexus Lesion: Klumpke's Paralysis
• Usually occurs when the upper limb is forcefully abducted above the head (e.g., grabbing an object when falling, thoracic outlet syndrome, or birth injury) • Trauma will injure the **C8** and **T1** spinal nerve roots of the inferior trunk • Primarily affects the ulnar nerve and the intrinsic muscles of the hand with weakness of the median-innervated muscles of the hand • Sign is combination of **"claw hand" (ulnar nerve)** and **"ape hand" (median nerve)**. • May include a Horner syndrome • Sensory loss on medial forearm and medial 1½ digits

► Lesions of Nerves of the Brachial Plexus

Radial Nerve (C5, C6, C7, C8)		
Axilla: (Saturday night palsy or using crutches)	**Mid-shaft of humerus at radial groove or lateral elbow (lateral epicondyle)**	**Wrist: (laceration)**
• Loss of extension at the elbow, wrist and MP joints • Weakened supination • Sensory loss on posterior arm, forearm, and dorsum of thumb • Distal sign is **"wrist drop"**	• Loss of forearm extensors of the wrist and MP joints • Weakened supination • Sensory loss on the posterior forearm and dorsum of thumb • Distal sign is **"wrist drop"**	• No **motor loss** • Sensory loss only on dorsal aspect of thumb (first dorsal web space)

Median Nerve (C6, C7, C8, T1)	
Elbow: (Supracondylar fracture of humerus)	**Wrist: (carpal tunnel or laceration)**
• Weakened wrist flexion (with ulnar deviation) • Loss of pronation • Loss of flexion of lateral 3 digits, resulting in the inability to make a complete fist; sign is **"hand of benediction"** • Loss of thumb opposition (opponens pollicis muscle); sign is **ape (simian) hand** • Loss of first two lumbricals • Thenar atrophy • Sensory loss on palmar surface of the lateral hand and the palmar surfaces of the lateral 3½ digits ***Note:* A lesion of median nerve at the elbow results in the "hand of benediction" and "ape hand."**	• Loss of thumb opposition (opponens pollicis muscle); sign is **ape or simian hand** • Loss of first two lumbricals • Thenar atrophy • Sensory loss on the palmar surfaces of lateral 3½ digits. Note sensation on lateral palm may be spared (see figure on next page). ***Note:* Lesions of median nerve at the wrist present without hand of benediction and with normal wrist flexion, digital flexion, and pronation.**

(Continued)

► Lesions of Nerves of the Brachial Plexus (*Cont'd.*)

Ulnar Nerve (C8, T1)
Elbow (medial epicondyle), wrist (lacerations), fracture of hook of hamate, midshaft clavicle fracture
• Loss of hypothenar muscles, third and fourth lumbricals, all interossei and adductor pollicis • With elbow lesion, there is minimal weakening of wrist flexion with radial deviation • Loss of **abduction** and **adduction of digits 2–5** (interosseus muscles) • Weakened IP extension of digits 2–5 (more pronounced in digits 4 and 5) • Loss of thumb adduction • Atrophy of the hypothenar eminence • Sign is **"claw hand"** (note that clawing is greater with a wrist lesion) • Sensory loss on medial 1½ digits
Axillary Nerve (C5, C6)
Fracture of the surgical neck of the humerus or inferior dislocation of the shoulder
• Loss of abduction of the arm to the horizon • Sensory loss over the deltoid muscle
Musculocutaneus Nerve (C5, C6, C7)
• Loss of elbow flexion and weakness in supination • Loss of sensation on lateral aspect of the forearm
Long Thoracic Nerve (C5, C6, C7)
• Often damaged during a radical mastectomy or a stab wound to the lateral chest (nerve lies on superficial surface of serratus anterior muscle) • Loss of abduction of the arm above the horizon to above the head • Sign of **"winged scapula"**; patient unable to hold the scapula against the posterior thoracic wall
Suprascapular Nerve (C5, C6)
• Loss of shoulder abduction between 0 and 15 degrees (supraspinatus muscle) • Weakness of lateral rotation of shoulder (infraspinatus muscle)

► Back Muscles

Action	Muscles Involved	Innervation
Extend/Rotate vertebrae	1. Splenius capitis, splenius cervicis	Dorsal rami of spinal nerves
	2. Erector spinae: • Iliocostalis • Longissimus • Spinalis	Dorsal rami of spinal nerves
	3. Transversospinalis: • Semispinalis • Multifidus • Rotatores	Dorsal rami of spinal nerves

► Effects of Lesions to Roots and Nerves of the Lumbosacral Plexus

The **lumbosacral plexus** is formed by an intermingling of the ventral rami of the L2 through S3 spinal nerves. The ventral rami of the lumbosacral plexus exhibit a proximal to distal gradient of innervation. Nerves that contain fibers from the superior rami of the plexus (L2 through L4) innervate muscles in the anterior and medial thigh that act at the hip and knee joints. Nerves that contain fibers from the inferior rami of the plexus (S1 through S3) innervate muscles of the leg that act at the joints of the ankle and foot.

Four major nerves arise from the lumbosacral plexus:

The **obturator** and **tibial** nerves contain anterior division fibers and innervate muscles in the medial and posterior compartments of the thigh, the posterior compartment of the leg, and in the sole of the foot.

The **femoral** and **common fibular** nerves contain posterior division fibers and innervate muscles in the anterior compartment of the thigh, in the anterior and lateral compartments of the leg, and in the dorsum of the foot.

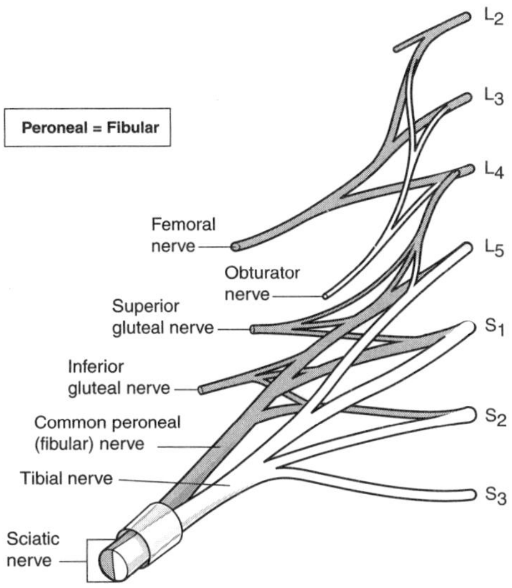

Lesioned Root	L3	L4	L5	S1
Dermatome paresthesia	Anterior thigh	Medial leg	Anterior leg, dorsum of foot	Lateral foot, sole
Reflex test	—	Patellar tendon	—	Achilles tendon
Muscles affected	Hip flexors Hip adductors	Knee extensors Hip adductors	Dorsiflexors Toe extensors	Plantar flexors Toe flexors
Causes of lesions	Osteoarthritis	Osteoarthritis	Herniation of L4/L5 disc	Herniation of L5/S1 disc
Lesioned Nerve	**Obturator (L2–L4)**	**Femoral (L2–L4)**	**Common Fibular (L4, L5, S1, S2)**	**Tibial (L4, L5, S1–S3)**
Altered sensation	Medial thigh	Anterior thigh, medial leg to medial malleolus	Anterior leg, dorsum of foot	Posterior leg, sole, and lateral border of foot
Reflex test	—	Patellar tendon	—	Achilles tendon
Motor weakness	Adduction of thigh	Extension of knee	Dorsiflexion, eversion of the foot	Plantar flexion Toe flexion
Common sign of lesion	—	—	Footdrop	—
Causes of lesions	Pelvic neoplasm Pregnancy	Diabetes Posterior abdominal neoplasm Psoas abscess	Compression at fibula neck Hip fracture/dislocation Misplaced gluteal injection Piriformis syndrome	Hip fracture/dislocation Penetrating trauma to buttock

Musculoskeletal Disorders

▶ Skeletal Disorders

Achondroplasia	• Autosomal dominant form of dwarfism; mutation of the fibroblast growth factor receptor 3 (FGFR3) • Abnormal cartilage synthesis • Decreased epiphyseal bone formation • Short limbs, proportionately large body and head (disease spares the cranium and vertebral bones), "saddle nose"
Enchondromatosis	• Multiple cartilaginous masses (enchondromas) within the medullary cavity of bone • **Ollier disease:** nonhereditary, multiple, most commonly hands and feet • Patients present with pain and fractures; may undergo malignant transformation • **Maffucci syndrome:** Familial; enchondromas and hemangiomas of the skin
Fibrous dysplasia	• Trabeculae of woven bone in a background of fibrous tissue • Incidence higher in male teenagers • Usually monostotic; often asymptomatic or may lead to pathologic fracture • Affects long bones, ribs, skull, and facial bones • Fibrosis starts within the medullary cavity and remains encased in cortical bone • **McCune-Albright syndrome:** Association of polyostotic fibrous dysplasia, café-au-lait spots, and sexual precocity in women
Hyperparathyroidism (osteitis fibrosa cystica)	• Osteoclasts resorb bone • Kidney wastes calcium • Osteitis fibrosa cystica more common in primary hyperparathyroidism • Bone pain and fractures • Fibrous replacement of marrow, causing cystic spaces in bone and "brown tumors"
Hypertrophic osteoarthropathy	• Idiopathic painful swelling of wrists, fingers, ankles, knees, or elbows • Periosteal inflammation, new bone forms at the ends of long bones, metacarpals, and metatarsals • Arthritis commonly seen, often with digital clubbing • Etiology: Intrathoracic carcinoma, cyanotic congenital heart disease, and inflammatory bowel disease • Regresses when underlying disease treated
Osteochondromatosis	• Bony metaphyseal projections capped with cartilage • Gardner syndrome: Exostoses and colonic polyps—may become carcinomas
Osteogenesis imperfecta	Defect in type I collagen characterized by fragile bones, blue sclera, and lax ligaments • *Type I*: autosomal dominant mild-to-moderate disease • *Type II*: autosomal recessive stillborn infant; generalized crumpled bones • *Type III*: autosomal recessive progressive severe deformity; white sclera • *Type IV:* autosomal dominant variable severity; normal sclera

(Continued)

► Skeletal Disorders *(Cont'd.)*

Osteomalacia and rickets	• **Vitamin D deficiency** due to chronic renal insufficiency, intestinal malabsorption, or dietary deficiency; osteoid produced in normal amounts but not calcified properly (diffuse radiolucency on bone films); low calcium and phosphorus and high alkaline phosphatase • *Rickets:* children, prior to closure of the epiphyses. Bone deformities, "rachitic rosary" (deformity of the chest wall), bowing of legs, and fractures • *Osteomalacia:* impaired mineralization of normal osteoid matrix; fractures, deformities
Osteomyelitis	• Spread by direct inoculation of bone or hematogenous seeding • *Staphylococcus aureus, Streptococcus, Haemophilus influenzae*, *Salmonella* (sickle cell disease), *Pseudomonas* (intravenous drug users and diabetics), *Mycobacterium tuberculosis* (Pott disease): tuberculous osteomyelitis of spine • Patients present with fever, localized pain, erythema, and swelling • X-ray may be normal for up to 2 weeks, then may show periosteal elevation • **Specific findings** include: – Sequestrum, a necrotic bone fragment – Involucrum, new bone that surrounds the area of inflammation – Brodie abscess, localized abscess formation in the bone
Osteopetrosis	• Osteoclasts unable to resorb bone • Increased density of cortex with narrowing of erythropoietic medullary cavities • Brittle bones, anemia, blindness, deafness, hydrocephalus, cranial nerve palsies • *Autosomal recessive:* affects children, causing early death due to anemia and infections (no bone marrow) • *Autosomal dominant*: adults—fractures
Osteoporosis	• Decrease in bone mass; postmenopausal women • Estrogen deficiency, low density of original bone, lack of exercise • Bone formed normally but in decreased amounts (thinned cortical bone, enlarged medullary cavity) • All bones are affected; x-ray shows generalized radiolucency • Weight-bearing bones predisposed to fractures
Paget disease	• Excessive bone resorption with replacement by soft, poorly mineralized matrix (woven appearance microscopically); x-ray: enlarged, radiolucent bones • Patients present with pain, deformity, fractures • Laboratory tests: extremely elevated alkaline phosphatase • Polyostotic: skull, pelvis, femur, and vertebrae • Progresses from an osteolytic to an osteoblastic phase • May cause bone hypervascularity with increased warmth of the overlying skin and eventually leading to high output cardiac failure

▶ Microbiology of Osteomyelitis

Type Infection	Case Vignette/Key	Most Common Causative Agent	Mechanism of Pathogenesis	Diagnosis	Treatment
Fever, bone pain with erythema and swelling; some patients (particularly those with diabetes) may have associated cellulitis	Adults, children, and infants without major trauma or special conditions	*Staphylococcus aureus*	Hematogenous spread → lytic bone lesions, lytic toxins	Blood culture or bone biopsy, Gram ⊕, catalase ⊕, coagulase ⊕, coccus	Nafcillin, 3rd gen cephalosporin, IV vancomycin
	Sickle cell anemia	*Salmonella* spp.	HbS patients are functionally asplenic and cannot kill bloodborne pathogens	Gram ⊖, oxidase ⊖, nonlactose fermenting	3rd gen cephalosporin, fluoroquinolones, chloramphenicol
	Trauma	*Pseudomonas aeruginosa*	Capsule protects against phagocytosis	Gram ⊖, oxidase ⊕, blue-green pigments; grape odor	Antipseudomonal beta-lactam + aminoglycoside, or carbapenem + antipseudomonal fluoroquinilone + aminoglycoside
	Spine, hip, knee, hands. Immigrants—Indian subcontinents	*Mycobacterium tuberculosis*	Tuberculous granuloma erodes into bone	Acid-fast bacilli or auramine stain	Multiple drug therapy

▶ Musculoskeletal Tumors

Osteoblastic Tumors	
Osteoblastoma	Similar to an osteoid osteoma, but is large and painless; often involves vertebrae; may be malignant
Osteoid osteoma	Benign; affects diaphysis of long bones; often tibia or femur Causes pain that is worse at night and relieved by aspirin X-ray findings—central radiolucency surrounded by a sclerotic rim Pathology: brown nodule surrounded by dense sclerotic cortical bone
Osteoma	Benign; frequently involves skull *Hyperostosis frontalis interna*: osteoma that extends into the orbit or sinuses Pathology: dense normal bone
Osteosarcoma	**Most common malignant bone tumor** Produces osteoid and bone Men are affected more often than women; usually second and third decade of life Associated with Paget disease in older patients Present with localized pain and swelling, weight loss, and anemia Classic x-ray findings—Codman triangle (periosteal elevation) and bone destruction Pathology: large, necrotic, and hemorrhagic mass Poor prognosis; patients are treated with amputation and chemotherapy Metastasis to the lungs common
Chondromatous Tumors	
Chondromyxoid fibroma	Benign, rare; affects young men Firm mass within the metaphyseal marrow cavity of the tibia or femur Contains fibrous and myxomatous tissue; must be differentiated from a malignant lesion
Chondrosarcoma	Malignant tumor; age range 30–60; men affected more than women May arise de novo or secondarily from pre-existing enchondroma Slower growing than osteosarcomas Typically presents with pain and swelling Involves the spine, pelvic bones, and upper extremities
Enchondroma	Solitary cartilaginous growth within the spongiosa of bone Solitary growths are similar to those in the multiple form (Ollier disease)
Osteochondroma	Benign metaphyseal growth; may be solitary; lesions identical to those in multiple form
Miscellaneous Tumors	
Ewing sarcoma	Malignant, rare; usually affects adolescents; often males Arises from mesenchymal cells Presents as pain, tenderness, and early widespread dissemination Commonly affects the pelvis and metaphysis of long tubular bones
Giant cell tumor	Usually benign, locally aggressive; uncommon; affects ages 20–50; arises in the epiphyseal region of long bones Presents as a bulky mass with pain and tenderness X-ray findings—expanding area of radiolucency without a sclerotic rim
Lipoma	Very common, soft, yellow, benign fatty tumor Often found subcutaneously; simple excision is curative
Liposarcoma	Malignant tumor of fatty tissue typically seen in middle-aged or older adults Typically found in deep subcutaneous tissues, deep fatty tissue of legs, or retroperitoneal areas

► Joint Pathology

Ankylosing spondylitis	Occurs predominantly in young men with HLA-B27 Also associated with inflammatory bowel disease Involves the sacroiliac joints and spine
Gout	**Hyperuricemia** leads to deposition of monosodium urate crystals (**needle-shaped and negatively birefringent**) in joints, leading to recurrent bouts of acute arthritis • Caused by overproduction of uric acid (under 10%) or underexcretion of uric acid (over 90%) • Joints are affected asymmetrically; **great toe** (first metatarsal joint) is classically affected (podagra) • Later stages → chronic arthritis and **tophi** in affected joints • Uric acid kidney stones develop in up to 25% of patients **Primary gout** (90% of cases): due to inborn error of purine metabolism, usually from an unknown enzyme deficiency **Secondary gout:** hyperuricemia unrelated to purine metabolism (Lesch-Nyhan syndrome is a rare cause due to HGPRT deficiency)
Juvenile rheumatoid arthritis (Still disease)	Peak incidence from 1–3 years; girls affected more frequently Often preceded by acute febrile illness Periarticular swelling, lymphadenopathy, hepatosplenomegaly, and absence of rheumatoid factor Variable course; resolution may occur
Osteoarthritis (degenerative joint disease)	Incidence ↑ with age; women more affected than men Affects 80% of people over 70 years old in at least one joint Aging or wear and tear (biomechanical) most important mechanism Insidious onset with joint stiffness, ↓ range of motion, and effusions X-ray findings—narrowing of the joint space due to loss of cartilage and osteosclerosis Joint fluid—few cells and normal mucin Most commonly affected joints—vertebrae, hips, knees, and distal interphalangeal (DIP) joints of fingers
Pseudogout (chondrocalcinosis)	Calcium pyrophosphate crystal deposition Associated with multiple diseases (e.g., Wilson disease, hypothyroidism, diabetes mellitus)
Psoriatic arthritis	Similar to rheumatoid arthritis, but absence of rheumatoid factor Associated with HLA-B27
Reactive arthritis (Reiter syndrome)	Triad of arthritis, conjunctivitis, urethritis possibly triggered by infections (e.g., *Chlamydia* and *Shigella*) Typically affects young men who are HLA-B27 positive
Rheumatoid arthritis	Progressive arthritis, associated with HLA-DR4 More common in women, ages 20–60 years Autoimmune reaction with the formation of IgM against Fc of IgG, anti-cyclic citrullinated peptide (CCP) antibodies (rheumatoid factor) Type IV hypersensitivity Symptoms—low-grade fever, malaise, fatigue, and morning stiffness Physical examination—joint swelling, redness, and warmth Synovial fluid—increased cells (usually neutrophils) and poor mucin Elevated sedimentation rate and hypergammaglobulinemia X-ray findings—erosions and osteoporosis Starts in the small joints of the hands and feet but may involve any joint; usually symmetric involvement **Felty syndrome:** polyarticular rheumatoid arthritis, splenomegaly, leukopenia
Suppurative arthritis	Tender, red, swollen joint (e.g., "a hot knee") Monoarticular; high neutrophil count in joint fluid Due to *Staphylococcus*, *Streptococcus*, and gonococci

▶ Infectious Arthritis

Presentation	Case Vignette/ Key Clues	Most Common Causative Agent	Mechanism of Pathogenesis	Diagnosis	Treatment
Pain, redness, low-grade fever, tenderness, swelling, reduced joint mobility	#1 overall, except in the 15–40 age group, where gonococcal is more prevalent	*Staphylococcus aureus*	Coagulase inhibits phagocytosis	Gram ⊕, coagulase ⊕ cocci, catalase ⊕	Nafcillin, 3rd gen cephalosporin, IV vancomycin
	15–40 years; mono- or polyarticular	*Neisseria gonorrhoeae*	Pili mediate adherence and inhibit phagocytosis	Gram ⊖ diplococcus; ferments glucose but not maltose	Ceftriaxone
	Prosthetic joint	Coagulase-negative staphylococci	Biofilm allows adherence to Teflon®	Gram ⊕, catalase ⊕ cocci	Nafcillin, 3rd gen cephalosporin
	Viral, polyarteritis nodosa	Rubella and hepatitis B, parvovirus	Immune complex mediated (type III hypersensitivity)	Detect immune complexes	Immunosuppressive therapy
	Chronic onset, monoarticular, weightbearing joints	*M. tuberculosis* or fungal	Granulomas erode into bone	Acid-fast bacillus or auramine stain, fungus stain	Multiple drug therapy

► Rheumatoid Arthritis Drugs

The rheumatoid arthritis (RA) **medications** can be divided into **three major classes**: anti-inflammatory drugs, bridging therapy, and disease-modifying antirheumatic drugs (DMARDs). Pharmacologic goals of therapy are to decrease pain, maintain "normal" functional status, reduce inflammation, decrease disease progression, and facilitate healing.

Drug	Mechanism/Other Uses	Adverse Effects
	Anti-inflammatory Drugs	
Salicylates (aspirin)	**Irreversibly** inhibit COX-1 and -2, decreasing PG synthesis • Low dose: ↓ platelet aggregation • Intermediate dose: antipyretic, analgesic • High dose: anti-inflammatory	• Chronic use associated with gastric ulcers, upper GI bleeding, acute renal failure, and interstitial nephritis • Large doses can produce tinnitus, vertigo, respiratory alkalosis • Overdose → metabolic acidosis, hyperthermia, dehydration, coma, death
NSAIDs (ibuprofen, naproxen, diclofenac, ketoprofen, indomethacin)	**Reversibly** inhibit COX-1 and -2, leading to decreased production of PGs Anti-inflammatory, analgesic, antipyretic; indomethacin used to close PDA	• Abdominal distress, bleeding, ulceration • Renal damage (especially in patients with renal disease) due to clearance by kidney
COX-2 inhibitors (celecoxib)	Selectively inhibit COX-2 **COX-1 pathway:** produces PGs that protect the GI lining, maintain renal blood flow, and aid in blood clotting **COX-2 pathway:** produces PGs involved in inflammation and pain	• Beneficial because of reduced GI side effects • This drug class is under scrutiny due to ↑ incidence of stroke and MI.
DMARDs	• May slow or reverse joint damage • Indicated for the treatment of RA when anti-inflammatory therapy insufficient to control patient's symptomatology • DMARDs usually do not show benefit for 6–8 weeks or longer; so, **bridging therapy** (corticosteroids) may be used until a full therapeutic effect is obtained. • DMARDs have severe and potentially fatal side effects.	
Hydroxychloroquine	• Stabilizes lysosomes, ↓ chemotaxis • Also an antimalarial	Ophthalmic abnormalities, dermatologic reactions, hematotoxicity, GI reactions
Methotrexate	• Inhibits dihydrofolate reductase, immunosuppressant • Also an antineoplastic	Hemotoxicity, ulcerative stomatitis, renal toxicity, elevated LFTs
Sulfasalazine	• Metabolized to 5-aminosalicylic acid (5-ASA) and sulfapyridine; parent drug and/or metabolites have anti-inflammatory and/or immunomodulatory properties • Used in inflammatory bowel disease	Rash, GI distress, headache, hematotoxicity
Azathioprine	• ↓ purine metabolism and nucleic acid synthesis; immunosuppressant	Hematologic, GI disturbance, secondary infection, increased risk of neoplasia
Etanercept	Binds TNF	Injection site reactions
Leflunomide	Inhibits cell proliferation and antiinflammatory	Hepatotoxicity, immunosuppression, GI disturbance, alopecia, rash, teratogen
Infliximab	• Monoclonal antibody to TNF-α • Also used in inflammatory bowel disease	Infusion reactions, infections, activation of latent TB

Definition of abbreviations: COX, cyclooxygenases; DMARDs, disease-modifying, slow-acting antirheumatic drugs; LFTs, liver function tests; PGs, prostaglandins; TNF, tumor necrosis factor; TB, tuberculosis.

► Drugs Used in the Treatment of Gout

There are **three** primary ways of treating gout: *1*) decreasing inflammation in acute attacks (NSAIDs, colchicine, intra-articular steroids), *2*) using uricosuric drugs to increase renal acceleration of uric acid, and *3*) decreasing conversion of purines to uric acid by inhibiting xanthine oxidase (allopurinol).

Agents	Mechanism	Comments
Acute treatment of gout	Acute treatment measures include NSAIDs (primarily indomethacin), colchicine, and corticosteroids (used only in resistant cases).	
NSAIDs	(*See* Rheumatoid Arthritis Drugs table.)	**Indomethacin** is drug of choice for acute gouty arthritis, although other NSAIDs also effective
Colchicine	**Binds tubulin and prevents microtubule assembly** Reduces the inflammatory response by decreasing leukocyte migration and phagocytosis	Previously considered drug of choice for gouty arthritis; however, its side effect profile limits its usage **Adverse effects:** severe diarrhea and abdominal distress, hematologic (bone marrow suppression, aplastic anemia, or thrombocytopenia), renal failure, hepatic failure, peripheral neuropathy, alopecia
Chronic/prophylactic treatment of gout	These agents are used for the treatment and/or prevention of hyperuricemia with gout and gouty arthritis.	
Uricosuric agents (probenecid, sulfinpyrazone)	**Inhibits reabsorption of uric acid**, thus ↑ its excretion	Inhibits the secretion of many weak acids (e.g., penicillin, methotrexate) **Adverse reactions:** may precipitate acute gouty arthritis, which can be prevented by concurrent NSAIDs; cross-allergenicity with other sulfonamides
Allopurinol	**Inhibits xanthine oxidase**, the enzyme responsible for conversion of hypoxanthine and xanthine to uric acid	Also used as an adjunct to cancer chemotherapy Inhibits metabolism of 6-mercaptopurine and azathioprine (which are metabolized by xanthine oxidase) **Adverse reactions:** GI distress, rash

► Tumors Involving Joint Space

Malignant fibrous histiocytoma	Relatively common, affecting adult men > women Arise in soft tissue or bones Lower extremities > upper; also abdominal cavity
Pigmented villonodular synovitis	Villous proliferation of synovium colored brown by hemosiderin deposition Probably a reactive response to recurrent trauma or possibly a neoplastic process that does not metastasize
Synoviosarcoma	Rare tumor, early adulthood; affects males and females equally Slow growing, painless masses Aggressive, early metastases to the lung and pleura Two-thirds occur in lower extremities and one-third in upper extremities

▶ Muscle Disorders

Muscular Dystrophies	
Becker muscular dystrophy	X-linked recessive inheritance or spontaneous Milder; patients may walk until age 20 or 25 Cardiac lesions are mild
Duchenne muscular dystrophy	Severe, **X-linked**, abnormal **dystrophin** protein, loss of muscle cell membrane stability Elevation of creatine kinase and histologic degeneration precedes clinical features Pelvic girdle weakness and ataxia Course is progressive; children unable to walk by the age of 10 Pseudohypertrophy of the calves characteristic Myocardial muscle involvement accompanies other muscle degeneration; may cause death Heterozygous female carriers have subclinical degeneration of muscle fibers
Facioscapulohumeral muscular dystrophy	Autosomal dominant, but spontaneous mutation relatively common Usually involves the face, neck, and shoulder muscles; pelvic muscles in later stages
Limb-girdle muscular dystrophy	Autosomal recessive Weakness begins in pelvic or shoulder girdle; may retain ambulation for 25 years
Myotonic dystrophy	Autosomal dominant pattern or spontaneous mutations Trinucleotide repeat (CTG) in a protein kinase Clinically unique: weakness, atrophy, and myotonia (tonic contractions) Head and neck muscles frequently weak and atrophic
Additional Muscular Disorders	
Myasthenia gravis	**Autoimmune** disease; antibodies against **neuromuscular junction acetylcholine receptors** (nicotinic AChR) Typically affects young women with **fluctuating weakness** but **no sensory** abnormalities; worsens with increased use of muscles Diagnosis—decremental response on EMG or improvement with **edrophonium** May have **thymic abnormalities**, including thymoma (10–20%) or thymic hyperplasia (70–80%)
Lambert-Eaton myasthenic syndrome	• Closely related to myasthenia gravis with similar symptoms • Autoantibodies are directed against NMJ Ca^{2+} channels • May occur in a paraneoplastic setting
Myositides	**Polymyositis** and **dermatomyositis**; autoimmune or collagen vascular diseases Polymyositis more common in females Neck and proximal limb muscle weakness, dysphagia, and muscle pain Dermatomyositis: purple discoloration of the eyelids (heliotrope rash) and ↑ risk of internal malignancies
Myositis ossificans	Ossification at the site of traumatic hemorrhage Pain, swelling, and tenderness
Rhabdomyosarcoma	Most common soft tissue sarcoma in children 40% have metastases at the time of diagnosis **Embryonal rhabdomyosarcoma:** • Most often located in head and neck tissues • Sarcoma botryoides: embryonal rhabdomyosarcoma with a grape-like, soft, polypoid appearance usually located in the genitourinary or upper respiratory tract

Definition of abbreviation: EMG, electromyogram; NMJ, neuromuscular junction.

Skin

▶ Skin and Skin Appendages

The integument consists of the skin (epidermis and dermis) and associated appendages (sweat and sebaceous glands, hairs, and nails). The epidermis is devoid of blood vessels and contains a stratified squamous epithelium derived primarily from ectoderm.

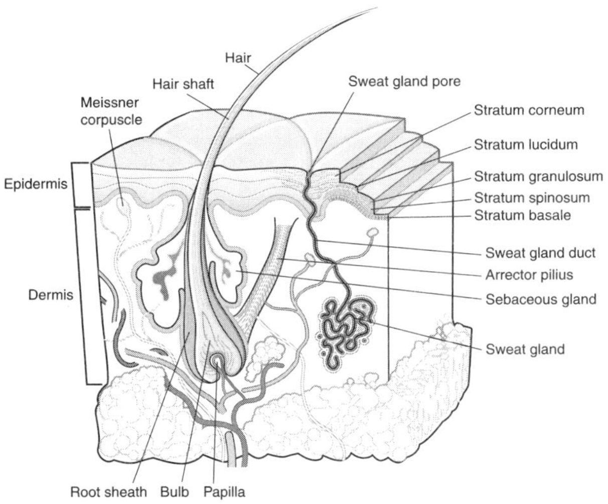

The **epidermis** is composed of five layers in thick skin:

- **Stratum basale:** a proliferative layer of columnar/cuboidal cells
- **Stratum spinosum:** a multilaminar layer of cuboidal/polygonal cells
- **Stratum granulosum:** has more flattened polygonal cells containing basophilic granules
- **Stratum lucidum:** a thin, eosinophilic layer of squamous cells
- **Stratum corneum:** a thick layer containing anucleate keratinized cells

- The **epidermis** contains four cell types: **keratinocytes**, which produce keratin; **melanocytes** (derived from neural crest) that produce melanin; **Langerhans cells**, which are antigen-presenting cells; and **Merkel cells**, associated with nerve fibers.
- The **dermis** is a connective tissue layer mainly of mesodermal origin.
- **Sweat glands** may be eccrine or apocrine.
- **Sebaceous glands** are branched, holocrine acinar glands that discharge their secretions onto hair shafts within hair follicles. They are absent in the palms and soles.
- **Hair** is composed of keratinized epidermal cells. Hair follicles and the associated sebaceous glands are known as pilosebaceous units.

▶ Skin Pathology

Acanthosis nigricans	Epidermal hyperplasia producing velvety hyperpigmentation of body folds in areas such as axilla, neck, and groin Can be associated with hyperlipidemia, diabetes, and visceral malignancies.
Actinic keratosis	Premalignant and may develop into squamous cell carcinoma Fair-skinned people of middle age associated with chronic sun exposure
Atopic dermatitis (eczema)	Itchy eruption that often preferentially involves the flexural areas Typically diagnosed at about 6 months of age — often a lifetime illness with a remitting/flaring course; thought to be due to an immediate hypersensitivity (Type I) reaction with elevated serum IgE May be associated with asthma, allergic rhinitis, and food allergy
Basal cell carcinoma	Pearly papules with telangiectasias Invasive, but rarely metastasizes Occurs on sun-exposed areas in middle-aged or elderly individuals with fair complexions Complete excision is usually curative; 50% recurrence rate
Bullous pemphigoid	Autoantibodies to dermoepidermal junction antigens Pemphigus vulgaris is due to autoantibodies to keratinocyte intercellular junction antigens
Capillary hemangiomas	Arise within the first weeks of life and usually resolve spontaneously; starting at 1–3 years of age; most completely gone by age 5 Soft, red, lobulated mass, 1–6 cm in diameter, composed of thick-walled capillaries

(Continued)

▶ Skin Pathology *(Cont'd.)*

Contact dermatitis	Localized skin rash caused by contact with a foreign substance Rash is typically bright red, sometimes with blisters, wheals, or urticaria; may have intense itchiness and burning sensation Can be due to chemical irritation (with or without light exposure), true allergic reaction, or physical irritation Often resolves spontaneously; treated with oral antihistamines or hydrocortisone cream; systemic corticosteroids can be used in severe, persistent cases
Dermatitis herpetiformis	Vesicular, pruritic disease often associated with celiac sprue IgA is found at the dermoepidermal junction
Erythema multiforme	Hypersensitivity reaction to drugs Stevens-Johnson syndrome is the severe form.
Erythema nodosum	Hypersensitivity reaction that causes inflammatory nodules in adipose tissue (panniculitis), typically on the anterior shins Peak age in the 20s to 30s; female predominance Can be associated with diseases that stimulate the immune system, including tuberculosis, coccidiomycosis, histoplasmosis, leprosy, sarcoidosis, and streptococcal infections
Kaposi sarcoma	Malignant mesenchymal tumor characterized by an aggressive course in patients with AIDS and by a slower course in elderly men without HIV Caused by human herpes virus type 8 (HHV8)
Lichen planus	Small, itchy, purple, polygonal papules of the skin and oral mucosa Dense infiltrate of lymphocytes at the dermal epidermal junction accompanied by irregular, "saw-tooth" extensions of the dermis into the epidermis
Malignant melanoma	Peaks by ages 40–60 Melanoma grows horizontally first (radial growth), followed by vertical dermal invasion (nodular growth) and forms a large, brown-black patch best prognosis of all forms of melanoma **Lentigo maligna** best prognosis of all forms of melanoma **Nodular** melanoma shows extensive dermal invasion and rapid growth Raised brown-black lesions may be found anywhere on skin or mucosa Worst prognosis of the melanomas Prognosis related to **depth of invasion** (Breslow thickness)
Melasma	Hyperpigmentation occurring in pregnancy, sometimes called "mask of pregnancy" because it often involves the face
Nevocellular nevus	Common benign mole containing nevocytes derived from melanocytes • Junctional nevus: nevocytes are just at the dermoepidermal junction • Dermal nevus: nevocytes just in the dermis • Compound nevus: nevocytes are both at the junction and in the dermis
Nevus flammeus (port wine stain)	Common congenital lesion; composed of telangiectatic vessels Usually located on the neck or face as a large, flat, irregular pink patch that tends to resolve spontaneously
Pemphigus vulgaris	Potentially life-threatening blistering disease of skin and mucous membranes Autoimmune etiology involving antibodies directed against desmoglein 3 Blisters form within the epidermis
Pityriasis rosea	Self-limited skin eruption that characteristically starts with a single, isolated lesion called the "herald patch" and then 1 or 2 weeks later progresses to a generalized rash with large numbers of large, flaky, reddish skin lesions
Psoriasis	Silvery, scaly plaque that primarily affects knees, elbows, and the scalp
Seborrheic keratosis	Common benign (but often biopsied) skin lesion of elderly people - flat, greasy papules that appear "stuck on" on the head, trunk, and extremities Microscopically shows a thickened, benign epidermis composed of basaloid cells with horn cyst formation within the epidermis

(Continued)

▶ Skin Pathology *(Cont'd.)*

Squamous cell carcinoma	Malignant tumor; most frequently in sun-exposed areas with peak at 60 years of age Preponderance among women When on sun-exposed regions, rarely metastasizes When on unexposed skin, up to 50% metastasize
Toxic epidermal necrolysis (TENS; Lyell's syndrome)	Life-threatening dermatologic condition in which the epidermis detaches from the dermis all over the body, particularly involving the mucous membranes Considered to be a very severe form of Stevens-Johnson syndrome Typically occurs as a severe reaction to medications, notably including sulfonamides, non-steroidal anti-inflammatory drugs, allopurinol, anti-HIV drugs, corticosteroids, and anticonvulsants Patients are treated similarly to those with severe burns
Urticaria	Urticaria (hives) due to localized areas of allergic-based mast cell degranulation leading to dermal edema with intense itchiness
Vitiligo	Vitiligo is an acquired pigmentation disorder characterized by localized areas of complete skin depigmentation

▶ Infectious Diseases of the Skin, Mucous Membranes, and Underlying Tissues

Case Vignette/ Key Clues	Diagnosis	Common Causative Agents	Mechanism of Pathogenesis	Treatment
		Furuncles, carbuncles		
Neck, face, axillae, buttocks	Catalase ⊕, coagulase ⊕, gram ⊕ cocci in grape-like clusters	*Staphylococcus aureus*	Coagulase breaks fibrin clot Neutrophils + bacteria → pus	Nafcillin for methicillin-sensitive *S. aureus* (MSSA); vancomycin for methicillin-resistant *S. aureus* (MRSA)
Inflamed follicles from neck down	Oxidase ⊕, gram ⊖ rod, blue-green pigment, grape odor	*Pseudomonas aeruginosa* (hot tub folliculitis)	Capsule inhibits phagocytosis	Antipseudomonal beta-lactam + aminoglycoside
		Acne vulgaris		
Inflammation of follicles and sebaceous glands; adolescent	Gram ⊕ rod, identified by clinical clues	*Propionibacterium acnes*	Fatty acids and peptides produced from sebum cause inflammation	Tetracycline, macrolide
		Cutaneous lesions (scratching mosquito bites, cat scratches, etc.)		
Initially vesicular; skin erosion; honey-crusted lesions	Catalase ⊖, gram ⊕ cocci, bacitracin sensitive	*Streptococcus pyogenes*	Streptokinase A and B DNAse, hyaluronidase	Penicillin, macrolide
Initially vesicular but with longer-lasting bullae	Catalase ⊕, coagulase ⊕, gram ⊕ cocci, in clusters	*Staphylococcus aureus*	Exfoliatins produce bullae	Nafcillin for MSSA; vancomycin for MRSA
		Red, raised, butterfly-wing facial rash		
Dermal pain, edema, rapid spread	Catalase ⊖, gram ⊕ cocci, bacitracin-sensitive	*Streptococcus pyrogenes* (erysipelas)	M protein inhibits phagocytosis, erythrogenic exotoxins, hyaluronidase	Penicillin, macrolide

(Continued)

► Infectious Diseases of the Skin, Mucous Membranes, and Underlying Tissues *(Cont'd.)*

Case Vignette/ Key Clues	Diagnosis	Common Causative Agents	Mechanism of Pathogenesis	Treatment
Jaw area swelling with pain, sinus tract formation, yellow granules in exudate				
Carious teeth, dental extraction or trauma	Gram ⊕, anaerobic, filamentous branching rods, non-acid fast	*Actinomyces israelii*; "lumpy jaw"; actinomycosis	Unknown	Penicillin
Vesicular lesions				
Sometimes preceded by neurologic pain	Cell culture, intranuclear inclusion, multinucleated cells	Herpes	Virus-rich vesicles ulcerate dsDNA, enveloped (nuclear membranes)	Acyclovir, valacyclovir, famciclovir
Sometimes large	Catalase ⊕, coagulase ⊕, gram ⊕ cocci, in clusters	*Staphylococcus aureus*	Exfolatins produce bullae	Nafcillin for MSSA; vancomycin for MRSA
Subcutaneous granulomas/ulcers/cellulitis				
Tropical fish enthusiasts; granulomatous lesion (most commonly freshwater)	Biopsy, slow growing acid-fast bacilli	*Mycobacterium marinum*	Trauma + water exposure → granulomas form	Clarithromycin initially, then antimycobacterial therapy
Cellulitis following contact with saltwater or oysters	Green colonies on TCBS agar (alkaline), gram ⊖ rod, oxidase ⊕	*Vibrio vulnificus*	Cytolytic compounds, antiphagocytic polysaccharides	Tetracycline, aminoglycosides
Solitary or lymphocutaneous lesions; rose gardeners or florists; sphagnum moss	Cigar-shaped yeast in pus	*Sporothrix schenckii* (rose gardener's disease)	Ulceration or abscess	Potassium iodide, ketoconazole
Subcutaneous swelling (extremities, shoulders), sinus tract formation, granules (mycetoma)	*Actinomyces*—Gram ⊕, anaerobic, filamentous branching non-acid fast rods *Nocardia*—partially acid-fast, branching filaments, aerobic	*Actinomyces, Nocardia*	Unknown; granules are microcolonies	*Actinomyces*—penicillin, doxycycline, clindamycin *Nocardia*—sulfonamide, sulfa antibiotics; carbapenem for resistant cases
Malignant pustule				
Pustule → dark-red, fluid-filled, tumor-like lesion → necrosis → black eschar surrounded by red margin; postal worker or wool handler/ importer	Gram ⊕, spore-forming, encapsulated rods	*Bacillus anthracis*	Poly-D-glutamate capsule, exotoxin causes edema, cell death Three-component toxin	Ciprofloxacin, penicillin
As above, with pseudomonal septicemia	Blood culture, gram ⊖, oxidase ⊕, produces blue-green pigments, fruity odor	*Pseudomonas aeruginosa*, (**ecthyma gangrenosum**)	Endotoxin	Susceptibility testing necessary

(Continued)

► Infectious Diseases of the Skin, Mucous Membranes, and Underlying Tissues *(Cont'd.)*

Case Vignette/ Key Clues	Diagnosis	Common Causative Agents	Mechanism of Pathogenesis	Treatment
		Burns, cellulitis		
Blue-green pus; grape-like odor	Oxidase ⊕, gram ⊖ rod, blue-green pigments, grape odor	*Pseudomonas aeruginosa*	Capsule inhibits phagocytosis	Antipseudomonal beta-lactam + aminoglycoside
		Wounds		
Surgical wounds (clean)	Same as above for *S. aureus*	*Staphylococcus aureus*	Same as above for *S. aureus*	Nafcillin for MSSA, vancomycin for MRSA
Surgical wounds (dirty)	Gram ⊖ facultative anaerobes	Enterobacteriaceae, anaerobes	Contamination from fecal flora	3rd gen cephalosporin
Trauma with damage to blood supply	Nagler reaction, anaerobic, gram ⊕ rod, spore forming	*Clostridium perfringens* and others	Alpha toxin (lecithinase) gas production, edema, cytotoxicity	Debridement, clindamycin, chloramphenicol, tetracycline
Animal bites (various)	Gram ⊖ rods (bite wounds are not generally cultured)	*Pasteurella multocida*	Capsule	Amoxicillin/clavulanate
Human bites, fist fights	Gram ⊖ oral floral	*Eikenella corrodens*	Pili, phase variation	3rd generation cephalosporins, fluoroquinolones
Dog bites	Gram ⊖ fusiform	*Capnocytophaga canimorsus*	Sialidase allows adherence to host cells	As above
Rat bites	Gram ⊖ pleomorphic rod	*Streptobacillus moniliformis and Spirillum minus*	Endotoxin	Penicillin G or V
Cat scratches, resulting in lymphadenopathy with stellate granulomas	Gram ⊖ envelope	*Bartonella henselae*	Obligate intracellular	Various antibiotics (rifampin, ciprofloxacin, gentamicin, TMP-sulfamethoxazole)
Shallow puncture wound through tennis shoe sole	Oxidase ⊕, gram ⊖ rod, blue-green pigments	*Pseudomonas aeruginosa*	Capsule inhibits phagocytosis	Antipseudomonal beta-lactam + aminoglycoside
		Leprosy		
Blotchy, red lesions with anesthesia; facial and cooler areas of skin	Acid-fast, intracellular bacilli in punch biopsy, ⊕ lepromin test	*Mycobacterium leprae* (tuberculoid form)	Cell-mediated immunity kills intracellular organisms, damages nerves	Dapsone, clofazimine +/- rifampin
Numerous nodular lesions; leonine facies	Acid-fast, intracellular bacilli in punch biopsy, ⊖ lepromin test	*Mycobacterium leprae* (lepromatous form)	Humoral immunity elicited does not stop growth of organisms	Dapsone, clofazimine +/- rifampin

(Continued)

► Infectious Diseases of the Skin, Mucous Membranes, and Underlying Tissues *(Cont'd.)*

Case Vignette/ Key Clues	Diagnosis	Common Causative Agents	Mechanism of Pathogenesis	Treatment
		Keratinized area of skin (ringworm)		
Reddened skin lesion in growing ring shape, raised margin; infection nail bed or hair shaft	Wood's lamp (fluoresce), skin scraping and KOH; arthroconidia	*Trichophyton* spp. (skin, hair, nails) *Epidermophyton* spp. (skin, nails) *Microsporum* spp. (skin, hair)	Fungi germinate in moist areas, invade	Topical miconazole or oral imidazoles if hair shaft or nails infected
		Dermatitis		
Itching skin rash after swimming in fresh water lakes (swimmer's itch)	Clinical signs and history	Bird schistosomes	Skin penetration by cercariae → death in skin → hypersensitivity	Topical anti-inflammatory
Snake-like tracks on bare skin exposed to dog/cat feces (plumber's itch, cutaneous larva migrans)	Clinical signs and history	Dog and cat hookworms (*Ancylostoma* spp.)	Skin penetration by larvae → death in skin → hypersensitivity (type 1)	Topical anti-inflammatory, thiabendazole
		Warts		
Plantar surfaces	Intranuclear inclusion bodies	HPV 1 (dsDNA, naked icosahedral)	Virus infects basal layers of skin, stimulates cells to divide	Cryotherapy
Common warts		HPV serotypes 2, 4		
Umbilicated warts; wrestling teams; may be anogenital	Intracytoplasmic inclusions	*Molluscum contagiosum* (pox family, dsDNA, enveloped complex)	Infects epidermal cells to form fleshy lesion	Cryotherapy
Anogenital warts	Intranuclear inclusion bodies	HPV 6 and 11 (most common) HPV 16 and 18 (premalignant)	Virus stimulates cell division Cervical intraepithelial neoplasia Tumor suppressor gene inactivation	Imiquimod, interferon-α, cidofovir
		Mucocutaneous erosive lesions		
Foreign immigrant or military stationed in the Middle East, ulcers; chronic facial disfigurement; sandfly vector	Finding amastigotes with flagellar pocket inside phagocytic cells in biopsy	*Leishmania* spp.	Amastigotes intracellular in macrophages, proliferate and spread	Antimonials pentamidine

► Selected Rashes

Type of Rash	Progression	Other Symptoms	Causative Agent(s)	Pathogenesis	Diagnosis	Treatment
Scarlet fever						
Erythematous maculopapular (sandpaper-like)	Trunk and neck → extremities (spares palms and soles)	Sore throat, fever, nausea	*Streptococcus pyogenes*	Exotoxins A–C (superantigens)	Gram ⊕, catalase ⊖ cocci	Penicillin, clindamycin
Toxic shock syndrome						
Diffuse, erythematous, macular sunburn-like	Trunk and neck → extremities with desquamation on palms and soles	Acute onset, fever >102 F, myalgia, pharyngitis, vomiting, diarrhea; hypotension leading to multiorgan failure	*Staphylococcus aureus*	TSST-1 (superantigen)	Gram ⊕, catalase ⊕, coagulase ⊕ cocci	Nafcillin , oxacillin; vancomycin in penicillin allergic patients
Staphylococcal skin disease: scalded skin disease and scarlatina						
Perioral erythema, bullae, vesicles, desquamation	Trunk and neck → extremities, except tongue and palate; large bullae and vesicles precede exfoliation	Abscess or some site of infection	*Staphylococcus aureus*	Exotoxin	Gram ⊕, catalase ⊕, coagulase ⊕ cocci	Nafcillin , oxacillin; vancomycin in penicillin allergic patients
Lyme disease						
Erythematous concentric rings (Bull's eye)	Originates at site of tick bite	Fever, headache, myalgia, Bell's palsy	*Borrelia burgdorferi* (#1 vector-borne disease in U.S.)	Invades skin and spreads to involve heart, joints and CNS. Arthritis is type III hypersensitivity	Serology	Doxycycline, ceftriaxone
Epidemic typhus						
Petechiae → purpura	Trunk → extremities; spares palms, soles, and face	Fever, rash, headache, myalgias, and respiratory symptoms	*Rickettsia prowazekii*	Endotoxin	Serology, Weil-Felix	Doxycycline, chloramphen-icol
Rocky Mountain spotted fever (most common on East Coast)						
Petechiae	Ankles and wrists → generalized with palms and soles	Fever, rash, headache, myalgias, and respiratory symptoms	*Rickettsia rickettsii*	Endotoxin (overproduces outer membrane fragments)	Serology, Weil-Felix	Doxycycline, chloramphen-icol
Early meningococcemia						
Petechiae → purpura	Generalized	Abrupt onset, fever, chills, malaise, prostration, exanthem → shock	*Neisseria meningitidis*	Endotoxin	Gram ⊖ diplococcus on chocolate agar; LPA for capsular antigens	Ceftriaxone

(Continued)

► Selected Rashes *(Cont'd.)*

Type of Rash	Progression	Other Symptoms	Causative Agent(s)	Pathogenesis	Diagnosis	Treatment
Secondary syphilis						
Skin: maculopapular; mucous membrane: condylomata lata	Generalized bronze rash involving the palms and soles	Fever, lymphadenopathy, malaise, sore throat, splenomegaly, headache, arthralgias	*Treponema pallidum*	Endotoxin	Serology: VDRL (nonspecific), FTA-ABS (specific)	Penicillin, doxycycline, erythromycin
Measles						
Confluent, erythematous, maculopapular rash, unvaccinated child	Head → entire body Koplik's spots	Cough, coryza, conjunctivitis, and fever (prodrome); oral lesions, exanthem, bronchopneumonia, ear infections (unvaccinated individual)	Rubeola virus; negative sense RNA virus, non-segmented = Paramyxovirus	T-cell destruction of virus-infected cells in capillaries causes rash	Virus cultures, serology	Supportive
Chickenpox/Shingles						
Asynchronous rash, unvaccinated child	Generalized with involvement of mucous membranes	Fever, pharyngitis, malaise, rhinitis, exanthem	Varicella zoster virus (Herpesviridae, dsDNA)	Virus replicates in mucosa and is latent in dorsal root ganglia	Tzanck smear (find syncytia), Cowdry type A intranuclear inclusions, PCR	Supportive, avoid aspirin due to Reye syndrome
Unilateral vesicular rash following a dermatome, 50-60 year old patient	Restricted to one dermatome	Fever, severe nerve pain, pruritus	Varicella zoster virus (Herpesviridae, dsDNA)	Reactivation of latent infection	Tzanck smear (find syncytia), Cowdry type A intranuclear inclusions, PCR	Acyclovir, famciclovir, valacyclovir

The Hematologic and Lymphoreticular System

Chapter 9

Hematopoiesis

All of the different blood cells are derived from stem cells in the bone marrow, as shown below.

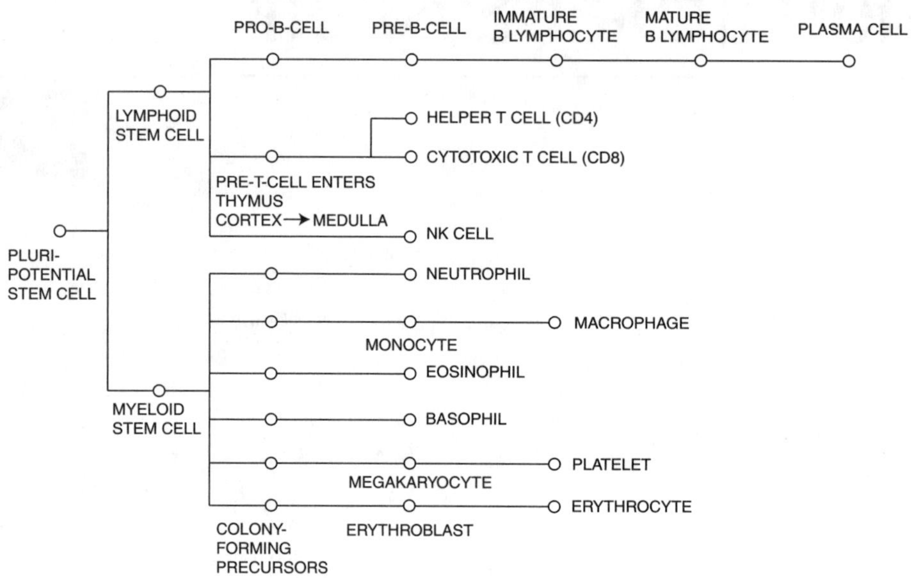

Hemostasis

Hemostasis is the sequence of events leading to the cessation of bleeding by the formation of a stable fibrin-platelet plug. It involves the vascular wall, platelets, and the coagulation system.

► Platelet Function and Dysfunction

Platelets are anuclear, membrane-bound cellular fragments derived from megakaryocytes in the bone marrow. They have a short lifespan of approximately 10 days. There are normally 150,000–400,000 platelets per mm^3 of blood. Platelet activity is measured by **template bleeding time**. Clinically, dysfunction is seen as **petechiae**. The platelet reaction consists of three steps. Dysfunction of each step is associated with different diseases:

- Adhesion (e.g., von Willebrand disease, Bernard-Soulier syndrome)
- Primary aggregation (e.g., thrombasthenia)
- Secondary aggregation and release (e.g., aspirin, storage pool disease)

► Formation of the Platelet Plug

Vascular wall injury	• Injury causes exposure of subendothelial extracellular collagen • Arteriolar contraction due to reflex neurogenic mechanisms, and the local release of **endothelin** occurs
Adhesion	• **von Willebrand factor (vWF)** binds exposed collagen fibers in the basement membrane • Platelets adhere to vWF via **glycoprotein Ib** and become **activated** (shape change, degranulation, synthesis of **thromboxane A_2, TxA_2**) • Deficiency of vWF → **von Willebrand disease**; deficiency of glycoprotein Ib receptor → **Bernard-Soulier syndrome**
Release reaction	• Release contents of platelet dense bodies (e.g., **ADP**, **calcium**, serotonin, histamine, epinephrine) and alpha granules (fibrinogen, fibronectin, factor V, vWF, platelet-derived growth factor) • Membrane expression of phospholipid complexes (important for coagulation cascade)
Aggregation	• **ADP** and **thromboxane A_2 (TxA_2)** is released by **platelets** and **promote aggregation** (TXA_2 production is inhibited by **aspirin**) • Cross-linking of platelets by **fibrinogen** requires the **GpIIb/IIIa receptor**, which is deficient in **Glanzmann thrombasthenia** • Decreased endothelial synthesis of antithrombogenic substances (e.g., prostacyclin, nitric oxide, tissue plasminogen activator, thrombomodulin)

▶ Disorders of Platelet Numbers

Thrombocytopenia	• **Decrease** in the platelet count (normal = 150,000–400,000/mm^3) • **Clinical features:** bleeding from small vessels, often skin, GI/GU tracts; **petechiae** and **purpura** are seen • **Classification:** decreased production (aplastic anemia, drugs, vitamin B_{12} or folate deficiency); increased destruction, (e.g., DIC, TTP, ITP, drugs, malignancy); abnormal sequestration
Idiopathic thrombocytopenic purpura (ITP)	• Spleen makes antibodies against platelet antigens (e.g., GpIIb–IIIa, GpIb–IX); platelets destroyed in the spleen by macrophages • Acute form (children): self-limited, postviral • Chronic form (adults): ITP may be primary or secondary to another disorder (e.g., HIV, SLE) • Smear shows enlarged, immature platelets; normal PT and PTT • Treatment: corticosteroids, immunoglobulin therapy, splenectomy
Thrombotic thrombocytopenic purpura (TTP)	• **Clinical features:** pentad (thrombocytopenic purpura, fever, renal failure, neurologic changes, microangiopathic hemolytic anemia); usually in young women • Inherited or acquired deficiency of **ADAMTSI3** • Smear shows few platelets, schistocytes, and helmet cells • **Hemolytic uremic syndrome (HUS):** mostly in children after gastroenteritis with bloody diarrhea; organism: verotoxin-producing *E. coli* O157:H7; similar clinical triad
Thrombocytosis (reactive)	Increase in count due to bleeding, hemolysis, inflammation, malignancy, iron deficiency, stress, or postsplenectomy
Essential thrombocythemia	Increase in count due to primary myeloproliferative disorder

▶ Disorders of Platelet Function Leading to Increased Bleeding

Bernard-Soulier disease	Defective platelet plug formation secondary to decreased Gp1b, which causes impaired platelet-to-subendothelial collagen aggregation
Glanzmann thrombasthenia	Defective platelet plug formation secondary to decreased GpIIb/IIIa, which causes impaired platelet-to-subendothelial collagen aggregation
von Willebrand disease	Defective platelet plug formation due to an autosomal dominant defect in quantity or quality of von Willebrand factor (vWF); increased bleeding time and increased PTT (because vWF stabilizes factor VIII)

► Coagulation

Coagulation begins anywhere from a few seconds to 1–2 minutes after an injury.

Intrinsic Pathway

- **Factor XII** (Hageman factor) is activated on contact with the collagen
- "a" indicates activated form

Extrinsic Pathway

Initiated by exposure to tissue thromboplastin

Common Pathway

Factors IXa, VIIa, VIIIa, platelet phospholipids, and calcium activate factor X

Thrombin (IIa):

- Able to catalyze own activation
- Increases platelet aggregation
- Activates **factor XIII** (fibrin-stabilizing factor) and potentiates binding of factors V and VIII to phospholipid/Ca^{2+} complex

Fibrinogen (I):

- Split into self-polymerizing fibrin monomers
- Initially bind via loose hydrogen and hydrophobic bonds
- **Factor XIII** catalyzes formation of strong covalent bonds

Vitamin K–Dependent Factors

Factors II (prothrombin), VII, IX, X, protein C, and protein S

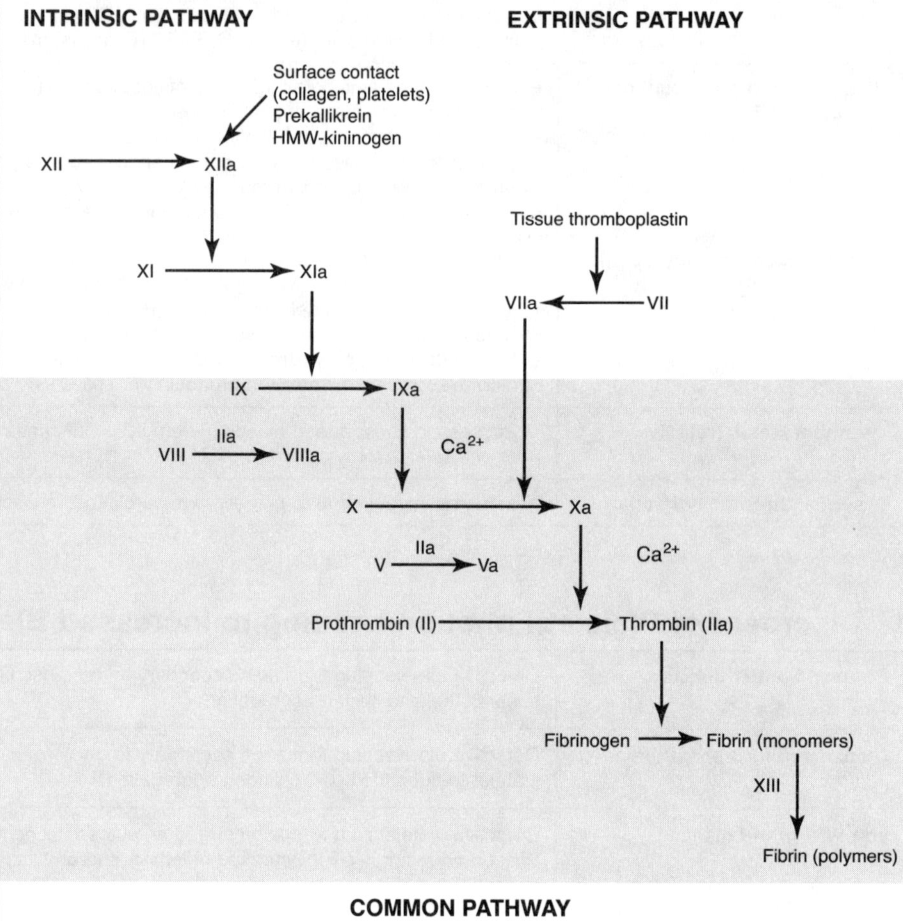

► Final Step: Clot Retraction and Dissolution

- After the clot is formed, it begins to shrink.
- Edges of small wounds are pulled together by platelet actinomyosin.
- Fibrinolysis (dissolution) requires activation of plasminogen.
- Clot releases plasminogen activator, which converts plasminogen to plasmin, which in turn proteolyses fibrinogen and fibrin.
- Urokinase and streptokinase are exogenous sources of plasminogen activation. Tissue plasminogen activator (t-PA) is endogenously produced, but can also be administered as a drug in the setting of acute myocardial infarction.

Erythropoiesis

Erythropoiesis is the process of RBC formation. Bone marrow stem cells (colony-forming units, CFUs) differentiate into proerythroblasts under the influence of the glycoprotein **erythropoietin**, which is produced by the kidney.

Proerythroblasts → **basophilic erythroblasts** → **normoblasts (nucleus extruded)** → **reticulocyte (still contains some ribosomes)** → **erythrocyte** (remain in the circulation approximately 120 days and are then recycled by the spleen, liver, and bone marrow)

Disorders of Red Blood Cells

► Polycythemia (Increase in Red Blood Cell Mass)

Polycythemia vera (primary)	• Myeloproliferative syndrome • Males age 40–60 • Vessels distended with viscous blood, congestive hepatosplenomegaly, and diffuse hemorrhages • Management is generally with therapeutic phlebotomy
Secondary polycythemia	• Increased erythropoietin levels • Etiologies: high altitude, cigarette smoking, respiratory, renal and cardiac disease and malignancies (e.g., renal cell carcinoma, hepatoma, leiomyoma, adrenal adenoma, cerebellar hemangioblastoma)
Relative polycythemia	Fluid loss with stable RBC mass (vomiting, diarrhea, burns)

► Anemia

Secondary to decreased production, increased destruction, sometimes both
Symptoms: palpitations, high-output heart failure, pallor, fatigue, dizziness, syncope, and angina

Decreased Production (Low Reticulocyte Count)	
Decreased production (low reticulocyte count) **Iron deficiency** (smear: hypochromic, microcytic)	• An important differential feature between the thalassemia traits and iron deficiency is that thalassemia traits result in an elevated number of microcytes, whereas iron deficiency results in a decreased number of microcytes. • Serum iron, total iron-binding capacity (TIBC), and ferritin confirm the diagnosis.
Megaloblastic—B_{12}/folate (smear: macrocytic, hypersegmented neutrophils)	• Impaired DNA synthesis • Vitamin B_{12} deficiency neurologic (subacute combined degeneration) and hematologic sequelae • **Vitamin B_{12}:** copious body stores, years to develop deficiency *Causes:* dietary deficiency, malabsorption, tapeworm, bacterial overgrowth, deficiency of intrinsic factor (pernicious anemia) • **Folate:** deficiency develops much more quickly (months) *Causes:* deficient intake (poor diet, alcoholism, malabsorption), increased need (pregnancy, malignancy, increased hematopoiesis), or impaired use (antimetabolite drugs) • Must treat patient with both folate and B_{12}. Folate may reverse anemia in a B_{12} deficiency but not neurologic complications
Aplastic	• Pancytopenia • *Multiple etiologies:* idiopathic, drugs, including alkylating agents, chloramphenicol, radiation, infections, and congenital anomalies (i.e., Fanconi anemia) • Prognosis is poor • Bone marrow transplant may be curative
Myelophthisic	Displacement of hematopoietic bone marrow by infiltrating tumor
Myeloid metaplasia with myelofibrosis	• Chronic myeloproliferative disorder with small numbers of neoplastic myeloid stem cells • Resultant bone marrow fibrosis leads to pancytopenia

Thalassemias		
Types	**Key Points**	**Clinical Picture**
ALPHA	Secondary to gene deletion: **four** genes can be deleted: **1 deleted:** silent carrier **2 deleted:** trait **3 deleted:** HbH disease **4 deleted:** hydrops fetalis, Bart Hb	• Variable clinical severity • Non α-chain aggregates less toxic • Mild hemolysis and anemia tend to be milder; Bart's in the neonate leads to anoxia and intrauterine death
BETA	• Defects in mRNA processing. • Homozygous: β-thalassemia major • Heterozygotes: β-thalassemia minor	• Mediterranean countries, Africa, and Southeast Asia • Relative excess of α chains; Hb aggregates and becomes insoluble • Intra- and extramedullary hemolysis • Extramedullary hematopoiesis • Secondary hemochromatosis
HB ELECTROPHORESIS	• α-Thalassemia: normal HbA_2 and HbF • β-Thalassemia minor (trait): elevated HbA_2, HbF	

Increased Destruction (Normal–High Reticulocyte Count)	
Blood loss	Loss rather than destruction Clinical features depend on rate and severity of blood loss Chronic loss better tolerated, regenerate by increasing erythropoiesis Acute blood loss: possible hypovolemia may lead to shock and death Hematocrit may be initially normal because of equal plasma and RBC loss; will decrease as interstitial fluid equilibrates
	Extravascular—premature RBC destruction, hemoglobin (Hb) breakdown, and a compensatory increase in erythropoiesis *Intravascular*—elevated serum and urinary Hb, jaundice, urinary hemosiderin, and decreased circulating haptoglobin. Bile pigment gallstones arise from chronic, not acute hemolysis
Warm hemolytic anemia	IgG Secondary to drugs, malignancy, and SLE
Cold hemolytic anemia	IgM Functions below body temperature in the periphery Associated with mononucleosis, *Mycoplasma* infection, idiopathic hemolytic anemia, and hemolytic anemia associated with lymphoma
Paroxysmal hemolytic anemia	IgG Functions in the periphery
Hereditary spherocytosis *Presplenectomy smear:* spherical cells lacking central pallor and reticulocytosis *Postsplenectomy smear:* more spherocytes and Howell-Jolly bodies	Autosomal dominant defect in spectrin Less pliable; vulnerable to destruction in the spleen Anemia, jaundice, splenomegaly, cholelithiasis Exhibit characteristically increased osmotic fragility Treatment: splenectomy
G6PD deficiency *Smear:* reticulocytosis and Heinz bodies (Hb degradation products)	X-linked deficiency of the enzyme (hexose monophosphate shunt) Decreased regeneration of NADPH, therefore glutathione Older cells unable to tolerate oxidative stress Associated with drugs (e.g., sulfa, quinine, nitrofurantoin), infections (particularly viral), or certain foods (fava beans)
Paroxysmal nocturnal hemoglobinuria	Acquired deficiency of membrane proteins: decay accelerating factor (CD55) and membrane inhibitor of reactive lysis (CD59) Chronic intravascular hemolysis Predisposes to stem cell disorders (e.g., aplastic anemia, acute leukemia) Most frequently die of infection or venous thrombosis Diagnosis: flow cytometry shows absence of CD55 and CD59

* See **Appendix D** for Abnormal Erythryocytes on Peripheral Smear

Sickle Cell Disease		
Incidence	**Key Points**	**Clinical Picture**
• 0.2% of the U.S. African-American population has disease • 8% carry trait	• Substitution of valine for glutamic acid at position 6 of the beta chain • Sickle trait: 40% HbS-sickle in extreme conditions • "Sickle prep" is a blood sample treated with a reducing agent, such as metabisulfite; sickled cells may be seen • Definitive diagnosis made by Hb electrophoresis • HbS aggregates at low oxygen tension; leads to sickling • Heterozygote is protected from *Plasmodium falciparum* malaria	• Microvascular occlusion and hemolysis • Recurrent splenic thrombosis and infarction; autosplenectomy usually by age 5 • Also affects liver, brain, kidney, bones, penis (painful prolonged erection—priapism) • Vaso-occlusive crises ("painful crises") may be triggered by infection, dehydration, acidosis • Aplastic crises: Parvovirus • Functional asplenia: vulnerable to *Salmonella* osteomyelitis and infections with encapsulated organisms, such as *Pneumococcus* • Most patients die before age 30

Agents Used to Treat Anemia		
Class	**Mechanism**	**Indications**
Iron	Needed to form heme, the oxygen-carrying component of hemoglobin	Iron deficiency (microcytic hypochromic) anemia
Vitamin B_{12} (cyanocobalamin, hydroxocobalamin)	Required for DNA synthesis, RBC production, and nervous system function	Pernicious anemia and anemia resulting from gastric resection
Folate	Essential for DNA synthesis and maintenance of normal erythropoiesis	Folic acid deficiency secondary to malabsorption syndrome and dietary insufficiency; macrocytic/megaloblastic anemias
Hydroxyurea (HU)	An antimetabolite that inhibits ribonucleotide reductase HU reactivates HbF synthesis and increases the number of reticulocytes containing HbF in sickle cell patients	Sickle cell anemia, polycythemia vera, and chronic myelogenous leukemia
Erythropoietin (EPO) **Darbepoetin alpha**	EPO is normally produced by the kidney Stimulates RBC production	Used for a variety of anemias, including anemia of renal failure Hypertension a common and severe side effect Erythropoiesis-stimulating agents increase the risk of tumor progression or recurrence; severe caution when used in patients with cancer

White Blood Cells

Leukocytes can be divided into **granulocytes** and **agranulocytes** (mononuclears) based on the presence of cytoplasmic granules.

▶ Granulocytes

Granulocyte Type	Features	Functional Role	Relative Abundance
Neutrophils	• 3–5 nuclear lobes • Contain **azurophilic granules** (lysosomes) • Specific granules contain bactericidal enzymes (e.g., lysozyme)	First cells in **acute inflammation**	54–62% of leukocytes Normal value: 1800–7800/µl
Eosinophils	• Bilobed nucleus • Acidophilic granules contain hydrolytic enzymes and peroxidase	More numerous in the blood during **parasitic infections and allergic diseases**	1–3% of leukocytes Normal value: 0–450/µl
Basophils	Large basophilic and metachromatic granules, which contain proteoglycans, heparin, and histamine. Note that **mast cells are essentially tissue basophils.**	Degranulate in **type I hypersensitivity**, releasing granule contents and producing slow-reacting substance (SRS-A) = leukotrienes LTC_4, LTD_4, LTE_4	1% of leukocytes Normal value: 0–200/µl

▶ Granulopoiesis

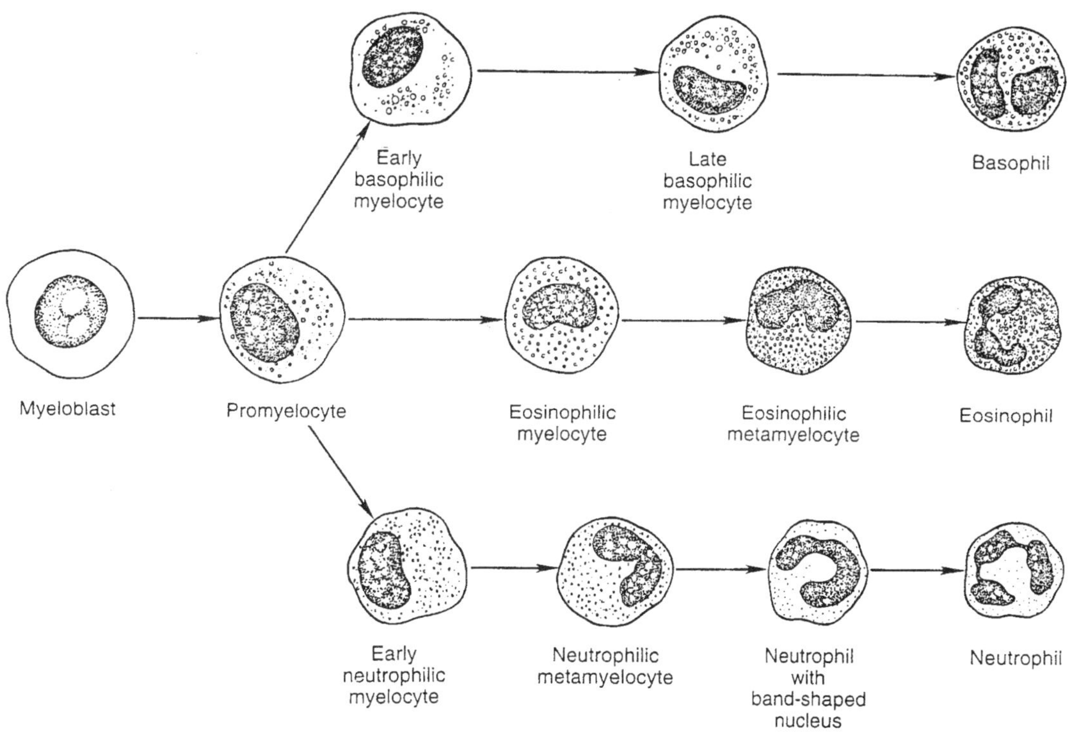

▶ Agranulocytes (Mononuclears)

Agranulocyte Type	Features	Functional Role	Relative Abundance
Lymphocytes	Dark blue, round nuclei; scant cytoplasm	T cells, B cells, null cells in immune system	25–33% of leukocytes Normal value: 1000–4000/µl
T cells	Differentiate in thymus	Helper and suppressor cells modulate the immune response	—
B cells	Differentiate in bone marrow	Humoral immunity—antibodies produced by plasma cells	—
NK (Natural Killer) cell	Produced in bone marrow	Destroy some tumor cells and some virus-infected cells on which MHC class I antigens are not expressed	10% of total lymphocyte count
Monocytes/macrophages	• Largest peripheral blood cells • Kidney-shaped nuclei, stain lighter than lymphocytes	Monocytes are precursors of tissue macrophages (histiocytes), osteoclasts, alveolar macrophages, and Kupffer cells of the liver	3–7% of leukocytes Normal value: 0–900/µl

Disorders of Leukocytes

▶ Nonneoplastic White Blood Cell Disorders

<table>
<tr><td>Neutropenias: decreased production (most common)</td><td>• Megaloblastic anemia
• Aplastic anemia
• Leukemia/lymphoma
• Autoimmune destruction of stem cells</td><td rowspan="2">• Lack of innate immune defense
• Constitutional symptoms and a high susceptibility to infection, particularly gram-negative septicemia
• Poor prognosis: death from overwhelming infection
• Infected, necrotic ulcers may occur in mucosa (oral cavity, skin, vagina, anus, gastrointestinal tract)
• Granulocyte-macrophage colony-stimulating factor (GM-CSF) and granulocyte-stimulating factor (GSF) are now used to treat postchemotherapy neutropenias</td></tr>
<tr><td>Neutropenias: increased destruction</td><td>Splenic sequestration, often immune-mediated (e.g., Felty syndrome)</td></tr>
<tr><td>Drug-induced neutropenia</td><td>Alkylating agents, chloramphenicol, sulfonamides, chlorpromazine, and phenylbutazone</td><td>• Usually reversible
• Chloramphenicol: dose-related marrow suppression in all patients; aplastic anemia in rare individuals</td></tr>
<tr><td>Polymorphonuclear leukocytosis (most common)</td><td>• Acute bacterial infection, tissue necrosis, and “stress”
• Increased bands and left shift</td><td>• Döhle bodies (round, blue, cytoplasmic inclusions, product of rough endoplasmic reticulum)
• Toxic granulations: coarse, dark, granules (lysosomes)</td></tr>
<tr><td>Monocytosis</td><td colspan="2">Tuberculosis, endocarditis, malaria, brucellosis, rickettsiosis</td></tr>
<tr><td>Lymphocytosis</td><td colspan="2">Tuberculosis, brucellosis, pertussis, viral hepatitis, cytomegalovirus infections, infectious mononucleosis</td></tr>
<tr><td>Mononucleosis</td><td colspan="2">• Increase in mononuclear cells: lymphocytes and monocytes
• Viral infections, EBV, CMV</td></tr>
<tr><td>Eosinophilic leukocytosis</td><td colspan="2">Neoplasms, allergy, asthma, collagen vascular diseases, parasitic infections, skin rashes</td></tr>
</table>

► Hematopoietic Growth Factors

Granulocyte colony-stimulating factor (G-CSF; filgrastim)	A glycoprotein that stimulates the bone marrow to produce granulocytes while promoting their survival and differentiation	Accelerates neutrophil recovery following chemotherapy; used for primary and secondary neutropenia
Granulocyte-monocyte colony-stimulating factor (GM-CSF, sargramostim)	A glycoprotein growth factor for erythroid megakaryocyte and eosinophil precursors. It also enhances the survival and function of circulating granulocytes, monocytes, and eosinophils	

► Nonneoplastic Lymph Node Disorders

Nonspecific lymphadenitis	Drugs, toxins, or infection	• In neck following dental or tonsillar infection • In axillary/inguinal regions after infections of the extremities • Enlarged abdominal lymph nodes (mesenteric adenitis) may cause abdominal pain resembling acute appendicitis
Generalized lymphadenopathy	Systemic viral or bacterial infections	• May be a precursor to AIDS • Associated with hyperglobulinemia and normal CD4 lymphocyte counts
Acute lymphadenopathy	• Swollen, red-gray nodes with prominent lymphoid follicles • Older patients have fewer germinal centers than children	
Chronic lymphadenopathy	Most common in axillary and inguinal nodes; nodes large and nontender	
Microscopic Findings: Three Basic Patterns		
Follicular hyperplasia **B-cell antibody response**	• Large germinal centers, containing mostly B cells, helper T cells, and histiocytes • Seen in bacterial infections or with exposure to new antigens	
Paracortical hyperplasia **T-cell reaction**	• Reactive changes in cortex • Seen with phenytoin use, viral infections, or secondary immune responses	
Sinus histiocytosis	• Lymphatic sinusoids prominent and distended with macrophages • Seen in nodes draining carcinomas or any chronic inflammation	

► Neoplastic Leukocyte Disorders

Hodgkin Disease
• Contiguous spread (from one node to the next) with spleen involved before liver • High cure rate, rarely has leukemic component • **Reed-Sternberg (RS)** cells (large, containing large "owl-eyed" nucleoli with a clear halo; abundant cytoplasm) are necessary, but not sufficient, to make diagnosis • Bimodal age distribution (high peak: 15–35; low peak: 50+) in both men and women • Clinical: painless cervical adenopathy +/– constitutional symptoms

Four Variants of Hodgkin Disease (Worsening Prognosis ↓)	
Lymphocyte predominance	Sea of lymphocytes, few RS cells, variable number of histiocytes, little fibrosis, and no necrosis
Nodular sclerosis	• More common in women • Mediastinal, supraclavicular, and lower cervical nodes • Mixture of lymphocytes, histiocytes, a few eosinophils, plasma cells, and RS cells. Collagen bands create nodular pattern; RS cells called lacunar cells
Mixed cellularity	• Mixture of neutrophils, lymphocytes, eosinophils, plasma cells, and histiocytes • Large number of RS cells
Lymphocyte depletion	• Rare lymphocytes, many RS cells with variable eosinophils, plasma cells, and histiocytes • Diffuse fibrosis may be seen

▶ Non-Hodgkin Lymphomas (NHL)

- Lymphadenopathy and hepatosplenomegaly. In 30% of cases, initial involvement extranodal
- Usually discovered in only one chain of nodes—usually cervical, axillary, inguinal, femoral, iliac, or mediastinal
- Patients present with local or generalized lymphadenopathy, abdominal or pharyngeal mass, abdominal pain, or GI bleeding
- Involve lymph nodes or lymphoid tissue in the gut, oropharynx, liver, spleen, and thymus
- **Do not produce Reed-Sternberg cells**, do not spread in contiguity, and frequently have a leukemic or blood-borne phase
- Occur in late 50s (rare and more aggressive in children and young adults)
- Weight loss common sign of disseminated disease
- Common in immunosuppressed patients

Two main categories: **nodular** (better prognosis) and **diffuse**

Staging similar to Hodgkin disease but staging less clinically significant in NHL because prognosis is more affected by histology, and the disease is often disseminated at time of diagnosis

Disease	Characteristics	Pathology
Follicular lymphoma	Median age 60–65; median survival 8–10 years Painless adenopathy t(14;18) translocation brings bcl-2 close to heavy chain immunoglobulin gene May be associated with immunodeficiency states	Follicular or nodular pattern of growth with areas resembling germinal centers but lacking normal germinal center architecture
Well-differentiated lymphocytic lymphoma (diffuse)	Older patients Generalized lymphadenopathy, hepatosplenomegaly Often seeds the blood late in the disease similar to CLL Bone marrow almost always involved Survival: 5–7 years	Lymph nodes replaced by small round lymphocytes with scant cytoplasm, dark nuclei, and rare mitoses
Mixed lymphocytic-histiocytic lymphoma (nodular)	Prognosis fair; remission may be achieved with combination chemotherapy	Cells with atypical lymphocytes and large histiocytes
Lymphoblastic lymphoma (diffuse) Cells similar to ALL	Bimodal—high peak: adolescents/young adults, low peak: 70s; male:female ratio, 2.5:1 Associated with a mediastinal mass, particularly in boys Often express T-cell markers Prognosis uniformly poor; T-cell lymphomas worse	Uniform size, scant cytoplasm, delicate chromatin, and absent nucleoli Nuclear membrane is loculated or convoluted Frequent mitoses
Burkitt undifferentiated lymphoma	Endemic in Africa (mandible or maxilla) and sporadic in the United States (abdomen) Children or young adults Tied to **Epstein-Barr virus (EBV),** especially the African form Leukemic phase is rare; prognosis is fair African Burkitt: translocations (8;14, 2;8, or 8;22) bring c-myc gene close to enhancers of heavy or light chain synthesis in B cells	Sea of intermediate size lymphocytes with lipid-containing vacuoles interspersed with macrophages to produce **"starry sky pattern."**
Mantle cell lymphoma	Median age 60; median survival 3 years t(11;14) translocation links immunoglobin heavy chain to bcl-1 Can present with lymphadenopathy, fever, night sweats, massive splenomegaly, or hepatomegaly	Expansion of the mantle zone surrounding germinal centers with small to medium atypical lymphocytes

▶ Cutaneous T-Cell Lymphomas

Mycosis fungoides	Three phases of skin lesions: inflammation, plaque, and tumor. Epidermal and dermal infiltrates by neoplastic T (CD4) cells with cerebriform nuclei. Nodules and fungating tumors may develop later in the disease. Nodal and visceral dissemination can occur.
Sézary syndrome	Rare chronic disease with progressive, pruritic erythroderma, exfoliation, and lymphadenopathy. "Sézary cells," T cells with cerebriform nuclei (similar to those seen in mycosis fungoides) infiltrate the peripheral blood. May be considered a preterminal phase of mycosis fungoides.

▶ Leukemias

Disease	Characteristics	Pathology
Acute lymphocytic leukemia (ALL)	• 60–70% of cases occur in childhood; peak age 4; rare over 50 • 75% of children are cured; prognosis for adults is very poor • Fatigue, fever, epistaxis, gingival petechiae, ecchymoses 2° to thrombocytopenia; may have subarachnoid or cerebral hemorrhage • Present with lymphadenopathy, bone pain, hepatosplenomegaly • Most likely leukemia to involve CNS • Prognosis: death often from infection or bleed • Most cells pre-B cells; T-cell variants occur, usually affecting boys and causing a thymic mass that may compress the trachea	Smear: lymphoblasts are prominent; mature WBCs rare **CD10 (CALLA)** is the diagnostic surface marker; terminal deoxynucleotidyl transferase (TDT) positive in both B-cell and T-cell ALL and negative in AML
Acute myelogenous leukemia (AML)	20% of acute leukemia in children, most common acute leukemia in adults Signs and symptoms resemble ALL, except usually also present with lymphadenopathy or splenomegaly AML: t(15;17); acute promyelocytic leukemia: t(1;12)	Primary cell type variable; see the French, American, and British (FAB) Classification of Myelogenous Leukemias, page 475.
Chronic myelogenous leukemia (CML)	• Middle age but may occur in children/young adults • Fatigue, fever, night sweats, and weight loss • Splenomegaly (up to 5 kg) giving abdominal discomfort • Variable remission period, may develop blast crisis • Two-thirds convert to AML; one-third to B-cell ALL • **Philadelphia chromosome (Ph1), t(9;22):** ***bcr:abl*** translocation is pathognomonic; present in 95% of cases • Prognosis in CML is worse in Ph1-negative patients	• Marked leukocytosis • Low-to-absent leukocyte alkaline phosphatase • Elevated serum vitamin B_{12} and vitamin B_{12}–binding proteins • High uric acid levels (due to rapid cell turnover)
Chronic lymphocytic leukemia (CLL)	• Over 60 years of age • Asymptomatic or fatigue and weight loss; lymphadenopathy and hepatosplenomegaly later findings • Higher incidence of visceral malignancy • Median survival with treatment is 5 years but varies widely; prognostic factor is extent of disease	Lymph node histology indistinguishable from diffuse, well-differentiated lymphocytic lymphoma Classic cell: CD5 B cell Cells do not undergo apoptosis
Hairy cell leukemia	• Rare disease; cells express tartrate-resistant acid phosphatase • Present with hepatosplenomegaly; pancytopenia common • Prognosis: may now be cured with 2-chloro-deoxyadenosine (2CdA), an apoptosis inducer	Leukemic cells have "hair-like" cytoplasmic projections visible on phase-contrast microscopy Cells express some B-cell antigens
Adult T-cell leukemia/ lymphoma (CD4 T cell)	• Endemic in Japan • Lymphadenopathy, hepatosplenomegaly, skin involvement, and hypercalcemia • Poor prognosis; however, many infected patients do not progress to disease	Caused by human T-cell leukemia/lymphoma virus (HTLV1); exposure to the virus may be decades earlier
Myelodysplastic syndromes	Proliferative stem cell disorders—maturation defect Gray zone between benign proliferation and frank acute leukemias One-third of these patients later develop frank acute myelocytic leukemia	Presents as pancytopenia in elderly patients

* See **Appendix D** for Abnormalities of White Blood Cells and Platelets on Peripheral Smear

Leukemia Clues	
Children	ALL
Myeloblasts	AML
Auer rods	AML, promyelocytic
DIC	Promyelocytic
Elderly	CLL
Splenomegaly	CML
Philadelphia chromosome	CML
Tartrate-resistant acid phosphatase	Hairy cell
HTLV-1	Adult T cell

French, American, and British (FAB) Classification of Myelogenous Leukemias		
M0	Undifferentiated	—
M1	Myeloblasts without maturation	Myeloblasts have round-oval nuclei Auer rods
M2	Granulocyte maturation	—
M3	Promyelocytic	Auer rods DIC
M4	Mixed myeloid and monocytic	Features of both myelocytes and monocytes
M5	Monoblastic or monocytic	—
M6	Erythroid differentiation	Di Guglielmo disease Atypical multinucleated RBC precursors Usually converts to AML
M7	Megakaryocytic differentiation	—

▶ Plasma Cell Dyscrasias

Polyclonal hypergammaglobulinemia	1–2 weeks after an antigen stimulus (e.g., bacterial infection); also associated with granulomatous disease, connective tissue disorders, and liver failure Elevated serum globulins, elevated ESR Polyclonal Bence-Jones proteins in serum or urine Hyperviscosity of blood may lead to sludging and rouleaux formation with subsequent thrombosis, hemorrhage, renal impairment, and right-sided congestive heart failure
Lymphoplasmacytic lymphoma (Waldenström macroglobulinemia)	Age 60–70 years in both men and women Monoclonal IgM resembles lymphocytic lymphoma with M-protein spike on serum protein electrophoresis Symptoms due to hypergammaglobulinemia and tumorous infiltration Hepatosplenomegaly, lymphadenopathy, bone pain, and hyperviscosity Blindness and priapism due to hyperviscosity may be seen 2–5-year survival rate with chemotherapy
Monoclonal gammopathy of undetermined significance (MGUS)	Asymptomatic M-protein spike on serum electrophoresis Prognosis: initially thought benign, but approximately 2% may later develop myeloma, lymphoma, amyloidosis, or Waldenström macroglobulinemia
Multiple myeloma	Peak incidence is 50–60 years old; male = female Multifocal plasma cell neoplasms in the bone marrow, occasionally soft tissues Monoclonal immunoglobulin (IgG) Signs and symptoms result from excess abnormal immunoglobulins (causing hyperviscosity) and from infiltration of various organs by neoplastic plasma cells Proteinuria may contribute to progressive renal failure Infiltration of bone with plasma cell neoplasms may lead to bone pain and hypercalcemia Over 99% of patients have elevated levels of serum immunoglobulins or urine Bence-Jones proteins, or both Serum protein electrophoresis (SPEP) shows homogeneous peak or "spike" Marrow is infiltrated with plasma cells (usually over 30%) in various stages of maturation, called "myeloma cells"; contain cytoplasmic inclusions (acidophilic aggregates of immunoglobulin) called Russell bodies Multiple osteolytic lesions throughout the skeleton; appear as "punched-out" defects on x-ray Kidney: protein casts in distal tubules Prognosis: less than 2-year survival without therapy; death usually results from infection, bleeding, or renal failure **(Bence-Jones proteins)**

Hematologic Changes Associated with Infectious Disease

► Changes in Blood Cells

Signs and Symptoms	Case Vignette/ Key Clues	Most Common Causative Agents	Pathogenesis	Diagnosis	Treatment
Anemia	Megaloblastic Ingestion of raw fish	*Diphyllobothrium latum*	Parasite absorbs B_{12}	Operculated eggs in stool	Niclosamide
	Normocytic	Chronic infections	Bacteria chelate iron	Culture, Gram stain	Depends on agent
	Microcytic and hypochromic (iron-deficiency anemia)	*Ancylostoma*, *Necator* *Trichuris*	Hookworms suck blood; trichuris damages mucosa	Golden brown, oval eggs; eggs with bipolar plugs	Mebendazole
Patient with cyclic or irregular fever, ↓ hemoglobin and hematocrit	Travel to tropics, parasites in RBCs	*Plasmodium* spp.	Parasite lyses RBC Autoimmune RBC destruction	Rings/trophozoites in blood film	Chloroquine, etc. (considerable drug resistance), followed by primaquine if *P. vivax* or *P. ovale*
↓ CD4 cell count	Lymphadenopathy Opportunistic infections	HIV	Virus infects and destroys CD4 ⊕ T cells, and macrophages	ELISA, Western blot	NRTIs, NNRTIs, protease inhibitors, fusion inhibitors, CCR5 antagonists, integrase inhibitors
↑ PMNs (neutrophilia)	—	Generally found in many extracellular bacterial infections	*N*-formyl methionyl peptides are chemotactic for PMNs	Culture, Gram stain	Depends on agent
↑ eosinophils (eosinophilia)	—	Allergy	ECF-A released by mast cells attracts eosinophils	Skin testing: wheal and flare	Antihistamines
		Helminths during migrations	Parasites release allergens	Depends on agent	Depends on agent
↑ monocytes and/or lymphocytes	—	Intracellular organisms: viruses, *Listeria*, *Legionella*, *Leishmania*, *Toxoplasma*	Intracellular organisms elicit TH1 cells and CMI	Depends on agent	Depends on agent
Above plus fever, fatigue, lymphadenopathy, myalgia, headache	Infectious mononucleosis Downey type II cells (reactive T cells), sore throat, lymphadenopathy, young adult	Epstein-Barr virus	Virus infects B lymphocytes via CD21; CTLs respond to kill virus-infected cells	Monospot ⊕ Complete blood count, 70% lymphocytosis	Supportive
	Heterophile ⊖	CMV	Virus infects fibroblasts; CTLs respond to kill virus-infected cells	Monospot ⊖ Virus culture	Ganciclovir (severe cases)
Lymphocytosis with hacking cough	Unvaccinated child, hypoglycemic	*Bordetella pertussis*	Tracheal cytotoxin, fimbrial antigen, endotoxin, ↓ chemokine receptors	Gram ⊖ rod Culture Bordet-Gengou agar or serology	Erythromycin, antitoxin

Section III

Dental Anatomy, Occlusion, and Histology

Contents

General Characteristics

▶ Definitions

General	**Exfoliation**	Process of shedding or losing deciduous teeth
	Mixed dentition	Containing a combination of both primary and permanent teeth

Arrangement	**Maxilla**	Stationary, upper jaw
	Mandible	Lower, moveable jaw
	Arch trait	Characteristics of the teeth of 1 arch (3 roots in a maxillary molar versus 2 in a mandibular molar)
	Type trait	Differences between the arch components of each class that make them easily identifiable (difference between manibular central incisor and mandibular lateral incisor)
	Set trait	Characteristic that identifies what dentition the tooth belongs to

Types of Teeth	**Deciduous**	Primary teeth 20 teeth in all Must be exfoliated
	Permanent	Adult dentition 32 teeth in all Usually erupt between 6–18 years
	Succedaneous	Take the place of the exfoliated primary teeth

▶ Anatomy of a Tooth

Crown	Surface portion that erupts through the gingiva Composed of enamel, dentin, and pulp
Root	Anchoring portion of the tooth Composed of cementum, dentin, and pulp
Clinical crown	Portion visible in the oral cavity
Gingiva	Soft tissue surrounding crown and boundary between clinical crown and root
Alveolus	Bony socket anchoring tooth
Cervical line	Boundary between anatomic crown and root (cementoenamel junction)

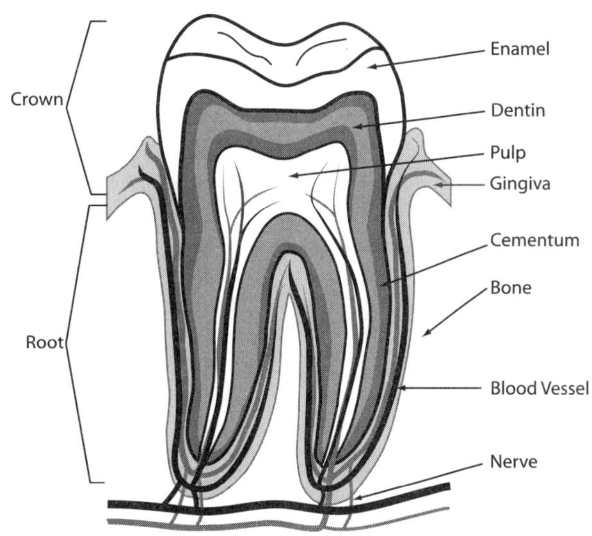

Root Structure

Single-rooted teeth: all anteriors, maxillary second premolar, mandibular first and second premolars)

Bifurcation—**2** terminal roots (maxillary first premolar, mandibular molars)

Trifurcation—**3** terminal roots (maxillary molars)

Root trunk—common part of the tooth root before the root separates

Cervical line—boundary between the enamel of the anatomical crown and the cementum of the anatomical root (cementoenamel junction)

Each root usually has one canal, *except*:*

Maxillary	second premolar (occasionally)
	molars (mesiobuccal can have 2)
Mandibular	central (occasionally)
	lateral (occasionally)
	canine (occasionally)
	first premolar (occasionally)
	second premolar (occasionally)
	molars (mesial root has 2 canals; distal may have 2)

*Note that there are rare exceptions to rules about roots.

Pulp Cavity

Pulp chambers and **pulp canals** make up the pulp cavity.

The **pulp chamber** is generally in the crown portion of the mouth. It is a singular chamber in all teeth and extends into the root trunk, generally 1–2 mm below the cervical line. The chamber outline follows the outline of the tooth.

Pulp horns are projections of the pulp chamber into the major cusps of the teeth. They are also found in mammelons of the maxillary incisors when teeth are young.

Tissue

	Composition	Characteristics	Function	Location	Strength
Enamel	96–98% inorganic material (mineral)	Hard, translucent Cannot repair itself Complete at time of eruption	Protects biting surface of tooth	Covers anatomic crown	Hardest substance in body
Cementum	50% organic 50% inorganic	2 types: cellular, acellular Blood supply through the cementum (nourishment from outside tooth)	Provides anchoring mechanism to tooth (periodontal ligament between cementum and alveolar bone)	Covers surface of anatomic root	Less dense than enamel
Dentin	22% organic* 65% inorganic* 13% water* Composed of tubules (extension of nerve tissue from pulp extend into these tubules)	Makes up bulk of tooth **2 types:** primary (produced during development) and secondary (formed to protect the pulp)	Provides elasticity to tooth	Beneath the enamel and cementum	Softer and less brittle than enamel
Pulp	Nerves, blood vessels, lymph	Formative (will produce dentin throughout life) Contains odontoblasts	Provides nutrients to tooth Sensory (pain from heat, cold, decay, etc.)	Innermost portion of the tooth	Soft tissue

*Values vary in some texts; it has been stated that as much as 60–65% of dentin may be inorganic.

▶ Characteristics of Classes

Class	Number per Quadrant	Characteristics	Function	Position
Incisors (I)	2	Front teeth, single rooted Straight incisal edge	Cutting, aesthetics, phonetics, biting	Central—closest to midline Lateral—2nd position from midline
Canines (C)	1	Canine prominence of tooth seen at corner of mouth Long rooted	Cutting, shearing, tearing	3rd position from midline
Premolars (PM)	2	Single roots, except for maxillary first premolar (2 roots)	Mastication	4th and 5th position from midline
Molars (M)	3	Grinding, chewing 4 cusps or more Wide masticating surface	Mastication	6th, 7th, and 8th position from midline

▶ Anatomic Divisions and Orientations

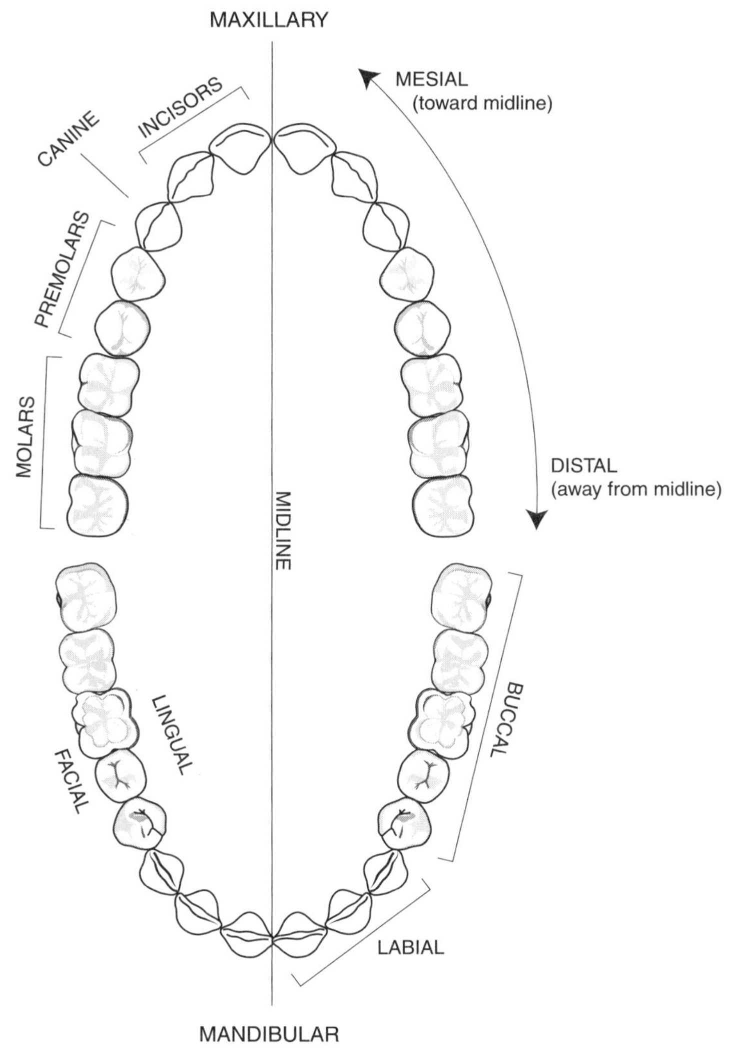

Surfaces

Occlusal—biting surface of posterior teeth

Incisal—biting surface of anterior teeth

Gingival/Cervical—area near gingiva

Contact area—area that contacts an adjacent tooth on the proximal surface of the tooth

Definitions

Mesial—closer to midline

Distal—away from midline

Proximal—area between two teeth

Lingual—surface facing the tongue also **palatal** in maxilla)

Facial—outer surface facing toward cheek

Labial—surface facing check in anterior teeth

Buccal—surface facing check in posterior teeth

Imaginary Thirds

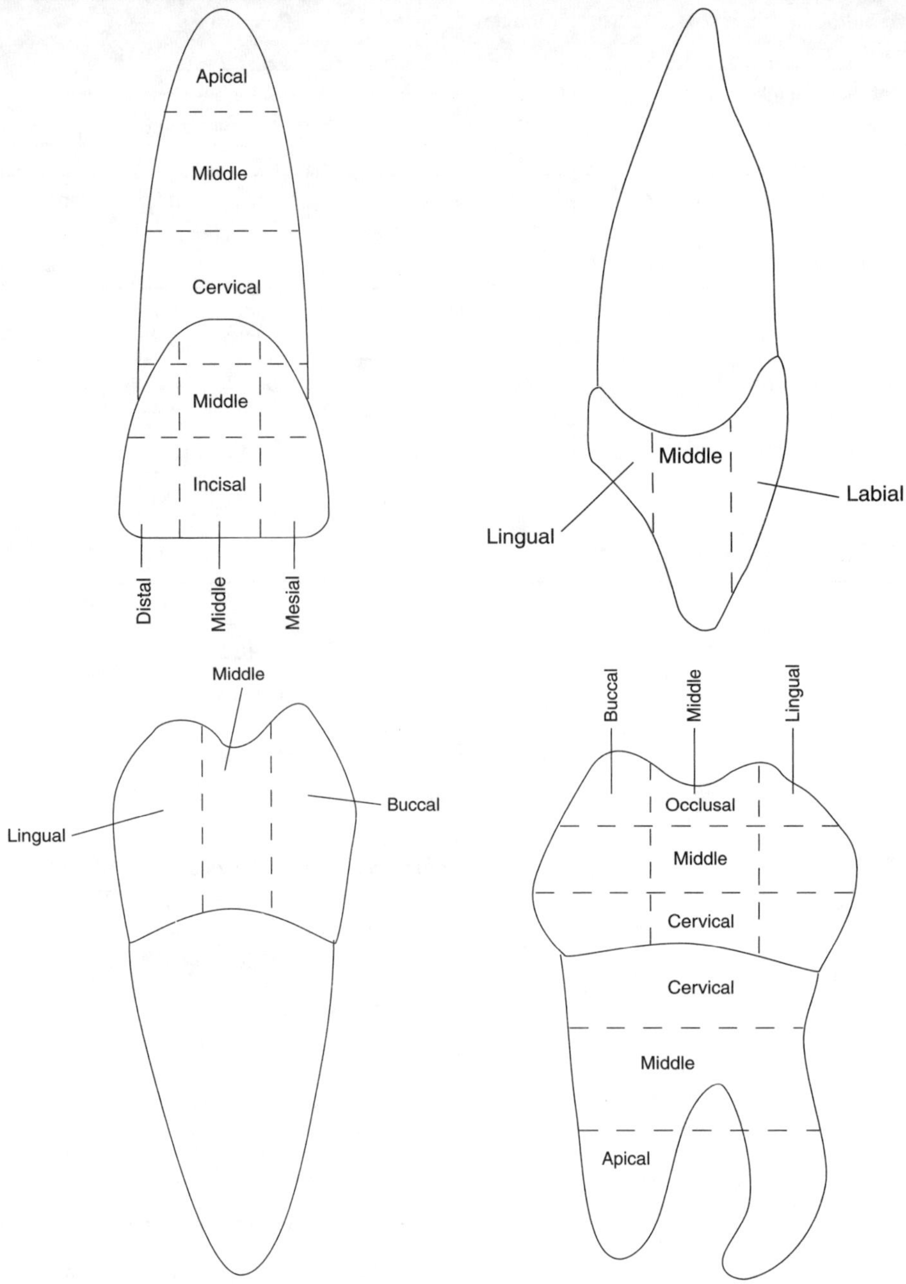

Examples
Incisal Third
Horizontal third closest to the working surface
Cervical Third
Horizontal third closest to the neck of the tooth and gingiva
Middle Third
Middle of the crown

▶ Nomenclature

Shorthand

Permanent Dention

UNIVERSAL SYSTEM

Teeth are numbered from 1–32 starting with the permanent maxillary right third molar, i.e., perm/max/right/central incisor = #8.

MAXILLARY

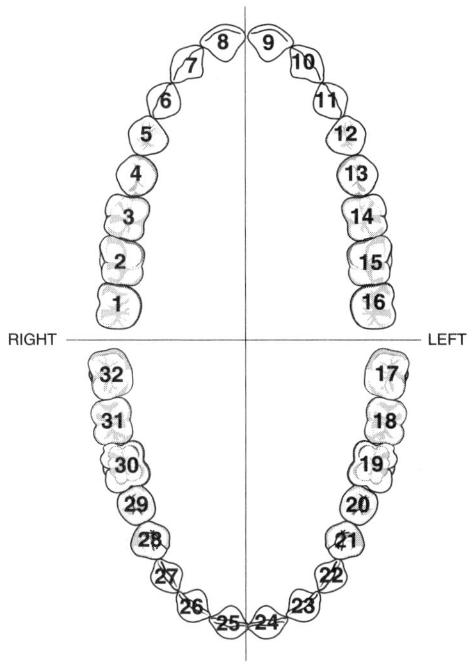

MANDIBULAR

1	2	3	4	5	6	7	8	9	10	11	12	13	14	15	16
32	31	30	29	28	27	26	25	24	23	22	21	20	19	18	17

FDI (FEDERATION DENTAIRE INTERNATIONALE)

Uses quadrant system

MAXILLARY

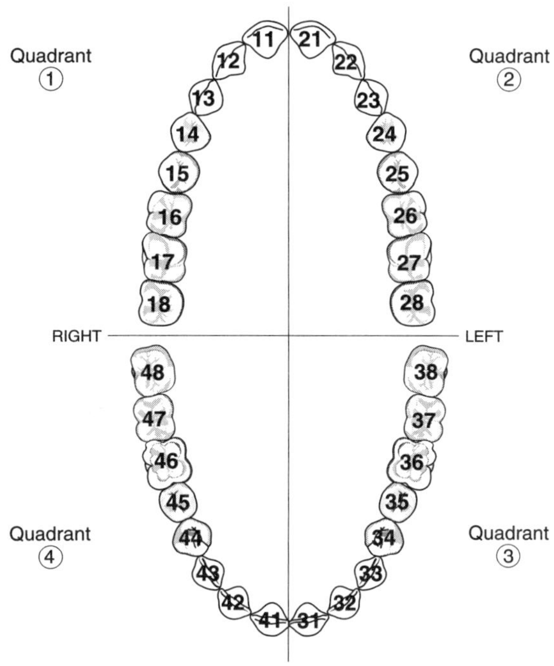

MANDIBULAR

18	17	16	15	14	13	12	11	21	22	23	24	25	26	27	28
48	47	46	45	44	43	42	41	31	32	33	34	35	36	37	38

Primary Dentition

UNIVERSAL SYSTEM

Teeth are numbered from A–T starting with the primary maxillary right second molar, i.e., perm/max/right/central incisor = E.

MAXILLARY

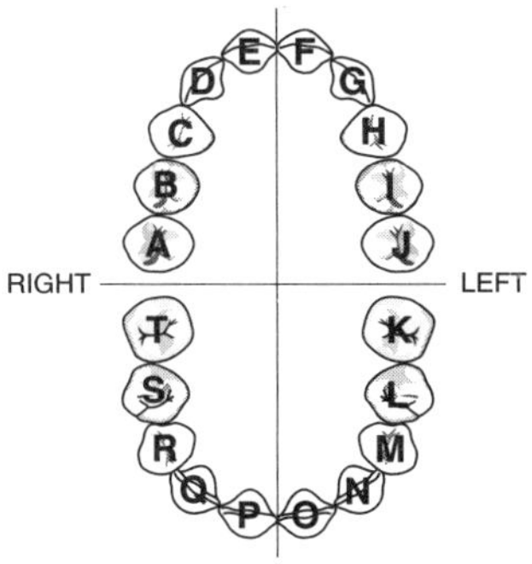

MANDIBULAR

A	B	C	D	E	F	G	H	I	J
T	S	R	Q	P	O	N	M	L	K

FDI (FEDERATION DENTAIRE INTERNATIONALE)

Uses quadrant system

MAXILLARY

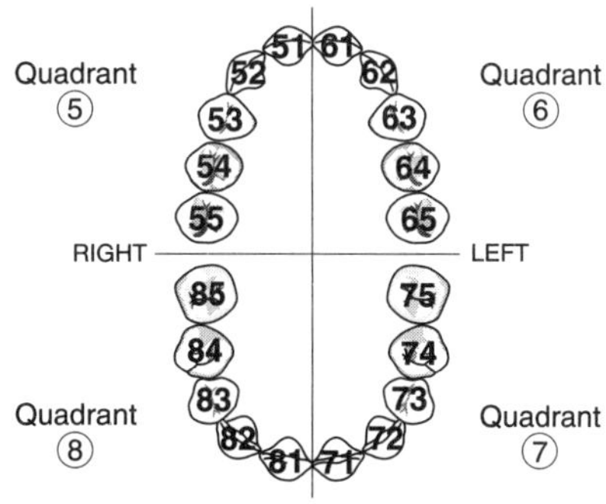

MANDIBULAR

55	54	53	52	51	61	62	63	64	65
85	84	83	82	81	71	72	73	74	75

Dental Formula

The number of teeth in each class constitutes the dental formula. The number of teeth on one quadrant of the upper jaw is indicated over the number of the same class on the lower jaw. You must multiply the sum by two to get the total number of teeth.

Anterior teeth — incisors and canines
Posterior teeth — premolar and molars

Permanent Teeth

$\mathbf{I}\ ^2/_2 + \mathbf{C}\ ^1/_1 + \mathbf{PM}\ ^2/_2 + \mathbf{M}\ ^3/_3 = 16 \times 2 = \mathbf{32}$

Primary Teeth (No Premolars)

$\mathbf{I}\ ^2/_2 + \mathbf{C}\ ^1/_1 + \mathbf{M}\ ^2/_2 = 10 \times 2 = \mathbf{20}$

Naming Teeth	
Standard order:	1. Set
	2. Arch
	3. Quadrant
	4. Type and class

i.e., "permanent/mandibular/right/first molar"

▶ Development of Cusps and Lobes

Tooth germs (or tooth buds) are small groupings of cells that develop during the eighth week of embryonic development. **Calcification**, the hardening of tooth tissues by the deposition of minerals found within, begins at the fourth to fifth month of fetal life. Calcification begins in permanent teeth just after birth.

Lobes

All anterior teeth develop from **four major growth centers** called **lobes**, i.e., **mammelons** and **cingula**.

The posterior teeth develop from four to five lobes. Cusps develop from the lobes, and the coalescence of lobes is marked by developmental grooves.

Lobes

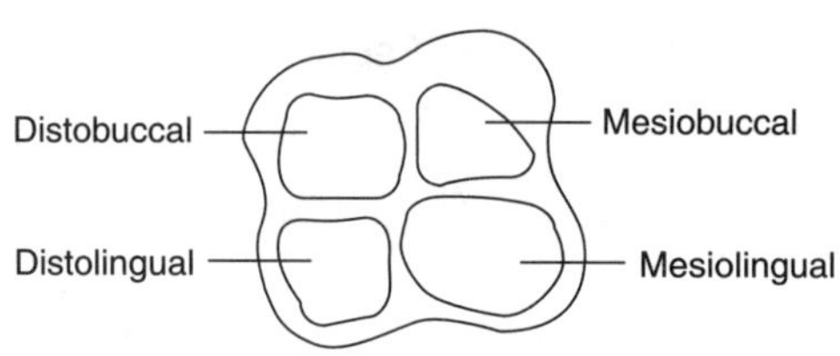

Mammelons

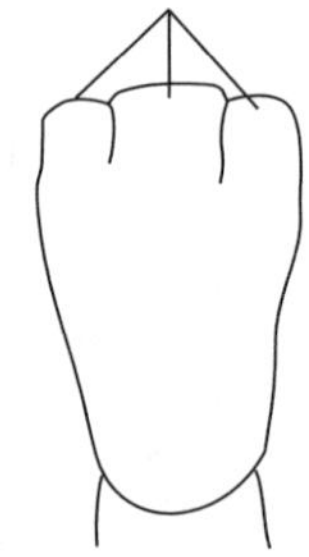

The lobes of a tooth act as the major center of the formation of enamel. In the fully developed tooth, these lobes give rise to the formation of **cusps, mammelons, and cingula**. The coalescence of the lobes is marked by the formation of developmental depressions (anterior teeth) and developmental grooves (posterior teeth).

Anterior teeth (incisors and canines) have four facial lobes: distolabial, middlelabial, mesiolabial, and one lingual lobe, cementum.

Premolars have four lobes: distobuccal, middlebuccal, mesiobuccal, and one lingual lobe, lingual cusp.

Molars have **four lobes:** distolingual, distobuccal, and mesiolingual, mesiobuccal. The maxillary first molar has the cusp of Carabelli (a small fifth cusp), and the mandibular first molar has a fifth cusp (distal cusp).

▶ Dental Terminology

MAXILLARY RIGHT CANINE

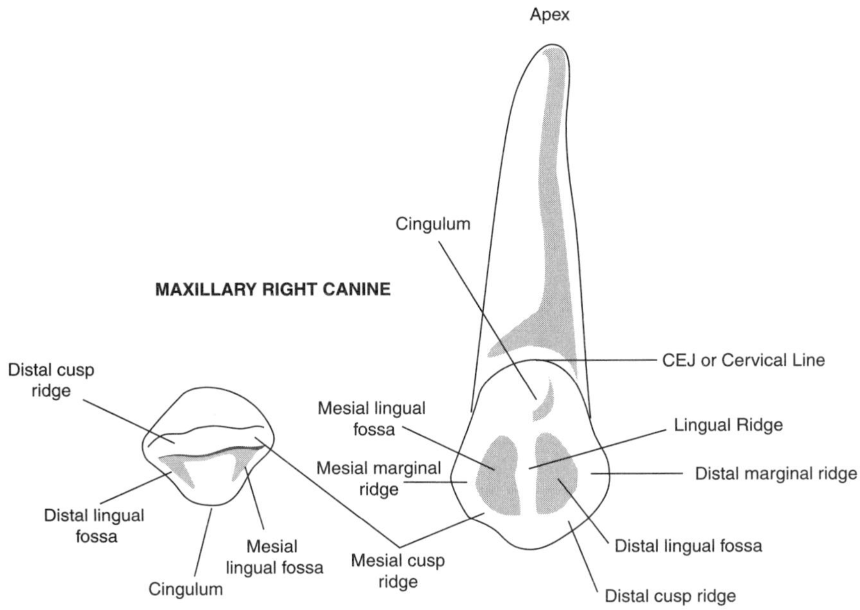

INCISAL LINGUAL

Fossa: irregular rounded depression on surface of crown

Lingual fossa: broad shallow depression on lingual surface of anterior teeth

Central fossa: deep depression in central portion of anterior or posterior

Triangular fossa: triangular fossa located in the marginal ridges of the posterior teeth

Cusp: elevation on the crown portion of tooth; forms the bulk of the occlusal surface

Cingulum: rounded eminence or bulge on lingual side of anterior teeth

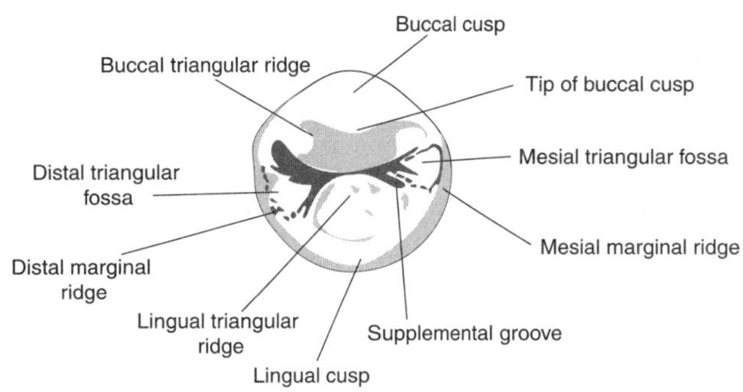

MAXILLARY RIGHT SECOND PREMOLAR

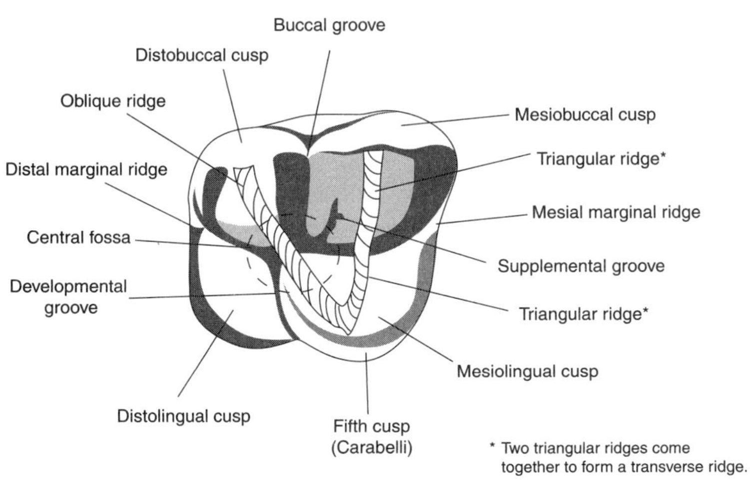

* Two triangular ridges come together to form a transverse ridge.

[hatched box] represents triangle formed by the major ridges of the maxillary first molar.

MAXILLARY RIGHT FIRST MOLAR

Ridge: any linear elevation on surface of tooth; named according to location

Marginal ridge: rounded borders of enamel; form mesial and distal margins of occlusal surfaces of premolars and molars; form mesial and distal margins of lingual surfaces of incisors and canines

Triangular ridge: prominent elevation, triangular in cross-section

Transverse ridge: union of two triangular ridges crossing the occlusal surface of posterior tooth

Incisal ridge: found on newly erupted anterior teeth (mammelons)

Oblique ridge (maxillary molars only): transverse ridge that runs from distal buccal to mesial lingual cusp

► Maxillary Versus Mandibular Teeth

Although there are general rules for cusp and root numbers, numerous anomalies exist.

All teeth are wider faciolingually than mesiodistally, except for:

- maxillary central and lateral incisors
- mandibular first, second, and third molars.

Smallest tooth—mandibular central incisor
Longest tooth—maxillary canine

	Maxillary	Mandibular
Anterior	Wider, less symmetrical crown	Long, narrow symmetric crown
Molars	Wider in a faciolingual direction 3 roots—2 facial, 1 lingual (palatal)	Wider in a mesiodistal direction 2 roots—1 mesial, 1 distal
Premolars	First premolar has 2 roots; others are single roots	All single roots
Posteriors		
Occlusal tables	More centered in a faciolingual direction Centered over root trunk	Somewhat lingually placed
Buccal cusps	Displaced from midline in faciolingual direction; height of contour low	Buccal cusp more toward middle of tooth in the faciolingual direction
Lingual cusps	Displaced from midline in faciolingual direction	Lingual almost in line with lingual profile of root
Occlusal view	Equal amounts of buccal and lingual surfaces seen	More buccal (up to 1/3) than lingual surface seen
Contours	Buccal height is low; lingual heights relatively high on crown	Buccal height of contour very low, near cervical

► Fundamental Geometric Shapes of Crowns

Axial Views			
Facial or Lingual View of All Teeth	**Mesial or Distal View of Anterior Teeth**	**Mesial or Distal View of Maxillary Posterior Teeth**	**Mesial or Distal View of Mandibular Posterior Teeth**
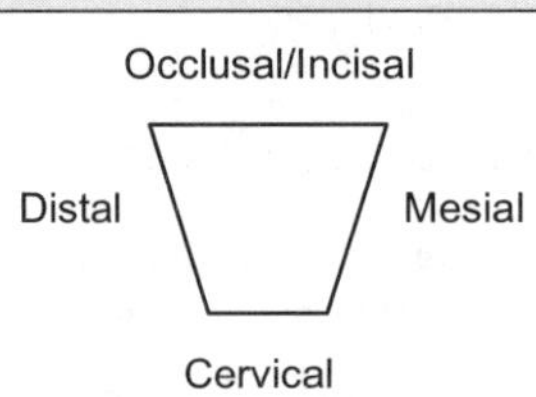	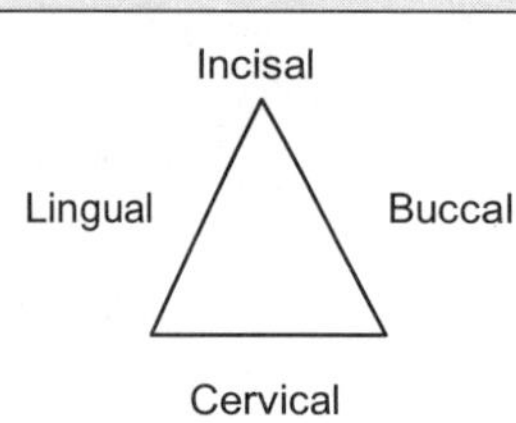	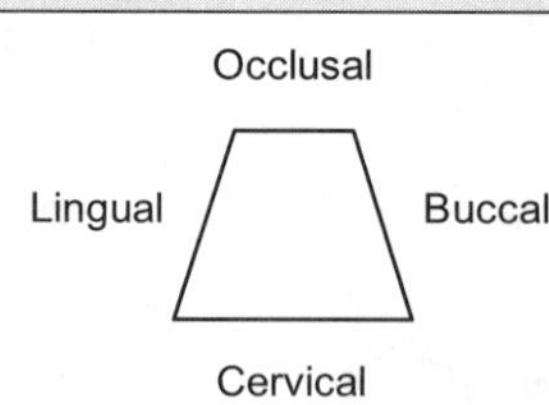	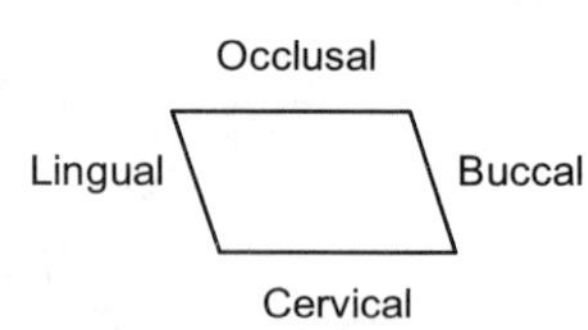
All teeth are fundamentally **trapezoidal** when viewed **facially or lingually**. The long side of the trapezoid is the occlusal or incisal, and the short side is the cervical.	**Incisors and canines**, when viewed from **mesial** or **distal**, are **triangular** in shape.	**Maxillary posteriors**, when viewed from **mesial** or **distal**, are fundamentally **trapezoidal**. The long side is the cervical.	**Mandibular posteriors**, when viewed from **mesial** or **distal**, are **rhomboidal**. The lingual occlusal and the buccocervical angles are acute.

► Heights of Contours and Contacts

The **height of contour, or the crest of curvature,** is the greatest elevation of the tooth. The contact areas are also considered the location of the height of contour on the proximal surfaces.

Knowing the heights of contour helps to understand contact relationships.

- Generally, the **mesial height of contour** is more incisal or occlusal than is the distal, except for the mandibular central incisor, premolars, and possibly molars.
- The **lingual height of contour** of the mandibular posteriors is much more occlusal than that of the maxillary posteriors.
- The **facial height of contour** of the maxillary posteriors is generally more occlusal than that of the mandibular posteriors.
- The **facial and lingual heights of contour** generally have a convexity of approximately 0.5 mm, except for the lingual of the mandibular posteriors, where it may measure up to 1 mm.

Maxillary Heights of Contours/Contacts				
	Lingual	**Facial**	**Mesial Contact**	**Distal Contact**
Central incisor	Cervical 1/3	Cervical 1/3	Incisal 1/3	Junction of middle and incisal 1/3
Lateral incisor	Cervical 1/3	Cervical 1/3	Junction of middle and incisal 1/3	Middle 1/3
Canine	Cervical 1/3	Cervical 1/3	Junction of middle of incisal 1/3	Middle 1/3
First premolar	Middle 1/3	Cervical 1/3	Middle 1/3	Middle 1/3
Second premolar	Middle 1/3	Cervical 1/3	Middle 1/3	Middle 1/3
First molar	Middle 1/3	Cervical 1/3	Middle 1/3	Middle 1/3
Second molar	Middle 1/3	Cervical 1/3	Middle 1/3	Middle 1/3
Third molar	Middle 1/3	Cervical 1/3	Middle 1/3	No distal contact

Mandibular Heights of Contours/Contacts				
	Lingual	**Facial**	**Mesial Contact**	**Distal Contact**
Central incisor	Cervical 1/3	Cervical 1/3	Incisal 1/3	Incisal 1/3
Lateral incisor	Cervical 1/3	Cervical 1/3	Incisal 1/3	Incisal 1/3
Canine	Cervical 1/3	Cervical 1/3	Incisal 1/3	Middle 1/3
First premolar	Junction of cervical and middle 1/3	Cervical 1/3	Middle 1/3	Middle 1/3
Second premolar	Middle 1/3	Cervical 1/3	Junction of middle and occlusal 1/3	Junction of middle and occlusal 1/3
First molar	Middle 1/3	Cervical 1/3	Junction of middle and occlusal 1/3	Middle 1/3
Second molar	Middle 1/3	Cervical 1/3	Middle 1/3	Middle 1/3

▶ Contact Areas

Contact areas are influenced by the **size**, **form**, and **alignment** of the teeth. They are located at the **widest portion of a tooth** and correspond to the height of the contour. They function to:

- Stabilize the arch
- Prevent food impaction
- Protect the interproximal gingival tissue

Interproximal caries typically form immediately apical to the contact area.

Contact areas are described by **two coordinates: incisocervical** (occlusocervical) and **faciolingual.**

Incisocervical (occlusocervically)	Faciolingual
At the mesial and distal heights of contour Mesial contact area is more occlusal or incisal than the distal (except for mandibular central incisors, premolars, possibly molars.	Anterior teeth centered faciolingually Posterior teeth placement may be more facial in the buccal third.

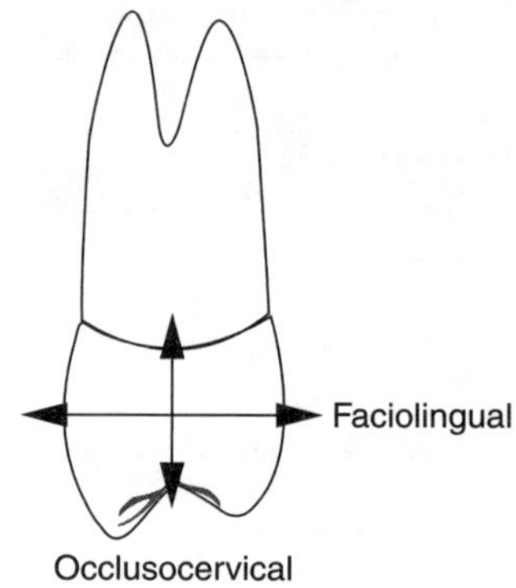

▶ Junctions

DEJ (Dentinoenamel)	CEJ (Cementoenamel)	CDJ (Cementodentinal)
Dentin meeting enamel	Between cementum and enamel; border of anatomic crown	Cementum meets dentin
Found only in crown	Mesial curvature greater than on distal of same tooth Curvature becomes less distinct as you move toward posterior Molar's CEJ relatively straight Greatest mesial CEJ curvature of all teeth on maxillary central incisor (~3.5 mm; mesial surface)	Found only in root

The greatest curvature of cervical line is on the mesial surface.

Line angle—where two surfaces come together to form a line, e.g., anterior teeth: mesiolabial, distolabial

Point angle—where three surfaces come together to form a point; takes name of surfaces involved, i.e., posterior teeth: mesiolingual/occlusal, mesiobuccal/occlusal

▶ Embrasures

Definition	Gap between two adjacent teeth, as teeth curve away from contact area Form is dependent upon size, shape, and form of teeth Four embrasures per contact area: lingual, facial, incisal/occlusal, gingival
Functions	Act as spillways for food from occlusal surfaces Make teeth more self-cleansing
Characteristics	
Maxillary anteriors	Lingual is greater than facial
Mandibular anteriors	Facial is greater than lingual
Posteriors	Lingual is generally greater than the facial (except maxillary molars)
Incisals	Incisal/occlusal is smaller than the gingival Incisal may be missing between the mandibular central incisors because of high placement of mesial contact areas

Adult Dentition

General

Incisors are involved with all of the main functions: **mastication, aesthetics, and phonetics.**

There are **8** permanent incisors (2 per quadrant). The central incisors are at the midline with the lateral incisors distal to the centrals.

Incisors are the **first succedaneous teeth to erupt.**

All incisors except the mandibular central have rounder distoincisal angles than mesioincisal angles (mandibular central is symmetric).

Smallest tooth—mandibular central incisor
Bilaterally symmetric—mandibular central incisor
Most distinct lingual anatomy—maxillary lateral incisor
Incisal edge not perpendicular to labiolingual bisecting line—mandibular lateral incisor

▶ INCISORS

Maxillary	Mandibular
Larger	Smaller
Wider mesiodistal diameter **(arch trait)**	Wider labiolingual diameter
More distinct lingual anatomy	Less distinct lingual anatomy
May have lingual pits	Does not have lingual pits
Incisal edge is centered labiolingually	Incisal edge is lingual to labiolingual midpoint
Heights of contour more toward middle/incisal	Heights of contour more incisal
Lingual embrasure is greater than facial	Facial embrasure is greater than lingual
Contacts more cervically located	Contacts near incisors
More rounded distoincisal angles	Labial surface is straighter and flatter

▶ Summary of Lateral Versus Central Maxillary Incisors

	Maxillary Central Incisor	Maxillary Lateral Incisor
Crown	Not as rounded as lateral	Characterized by roundness; slightly more round on mesioincisal (distinctly so on distoincisal angles)
Root Cross-Section	Round	Ovoid
Other Features	Distinct lingual anatomy Distinct mammelons on incisal edge	More distinct lingual anatomy Mammelons may be present only on newly erupted tooth

▶ Summary of Lateral Versus Central Mandibular Incisors

Mandibular Central Incisor	Mandibular Lateral Incisor
Smallest tooth	Not as small as central
Bilaterally symmetric	Not symmetric
Mirror mesial and distal axial surfaces	Distoincisal angle more round
Incisal edge perpendicular to a labiolingual bisecting line	Incisal edge not perpendicular to a labiolingual bisecting line

► Maxillary Central Incisor

Position		
	Right	Left
Universal	8	9
International	11	21

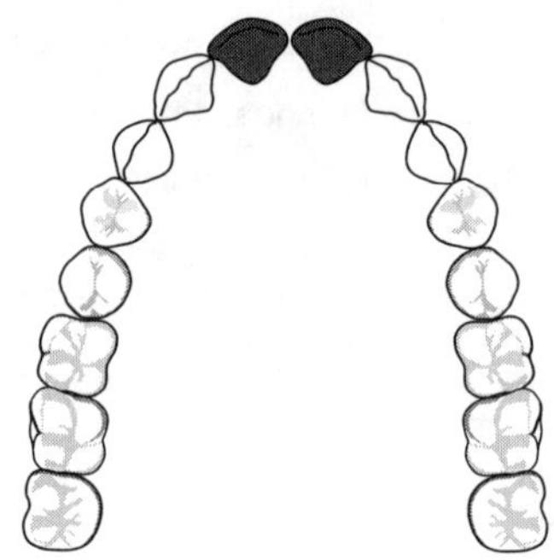

Developmental Data	
First evidence of calcification	3–4 months after birth
Enamel completed	4–5 years
Eruption	7–8 years
Root completed	10 years
Number of roots	1
Number of pulp horns	3
Developmental lobes	4

Maxillary Right Central Incisor				
Labial	Lingual	Mesial	Distal	Incisal
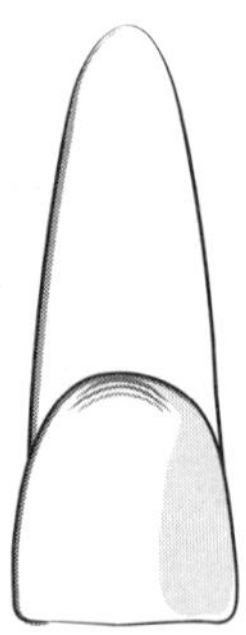	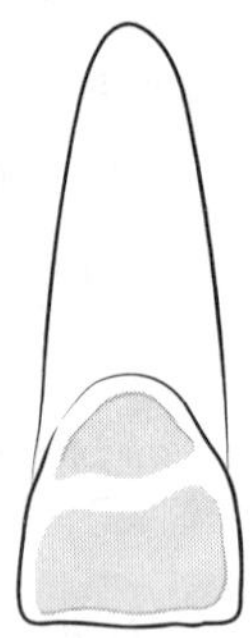	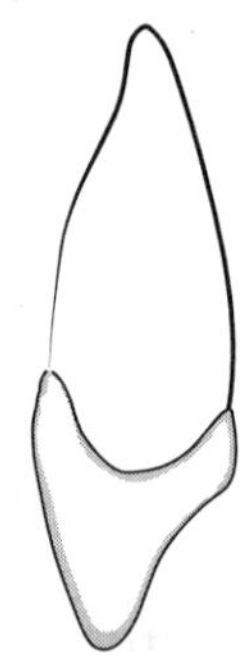	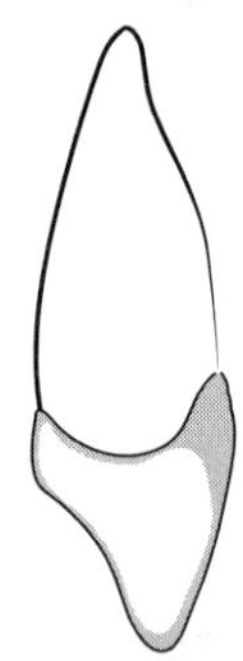	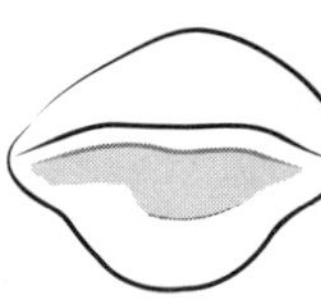
Surface convex in both directions Developmental depressions, lobulated appearance Mammelons at time of eruption Trapezoid Incisal outline straight Root cone-shaped Imbrication lines (faint curved lines parallel to CEJ)	Slightly more narrow than labial Trapezoid Lingual fossa scoop-like Tendency for lingual fossa and cingulum to have central pit Distinct mesial and distal marginal ridges and lingual fossa	Triangular (wedge-shaped) Apex of root toward labial Crest of curvature in cervical third Greatest cervical line curvature Contour relatively straight	Similar to mesial Wedge-shaped, more rounded	Triangular Incisal edge centered, straight, three mammelons Cingulum toward distal Cross section at the cervical line is roundish

Variations on the Central Incisor

- Microdontia
- Macrodontia
- Hypercementosis—excessive amount of cementum
- Gemination (split)—
  Partial (1 pulp, 1 large tooth)
  Complete (results in twin teeth)
- Fusion—two teeth fused together along cementum; each tooth has own pulp
- Dilaceration—sharp angle of the root of tooth
- Plexion—sharp bend

▶ Maxillary Lateral Incisor

The maxillary lateral incisor is the **most variable** of teeth, ranging from absent to peg-shaped to normal incisor shape. Its lingual surface can be flat, bulbous, or deeply pitted. It is characterized also by the **roundness of its distoincisal and mesioincisal angles** and is the incisor **most likely to need a lingual restoration**.

The lateral incisors complement the central incisors. They are **smaller** in dimension, **except in root length**, and the **features** of the **lateral** are more **prominent**.

Position		
	Right	**Left**
Universal	7	10
International	12	22

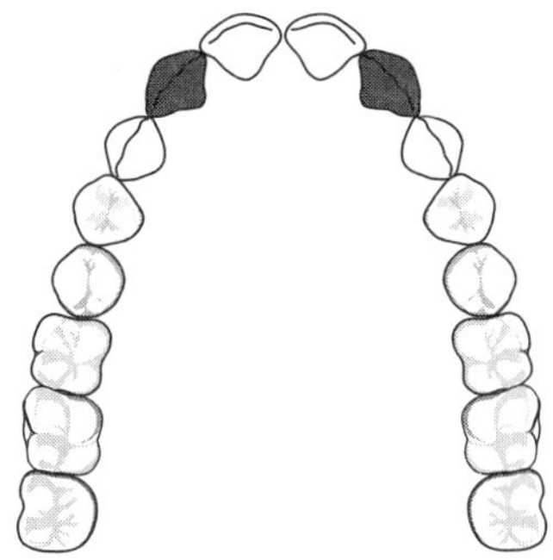

Width	Wider mesiodistally than labiolingually
Root	Conical in shape
Angle	Distoincisal angle more rounded than the mesioincisal

Developmental Data	
First evidence of calcification	1 year
Enamel completed	4–5 years
Eruption	8–9 years
Root completed	11 years
Number of roots	1
Number of pulp horns	1–3
Developmental lobes	4

Variations on the Lateral Incisor

- Missing altogether—partial anodontia
- Extra lateral incisor—supernumerary (accessory tooth between two maxillary central incisors called **mesiodens**)
- Incomplete development of mesial and distal lobe—"peg lateral"
- Lingual surface—deep pit, dens en dente

Maxillary Right Lateral Incisor				
Labial	**Lingual**	**Mesial**	**Distal**	**Incisal**
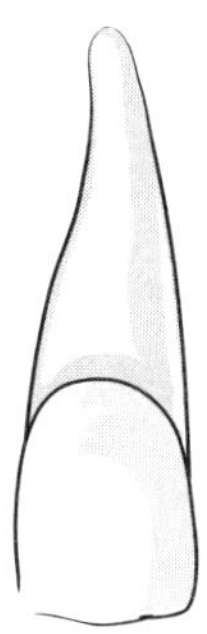	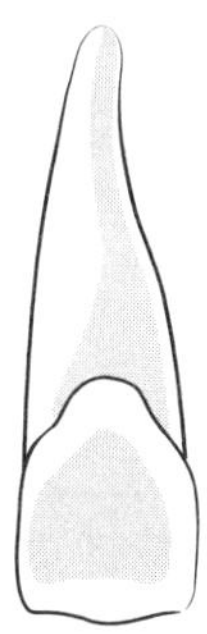	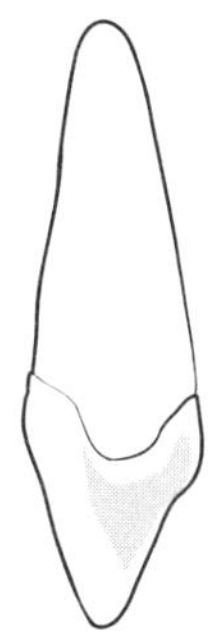	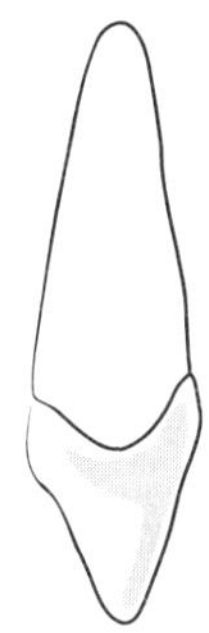	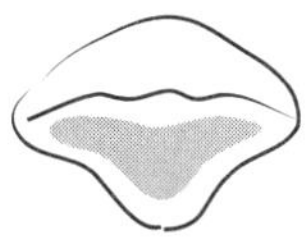
Surface has more curvature than central Distal outline more rounded Root surface length greater in proportion to crown than in central	Smaller than central Distinct anatomy: **mesial** and **distal marginal ridges, cingulum, lingual fossa, central pit** Incisal edge well developed Lingual fossa more concave Tendency to have pit Cingulum appears more prominent Surface may be lobulated and slightly convex	Crest of curvature in cervical third Cervical line deeper than on distal	Cervical line not as deep as in mesial	More ovoid in shape Mesiolabial and distolabial line angle more rounded Evidence of lobes seen

► Mandibular Central Incisor

The mandibular central incisor is the **narrowest** and **most symmetric** of all teeth. **Mesial and distal profiles mirror one another.**

Position		
	Right	**Left**
Universal	25	24
International	41	31

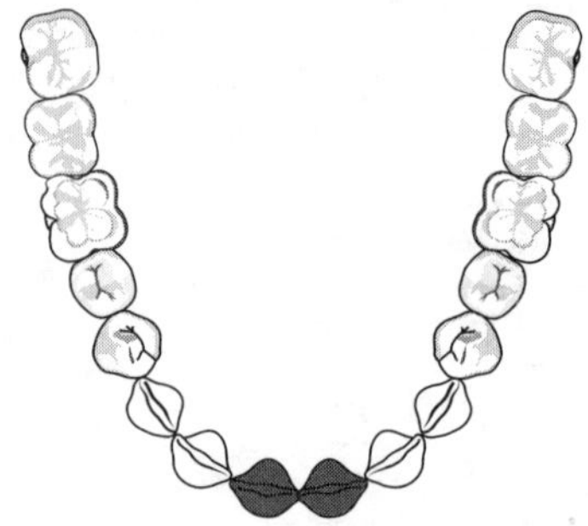

Developmental Data	
First evidence of calcification	3–4 months after birth
Enamel completed	4–5 years
Eruption	6–7 years
Root completed	9 years
Number of roots	1
Number of pulp horns	1–3
Developmental lobes	4

Width	Narrowest of all teeth
Root	Ovoid on cross section; wider labiolingually than mesiodistally; symmetry
Angles	Mesioincisal and distoincisal angles very sharp

Mandibular Right Central Incisor				
Labial	**Lingual**	**Mesial**	**Distal**	**Incisal**
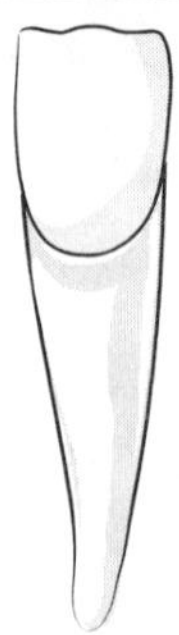	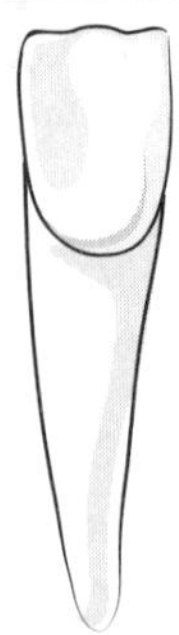	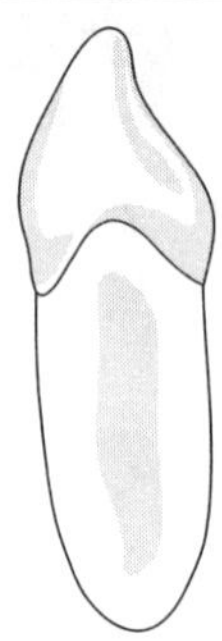	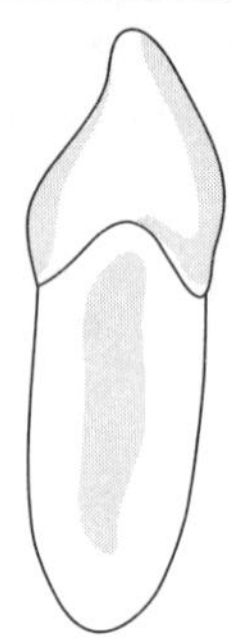	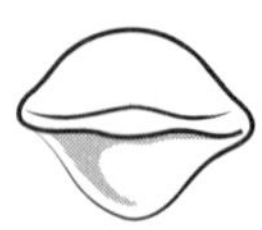
Root relatively long and straight Cervical line more rounded than on lingual Smooth surfaces (no marginal ridge) Almost perfectly symmetrical crown	Indistinct lingual anatomy Root relatively long and straight Small cingulum Almost perfectly symmetrical crown	Roots are wide faciolingually with depressions on both sides Incisal edge on or lingual to root axis	Distal surface of crown and root very similar to mesial view Distal contact area more toward cervical than mesial contact	Symmetry between mesial and distal Incisal edge toward lingual

▶ Mandibular Lateral Incisor

Mandibular lateral incisors are similar to mandibular central, except for the following:

- Lingual anatomy is indistinct.
- Mesial contour is straight with a height of contour at incisal edge.
- Incisal edge is **lingual to the labiolingual midpoint of the crown**, but the edge itself is not at right angles to a line bisecting the crown. However, it does follow arch curvature, making the distal end more lingually placed. The incisal edge appears to be rotated on the root.
- The root itself is very ovoid, being wider labiolingually than mesiodistally and may have mesial and distal depressions.

Position		
	Right	**Left**
Universal	26	23
International	42	32

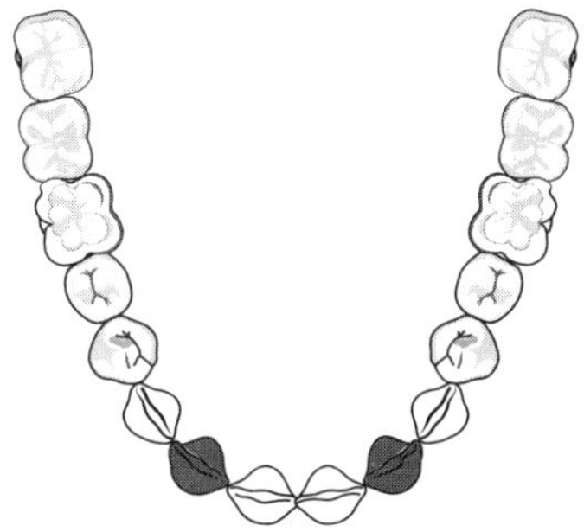

Developmental Data	
First evidence of calcification	3–4 months after birth
Enamel completed	4–5 years
Eruption	7–8 years
Root completed	10 years
Number of roots	1
Number of pulp horns	1–3
Developmental lobes	4

Width
Wider mesiodistally than central incisor

Mandibular Right Lateral Incisor				
Labial	**Lingual**	**Mesial**	**Distal**	**Incisal**
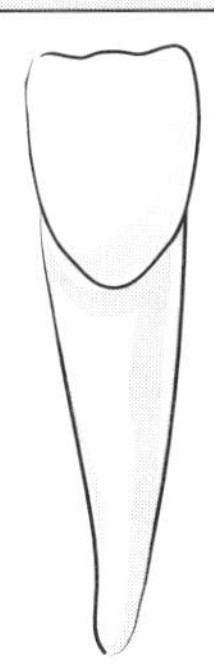	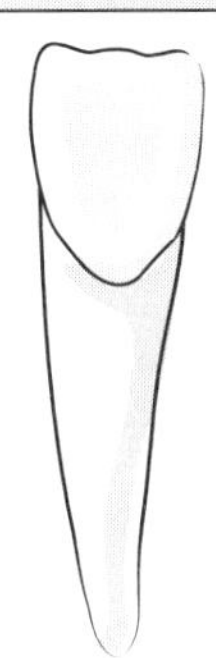	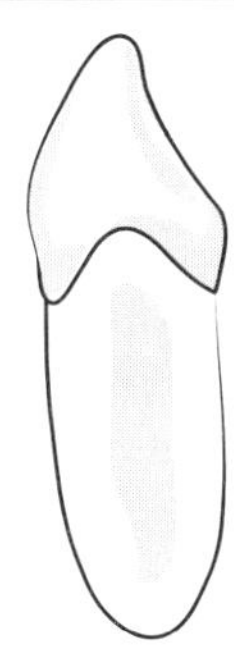	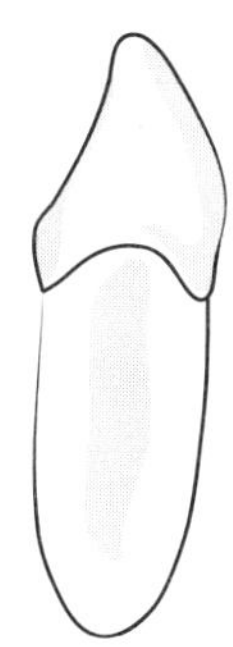	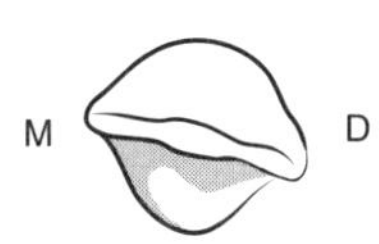
Asymmetric crown	Anatomy indistinct Cingulum distal to the long axis of tooth	Greater height of curvature of the CEJ From mesial, more of the lingual is visible (distal tilt)	Distal portion of incisal edge has a lingual turn	Incisal edge not straight mesiodistally and curves toward lingual on distal edge Cingulum is slightly toward distal Marginal ridge longer on mesial than distal side

► CANINES

There is only **one canine per quadrant** in the human. They are only teeth with a **single cusp**. The canines are the **longest** and **most stable teeth** in the adult permanent dentition and have an **oversized root**.

Maxillary	Mandibular
Wider mesiodistally	Narrower mesiodistally
Distinct lingual anatomy (lingual cingulum)	Less distinct anatomy on lingual (cingulum less pronounced)
Contact point more cervical	Contact areas and heights of contour higher; contact points more incisal
Anomalies rare (maybe tubercle between cusp tip and lingual ridge); very stable	One anomaly is a bifurcated root
Longest tooth in mouth	Anatomic crown longer
Incisal edge centered labiolingually	Incisal edge lingual to the labiolingual midpoint
Buccal tip centered in the long axis of the tooth	Cusp tip distally displaced
Wider mesiodistally	Narrower mesiodistally
Longer total length	Shorter total length
Distinct lingual anatomy; may have lingual pit	Lingual anatomy less distinct
Crown generally in line with root and is shorter, fatter	Longer, slimmer crown that appears distally bent
Incisal edge in labiolingual midpoint	Incisal edge lingual to labiolingual midpoint
Prominent distal and mesial marginal ridge	Less prominent marginal ridges
Lingual ridge from cusp to cingulum	Less prominent lingual ridge
Labial surface has prominent middle lobe running from cusp tip to cervical line	
Buccal surface marked by three-lobed appearance	

► Maxillary Canine

The maxillary canine is pointed and the **longest tooth in the mouth.**

Position		
	Right	**Left**
Universal	6	11
International (FDI)	13	23

Developmental Data	
First evidence of calcification	4–5 months after birth
Enamel completed	6–7 years
Eruption	11 to 12 years
Root completed	14 to 15 years
Number of roots	1
Number of pulp horns	1–3
Developmental lobes	4

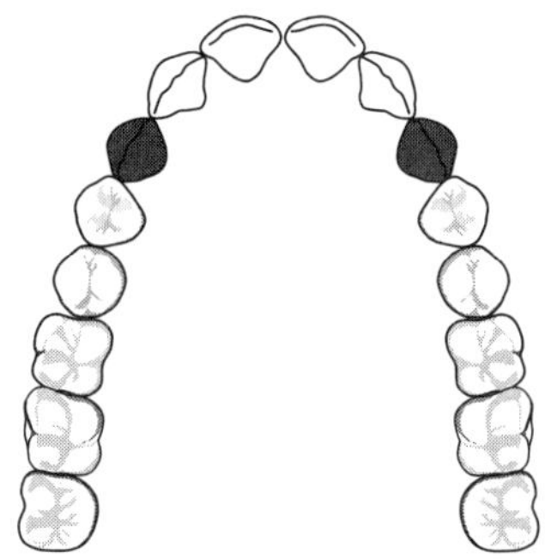

Maxillary Right Canine				
Labial	**Lingual**	**Mesial**	**Distal**	**Incisal**
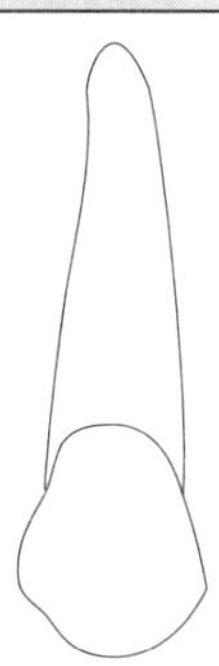	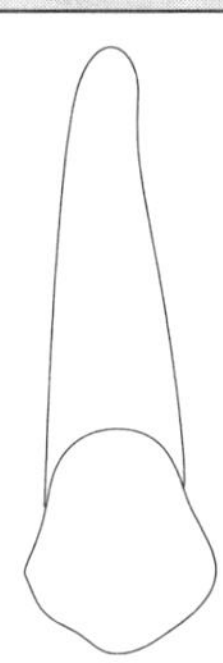	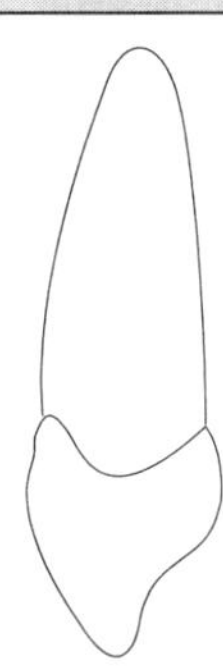	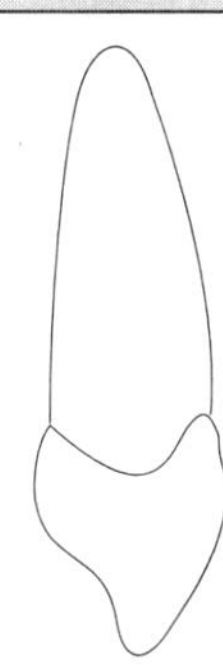	D 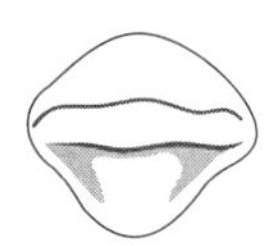 M
Root is long and tapers evenly Mesial ridge longer than distal Mesial incisal angle sharp One-cusp tip	Outline similar to facial Pronounced cingulum Marginal ridges Lingual fossae (mesial and distal) Possible lingual pit	Root is straight (wider labial lingually than mesial distally) Mesial cervical line more curved than distal	Distal contour is very bulbous or convex	**Triangular** Cusp tip is facial and mesial in placement Cingulum is slightly distal Pulp cavity centered in root Root is wider faciolingually than mesiodistally
Anomalies				
One anomaly associated with the mandibular canine is a bifurcated root.				

► Mandibular Canine

The mandibular canine is also a long, pointed tooth in which the total length is less than the maxillary canine, but the crown is longer. It has a **trilobed buccal surface**.

Position		
	Right	**Left**
Universal	27	22
International (FDI)	43	33

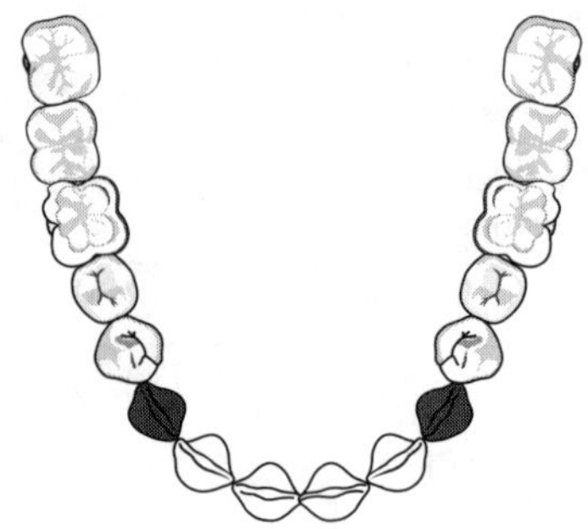

Developmental Data	
First evidence of calcification	4–5 months after birth
Enamel completed	6–7 years
Eruption	9–10 years
Root completed	12–14 years
Number of roots	1
Number of pulp horns	1–3
Developmental lobes	4

Manibular Right Canine				
Labial	**Lingual**	**Mesial**	**Distal**	**Incisal**
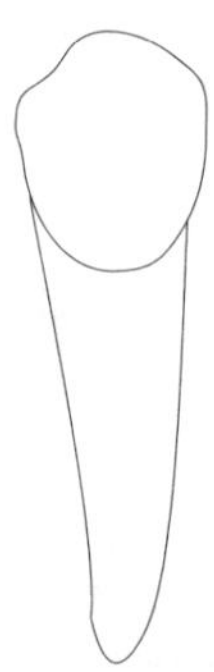	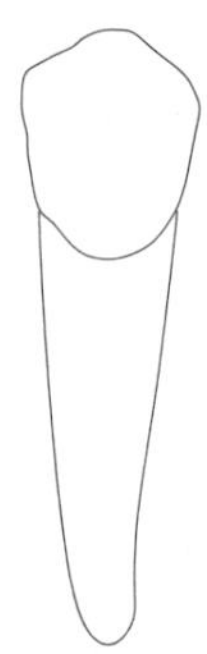	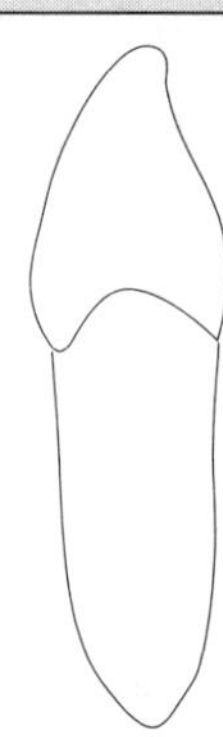	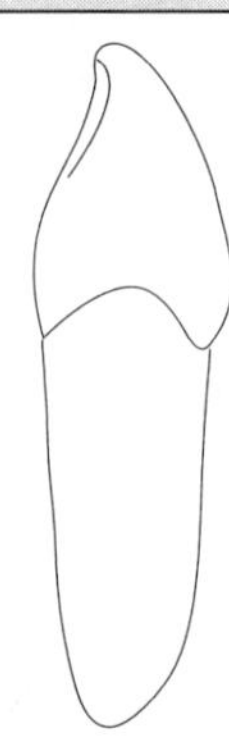	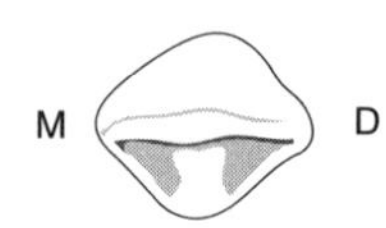
Mesial cusp ridge is shorter than distal	Anatomy is less distinct than maxillary canine Lingual pit is rare	Profile straight Possible root concavity Mesial cervical line more curved than distal	Similar to mesial view	Occlusal outline Crown is distally inclined with cusp tip slightly distally displaced Incisal edge is lingual to labiolingual midpoint Cingulum is distally positioned More symmetric than maxillary canine

▶ PREMOLARS

General

There are two premolars per quadrant. The buccal cusp is more predominant than the lingual, and each premolar has **two cusps**. Premolars are also known as bicuspids.

Maxillary and mandibular premolars are **approximately the same size mesiodistally and in total length**.

Know the premolars well. A surprisingly large number of dental anatomy questions involve these teeth.

Maxillary	Mandibular
Greater faciolingual diameter	Smaller faciolingual diameter
More distinct lingual cusps	Less distinct lingual cusps
Occlusal table centered faciolingually	Occlusal table lingually displaced
Two roots (buccal and lingual)	Buccal cusps more toward faciolingual midpoint
Buccal surface is straighter from height of contour to cusp tip	Buccal surface more convex
Prominent mesial root concavities	Rounder roots on cross-section

Comparison of Developmental Data of Premolars

	Maxillary First	Maxillary Second	Mandibular First	Mandibular Second
First evidence of calcification	1½–1¾ years	1–2½ years	1¾–2 years	2¼–2½ years
Enamel completed	5–6 years	6–7 years	5–6 years	6–7 years
Eruption	10–11 years	10–12 years	10–12 years	11–12 years
Root completed	12–13 years	12–14 years	12–13 years	13–14 years
Number of lobes	4	4	4	4–5
Number of roots	2	1	1	1

Comparison of the Premolars				
	Maxillary First	**Maxillary Second**	**Mandibular First**	**Mandibular Second**
Root	2 roots	1 root	1 root Relatively round and conical	1 root Roundest and conical root on cross section
Cusps	Distally displaced buccal cusp and mesially displaced lingual cusp	Buccal and lingual cusps equal and centered mesiodistally	Large buccal cusp dominates	**2 to 3 cusps** If 3, 2 are lingual, with mesiolingual larger than distolingual "Y" occlusal pattern for 3 cusps; "H" occlusal pattern for 2 cusps
Occlusal table	Trapezoidal	Rectangular	**Lingually inclined**	Square-shaped Less inclined than first premolar
Occlusal outlines	Hexagonal	Ovoid	Diamond	Square
Grooves	Mesial intraradicular groove Mesial marginal developmental groove	Short central groove Numerous supplemental grooves	**Mesiolingual developmental groove**	Lingual groove with 2 lingual cusps (3-cusp type)
Ridges	Lingual convergence Buccal cusp ridge inclines toward mesiolingual (twisted appearance)	Little lingual convergence	**Transverse ridge** Well-developed buccal ridge Mesial ridge less distinct than distal marginal ridge Lingual convergence	Little lingual convergence
Other distinguishing features	"Broad-shouldered" Prominent mesial concavity Prominent buccal lobes	"Narrow shouldered" Less prominent mesial axial concavity than maxillary first	Most resembles **canine** **Lingual cusp that resembles a cingulum** Transitional tooth Greatest discrepancy in size of buccal and lingual cusps and width (buccal dominant) Mesial/distal fossae with pits Prominent mesial bulge	Central pit Equal buccal and lingual surfaces

► Maxillary First Premolar

The maxillary first premolar has a **prominent buccal ridge**, and its buccal surface is wider than the lingual surface. It is the **only premolar that has two roots** (one buccal and one lingual) and **two cusps**.

The maxillary first premolar and its **intraradicular groove** is important to know for the **NBDE Part I**. Root planing of the mesial side and adapting a matrix band on the mesial side can both be difficult because of this groove.

Position		
	Right	**Left**
Universal	5	12
International (FDI)	14	24

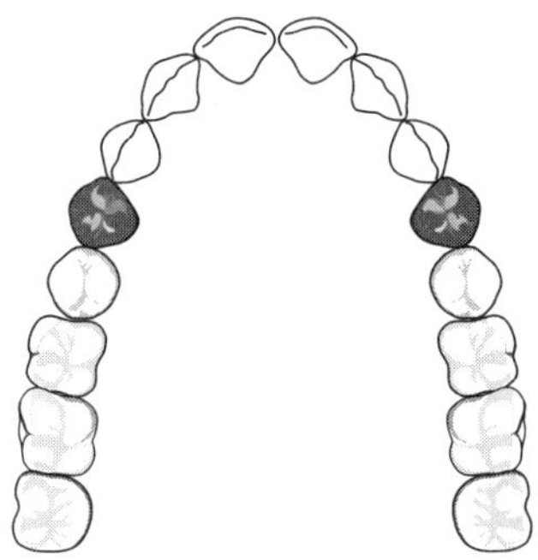

Maxillary First Right Premolar				
Buccal	**Lingual**	**Mesial**	**Distal**	**Occlusal**
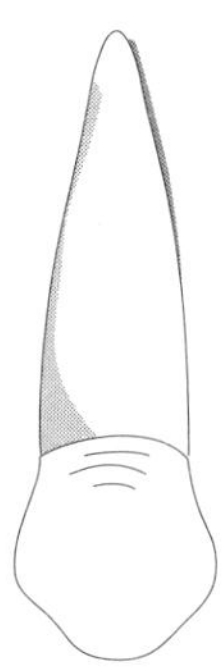	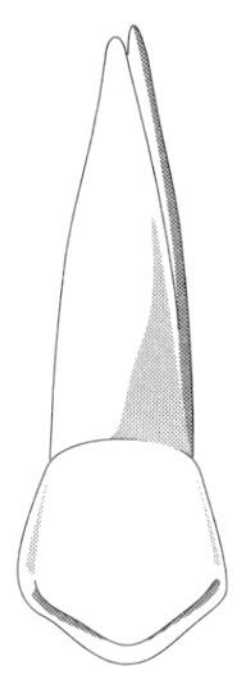	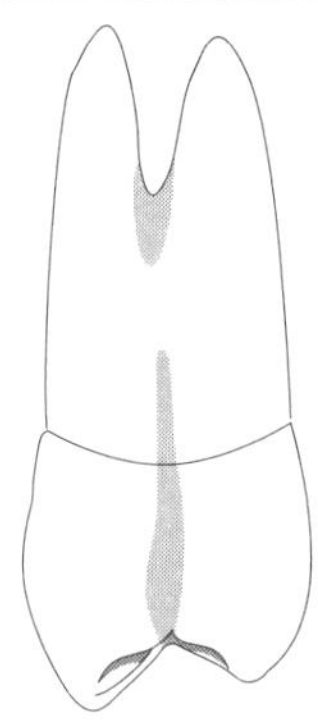	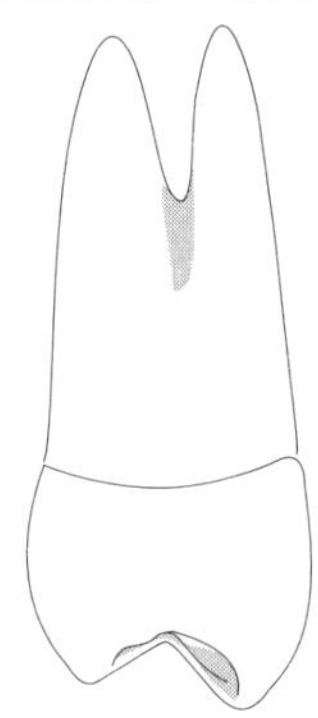	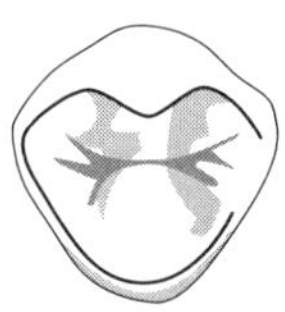
Rounded, long cusp Prominent buccal ridge running axially and bordered by depressions that give the surface a 3-lobed appearance Surface wider than lingual surface ("broad-shouldered")	Lingual cusp smaller Lingual cusp slightly mesial to midpoint and smaller than buccal cusp Surface rounded	Marked mesial concavity runs onto mesial root surface (**mesial interradicular groove**) **Mesial marginal developmental groove** (extension of central groove) interrupts mesial marginal ridge and progresses down mesial surface	Buccal cusp distally placed and larger than lingual cusp Also has developmental depression	**Hexagonal crown profile** (mesial and distal surfaces converge toward lingual) **Trapezoidal occlusal table** 2 cusps that are well defined: buccal is larger, and lingual is shifted mesially

Variants and Anomalies
• Single root • Occasionally 3 rooted

► Maxillary Second Premolar

The maxillary second premolar is a **"narrow-shouldered"** tooth from the buccal and is **slightly smaller** than the first premolar. It has **indistinct lobes**; a slight mesial concavity or even convexity may be seen on the mesial surface. **The mesial marginal ridge is not interrupted by a groove**. **Cusps** are more of an **equal height and lengths**, and the **tips are centered** on the tooth in a mesiodistal direction.

Position		
	Right	**Left**
Universal	4	13
International (FDI)	15	25

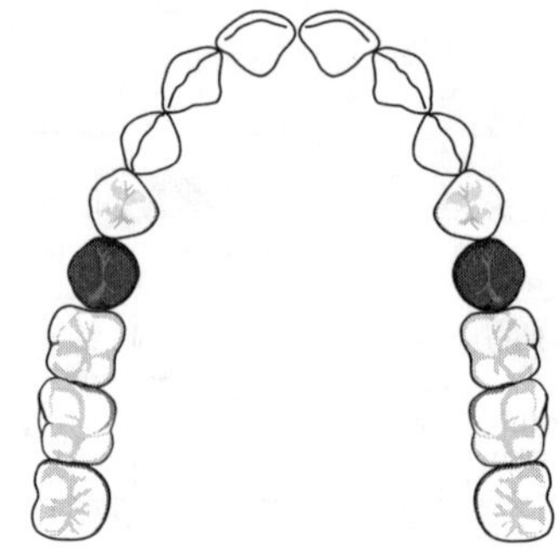

Maxillary Second Right Premolar				
Buccal	**Lingual**	**Mesial**	**Distal**	**Occlusal**
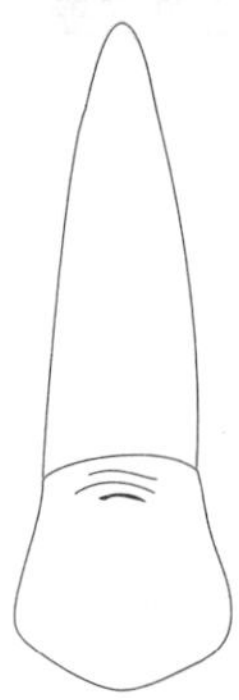	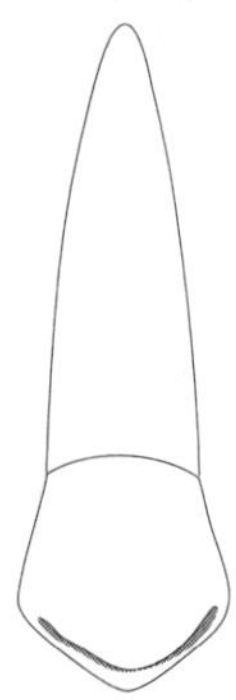	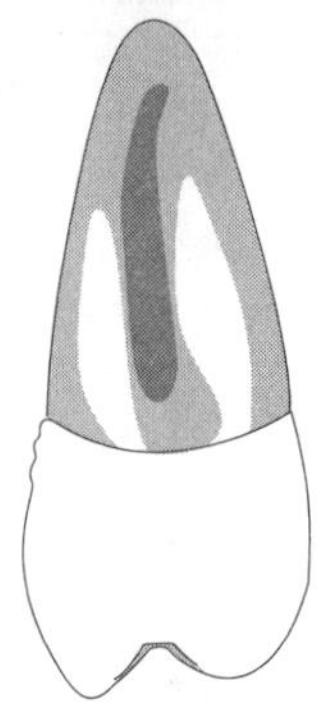	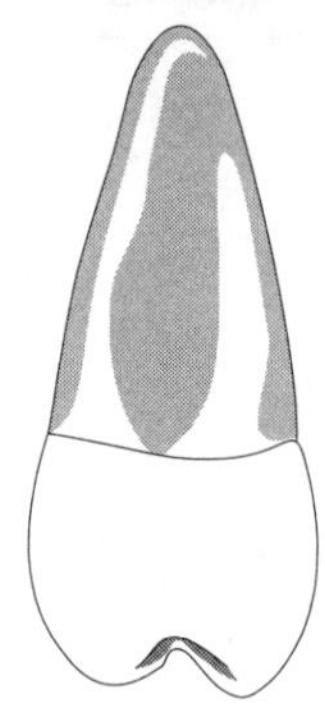	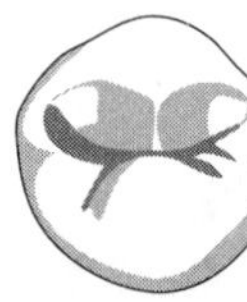
Indistinct lobes Buccal cusp is **shorter and rounder** than first premolar	Lingual cusp almost as big as buccal cusp Lingual cusp tip shifted mesially Smallest and most indistinct	Surface round Mesial marginal ridge is **not** interrupted by groove	Surface round	**Ovoid to round** shape **Rectangular** occlusal table Little lingual convergence

Variants and Anomalies
More variability than in first maxillary premolar

▶ Mandibular First Premolar

The mandibular first premolar may be viewed as a **transitional tooth, resembling a canine**. Its buccal cusp is much larger than is the lingual cusp, which may resemble a cingulum. It is the **only posterior tooth with a lingually inclined occlusal table.**

Position		
	Right	**Left**
Universal	28	21
International (FDI)	44	34

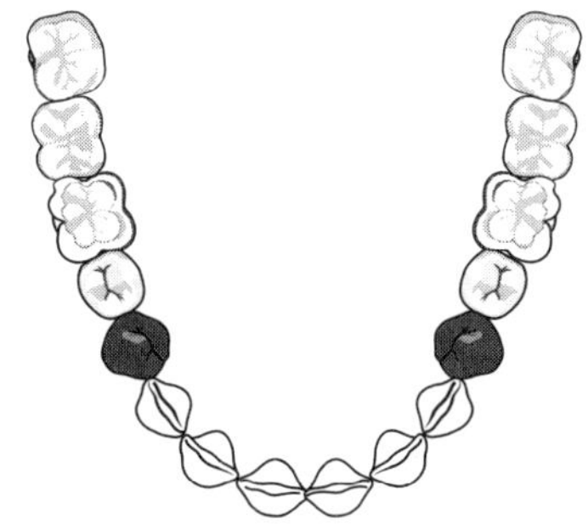

Mandibular First Right Premolar				
Buccal	**Lingual**	**Mesial**	**Distal**	**Occlusal**
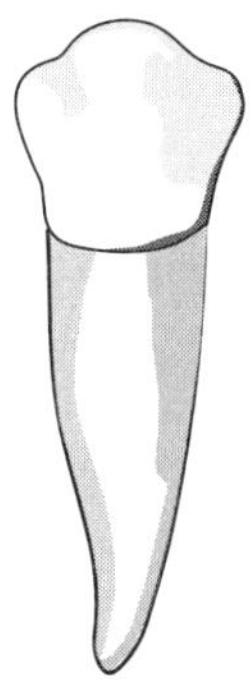	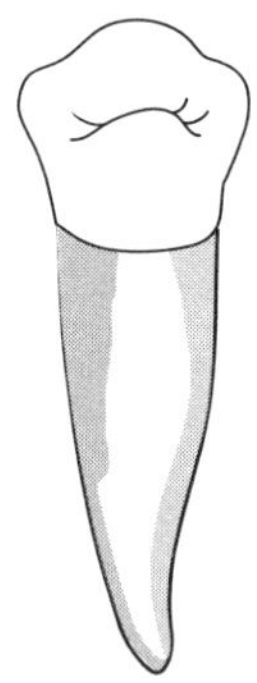	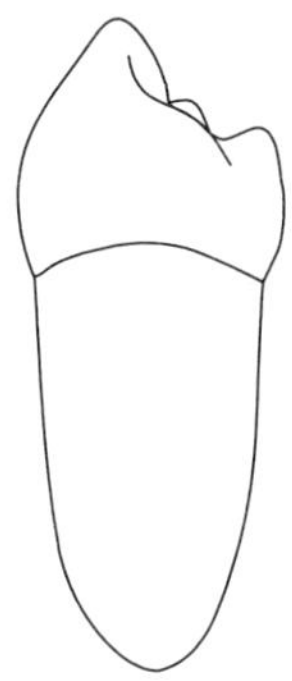	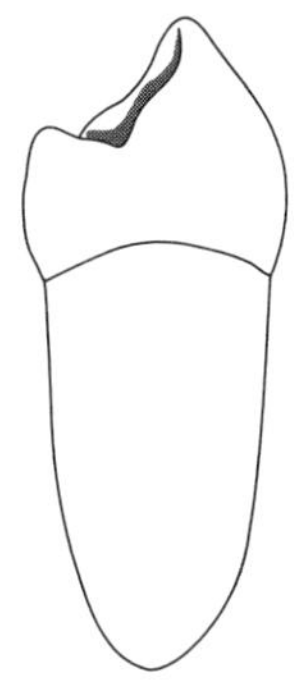	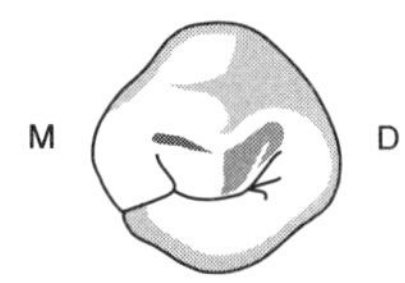
Outline is almost bilaterally symmetrical Large pointed buccal cusp Well-developed buccal ridge	**Smallest and indistinct cusp of all premolars** Lingual cusp may resemble a cingulum **Mesiolingual developmental groove** produces slight concavity at about the mesiolingual line angle	Prominent mesial bulge Very large buccal cusp tip centered over root tip Reduced lingual cusp Mesial/distal fossae with pits Marginal ridges well developed	Very large buccal cusp tip centered over root tip Reduced lingual cusp Mesial/distal fossae with pits Marginal ridges well developed	**Diamond shaped**, with convergence to the lingual Marginal ridges well developed Mesial and distal fossae with pits Mesiolingual developmental groove

Variants and Anomalies
• Grooved or bifurcated roots • Crown and root may be variable

▶ Mandibular Second Premolar

The mandibular second premolar is generally larger than the mandibular first premolar. It is distinguished by its **two variations of the lingual cusp.** If the mandibular second premolar has three cusps (more common) instead of two, the two appear on the lingual view and the mesiolingual is much larger than the distolingual. The mesiolingual cusp is also separated by a lingual groove extending from the central pit.

Position		
	Right	**Left**
Universal	29	20
International (FDI)	45	35

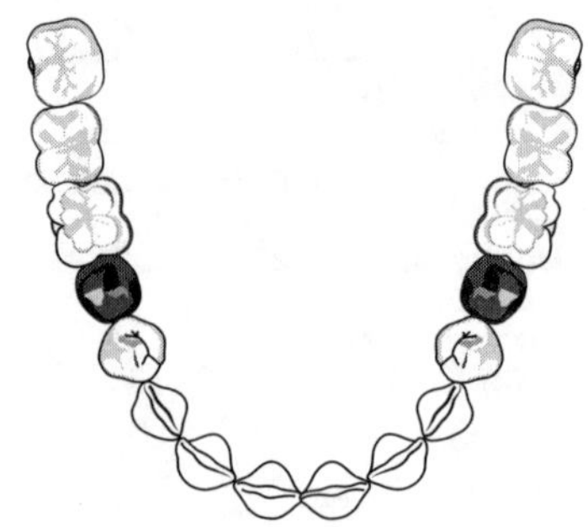

Manibular Second First Premolar				
Buccal	**Lingual**	**Mesial**	**Distal**	**Occlusal**
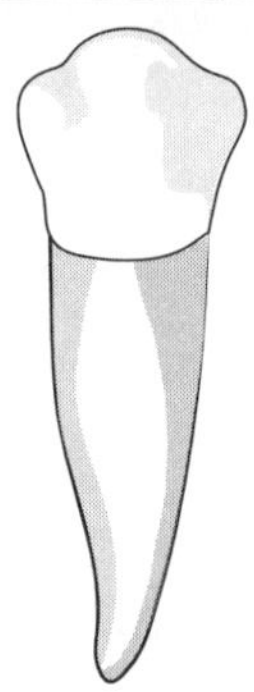	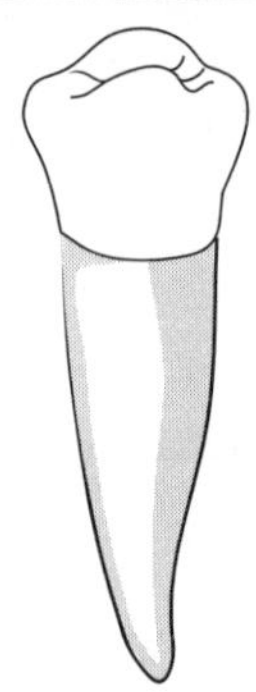	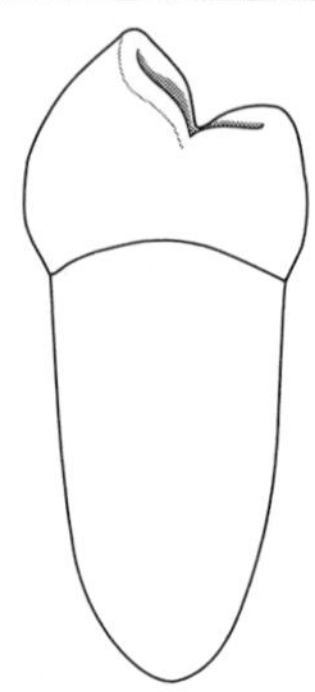	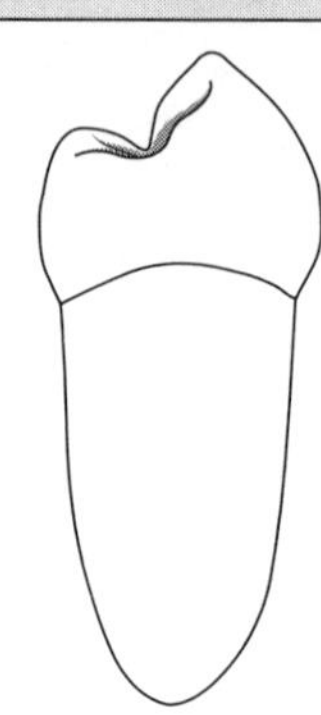	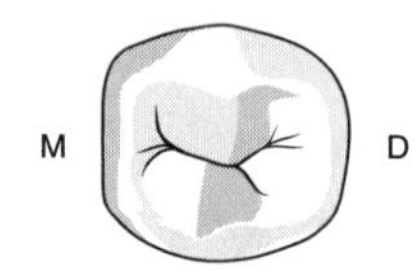
Buccal width nearly equal with lingual; buccal cusp size more equal with lingual cusp size	Lingual width nearly equal with buccal; lingual cusp size more equal with buccal cusp size If 3 cusps, 2 are lingual, with mesiolingual larger than distolingual Mesiolingual and distolingual cusp separated by lingual groove extending from central pit Little occlusal surface seen from the lingual In the single lingual cusp variant, its tip is shifted mesially	Buccal cusp is slightly shorter than first mandibular premolar Buccal cusp slightly longer than lingual cusp		Square in outline Central pit Variant groove patterns: • Y (3 cusps with central pit) • H (2 cusps with single developmental groove crossing transverse ridge from mesial to distal)

Variants and Anomalies
• One or two lingual cusps • Missing altogether

▶ MOLARS

General

The molar is derived from *mola*, Latin for "millstone." The main function of molars is to grind food, thus explaining their **large occlusal surfaces**. The most complicated of the adult human dentition, they can have from **three to five cusps** and **two to three roots**.

Questions on NBDE part I concerning molar anatomy will usually focus more on the first molar. This is because of increasing variation in the second and third molars.

Maxillary Molar	Mandibular Molar
3 roots	2 roots
4 pulp horns	2 pulp horns
4 cusps and extra variable Carabelli cusp (trait)	5 cusps
Buccal cusps unequal	Buccal cusps equal
Lingual cusps unequal; cusp of Carabelli mostly present	Lingual cusps equal; cusp of Carabelli absent
Oblique ridge diagonal	Oblique ridge not found on mandibular molars
Occlusal table centered labiolingually	Occlusal table lingually placed
Equal amounts of buccal and lingual surfaces may be seen from occlusal	More buccal surface than lingual surface may be seen from occlusal
Lingual height of contour in middle third just above junction of middle and cervical thirds	Lingual height of contour in middle third just below the junction of the middle and occlusal thirds
Wider faciolingually than mesiodistally	Wider mesiodistally than faciolingually
Distolingual groove	Buccal pit

Developmental Data						
	Maxillary			**Mandibular**		
	First	**Second**	**Third**	**First**	**Second**	**Third**
First evidence of calcification	Birth	2 ½ years	7–9 years	Birth	2½–3 years	8–10 years
Enamel completed	3–4 years	7–8 years	12–16 years	2½–3 years	7–8 years	12–16 years
Eruption	6 years	12–13 years	17–21 years	6–7 years	11–13 years	17–21 years
Root completed	9–10 years	14–16 years	18–25 years	9–10 years	14–15 years	18–25 years
Number of lobes	5	4	4	5	4	4
Number of roots	3	3	3 (may be fused into 1; highly variable)	2	2	2 (may be fused into 1; may be 3; highly variable)

Comparison of the Maxillary Molars			
	Maxillary First	**Maxillary Second**	**Maxillary Third**
Root	**3 roots** (2 buccal, 1 lingual) Buccal roots look like "pliers handles"; distobuccal smallest Large lingual root longest, "banana shaped" (almost straight) and centered between buccal roots 30% have fourth canal found in mesiobuccal root	**3 roots** (2 buccal, 1 lingual) Buccal roots distally inclined Roots are within crown profiles when seen from all angles	**3 roots** (2 buccal, 1 lingual) Often short Very distally inclined Tend to fuse (lingual to buccal)
Cusps	**4 major** (2 buccal, 2 lingual) **Fifth** minor cusp: **Carabelli** ML and MB cusps very large DB cusp large; DL cusp smaller 4 pulp horns (1 per major cusp)	**4 major** No Carabelli trait ML and MB cusps smaller than first DB cusp smaller; DL cusp even smaller (may be missing) 4 pulp horns (1 per major cusp)	**Usually 3** No Carabelli trait ML and MB cusps smaller than second DB cusp much smaller; DL cusp usually missing
Occlusal outlines	Rhomboidal	Rhomboidal or heart-shaped	Heart-shaped or triangular
Grooves	Lingual groove separates lingual cusps Buccal groove runs between buccal cusps Distal groove extends from central pit distolingually toward oblique ridge	Usually a short buccal groove; no buccal pit Similar to first molar	Variable pattern
Ridges	Oblique ridge most prominent, connects distobuccal cusp to mesiolingual cusp Mesial marginal ridge longer and more distinct than distal marginal ridge	Oblique ridge from distobuccal to mesiolingual Similar to first molar	Oblique ridges may be missing Variable pattern
Other distinguishing features	Looks like two premolars stuck together Distal and central fossa Distal triangular fossa contains distal pit Mesiolingual > mesiobuccal > distobuccal > distolingual	More exaggerated difference in cusp size: mesiolingual > mesiobuccal > distobuccal > distolingual	More variable morphology than any other tooth May be the most often congenitally missing

Comparison of the Mandibular Molars			
	Mandibular First	**Mandibular Second**	**Mandibular Third**
Root (for more details, see individual tooth)	2 roots Rounded apex Mesial root largest Roots less distally inclined than in second molar	2 roots More distinctly distally inclined Pointed apex Proximal root concavities not usually seen	2 roots Extremely distally inclined Short, often fused
Cusps	5 cusps	4 cusps	4 cusps (highly variable)
Occlusal outlines	Pentagonal	Rectangular	Ovoid
Grooves	2 buccal grooves (MB and DB) Mesial and distal marginal grooves	Single buccal groove No marginal grooves	Single buccal groove No marginal grooves
Ridges	Two transverse ridges, no oblique ridge	Two transverse ridges, no oblique ridge	Two transverse ridges, no oblique ridge
Other distinguishing features	Prove to misshapen enamel defect: mulberry molar Largest of the mandibular teeth	Most symmetric of the molars No distal cusp	Often has variable morphology May be the most often congenitally missing Common tooth to have enamel pearls

► Maxillary First Molar

The **Carabelli trait** is the most distinguishing feature of the maxillary first molar, and is highly variable, from being a full cusp to being barely visible.

Position		
	Right	**Left**
Universal	3	14
International (FDI)	16	26

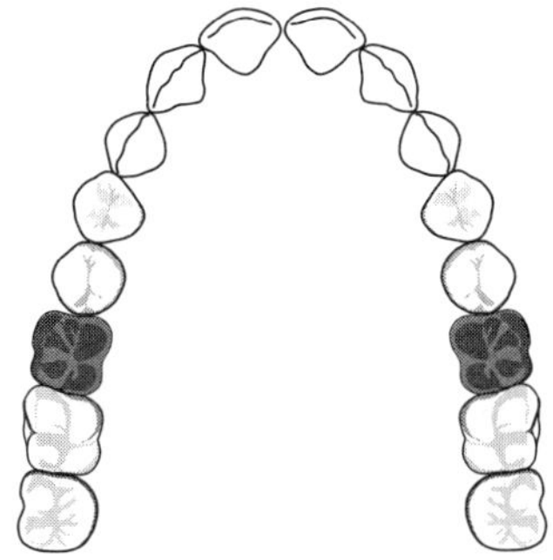

Maxillary First Right Molar				
Buccal	**Lingual**	**Mesial**	**Distal**	**Occlusal**
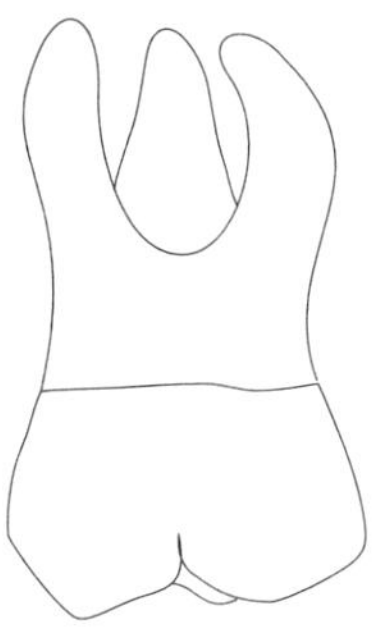	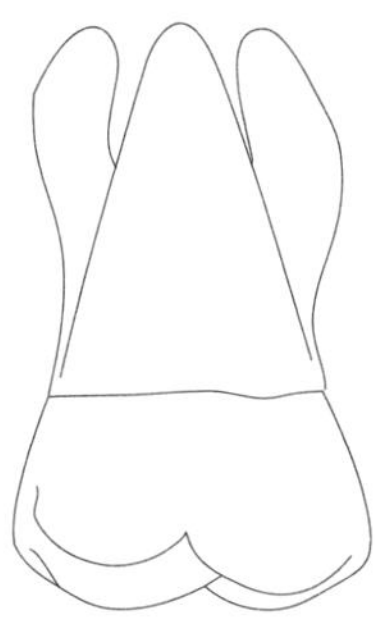	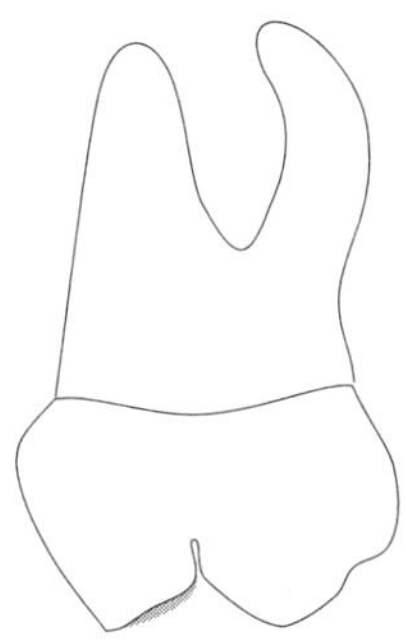	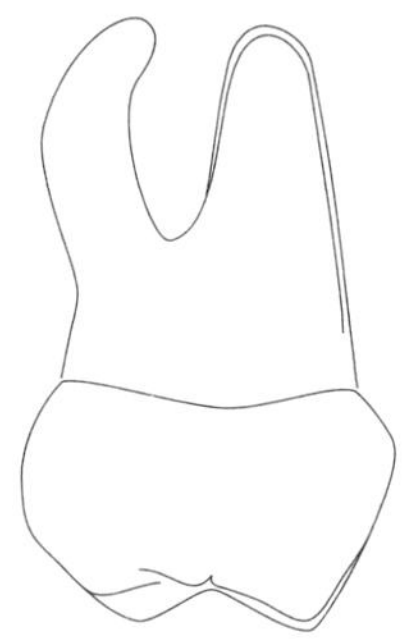	D 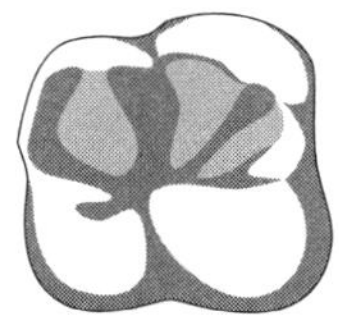 M
Larger mesiobuccal cusp Cervical line straight Mesiobuccal and distobuccal dominate Buccal developmental groove **Roots:** Buccal roots joined in common root trunk (extends 2.5–3.5 mm from cervical line) Root trunk may have deep developmental groove All roots can be seen from buccal view, with lingual root in between	Lingual surface convex throughout Lingual developmental groove (extension of distolingual groove) Larger mesiolingual cusp sometimes has Carabelli trait **Root:** Lingual is largest root (greatest diameter in mesiodistal direction) Massive root trunk Vertical depression on its lingual surface extending from cervical line Mesiobuccal has a mesial contour; distobuccal has distal contour	Flat to concave surface Cusp of Carabelli seen **Roots:** From mesial view, only mesiobuccal and lingual roots seen (distobuccal blocked by mesiobuccal)	Convex surface throughout, except for concave-to-flat area immediately above distobuccal root Distal marginal ridge shorter than mesial	**Rhomboid** shape **Angles:** Mesiobuccal and distolingual **acute**; distobuccal and mesiolingual **obtuse** 4 major cusps Cusp of Carabelli on mesiolingual cusp Lingual groove separates lingual cusps **Oblique ridge** (mesiolingual to distobuccal cusps) **Major** fossae: distal and central **Minor** fossa: mesial triangular, distal triangular **Distal pit** Largest crown of all maxillary molars

► Maxillary Second Molar

The maxillary second molar is very similar to the first molar, with the following exceptions: *1*) **the distobuccal cusp is relatively smaller or absent,** *2*) **the absence of the cusp of Carabelli,** *3*) the mesiobuccal and distolingual angles are more acute, whereas the mesiolingual and distobuccal angles are more obtuse, and *4*) there are **more supplemental grooves** on the occlusal surface.

Position		
	Right	**Left**
Universal	2	15
International (FDI)	17	27

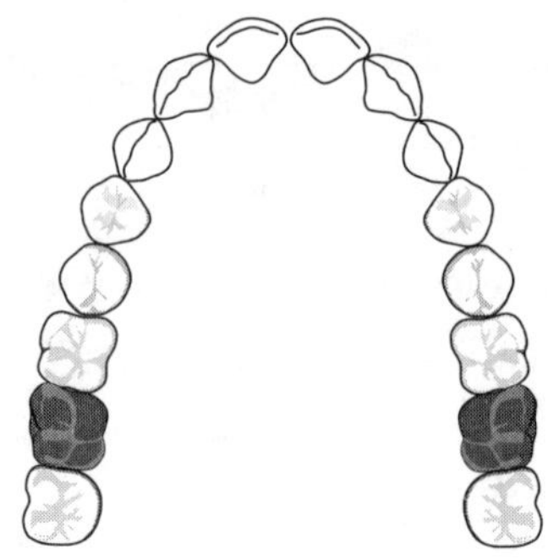

Maxillary Second Right Molar				
Buccal	**Lingual**	**Mesial**	**Distal**	**Occlusal**
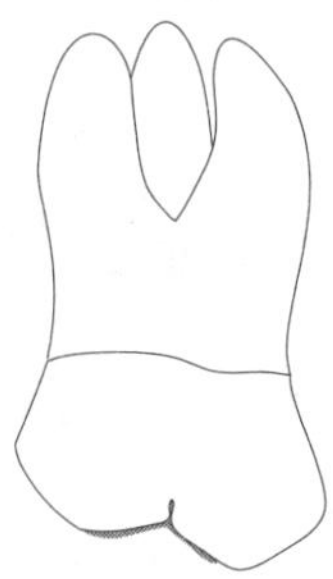	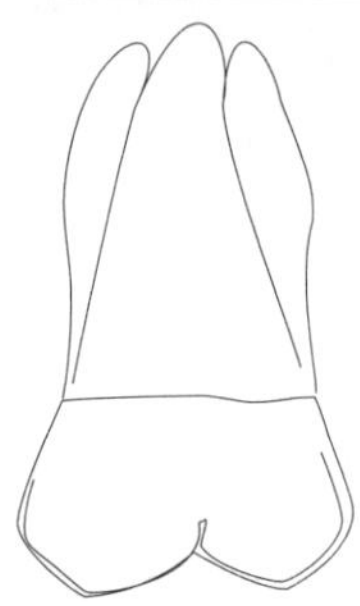	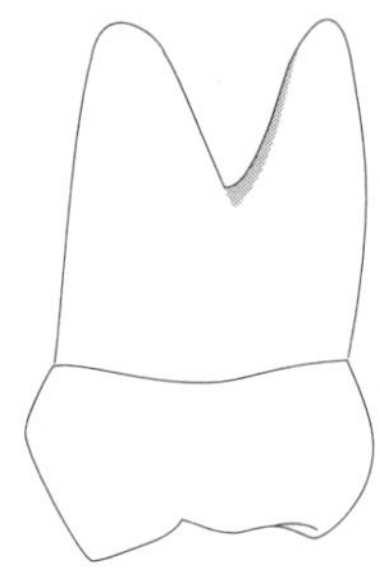	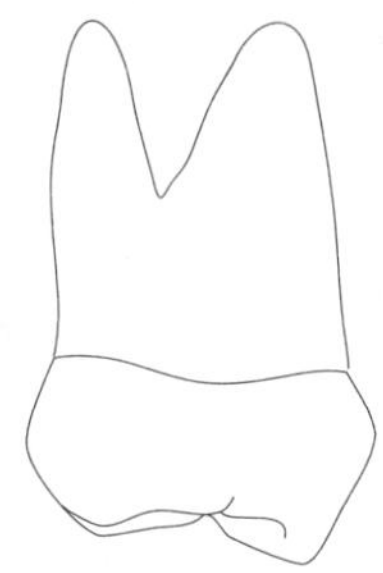	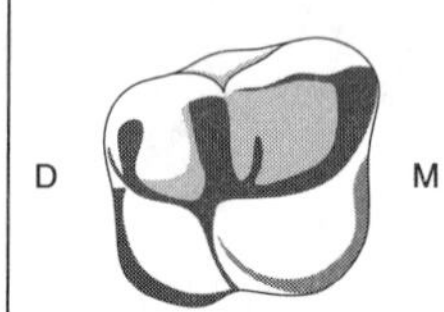
Crown is shorter occlusocervically and is narrower mesiodistally Distobuccal cusp is smaller **Root:** Mesiobuccal and distobuccal root are inclined distally and are more parallel and usually the same length	Distolingual cusp smaller No Carabelli cusp **Root:** Lingual root may be distally inclined (no "pliers handles")	Crown is shorter than first molar Roots confine themselves to width of crown		**Rhomboidal** (large distolingual cusp) or **heart-shaped** (smaller distolingual cusp) Distobuccal cusp smaller and less defined than first molar Oblique ridge less dominant Differences in cusp size is more exaggerated than on first molar

Variants and Anomalies
• Distolingual cusp absent • Occlusal shape rhomboidal or heart-shaped • Fused root

▶ Maxillary Third Molar

The maxillary third molar, as well as the maxillary lateral incisor, is known for **extreme variability of form.** Pointed, peg-like maxillary third molars are not uncommon. The sometimes fused, pointed roots can make extraction of these teeth easier than expected.

Position		
	Right	**Left**
Universal	1	16
International (FDI)	18	28

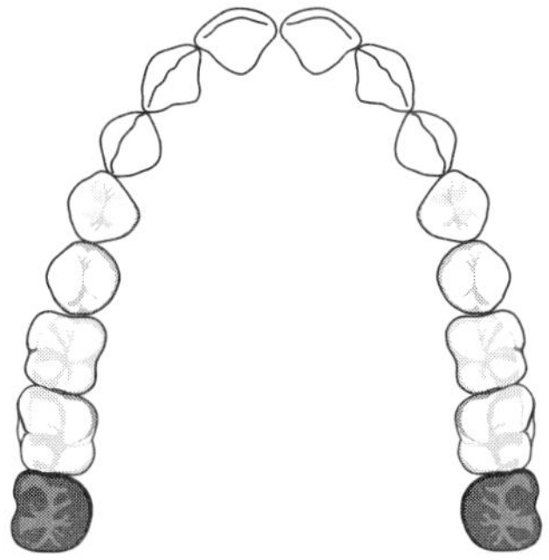

Maxillary Third Right Molar				
Buccal	**Lingual**	**Mesial**	**Distal**	**Occlusal**
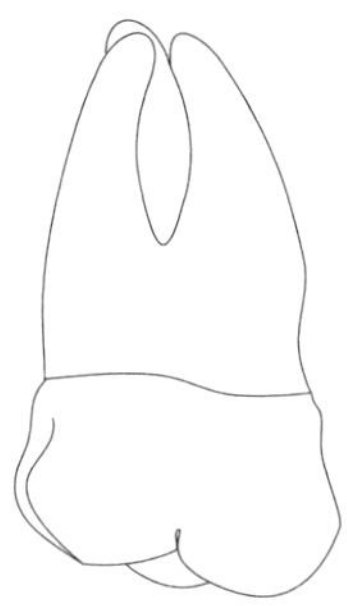	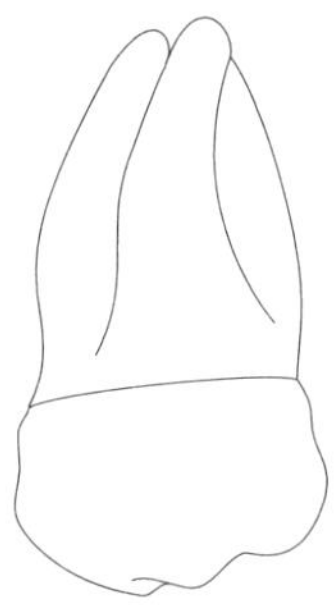	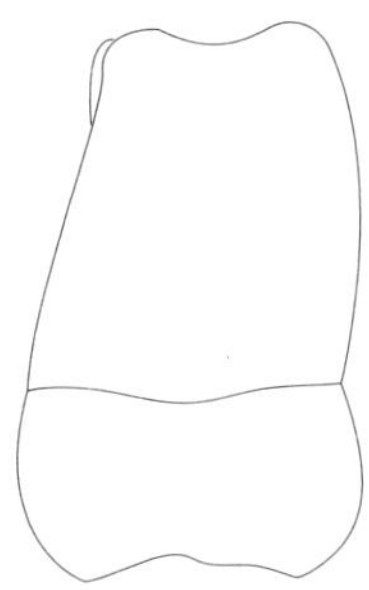	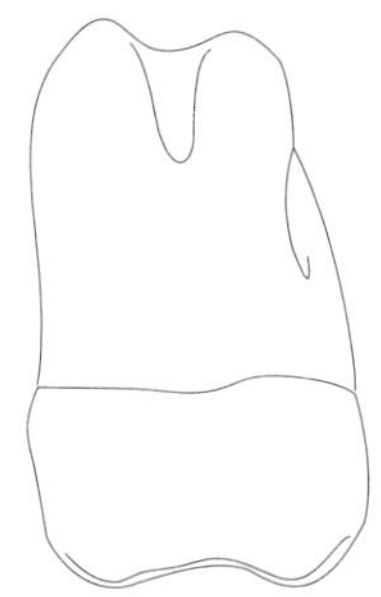	D 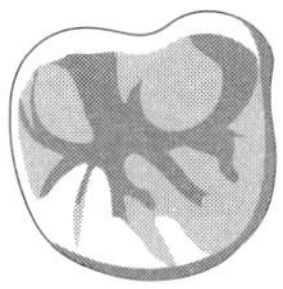 M
Distobuccal cusp smaller than mesiobuccal (sometimes missing) **Roots:** Buccal roots most often fused	Distolingual cusp often absent (mostly one large lingual cusp) **Root:** Lingual root often fused to buccal cusps	Crown outline rounded, bulbous	**No contact point** on distal surface Crown outline also rounded, bulbous	**Heart-shaped or triangular** Oblique ridge may be small or missing Smallest crown of the maxillary molars Mesiolingual cusp is largest; distobuccal is smallest (or distolingual, if present)

Variants and Anomalies
• Impaction common • Many cusps and grooves possible • Distobuccal cusp small • Distolingual cusp missing

► Mandibular First Molar

The mandibular first molar has a **distinctive pentagonal ("home plate") occlusal outline**, and two buccal and one lingual groove form the pattern distinctive to this tooth. The **buccal half is divided into three cusps, and the lingual is divided into two.**

Position		
	Right	**Left**
Universal	30	19
International (FDI)	46	36

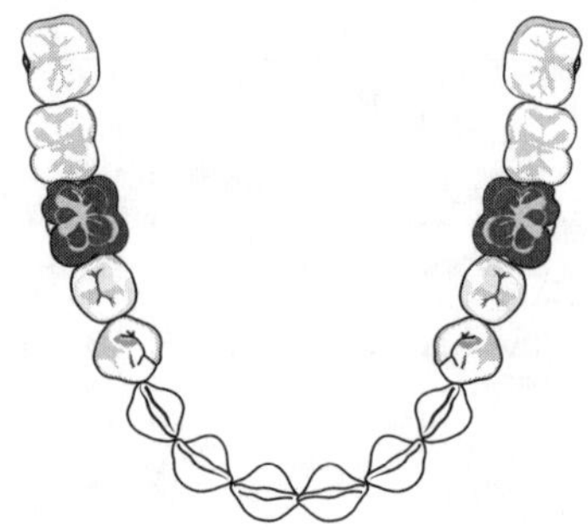

Mandibular First Right Molar				
Buccal	**Lingual**	**Mesial**	**Distal**	**Occlusal**
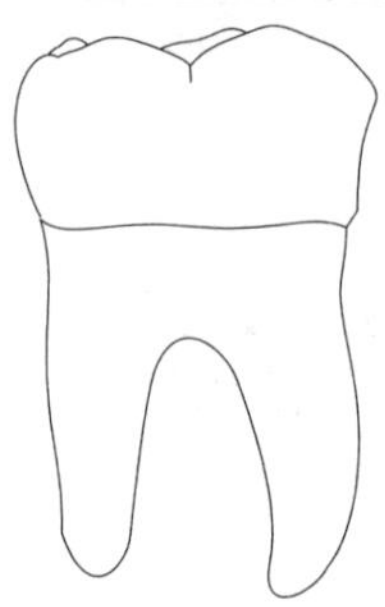	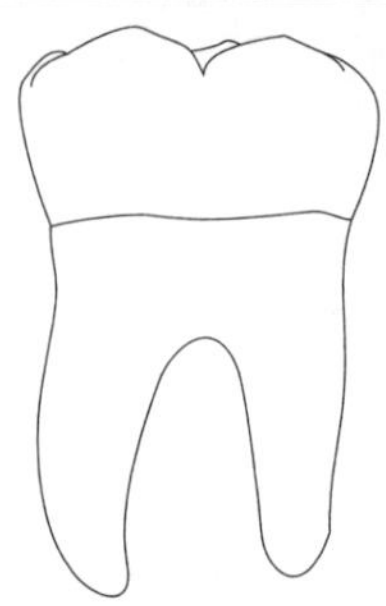	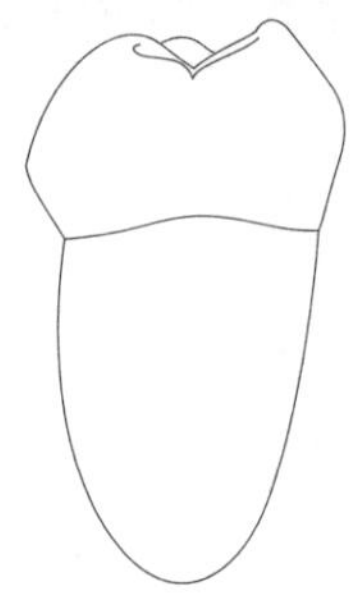	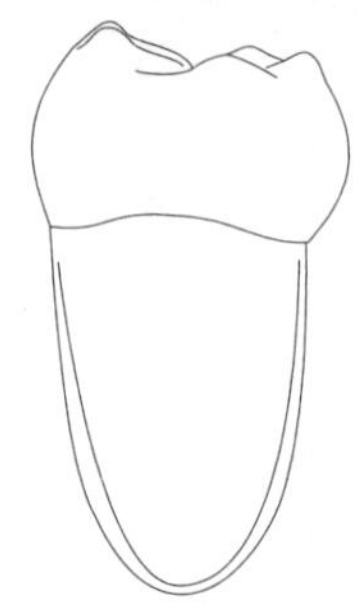	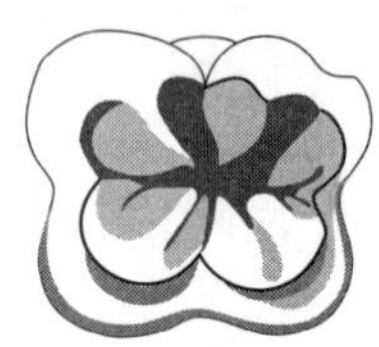
3 cusps seen 2 developmental grooves (mesiobuccal and distobuccal) Mesiobuccal groove ends in **buccal pit** on buccal surface Trapezoidal shape (wider at occlusal) Distal outline more rounded Mesiobuccal cusp widest; distobuccal smallest **Roots:** 2 clearly seen; distal root is less curved than mesial	3 cusps seen Developmental groove separates 2 lingual cusps Prominent cervical ridge height **Roots:** 2 visible	Rhomboid (tilted lingually) Lingual surface straighter than convex buccal surface Mesial marginal groove notches mesial marginal groove Buccal cervical ridge **Root:** Mesial root is the broadest root in the arch in a buccolingual direction; curves distally; distinct proximal root concavity on mesial surface; blunt; joined with distal at common root trunk	3 cusps seen (distobuccal, distal, distolingual) Tooth tapers toward distal Distal marginal ridge notched by distal marginal groove **Root:** Curves distally; blunt, distal smaller than mesial; may have shallow proximal root concavity; joined with mesial at common root trunk	**Pentagonal** ("home plate") shape **5** functional cusps **3 fossae, each with pit:** central, mesial, and distal Buccal outline divided into 3 (mesiobuccal and distobuccal grooves) Lingual outline divided into 2 (lingual groove) Distal marginal ridge smaller than mesial marginal ridge (both ridges cut through by developmental grooves)

Variants and Anomalies
• Distal cusp absent • Occasionally 2 mesial roots • Sixth cusp rare

► Mandibular Second Molar

The mandibular second molar is similar to the first molar except that it is *1*) smaller, *2*) the **distal cusp is missing**, *3*) the lingual and buccal surfaces are similar in length, *4*) there is **only one buccal groove**; *5*) the crown is also shorter, and *6*) there are **no developmental grooves interrupting the marginal ridges.** Finally, *7*) roots are more distally inclined than the first molar and have a more pointed apex.

Position		
	Right	**Left**
Universal	31	18
International	47	37

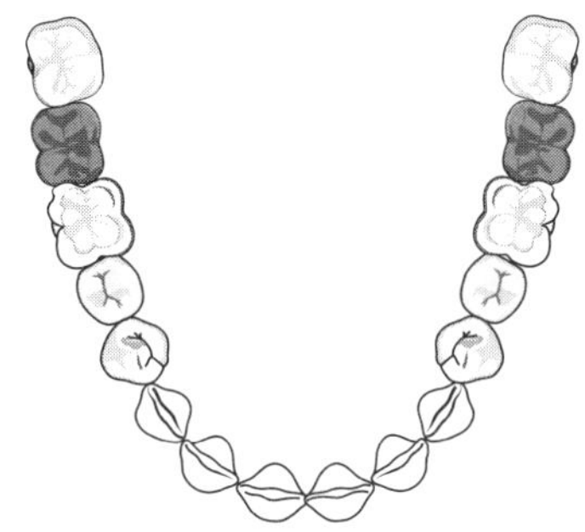

Mandibular Second Right Molar				
Buccal	**Lingual**	**Mesial**	**Distal**	**Occlusal**
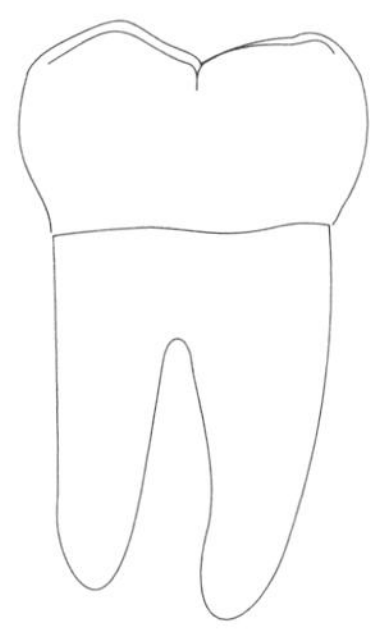	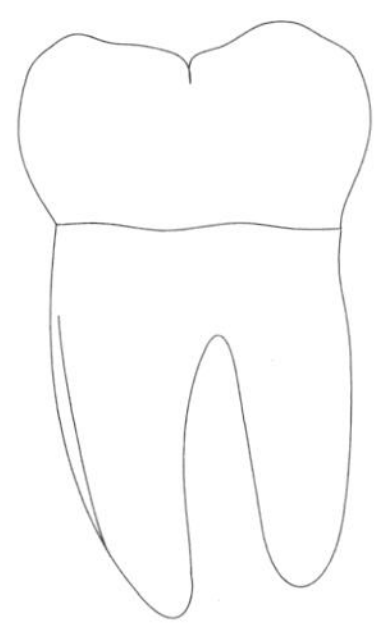	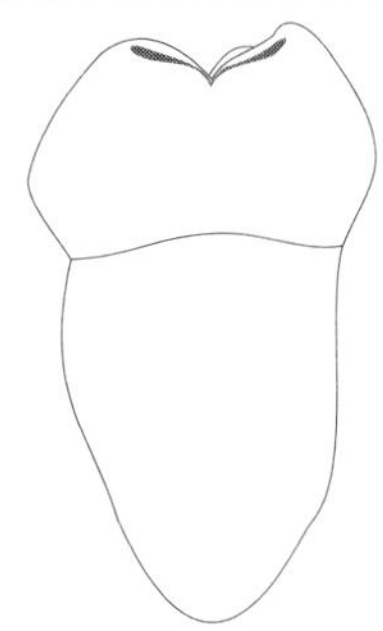	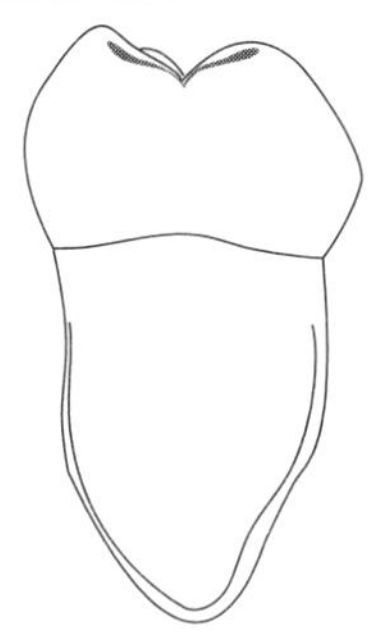	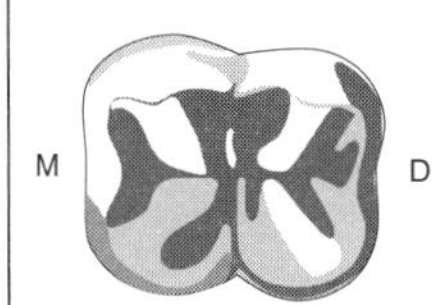
Buccal groove separates mesiobuccal from distobuccal cusps Trapezoidal shape No distal cusp (4 cusps) **Roots:** Closer together than first mandibular molar and are distally inclined	Trapezoidal shape Lingual groove **Roots:** Closer together than first mandibular molar and are distally inclined	Looks similar to first molar Cusps of equal height	Cusps of equal height Distal marginal ridge helps form profile Cervical line flat	**Rectangular** 4 cusps 3 grooves (buccal, lingual, central) 3 fossae, each with pit (central, medial, distal) Two transverse ridges

Variants and Anomalies
• 2 root canals for each root • Five cusps (rare)

▶ Mandibular Third Molar

Third molars vary in shape and **do not have a standard form**. They are usually smaller than the second molar.

Position		
	Right	**Left**
Universal	32	17
International (FDI)	48	38

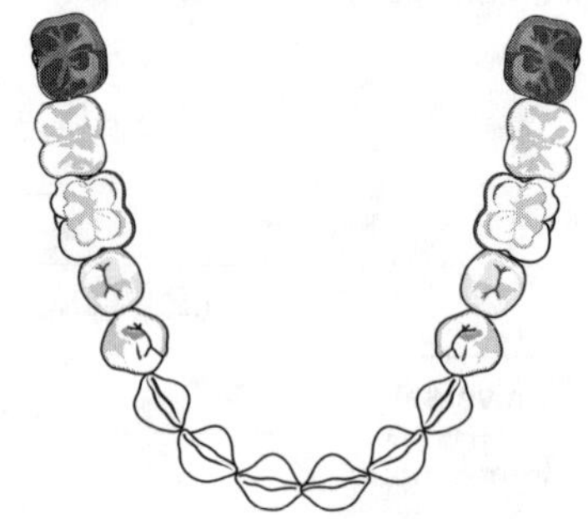

Mandibular Third Right Molar				
Buccal	**Lingual**	**Mesial**	**Distal**	**Occlusal**
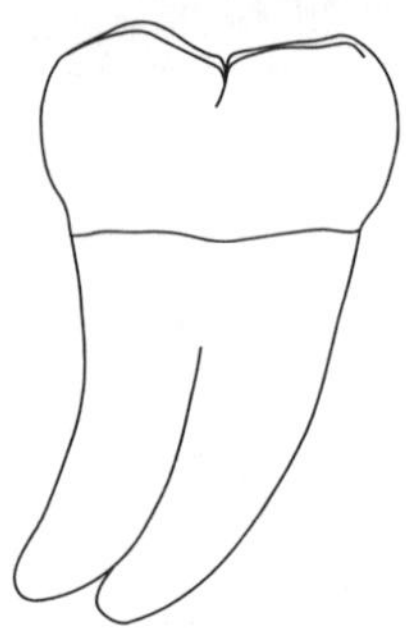	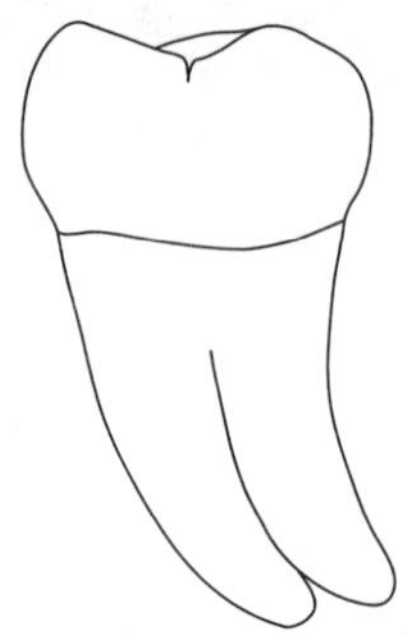	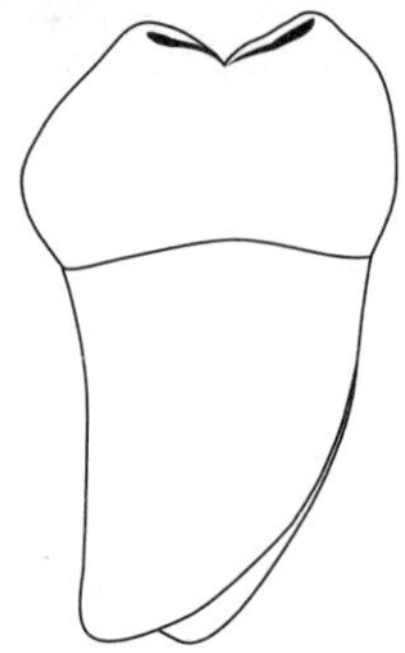	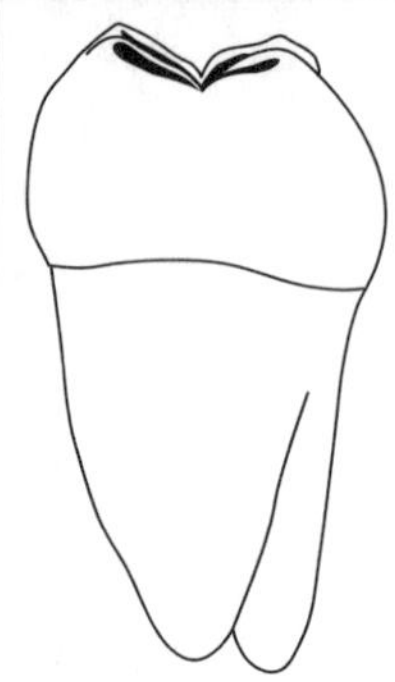	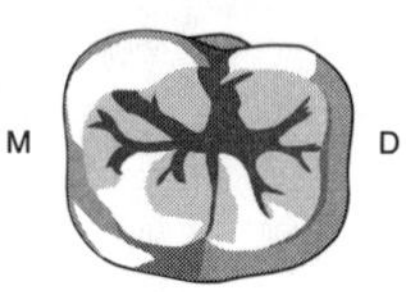
Crown short and bulbous **Roots:** distally inclined; poorly developed		Resembles first and second molars, but shorter crown		**Ovoid to round** 4–5 cusps May have indistinct grooves

Variants and Anomalies
• Most commonly missing permanent teeth • Often under- or oversized • Supernumerary (fourth molars) • May be partially erupted (susceptible to periodontal infections) • Occlusal surface may be crenulated (numerous grooves) • Often fail to erupt

Primary Dentition

▶ General

The deciduous dentition (also called "primary" or "baby" teeth) helps permanent teeth develop proper alignment, spacing, and occlusion. As stated in the first few pages of the General Characteristics section, there are 20 primary teeth in all (10 maxillary and 10 mandibular).

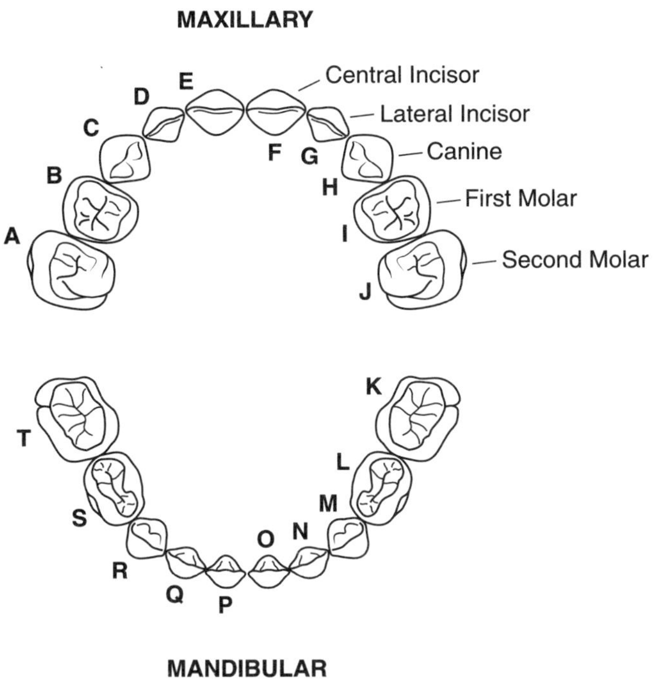

Maxillary	Eruption* (months)	Shedding (years)
Central incisor	8–12	6–7
Lateral incisor	9–13	7–8
Canine (cuspid)	16–22	10–12
First molar	13–19	9–11
Second molar	25–33	10–12
Mandibular		
Central incisor	6–10	6–7
Lateral incisor	10–16	7–8
Canine (cuspid)	17–23	9–12
First molar	14–18	9–11
Second molar	23–31	10–12

*Note that teeth tend to erupt in pairs.

Also, eruption and shedding patterns are seen earlier in girls.

Maxillary	Calcification (weeks in utero)	Root Formation Complete (months)
Central incisor	14	10
Lateral incisor	16	11
Canine (cuspid)	17	19
First molar	15	16
Second molar	19	26
Mandibular		
Central incisor	14	8
Lateral incisor	16	13
Canine (cuspid)	17	20
First molar	15½	16
Second molar	18	27

Primary Teeth Characteristics as Differing from Permanent Teeth

In general, the fewer primary teeth are **smaller and whiter** than permanent teeth and generally resemble the teeth that replace them, **except for the first molars**, which resemble nothing in the permanent dentition. **Primary molars** are replaced by **permanent premolars**.

Development of Primary Teeth

- Development begins at 6 weeks in utero
- Calcification begins at 18 weeks in utero (approx 4–6 months)
- By the age of 3, apices are completely formed

Features	Comparison with Permanent Teeth
Crowns	Crown-to-root ratio is smaller Shorter and fatter Rounded
Roots	Marked bowing and flaring Molars: long and slender with little or no trunk Incisors and canines: longer and slender
Enamel	Thinner
Surfaces	Lingual and facial cervical bulges Facial and lingual surfaces are flatter No mammelons on anterior teeth
Arch	More circular
Ridges	Cervical ridges more prominent

► Anterior Teeth

The primary incisors and canines resemble the permanent ones, **except for traits listed in the following table.** A notable trademark of the anteriors is **cervical constricture**.

Tooth	Position (Right/Left)	Replaced by	Differences from Permanent Replacement
Maxillary primary central incisor*	E/F 51/61	Maxillary permanent central incisor	Smooth labial surface No mammelons Cingulum may be prominent Cervical constricture: facial and lingual cervical bulges Height of crown smaller than mesiodistal diameter
Maxillary primary lateral incisor*	D/G 52/62	Maxillary permanent lateral incisor	Labial surface smoother than permanent No mammelons More distinct lingual anatomy Cervical constricture
Maxillary primary canine	C/H 53/63	Maxillary permanent canine	Diamond-shaped crown from facial Labial surface smoother Prominent cingulum (cusped appearance) Mesial and distal contacts are at same level Longer mesial incisal slope than distal incisal slope Height of crown less than mesiodistal diameter
Mandibular primary central	P/O 81/71	Mandibular permanent central incisor	Labial surface smooth, unmarked, flat Prominent cingulum on lingual Often, developmental groove or depression on distal of root Cervical contricture
Mandibular primary lateral	Q/N 82/72	Mandibular permanent lateral incisor	Prominent cingulum on lingual Cervical constricture
Mandibular primary canine	R/M 83/73	Mandibular permanent canine	Arrow-shaped from facial Smooth labial surface Longer distal incisal ridge than mesial incisal ridge

*These teeth are most damaged by baby bottle tooth decay (BBTD).

► Posterior Teeth

The primary first molar resembles nothing in the adult dentition. In general, **upper molars** have **3 roots**, whereas the **lower molars** have only **2**. First molars are also distinguished by a bulge on the buccal surface (cervical bulge).

Tooth	Position	Replaced by	Traits
Maxillary primary first molar	B/I 54/64	Maxillary permanent first premolar	Resembles nothing in permanent dentition Two-cusped (mesiobuccal and mesiolingual) **Nodule resembling small cusp** may be present on mesial ridge of the mesiobuccal cusp **Occlusal table outline is rectangular** with deep prominent **buccal developmental groove** (terminates in central pit) Frequently, **oblique ridge** from mesiolingual cusp to distobuccal cusp area Heights of contour low and prominent **Three roots very divergent, without trunk root;** looks like "elephant charging" when viewed from lingual and inverted
Maxillary primary secondary molar	A/J 55/65	Second maxillary premolar	Closely resembles maxillary permanent first molar (4 cusps, Carabelli trait), except: • Squatter and more bulbous • More prominent cervical bulges • Very little root trunk
Mandibular primary first molar	S/L 84/74	Mandibular permanent first premolar	Resembles nothing in permanent dentition **Looks more like a molar than maxillary primary first molar** 4 cusps (2 buccal, 2 lingual); mesiobuccal and mesiolingual largest **Transverse ridge** between mesiobuccal and mesiolingual (largest) cusps Mesial/distal profiles: highly convex Occlusal **outline rhomboidal** because of buccal cervical ridge Occlusal **table rectangular** Buccal profile: **low, prominent buccal cervical ridge** (unique; gives "pregnant" appearance) Deep buccal groove, shallow lingual groove; may have mesial marginal groove **2 roots: mesial larger** Central pit radiating a central groove (goes to mesial pit and buccal and lingual grooves)
Mandibular primary second molar	T/K 85/75	Mandibular permanent second premolar	Closely resembles mandibular permanent second molar, except: • 2 roots more divergent and without root trunk • Cervical bulges • All 3 buccal cusps equal in size (distal cusps smallest in permanent first molar)

Isomorphy of Primary Second and Permanent First Molars

In summary, there is remarkable resemblance between the maxillary and mandibular second primary molars and their first permanent molar counterparts, even down to the smallest detail.

This information about primary teeth is important to know for the NBDE Part I exam:

- The maxillary first primary molar somewhat resembles a premolar.
- The mandibular first primary molar has the most unique buccal cervical bulge or ridge.
- The mandibular first primary molar has prominent transverse ridge.
- The mandibular first and maxillary first primary molars resemble nothing in permanent dentition.
- The mandibular second and maxillary second primary molars resemble the mandibular first and maxillary first permanent molars, respectively.

Occlusion

Occlusion is the general contact relationship between the occlusal surfaces of the maxillary and mandibular arches and individual teeth.

► Arch-to-Arch Relationships

When the two arches come together, each tooth opposes two teeth in the opposite arch, with the exception of the **mandibular central incisor** and **the maxillary third molar**, each of which only opposes one tooth. Knowing the general relationships described below are critical when answering most occlusion questions.

The Maxillary Arch
Each tooth in the maxillary arch opposes two teeth in the mandibular arch—its counterpart in the mandibular arch, plus the tooth distal to its counterpart, except the maxillary third molar.
Example
The first maxillary premolar opposes the first mandibular premolar and second mandibular premolar.

Note: The tip of the maxillary canine is placed in the labial embrasure.

The Mandibular Arch
Each tooth in the mandibular arch opposes two teeth in the maxillary arch—its counterpart in the maxillary arch, plus the tooth mesial to its counterpart, except the mandibular central incisor.
Example
The first mandibular molar opposes the first maxillary molar (its counterpart), plus the second maxillary premolar (tooth mesial to its counterpart).

The arch form of the maxillae is larger compared with the mandibular arch, providing an overlapping of the maxillary teeth over the mandibular teeth. The **horizontal overlap** is referred to as **overjet,** and the **vertical overlap** is referred to as **overbite.** This overhanging provides a protective feature during opening and closing movements of the jaws. Soft tissues are displaced during the act of closure until the teeth have come together in occlusal contact. Therefore, the cheeks, lips, and tongue are less likely to be caught and injured during mandibular movements.

► Concepts and Definitions

The numbers in the first column of the table correspond with the figure.

	Area	Definition	Examples
1	**Guiding cusp**	Cusp of tooth **not in contact in occlusion** but **outside** occluding area Opposing embrasures or grooves in the opposing dentition	Buccal cusps of maxillary posteriors and lingual cusps of mandibular posteriors
2	**Supporting (holding) cusp**	Cusp of tooth that **contacts the opposing arch on marginal ridges or central fossa area** Responsible for **supporting the forces of occlusion**	Buccal cusps of mandibular posteriors and lingual cusps of maxillary posteriors
3	**Occlusal slope**		
4	**Guiding incline**	Inclines or slopes of the guiding cusps from the guiding cusp tip toward the center of tooth	Lingual inclines of buccal cusps of maxillary posteriors and buccal inclines of lingual cusps of mandibular posterior
5	**Functional outer aspect (FOA)**	The outside 1–2 mm of supporting cusp Makes contact with guiding inclines of guiding cusps of opposing dentition when in occlusion	1–2 mm wide strip from buccal cusp tips of mandibular posteriors on buccal surface, and 1–2 mm wide strip from lingual cusp tips of maxillary posteriors on lingual surface

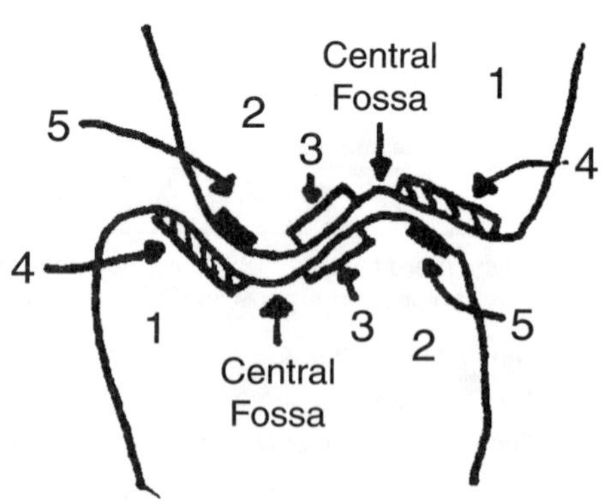

Posterior Teeth in General

The **buccal cusps of the mandibular posteriors** and **the lingual cusps of the maxillary posteriors** are the holding, supporting, or occluding cusps, and they contact marginal ridges and central fossae in the opposing arch.

The **buccal cusps of the maxillary posteriors** and the **lingual cusps of the mandibular posteriors** are the guiding cusps and oppose the embrasures and grooves of the opposing dentition.

Therefore, on each posterior tooth, we should expect **3 areas of contact** during occlusion:

1. The FOA of the holding cusp contacting the guiding incline(s) of the guiding cusp in the opposing dentition
2. The occlusal slope of the holding cusp contacting the occlusal slope of the opposing holding cusp
3. The guiding incline(s) of the guiding cusp contacting the FOA of the holding cusp of the opposing dentition

► Summary of Occlusal Contacts

Tooth Contacts in a Class I Normal Occlusion*

Maxillary Teeth	Mandibular Occlusal Contact	Mandibular Teeth	Maxillary Occlusal Contact
Central incisor	Central and lateral	Central incisor	Maxillary central incisor
Lateral incisor	Lateral incisor and canine	Lateral incisor	Central and lateral incisors
Canine	Canine and first premolar	Canine	Lateral incisor and canine
First premolar	First and second premolars	First premolar	Canine and first molar
Second premolar	Second and first molars	Second premolar	First and second premolar
First molar	First and second molars	First molar	Second premolar and first molar
Second molar	Second and third molars	Second molar	First and second molar
Third molar	Third molar	Third molar	Second and third molar

*The **mandibular central incisor** is the **only anterior tooth** that occludes with only one tooth.
The **maxillary third molar** is the only **posterior tooth** that occludes with only one tooth.

Tooth Guidance in Mandibular Movements

Canine guided	The maxillary and mandibular canine contact during working side mandibular movement, causing all posterior teeth to disocclude.
Group function	The maxillary canine and buccal cusps of the posterior teeth contact during working side mandibular movement, causing the disocclusion of the posterior teeth on the nonworking side.
Anterior guidance	Contact between the lingual surface of the maxillary teeth and the facial surfaces of the mandibular teeth during protrusive movement of the mandible disocclude all the posterior teeth.

► Arch (Angle) Classifications

Detailed information on angle classification is not needed until the NBDE Part II. Know the classes as described here.

Class I

In reality, the class I type of occlusion described by Angle is a **malocclusion**. Even though it has a normal cusp-groove relationship, there may be anterior crowding. Normal occlusion is not classified by Angle's system.

The mesiobuccal cusp of the first maxillary molar is **opposite** the mesiobuccal groove of the mandibular first molar. The maxillary canine is **in the labial embrasure** between the mandibular canine and the mandibular first premolar.

Class I occlusion is often called **neutroclusion.**

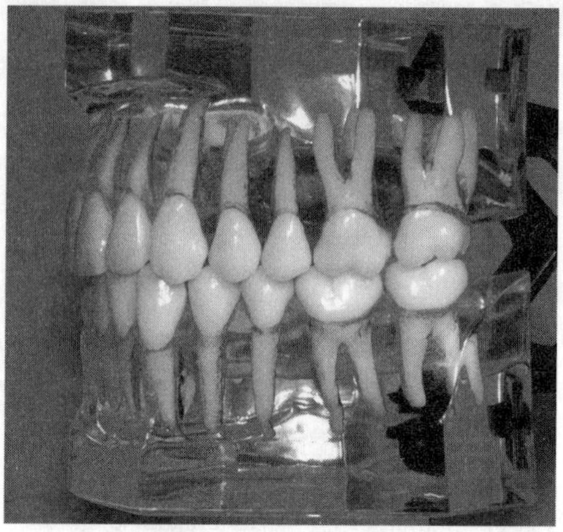

Class II

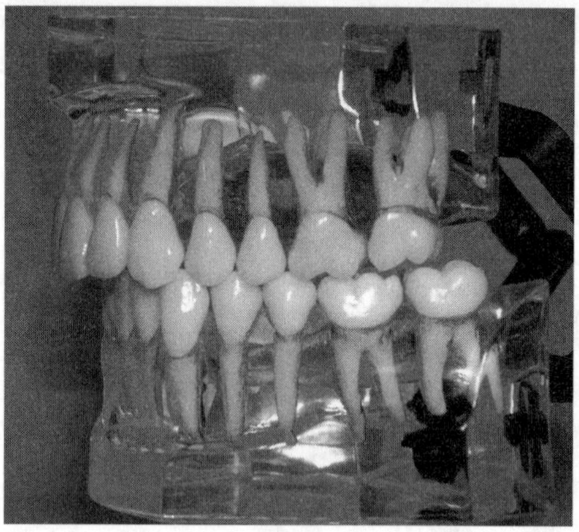

In class II occlusion, the mandible is small or **micrognathic**.

The mesiobuccal cusp of the first maxillary molar is **anterior** to the mesiobuccal groove of the mandibular first molar. The maxillary canine is **anterior** to the **labial embrasure** of the mandibular canine and the mandibular first premolar (often called **distoclusion**).

The lower arch is mesial to the upper arch.

Class III

In class III occlusion, the mandible is large or **prognathic**.

The mesiobuccal cusp of the first maxillary molar is **posterior** to the mesiobuccal groove of the mandibular first molar. The maxillary canine is **posterior** to the labial embrasure of the mandibular canine and the mandibular first premolar (often called **mesioclusion**).

The lower teeth are mesial to the upper teeth.

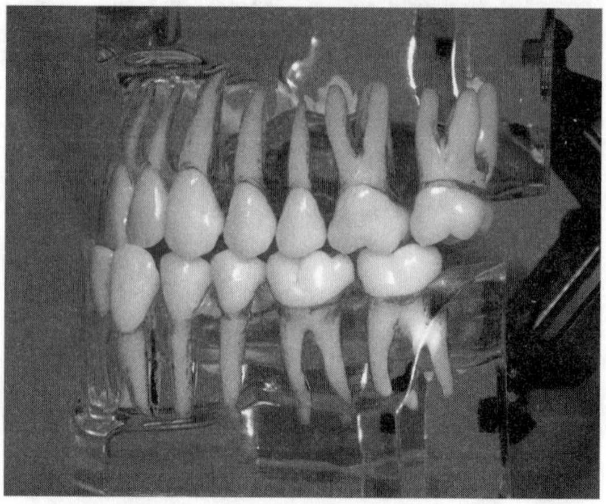

Curves	
Curve of Spree	**Curve of Wilson**
The anterior–posterior relation of the teeth viewed from the lateral, i.e., from the side. • The **maxillary** arch is **convex**. • The **mandibular** arch is **concave**.	The tilting of the mandibular posteriors lingually when the arches are viewed from the front (the maxillary posteriors tilt facially or buccally). • The **maxillary** arch is **convex**. • The **mandibular** arch is **concave**

Root Angulation

Roots	Angles
Mandibular	Anterior teeth angled distally Posterior teeth angled facially
Maxillary	Anterior teeth angled distally Posterior teeth angled lingually, except distobuccal root of first maxillary molar (inclined buccally)

► Temporomandibular Joint (TMJ)

The temporomandibular joint is both a **ginglymoarthrodial** joint **(hinge and gliding)** and a **diarthrosis** joint **(capable of free movement)**. It is located between the mandibular (glenoid) fossa of the temporal bone and the condylar head of the mandible.

The **mandibular condyle** is an oblong process wider mediolaterally than anteroposteriorly with a rounded posterior aspect and concave anterior aspect (**fovea pterygoidea**). Its articulating surface, the **superior anterior aspect**, is slightly convex. The condyle, as well as the articular tubercle, is covered by a rather thick layer of fibrous avascular tissue (fibrous connective tissue). The **articular eminence** is located anterior to the rather thin-boned articular fossa of the temporal bone.

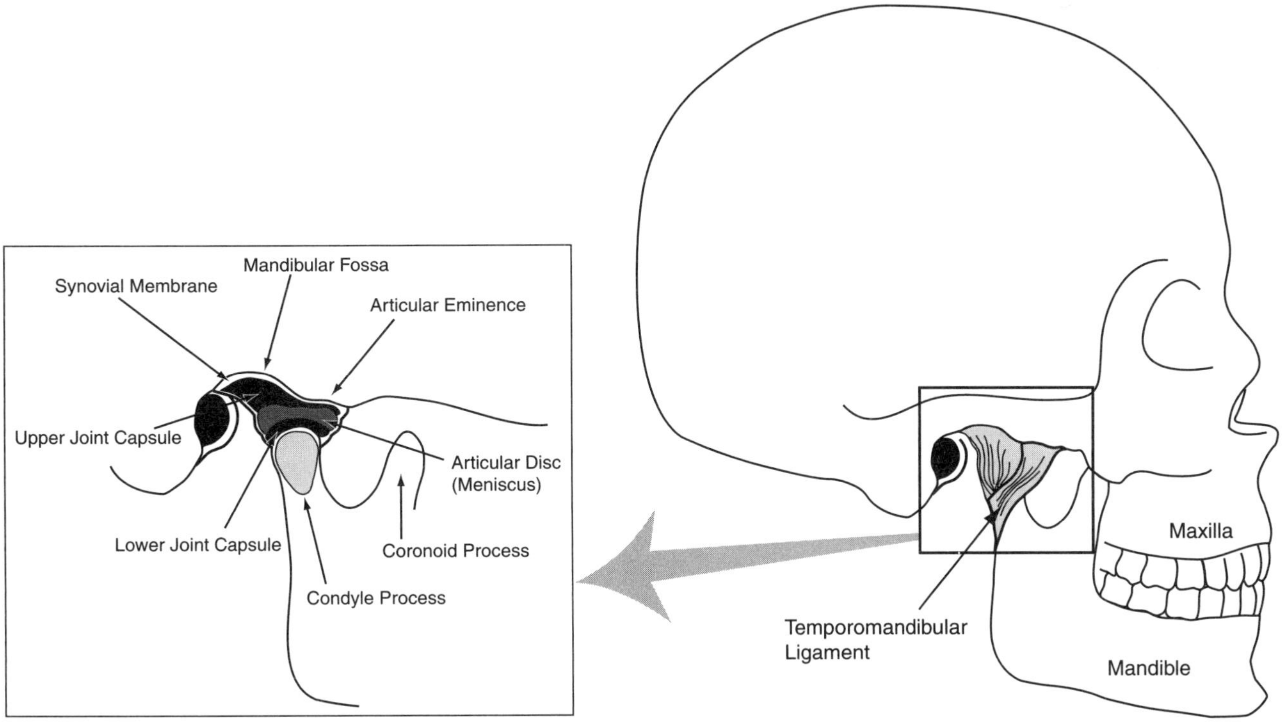

Breakdown of Structures		
Bone	**Condyle**	**Cancellous (spongy)** bone covered by a thin layer of compact bone Marrow is red, except in older persons, where it may be replaced by fatty marrow
	Glenoid (mandibular) fossa	Roof of fossa consists of thin layer of compact bone
	Articular tubercle	Consists of spongy bone covered with a thin layer of compact bone
Joint components	**Articular disc**	Dense, fibrous tissue with a few elastic fibers Center is very dense connective tissue; no blood vessels
	Articular space	Divided into two compartments: • **Lower**—between condyle and disc (hinge movement, rotation) • **Upper**—between disc and temporal bone (sliding movement, translation)
Ligaments	**Temporomandibular (lateral)**	Consists of two short, fibrous bands attached to: *(1)* the lateral surface of zygomatic arch and to the tubercle on its inferior border superiorly, and *(2)* the lateral surface and posterior border of the neck of the mandible inferiorly.
	Sphenomandibular	Thin band attached to spine of sphenoid bone and descends to the lingula of the mandibular foramen; gives support to mandible and helps limit the maximum opening of the jaw
	Stylomandibular	Extends from near the apex of the styloid process of temporal bone to the angle and posterior border of the ramus of the mandible; relaxed when the mouth is closed and when in extreme protrusion becomes tense
	Capsular ligament (fibrous capsule)	Surrounds entire joint; composed of fibrous tissue reinforced by accessory ligaments; restricts movement of mandibular condyle on wide opening
	Lateral ligament	Provides strong reinforcement of anterior lateral wall of capsule and helps prevent excess lateral and posterior displacement of mandible

Functional Contacting Movements	
Non-Working Side (Balancing Side)	**Working Side**
When the mandible is moved left or right, it is the side to which the mandible is moved.	When the mandible is moved to the left or right, it is the side to which the mandible is moved.

► Masticatory Muscle Function

Closing (elevating the mandible)	Masseter, medial pterygoid, temporalis
Opening (depressing the mandible)	Lateral pterygoid, mylohyoid, digastric, geniohyoid
Protruding	Lateral pterygoid
Lateral motion	Lateral pterygoid • **Right lateral pterygoid** moves the mandible to the **left** • **Left lateral pterygoid** moves the mandible to the **right**
Retruding	Temporalis, especially the posterior fibers

	Movement of the Mandible	Working Side Condyle	Non-Working Side Condyle
Protrusive	Mandible moves directly forward	Both condyles move simultaneously **forward and downward** along the articular eminence	
Lateral	Mandible moves to right or left without moving forward	Condyle **rotates**	Condyle moves **forward and downward**
Lateral protrusive	Combination of lateral and protrusive movements	Condyle **rotates** and moves **forward and down**	Condyle moves **anteriorly, downward, and medially**
Retrusive	Mandible moves directly backward	Both condyles move **upward and back** into mandibular fossa	

Mandibular Contacting Movement

When interpreting mandibular contacting movement, remember that the **maxillary teeth** are stationary and the **mandible** moves. If given a diagram of the maxillary arch with mandibular cusp pathways shown, the movement indicated would be the true movement of the mandible. If a diagram of mandibular teeth was shown, and maxillary cusps were illustrated, the movement of the maxillary cusps would be opposite the movement of the mandible.

The balancing side or nonworking side should not contact during the lateral contacting movements because of the mandibular condyles moving downward on the articular eminence.

The figures illustrate contacting movement.

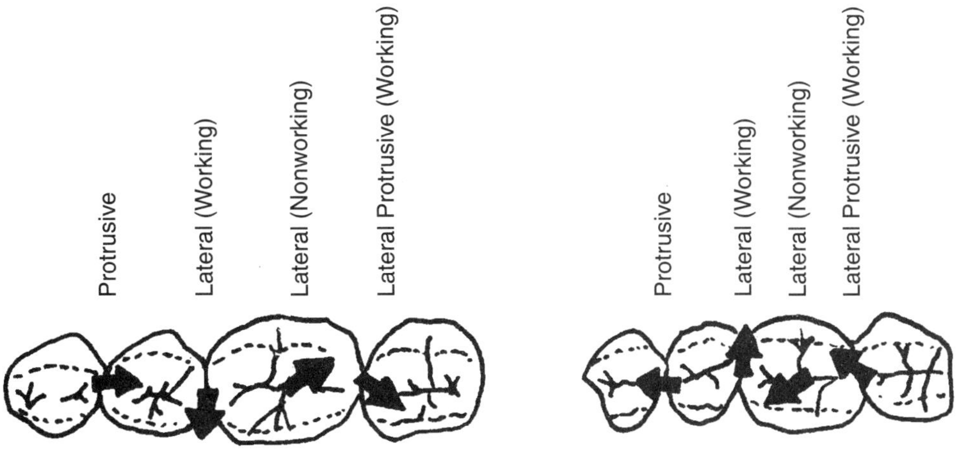

► Recording Mandibular Movements

Expect at least one question on the Posselt envelope of motion. Remember that the outline is the extreme position of all movements. The mandible can take any position within this outline.

Posselt Envelope of Motion

The **Posselt envelope of motion** defines the border movements of the mandible. To arrive at this diagram, one could place a tracer in the mandible between the two central incisors and record the position of the tracer when the mandible moves. The tracing records the **anterior–posterior** and **inferior–superior** positions. Remember that this is a recording of mandibular motion **viewed from the lateral**.

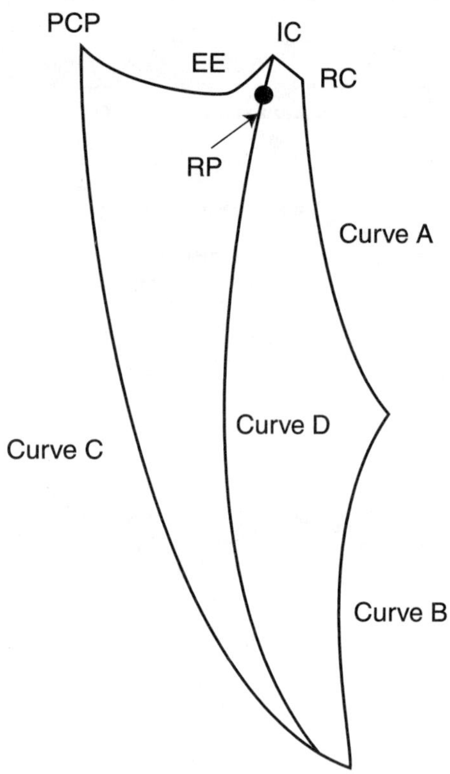

Sagittal View

Intercuspal (IC) Position

The **intercuspal *(IC)*** position is the **highest position of the mandible** and is seen when the teeth are in maximum intercuspation. Also known as **centric occlusion.**

Retruded Contract (RC) Position

Retruded contact (*RC*) is the most retruded position of the mandible (retruded contacting position, centric relation). In 90% of the population, the IC (or centric occlusion) is approximately 1.25 mm anterior to the **centric relation,** and in the other 10%, IC corresponds to RC. When going to this RC position, the mandible must move downward and posteriorly from its height in the intercuspal position. This is because of the holding cusps of the mandibular teeth sliding on the mesial inclines of maxillary cusps located posterior to them.

Opening Movements

The **mandibular condyles** are capable of two types of **opening** movement when in retruded contacting position:

- **Pure rotational movement (*curve A*** in figure)—The rotatory movement accounts for the first 20 or so millimeters of mandibular opening, and then ligaments become taut. For further opening, the ligaments must be loosened, and this is achieved by the mandibular condyles moving down the articular eminence.
- **Translational movement (*curve B*** in figure)—The mandible opens further (translational movement) to its maximal opening (40–50 mm separation of the anterior teeth).

The line that connects the position of maximal opening to protruded contact position **(*curve C*** in figure) is the **protrusive opening path**. This line describes the curve made if the mandible were placed as far forward as possible and then opened as far as possible.

Curve D represents normal chewing movement.

Posselt Envelope of Motion (*Cont'd.*)
Protruded Contact Position (PCP)
The protruded contact position (*PCP*) describes the most protruded or anterior position of the mandible. If the jaw is in this position, the incisors would not be in an edge-to-edge relationship, but instead the mandibular incisors would be more anterior than the maxillary incisors.
Edge to Edge (EE)
From PCP, remaining in tooth contact, the mandible is pulled backward until the incisors are edge to edge **(position EE, or "edge to edge").** The mandible must move down so that the incisors can come edge to edge. Moving from EE to IC, the mandibular cusps slide up the distal inclines of the maxillary cusps anterior to them. ***Curve D*** in the figure on the previous page illustrates the mandibular path when opening to the position of maximum opening. This curve is not pure rotatory motion, but rather **translational movement.** It is not a border movement because it occurs within the envelope of motion.
Normal Rest Position (RP)
Point RP is the normal **rest position** of the mandible. At rest, the teeth are not contacting. This position is also known as the **postural position** or **physiologic rest position.** The distance from RP to IC is called **freeway space.** That is, it represents the space between the teeth when the mandible is in the postural position (2–3 mm). Rest position is determined primarily by musculature.

Frontal View	
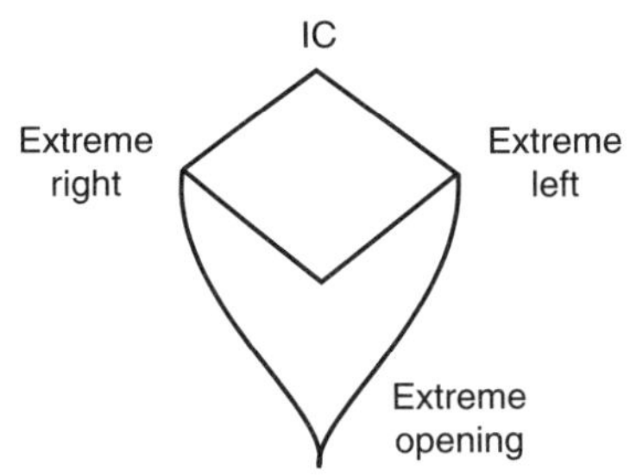	This figure represents the same movement as above, but here, in the lateral contacting positions, the mandible is opened to its maximum. The **chewing stroke**, or **masticatory stroke**, when seen from the anterior on the lateral, is well within the borders of the mandibular movement. It is described as a pear- or tear-shaped movement. When chewing, the chewing is usually unilateral, favoring a particular side. This accounts for the displacement towards one side of the inferior portion of this movement.
Horizontal View	
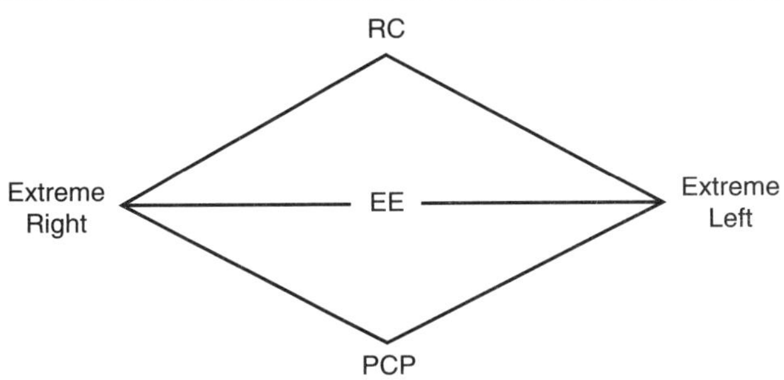	This diamond-shaped figure is a tracing of the mandible when starting in the RC position and then moving to the extreme right (right lateral contacting position), then moving to PCP (protruded contact position), then to the extreme left (left lateral contacting position), and finally back again to RC.

Oral Mucosa

The oral cavity is lined throughout with **oral epithelium (stratified, squamous epithelium)** and the underlying **lamina propria (connective tissue layer)**. Under the oral mucosa is the submucosa, which also differs from place to place, depending on the function of the particular area.

The surface epithelium may be categorized as **keratinized** or **nonkeratinized**. A full keratinized potential does not present in mucosal cells under normal conditions, except in the masticatory mucosa, although it may be expressed in any area under irritation. Because the keratinized potential does not present in the majority of mucosal cells, the stratum granulosum and the corneum are not seen.

► Layers of the Epithelium

Layer	Characteristics
Stratum basal layer (stratum germinativum)	Single layer of cuboidal to low columnar cells Basal layer provides new cells for the other epithelial layers Mitosis or cell division occurs at this level
Stratum spinosum (prickle cell layer)	A multilayer of polyhedral-like cells bound together by means of numerous desmosomal junctions Toward the surface, these cells flatten and widen considerably **No further changes occur in the nonkeratinizing epithelium**
Stratum granulosum	Flattened polygonal cells filled with basophilic keratohyalin granules This layer not seen in nonkeratinized epithelium
Stratum lucidum	Transitional zone This layer appears in the epidermis of thick shin (palms, soles) and not seen in oral
Stratum corneum	Anucleated (cells have lost their nuclei) Flat cells filled with keratin

The **lamina propria** is a dense layer of connective tissue. Its papillae indent the epithelium and carry both blood vessels and nerves. Between the connective tissue papillae are the epithelial rete pegs.

► Types of Stratified Squamous Epithelium

Three types of stratified squamous epithelium are found in the oral cavity.

Type	Location	Characteristics	Appearance
Nonkeratinized (nonmasticatory)	Buccal mucosa Cheeks Floor of the mouth Lips Soft palate Ventral surface of the tongue Alveolar mucosa	Basal cell, prickle cell, and outer most nonkeratinized layers	It appears as a soft, moist surface
Orthokeratinized (masticatory)	Gingival Dorsal surface of the tongue Hard palate	Basal cell, prickle cell, granular, and outer most keratinized layers	Coral-pink in color and highly vascular
Parakeratinized	Dorsum of the tongue Attached gingiva	Basal cell, prickle cell, and keratinized layers	Associated with lingual papillae of the tongue Taste buds present in this tissue

► Difference Between Skin of Lip and Mucous Membrane

The Skin of the Lip	The Transition Zone (Vermilion Border)
Keratinized epithelium—moderate thickness	Keratinized tissue ends in this area
Papillae of connective tissue—few and short	Long papillae carrying large capillary loops close to the surface
Sebaceous glands in association with hair	Few sebaceous glands
Sweat glands	

► Important Cells of the Epithelium

Keratinocytes	Responsible for the production of keratin Not found in oral mucosa
Melanocytes	Derivatives of neural crest ectoderm Responsible for production of pigment
Langerhans cells	Immune system cells Antigen-presenting cells
Merkel cells	Function in concert with nerve fibers Sensory cells

► Periodontium

The **gingival unit** consists of the **free gingiva, attached gingiva**, and **alveolar mucosa.** The gingival unit has a lining epithelium of either **masticatory mucosa**, which is thick keratinized epithelium with a dense collagenous connective tissue corium, or **lining mucosa**, which is thin, nonkeratinized epithelium with loose connective tissue corium containing elastic, and sometimes muscle, fibers.

Masticatory mucosa is found in the free and the attached gingiva, hard palate, and dorsum of the tongue, and lining mucosa is found elsewhere in the oral cavity.

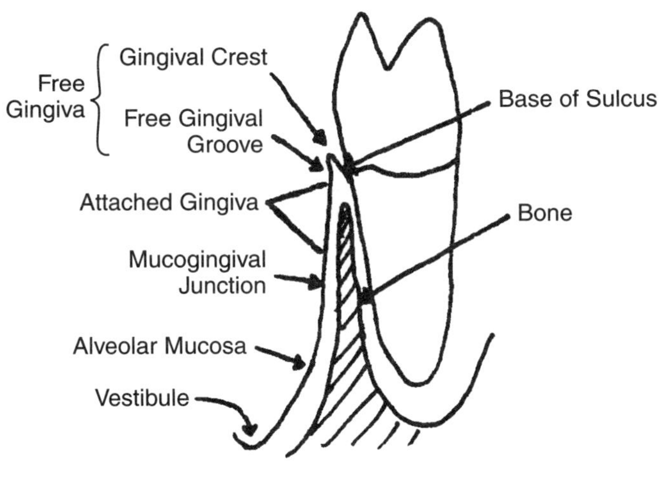

Free Gingiva
Gingival located above the base of the gingival sulcus
Gingival Sulcus
Area where the gingiva is attached to the tooth
Free Gingiva Groove
Extends from the base of the sulcus to the gingival crest
Attached Gingiva
Gingiva below the free gingival groove and above the mucogingival junction
Alveolar Mucosa
Below the mucogingival junction

► Attachment Apparatus

The attachment apparatus consists of the cementum, periodontal ligament, and alveolar bone. The periodontal ligament surrounds the tooth and connects to the bone, acting like a hammock. The attachment apparatus provides proprioceptive information to stimuli like pressure and pain. The bone and cementum can be resorbed when under controlled pressure, allowing for orthodontic movement of the teeth.

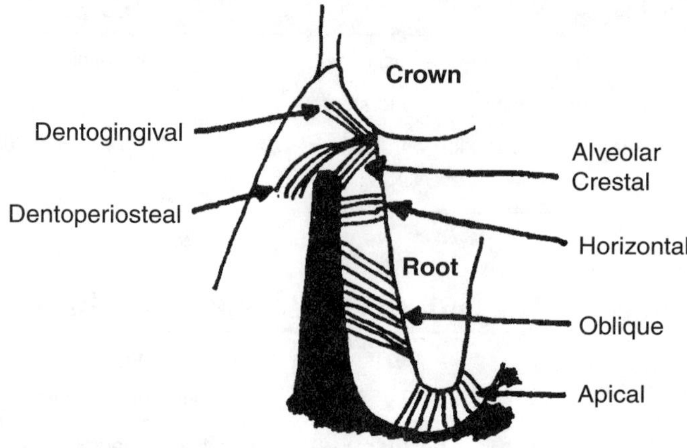

Principal Fiber Group

The principal fiber group comprises collagen fibers, which **do not attach to alveolar bone**.

Dentogingival	Runs from the cementum into the free gingiva
Dentoperiosteal	Runs from the cementum apically, over the alveolar crest of the bone, into the periosteum of the attached gingiva
Transseptal	Runs from the cementum of one tooth, over the alveolar crest bone, to the cementum of an adjacent tooth
Circular	Not attached to cementum; runs in the free gingiva around the tooth in a circular manner

Periodontal Fiber Group

The periodontal fiber group comprises collagen fibers, which **run from cementum to alveolar bone**.

Alveolar crestal	Runs from supra-alveolar cementum down to the alveolar crest
Horizontal	Runs from the cementum directly across to the alveolar bone
Oblique	Largest group of fibers Runs from the cementum, from the root to the bone, in a diagonal coronal direction
Apical	Runs from apex of root to alveolar bone in base of alveolus

► The Periodontal Ligament (PDL)

The periodontal ligament (PDL) is the connective tissue that surrounds the root of the tooth and attaches the root of the tooth to the bony alveolus.

Functions	**Formative:** cementoblasts, fibroblasts, and osteoblasts are derived from cells in the PDL **Supportive:** maintains the tooth in its position **Sensory:** extremely good innervation in PDL **Nutritive:** extremely good blood supply in the PDL
Blood supply	1. Periosteal blood supply from alveolar bone (**major source**) 2. Arteries of gingiva, which anastomose with the PDL (**minor source**) 3. Arteries of the periapical area, which arise from the vessels entering the pulp (**minor source**)
Nerve supply	Nerves follow path of blood vessels Free nerve endings are receptors for pain and proprioceptive stimuli*
Lymphatics	Follow path of blood vessels Flow of lymph is from ligament toward and into alveolar bone

*_Note:_ The proprioceptive information regulates the masticatory musculature and protects the tooth from sudden overload due to severe masticatory stresses.

Damage to the PDL	
In Loss of Function	**In Occlusal Trauma**
1. The PDL narrows. 2. The regular arrangement of fibers is lost. 3. The PDL becomes a thin membrane with irregularly arranged fibers. 4. Cementum may become thickened.	1. Alveolar bone is reabsorbed. 2. PDL is widened. 3. Tooth becomes loose. 4. When source of trauma removed, repair usually occurs.

▶ Innervation of Important Oral Structures

Tongue	**Function**	**Innervation**
Anterior 2/3	Sensory, nontaste	Lingual branch of the mandibular nerve **(CN V)**
Anterior 2/3	Taste	Chorda tympani of the facial nerve **(CN VII)**
Posterior 1/3	Taste, general sensory	Lingual branch of the glossopharyngeal nerve **(CN IX)**
Entire tongue	Motor innervation	Hypoglossal nerve **(CN XII)**
Teeth	**Type**	**Innervation**
	Lower molar and premolar	Inferior alveolar nerve of the mandibular nerve **(CN V3)**
	Lower incisors	Inferior alveolar nerve of the mandibular nerve (**CN V3**) incisal branch
	Maxillary third through first molar	Posterior superior alveolar nerve of the maxillary nerve (**CN V2**)
	Mesial buccal root of the maxillary first molar and the maxillary premolars	Middle superior nerve of the maxillary nerve
	Maxillary canines and incisors	Anterior superior alveolar nerve of the maxillary nerve
Supporting Tissues	**Tissue**	**Innervation**
Mandibular	Lingual gingiva and supporting tissue	Lingual nerve of the mandibular nerve (**CN V3**)
	Buccal molar region	Inferior alveolar nerve and the buccal nerve
	Anterior to molars	The mental nerve
Maxillary	Buccal tissues	Anterior, middle, and posterior superior alveolar nerve
	Posterior lingual	Greater palatine nerve
	Anterior lingual	Nasopalatine nerve

Note: The trigeminal nerve CN V supports both the dental (teeth) and the periodontal tissues. The maxillary nerve (CN V2) innervates the maxillary structures. The mandibular nerve (CN V3) innervates the mandibular structures.

► The Tongue

Papillae Types			
Papillae Type	**Vascular/ Nonvascular**	**Taste Buds?**	**Location**
Filiform	Nonvascular	No	Rows, anterior to middle
Fungiform	Vascular	Yes	Anterior only
Circumvallate (vallate)	Vascular	Yes	10 to 12 only, V-shaped row near anterior/posterior border
Foliate	Nonvascular	No	Lateral border of the tongue

Foramen Caecum

Remnant of thyroglossal duct; located at the apex of the "V" formed by the circumvallate

Other Papillae

Additional taste buds can be found on the posterolateral palate, epiglottis, and the pharynx

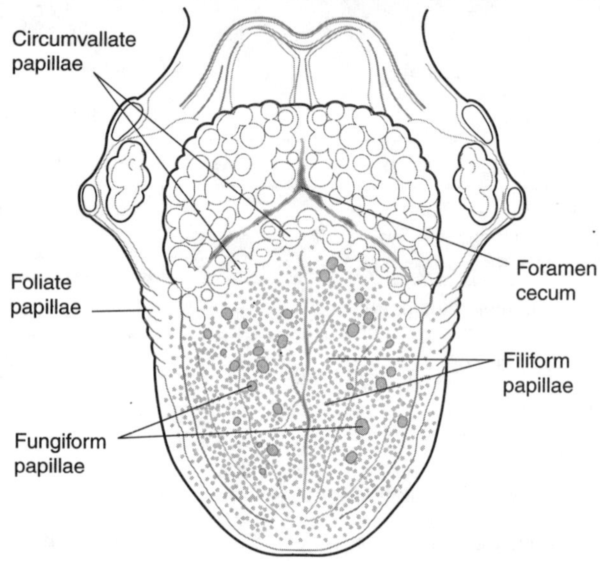

Tongue Innervation and Development	
Anterior two thirds	General sensation CN V (trigeminal) Taste by CN VII (facial)
Posterior third (including the circumvallate)	CN IX (glossopharyngeal)
Most posterior (valleculae and minor taste buds)	CN X (vagus)
Development of the tongue	Branchial arches 1–4 Lingual buds (bilateral swellings) Tuberculum impar Copula
Branchial arch and associated cranial nerve	Arch 1—CN V Arch 2—CN VII Arch 3—CN IX Arch 4—CN X

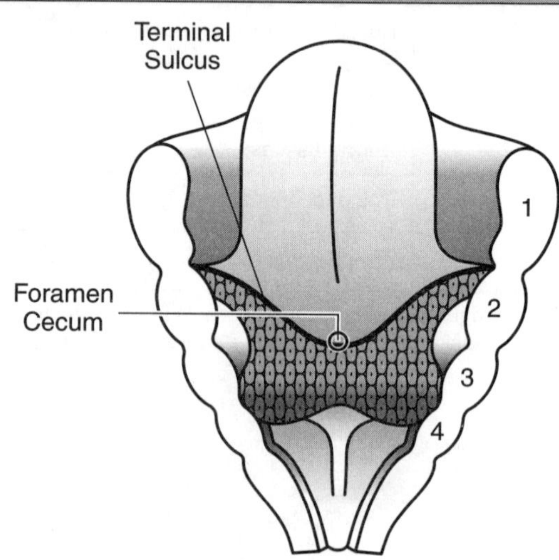